LIFE FORCE

WHAT THE WORLD'S GREATEST LEADERS IN SCIENCE & MEDICINE ARE SAYING ABOUT *LIFE FORCE* . . .

"*Life Force* is a tour de force. Tony Robbins and Peter Diamandis beautifully explain the latest scientific, medical, and lifestyle advances now available to maximize health- and lifespan. A must-read for anyone who desires to function optimally now and protect themselves from diseases in the future."

> —David Sinclair, PhD, professor of genetics at Harvard Medical School; codirector of the Paul F. Glenn Center for Biology of Aging Research at Harvard; author of the *New York Times* bestseller *Lifespan: Why We Age—and Why We Don't Have To*

"We are in the midst of a biotech revolution that has the potential to cure most diseases—adding decades to your healthspan. Tony Robbins and Peter Diamandis have authored a powerful and friendly road map for anyone to maximize their health and vitality. *Life Force* does a marvelous job of making technologies like CRISPR, gene therapy, and stem cells understandable, in a way that gives the reader a hopeful and compelling vision of the future."

> —George Church, PhD, professor of genetics at Harvard Medical School; professor of health sciences & technology at Harvard and MIT, and a founding member of the Wyss Institute for Biologically Inspired Engineering

"You will not regret buying this book. It is full of the latest, but importantly, scientifically grounded, facts aimed at extending one's lifespan and healthspan. Tony & Peter serve up a whole-body finger-buffet of essential information, written with a beautiful narrative arc. Perhaps most important, this isn't just a book about "here's what you should do," but in addition "how to do it." The book is actionable, practical. Bottom line: you will be changed by this book, and so, so much for the better."

> —Matthew Walker, PhD, professor of neuroscience at the University of California, Berkeley; sleep scientist at Google; author, *Why We Sleep: Unlocking the Power of Sleep and Dreams*

"*Life Force* is a visionary and extraordinary book—filled with the latest science-based information on health and healing that can help transform both the quality and quantity of your life. Highly recommended!"

—Dr. Dean Ornish, president and founder of the
Preventive Medicine Research Institute; clinical professor,
University of California, San Francisco School of Medicine;
author, *Reversing Heart Disease*, and *UnDo It!*

"Tony Robbins, long the master of helping others generate the right mindset for success, turns his attention in *Life Force* to providing us with useful lessons on whole-body health and a roadmap for how advances in precision medicine can help us improve and extend our wellness and overall healthspans."

—Dr. Michael Roizen, chief wellness officer emeritus
at Cleveland Clinic for Functional Wellness, award-
winning author of five *New York Times* bestsellers

"*Life Force* will help you find answers. It covers the most important innovators, inventions, and technologies that are transforming health and medicine today."

—Ray Kurzweil, famed inventor and futurist with a 30-year
track record of accurate predictions, awarded the National
Medal of Technology by President Bill Clinton, and the man
Inc magazine calls the "rightful heir to Thomas Edison"

"This remarkable biopsy of modern medicine's marvels takes us on a futuristic journey of hope and healing that is already at our fingertips and will have a seismic impact on readers."

—Mehmet Oz, MD, attending surgeon,
New York Presbyterian & Columbia University

"Tony Robbins gives you access to information that's not readily available. Story after story of medical breakthroughs will inspire you and provide you with effective solutions for greater health, wellness, and quality of life."

—Dr. Mark Hyman, head of strategy & innovation, Cleveland
Clinic Center for Functional Medicine, 14-time bestselling author,
internationally respected physician, researcher, educator, and activist

"You will find a treasure trove of the long-standing and emerging secrets to extending your healthspan and your lifespan in *Life Force*. In one place, Tony Robbins and Peter Diamandis have complied the insights from over 100 leading experts in the fields of health, medicine, and technology that readers can use to make better decisions to fuel a better heart, mind, and overall quality of life."

—Eric Verdin, MD, president and CEO, the Buck Institute; assoc. professor, University of California, San Francisco School of Medicine; fellow of the American Association for the Advancement of Science

"*Life Force* showcases the coming breakthroughs in treating and preventing dementia, cancer, and cardiovascular disease. This powerful book delivers actionable strategies to keep us healthier, longer. Tony and Peter make the promise of the precision medicine revolution understandable through compelling stories. This is a must-read for anyone who desires the healthiest possible future for themselves and the world!"

—Rudy Tanzi, PhD, bestselling author, *The Healing Self*; professor of neurology, Harvard University; co-director of the McCance Center for Brain Health, Mass. General Hospital

WHAT THE WORLD'S GREATEST ATHLETES ARE SAYING ABOUT TONY ROBBINS & *LIFE FORCE*

"In his new book Tony Robbins brings you the most important resources that can help anyone sustain peak performance, and lead a healthy and more vital life."

—Cristiano Ronaldo, top goal scorer of all time, 5-time Ballon d'Or winner, 33 career trophies, 7 league titles, and 5 UEFA Championship League titles

"In *Life Force* you'll find the latest breakthroughs and therapies available to help you heal and strengthen your body—the same nonsurgical solutions that helped me go from not being able to stand for longer than 10 minutes, to playing golf and hitting the tennis ball again without pain. They will dramatically enhance your life!"

—Jack Nicklaus, greatest golfer of all time with
120 professional tournament victories worldwide, and
winner of 18 professional major championship titles

"Tony Robbins helped me discover what I am really made of. With Tony's help, I've set new standards for myself, and I've taken my tennis game—and my life—to a whole new level!"

—Serena Williams, 23-time grand slam champion

WHAT THE WORLD'S GREATEST LEADERS ARE SAYING ABOUT TONY ROBBINS & *LIFE FORCE*

"When Tony Robbins focuses on a subject to help you, he speaks with the luminaries in the field to get the most important concepts, synthesizes them brilliantly, and lays them out in an easy-to-understand and entertaining way so it is a beautifully packed gift. *Life Force* is Tony Robbins at his best, dealing with the most important life question—how do we make our lives last longer and be of better quality? For those looking for answers to this question, this is a must-read. In this landmark book, Tony shows us the amazing scientific breakthroughs that are now being made and how you can take advantage of them to improve the quality and length of your life."

—Ray Dalio, founder & co-chief investment officer of
Bridgewater Associates, the largest hedge fund in the world,
#1 *New York Times* bestselling author of *Principles*

"Tony Robbins has been an enormous source of strength and insight for me both personally and professionally."

—Peter Guber, chairman & CEO of Mandalay Entertainment,
owner of the LA Dodgers and Golden State Warriors

"He has a great gift. He has the gift to inspire."

—Bill Clinton, former president of the United States

"Tony Robbins is a genius. . . . His ability to strategically guide people through any challenge is unparalleled."

—Steve Wynn, CEO and founder of Wynn Resorts

"Tony Robbins' strategies and tools have been at the core of our culture from the beginning. He has been one of the critical keys to Salesforce.com's leadership and growth into an over $25 billion company. Without Tony and his teachings, Salesforce.com would not exist today."

—Marc Benioff, founder, chairman, and CEO of Salesforce.com

"What Tony really gave me, a kid sitting on Venice Beach selling T-shirts, was to take risks, take action, and really become something. I'm telling you as someone who has lived with these strategies for 25 years: I'll come back for more again, and again, and again."

—Mark Burnett, five-time Emmy Award–winning television producer of *Survivor, Shark Tank*, and *The Voice*

"Tony's power is superhuman. . . . He is a catalyst for getting people to change. I came away with: It's not about motivation as much as it is allowing people to tap into what's already there."

—Oprah Winfrey, Emmy Award–winning media magnate

WHAT THE WORLD'S GREATEST FINANCIAL MINDS ARE SAYING ABOUT TONY ROBBINS

"Robbins is the best economic moderator that I've ever worked with. His mission to bring insights from the world's greatest financial minds to the average investor is truly inspiring."

—Alan Greenspan, former Federal Reserve chairman under four sitting presidents

"Tony came to my office for a 45-minute interview that ended up lasting four hours. It was one of the most thought-provoking interviews of my life. His energy and passion are contagious and energizing."

—The late John C. Bogle, founder, the Vanguard Group, which has more than $3 trillion in assets under management

"Tony Robbins is a human locksmith—using his unique insights into human nature, he knows how to open your mind to larger possibilities."

—Paul Tudor Jones II, founder, Tudor Investment Corporation, and one of the top ten traders in history

WHAT WORLD'S GREATEST ENTERTAINERS ARE SAYING ABOUT TONY ROBBINS

"No matter who you are, no matter how successful, no matter how happy, Tony has something to offer you."

—Hugh Jackman, Emmy– and Tony Award–winning actor, producer

"Tony Robbins is a genius, and only keeps on getting better. He inspires Rocky to keep punching."

—Sylvester Stallone

"I was afraid that my success would take something away from my family. Tony was able to turn it around and show me that I've helped millions of people. Probably the most intense feelings I've ever had."

—Melissa Etheridge, two-time Grammy Award–winning singer and songwriter

"If you want to change your state, if you want to change your results, this is where you do it; Tony is the man."

—Usher, Grammy Award–winning singer, songwriter, entrepreneur

LIFE FORCE

HOW NEW BREAKTHROUGHS IN PRECISION MEDICINE CAN TRANSFORM THE QUALITY OF YOUR LIFE & THOSE YOU LOVE

TONY ROBBINS

AND PETER H. DIAMANDIS, MD
with ROBERT HARIRI, MD / PhD

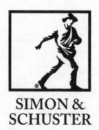

SIMON &
SCHUSTER

London · New York · Sydney · Toronto · New Delhi

First published in the United States by Simon and Schuster, Inc., 2022
First published in Great Britain by Simon & Schuster UK Ltd, 2022

Copyright © Anthony Robbins, 2022

The right of Anthony Robbins to be identified as the author
of this work has been asserted in accordance with the
Copyright, Designs and Patents Act, 1988.

3 5 7 9 10 8 6 4 2

Simon & Schuster UK Ltd
1st Floor
222 Gray's Inn Road
London WC1X 8HB

www.simonandschuster.co.uk
www.simonandschuster.com.au
www.simonandschuster.co.in

Simon & Schuster Australia, Sydney
Simon & Schuster India, New Delhi

The author and publishers have made all reasonable efforts
to contact copyright-holders for permission, and apologise for
any omissions or errors in the form of credits given.
Corrections may be made to future printings.

A CIP catalogue record for this book
is available from the British Library

Hardback ISBN: 978-1-4711-8836-7
Trade Paperback ISBN: 978-1-4711-8837-4
eBook ISBN: 978-1-4711-8838-1

Printed in the UK by CPI Group (UK) Ltd, Croydon, CR0 4YY

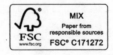

MIX
Paper from
responsible sources
FSC® C171272

This book is dedicated to those souls who will never settle for anything less than all they can be, do, share, and give in their lifetime. Most important, to God's greatest gift in my life, my wife of twenty-two years, my Sage, my children, grandchildren, and my extended chosen family, I am grateful beyond words to each of you.

—Tony Robbins

To my father, **Harry P. Diamandis, MD**, *a dear and glorious physician who made it to age to 89.*

And to my incredible mom, **Tula Diamandis**, *who at age 86 is going strong! May she make it to her 100th!*

—Peter H. Diamandis

I'd like to dedicate my contributions to this book to my family—Alex, Jack, Haley, and Maggie—with the hope that our ongoing work will add healthy years, even decades, to the lives of those who make our efforts meaningful.

—Dr. Robert Hariri

DISCLAIMER

This publication contains the opinions and ideas of its author(s). It is intended to provide helpful and informative material on the subjects addressed in the publication. It is sold with the understanding that the author and publisher are not engaged in rendering medical, health, or any other kind of personal professional services in the book. The reader should consult his or her medical, health, or other competent professional before adopting any of the suggestions in this book or drawing inferences from it. This book also is not intended to serve as the basis for any financial decision nor as a recommendation of a specific investment nor as an offer to sell or purchase any security.

Throughout this book, the author(s) may discuss several companies and entities in which the author(s) have a financial interest, and such interests are disclosed when those entities are first mentioned.

The author and publisher specifically disclaim all responsibility for any liability, loss or risk, personal or otherwise, which is incurred as a consequence, directly or indirectly, of the use and application of any of the contents of this book.

LIFE FORCE ADVISORY BOARD

We would like to thank the 11 members of our advisory board for their support on this book. They are all leaders in their field, and we are grateful for all of their collaboration.

- **Dean Ornish, MD**—president and founder of the Preventive Medicine Research Institute; Clinical Professor, University of California, San Francisco, School of Medicine; author, *Reversing Heart Disease* and *UnDo It!*
- **David Sinclair, PhD**—professor of genetics at Harvard Medical School; codirector of the Paul F. Glenn Center for Biology of Aging Research at Harvard; author of the New York Times bestseller *Lifespan: Why We Age—and Why We Don't Have To*
- **George Church, PhD**—professor of genetics at Harvard Medical School; professor of health sciences and technology at Harvard and MIT; and a founding member of the Wyss Institute for Biologically Inspired Engineering
- **Deepak Srivastava, MD**—president, Gladstone Institutes; professor, Department of Pediatrics and Department of Biochemistry and Biophysics, University of California, San Francisco, School of Medicine
- **Eric Verdin, MD**—president and CEO, the Buck Institute; associate professor, University of California, San Francisco, School of Medicine; fellow of the American Association for the Advancement of Science
- **Jennifer Garrison, PhD**—assistant professor at the Buck Institute and founder of the Global Consortium for Reproductive Longevity and Equality; assistant professor, cellular molecular pharmacology, University of California, San Francisco School of Medicine

- **Carolyn DeLucia, MD, FACOG**—practicing OB/GYN for more than 30 years and alternative therapy expert. Pioneer at the leading edge of noninvasive sexual wellness treatments
- **Rudy Tanzi, PhD**—professor of neurology, Harvard University; director of the Genetics and Aging Research Unit at Massachusetts General Hospital; vice chair of Neurology and codirector of the McCance Center for Brain Health
- **Rhonda Patrick, PhD**—published scientist and educator, creator of FoundMyFitness. Areas of expertise include research on aging (conducted at the Salk Institute), the role of genetics and epigenetics in health status, benefits of exposing the body to hormetic stressors, and the importance of mindfulness, stress reduction, and sleep.
- **Hector Lopez, MD**—cofounder of JUVN3 Holdings, LLC; founding partner and chief medical Officer, Supplement Safety Solutions, LLC, and Center for Applied Health Sciences, LLC; CEO of Ortho-Nutra and NutriMed Solutions
- **Matthew Walker, PhD**—professor of neuroscience at the University of California, Berkeley; sleep scientist at Google; author, *Why We Sleep: Unlocking the Power of Sleep and Dreams*

CONTENTS

SECTION 4: TACKLING THE TOP 6 KILLERS

SECTION 5: LONGEVITY, MINDSET & FULFILLMENT

PREFACE

Congratulations on picking up this book! We're thrilled to take you on a journey of scientific breakthroughs, many of which you can apply today to immediately improve the quality and perhaps the quantity of your life.

Here's just a taste of what you'll be learning in the pages ahead:

HOW TO GAIN PURE ENERGY, STRENGTH, AND MAXIMUM PERFORMANCE

- Learn how to immediately boost your energy by tapping into the power of a natural compound in your body that drives energy at a cellular level.
- Discover the four vitality ingredients that a world-renowned genetics professor has used to reverse his biological age by 20 years.
- Increase your strength and muscle mass, boost your metabolism, and increase your bone density up to 14 percent with a scientifically proven 10-minute workout (once a week!).
- Learn the third pillar of health—one of the simplest things you can do to increase your daily focus, boost your mood, and experience greater vitality without caffeine or other stimulants.
- Prime your body for peak performance by using the latest wearables and devices that give you 24/7 personalized fitness, sleep, and recovery data.

HOW TO ACCELERATE HEALING, REGENERATION, AND LONGEVITY (WITHOUT SURGERY)

- How stem cells have helped people regain the use of their arms and legs after strokes or severed spinal cords, recover from injuries like torn ligaments, and driven children with leukemia into remission.

- A novel gene therapy that's been shown to restore sight with just two injections.
- A new injection that's saving hundreds of lives by helping those suffering from anxiety and/or PTSD.
- Three new powerful and effective scientific breakthroughs for eliminating back pain.
- An incision-less brain surgery that uses ultrasound to significantly relieve Parkinson's symptoms in minutes, and is now being tested in its use to block the addictive pattern in the brain.
- A breakthrough molecule that could erase osteoarthritis by growing new, pristine cartilage within 12 months, with just a single injection.
- Exponential technologies such as artificial intelligence, CRISPR, and gene therapy are being used to unravel the mystery of aging, how to slow it, stop it, and perhaps even reverse aging.

HEALTHY WEIGHT LOSS AND INNOVATIVE ANTI-AGING REMEDIES

- Two FDA-approved solutions that help curb your appetite, one of which has delivered an average weight loss of 22 pounds.
- Accessible and affordable hair treatments that can increase hair growth, luster, and volume up to 60 percent without harsh chemicals or uncomfortable side effects.
- New anti-aging remedies customized specifically for your skin by taking into account your DNA, lifestyle, and environmental factors so you can have glowing skin regardless of age.
- A way to blast fat for good with a noninvasive technology that helps you lose fat and tightens your skin (without surgery or scarring).
- The building block your body naturally produces that can give you Botox without needles, plus a new head of hair.

NEW WAYS OF TACKLING THE TOP KILLERS

- **Cancer:** How to win the war on cancer with the most promising alternatives to chemotherapy and radiation and a revolutionary blood test that may detect more than 50 types of cancer before symptoms surface.

- **Heart Disease:** A new FDA-cleared artificial intelligence test that can predict heart disease five to ten years in advance and provide a road map to help prevent it.
- **Diabetes:** The pennies-per-dose medication that safely treats and helps prevent type 2 diabetes and may protect you from cancer, heart disease, and Alzheimer's.
- **Alzheimer's:** A company that's applying CRISPR gene-editing technology to relieve Alzheimer's symptoms such as anxiety and depression.
- **Stroke:** How virtual reality headsets, high-tech sensors, and video games improve stroke survivors' dexterity and mobility.

. . . and much more.

INTRODUCTION BY RAY KURZWEIL

Ray Kurzweil is one of the world's leading inventors, thinkers, and futurists, with a thirty-year track record of accurate predictions. Kurzweil was selected as one of the top entrepreneurs by Inc. *magazine, which described him as the "rightful heir to Thomas Edison." He was awarded the National Medal of Technology and Innovation, for pioneering and innovative achievements in computer science such as voice recognition, which have overcome many barriers and enriched the lives of disabled persons and all Americans.*

I have a very short list of people whom I will almost always say yes to when asked a request. Tony Robbins and Peter Diamandis are at the top of this list. So, when they asked me to write this foreword, I didn't hesitate. Tony and Peter share my belief that the power of human ideas can change the world, including how long we live. **No matter what quandaries we face— business problems, health issues, relationship difficulties, the great social and cultural challenges of our time—there exists an idea that will enable us to prevail.** We can and must find that idea. And when we find it, we need to implement it. *Life Force* **will help you find those answers. It covers the most important innovators, inventions, and technologies that are transforming health and medicine today.** We are on the cusp of profound medical advancements as Artificial Intelligence begins to unlock the mysteries of our bodies and brains. **Yet many conventional healthcare practitioners are still caught up in the old paradigm and don't practice medicine as an information technology. This means that each of us has to take control of our own healthcare.** I've had some experience with that. Let me explain.

My father had a heart attack when I was 15 and died of heart disease when I was 22 (he was 58) in 1970. I had confidence in my ability to solve problems that came my way, and I realized that I probably inherited my father's genes for heart disease, so I put this health challenge on my long-term to-do list. In 1983, when I was 35, **I was diagnosed with type 2 diabetes. The conventional treatment made it worse** (causing me to gain weight, which exacerbated the diabetes), so I decided the time had come to bring these personal health issues to the top of my to-do list. **I immersed myself in the health and medical literature, came up with my own approach involving nutrition, lifestyle, and supplements and <u>ultimately eliminated any indication of my diabetes by 1988.</u>** I wrote a bestselling health book about the experience, *The 10% Solution for a Health Life*, and have since written two more award-winning health books, *Fantastic Voyage* (2004) and *TRANSCEND: Nine Steps to Living Well Forever* (2009).

As I was going through this personal health revelation, I was also busy working on two inventions: the first music keyboard capable of accurately reproducing the sounds of a grand piano and other orchestral instruments and the first commercially marketed large-vocabulary speech recognition system. Today a descendant of that technology is Apple's voice-recognizing Siri. As an inventor, I realized that the key to success was timing. Most inventions and inventors fail, not because they are unable to get their gadgets to work, but because their timing is wrong. So, in the early 1980s I became an ardent student of technology trends, tracking the capacity and price performance of computing, and discovered that technology was advancing exponentially. This was a radical idea at the time because it turned our intuition—to think linearly—on its head.

It was around 1995 that I began to see that the exponential growth of technology applied to the **Genome Project**, which had begun in 1990. **Seven and a half years into the project, one percent of the Genome had been collected, which caused early critics to say that it was going to take seven hundred years to finish. My response was that the project was right on schedule and that one percent is only seven doublings away from 100 percent.** And indeed, the project continued to double each year and was done seven years later. The same rate of exponential progress has continued since the Genome Project ended. **Decoding that first**

genome cost more than $2.7 billion dollars. Today it costs less than $600. And every other aspect of what we call biotechnology—understanding the genome, modeling it, simulating it, and, most important, reprograming it, is progressing exponentially.

We now have the ability to prevent, treat, and (soon) cure diseases with biotechnology, guided by artificial intelligence. We are beginning to reprogram our biology in the same way that we reprogram our computers. Take for example the "turbocharged" flu vaccine created by researchers at Flinders University in Australia. They used a biology simulator to create trillions of chemical compounds and then used another simulator to see which compounds would be useful as immune-boosting drugs against the disease. They now have an optimal flu vaccine that is being tested on humans.

The trickle of current clinical biotechnology applications will become a flood by the end of the 2020s. **In the past three years we've reached a tipping point in computational power for artificial intelligence to quickly simulate, test, and solve biochemical problems.** The amount of computation devoted to training the best computer models since 2012 has doubled every three and a half months. **That's a 300,000-fold increase in the last nine years.** This has opened the door for AI to find medical solutions in a fraction of the time that it takes humans. Eventually, our trust in these AI driven simulations will grow and we will accept their results as sufficient without spending months on human trials. Soon we will be able to simulate trillions of possible solutions to every health problem and fully test them in hours or days.

This will bring us to the 2030s, when medical nanobots—blood cell–sized computers—will go into our bodies to combat disease from within our nervous system and travel into our brains through the capillaries where they will provide wireless communication between our neocortex and the cloud. Ideas and innovations will no longer be constrained by the size of our skulls. They will be free to grow exponentially in the cloud, expanding our intelligence a billionfold. But I am getting ahead of myself.

My point is that we must do everything we can today to be as healthy as possible, for as long as possible, in order to benefit from the fast-approaching merger of AI and medicine. Now is the time to make maximal use of the latest medical knowledge to help eliminate our chance of disease and to drastically slow down the aging process.

The tools to enhance and extend our lives are already in our hands. We just need the courage to question outdated assumptions that limit our ability to use them. Tony and Peter live by this philosophy and have written this book so that you can too.

THE LIFE FORCE REVOLUTION

Join me on a journey to answer some of life's most important questions and become the CEO of your own health. Learn **how stem cells are driving the regenerative medicine revolution,** discover the latest in preventative, predictive, personalized **diagnostics tools that could literally save your life or that of someone you love,** and discover the four **vitality ingredients that Harvard Geneticist and longevity expert David Sinclair, PhD, has used to reverse his biological age by 20 years!**

CHAPTER 1

LIFE FORCE: OUR GREATEST GIFT

Connect to the Supreme and Vital
Power of Your Life Force

"A healthy person has a thousand wishes, but a sick person has only one."
—INDIAN PROVERB

I'm walking through the open air of St. Peter's Square, past the immense dome of the Vatican, awed by the grandeur and beauty of this magnificent setting. As I walk up the white marble steps to the Vatican Hall, I see all heads suddenly turning. I follow their gaze, and I notice an older man with a benevolent smile and humble expression walking toward me. I look directly into his eyes as we reach out to shake hands . . . and then I realize it's the Holy Father, the Pope.

I've traveled to the Vatican for a landmark meeting with some of the greatest scientific minds in the world. They've flocked here for a conference hosted by Pope Francis himself. I've been invited to deliver the final speech to a roomful of pioneers in regenerative medicine—one of the great honors of my life.

Over three spellbinding days, we listen to a stream of brilliant scientists, doctors, and healthcare entrepreneurs. **They speak with urgency and passion about the solutions they're developing to combat deadly diseases and devastating medical disorders. They share mind-blowing revelations about new methods to restore the body at the cellular and molecular levels—therapies that can reinvigorate muscles and joints and blood vessels, revive damaged organs, conquer illnesses that previously seemed incurable. They take us on deep dives into stem cell** treatments, gene therapy, and other life-changing innovations that amplify the body's natural capacity to repair and renew itself. As you'll soon discover, many of these advances are so stunning that even a nonreligious person would describe them as miraculous!

As spiritual leader to 1.3 billion Catholics around the world, Pope Francis wants to nurture these scientific miracles for the good of all humanity. In his welcoming speech, he tells us how happy he is to have brought us together "from different cultures, societies, and religions" to serve our shared mission of helping "those who suffer" and exchanging knowledge "for the benefit of all."

The fact that the Pope himself is spearheading this historic event tells us just how far regenerative medicine has advanced. It speaks to the enormous potential of these trailblazing approaches to eliminating suffering, restoring our health, and enhancing our well-being.

In Rome we had a firsthand, front-row seat to see the impact of these unbelievable breakthroughs. **We met a 15-year-old who'd been given less than one chance in three of surviving leukemia—and was now, more than ten years later, in perfect health, thanks to a novel stem cell treatment.** We heard from people with advanced cancer who'd exhausted their options with chemo and radiation and were sent home to die. But they didn't give up. They tried some of the amazing new treatments you'll be reading about here—and two years later they weren't just surviving, but thriving!

I've written this book to help you understand what all this excitement is about. I want to empower you to take full advantage of this revolution in diagnostics, biotechnology, and regenerative medicine. It has already changed my life in ways I could never have imagined. It's transforming healthcare from top to bottom. It promises to expand our strength and vitality and potentially how long we can live. I want you to be among the first to benefit from these scientific discoveries, because I know from my own experience how dramatically they can improve the quality of *your* life. In fact, the practical knowledge that I'm about to share with you in these pages might actually *save* your life—or the life of someone you love.

The aim of this book is to give you the latest information on the astounding tools and therapies that are available RIGHT NOW, and others that could soon be approved by the U.S. Food and Drug Administration (FDA). These innovations will enable you to solve many of the most common health challenges before they get out of hand. **Imagine being able to find cancer at stage zero, when it's supremely treatable and ultimately curable. Wouldn't it be invaluable to understand your genetic risk factors, and some of the tools available that could lower or stop those risks from becoming reality? Think of the power of being able to change your lifestyle to avoid degenerative problems like heart disease and diabetes. Did you know that one company is in Phase 3 trials with a tool that could heal arthritis to help you regrow fresh cartilage like a teenager? Many of these developments are so astonishing that they sound like they'll be emerging in twenty or thirty years. In fact, <u>many of these are happening right now!</u>**

The speed of the biotech and healthcare revolution is geometrically *accelerating*, for two reasons. The first is a massive inflow of capital. While COVID-19 brought devastation to so many, it also served as a massive stimulus for investment. Despite the pandemic, more venture capital was invested in 2020—including a record $80 billion in healthcare startups alone—than at any other time in history. There are more dollars than ever before to drive more and more audacious medical and biotech innovations from research into the market.

The second reason is that biology is now an information technology, which means that the field of medicine is getting both better and cheaper at warp speed.

Thanks to technology, every phase of medical treatment is being reimagined. On the front end, sensors and networks are upending medical diagnostics. In the middle, robotics and 3D printing are reinventing traditional medical procedures. On the back end, artificial intelligence (AI), genomics, cellular medicine, gene therapies, and gene editing are transforming medicines themselves.

Taken altogether, biotech is remaking sick care into genuine healthcare. It's changing the medicine from the one-size-fits-all system we all grew up with to a totally new model: future-looking, proactive, personalized, precision medicine.

Not only is healthcare being transformed top to bottom by this geometric progression in technology, but costs are plummeting, as they are in other areas of daily life. For example: We forget how much cellphones used to cost. I actually had the first commercial model back in the 1980s, a Motorola that set me back $3,995—the equivalent of more than $10,000 today.[1] It was more than a foot long and weighed nearly two pounds! The battery charged for six hours, and it only gave you thirty minutes of talk time. Today you can get the latest Apple iPhone for free with most cell service contracts—and it has one hundred times more computational power than the computer that took the Apollo 11 astronauts to the moon.

Or think about this: Your computer runs on microchips—they're the brains of the machine. The first microchip contained 4,000 transistors that cost a dollar apiece. Today's state-of-the-art microchips feature more than six *trillion* transistors that cost an infinitesimal fraction of a penny. **They're 6,500 times faster and 4.2 million times cheaper!**

Our access to information, education, and entertainment has expanded exponentially as well. Every single day, **eighty-two *years'* worth of new video is uploaded to YouTube,** including entire courses from nearly every university in the world.

How do these trends relate to healthcare? Well, consider this: Less than **twenty-five years ago, it took more than a decade and cost $2.7 billion to read a complete human genome,** the full set of genetic instructions for a person's growth and development. **Today it's done for under $600—and completed overnight.**[2]

We now have the technology to "write over" a genome to *cure* sickle cell anemia and some forms of congenital blindness. Stem cells can regrow healthy lungs once thought to be damaged beyond repair. Other "living" medicines—using enhanced T cells or natural killer (NK) cells—can supercharge our immune system. Pharmaceutical-quality over-the-counter supplements exist today that can restore or enhance our energy and zest for the highest possible quality of life.

Do I have your attention? Are you ready to join me on this

---

1 McCusker, "How Much Is That in Real Money?"

2 Gertner, "Unlocking the Covid Code."

adventure? In fact, the innovations I've just mentioned are only a sliver of what you'll find in the chapters ahead!

But before we go any further into the marvels of regenerative medicine, before we share more about these life-changing, life-saving formulas, I need to tell you a story. I need to explain what brought me to the Vatican in the first place—what happened in my own life to make me rethink everything I thought I knew about health and healthcare. After all, if you'd told me ten years ago that I'd be rubbing shoulders with these scientific superstars, I'd have laughed!

So how did I, of all people, become an evangelist for these groundbreaking advances in cellular and molecular medicine? How did I learn that our bodies could self-renew and self-heal to the point that science fiction is turning into science fact?

In short, how did I end up here with you right now, preparing to tell you about all of these remarkable technological breakthroughs—advances that I'm convinced can help you and your loved ones live much healthier, longer, more vibrant, more energetic, and more joyful lives?

FROM PAIN TO POWER

*"Do not judge me by my successes, judge me by how
many times I fell down and got back up again."*

—NELSON MANDELA

Like all of us, I arrived at where I am today because of a series of decisions. Some of them were conscious and deliberate. But as I look back, I believe without a doubt in the element of grace, the times when I was guided to the right answer. When challenging circumstances reshaped my core beliefs and made me willing to seize an opportunity that changed everything. I'm sure you've experienced moments like this in your life. You know what I'm talking about. Where something terrible happened, something so painful that you'd never want to go through it again, or have anyone you care about go through it, but afterward, you realized that challenging time made you grow. It made you care more, produced a different level of drive that helped you improve the quality of your life or the lives of those you love. Many of these painful experiences are what prepared me to write this book. The sum of the darkest and most difficult times gave me the insights that I'm ready to share with you today—insights that can boost your health, happiness, and vitality. That can make life truly worth living.

It all began with the gift of growing up in a tough environment. Don't get me wrong. There was lots of love in my family. But my upbringing was also filled with violence, chaos, insecurity, and fear. My mom was wonderful in so many ways, but she struggled with addictions to alcohol and prescription drugs. Many times we were too broke to buy food or clothes. I was desperate for answers, desperate to learn anything that could ease my suffering.

For as long as I can remember, I also hated to see others suffer. That's why I've spent more than four and a half decades of my life working to help millions of people uncover the most effective strategies to get from where they are to where they truly want to be. To achieve their dreams and more—to live a life of meaning and fulfillment. I'm obsessed with helping people lift themselves up from pain to power. But when I was starting out, I didn't have a single role model for success or achievement. So what could I do? Where could I turn for insight and inspiration?

I turned to books—my great escape. I discovered that I could enter the world of philosophy by reading the essays of Ralph Waldo Emerson. I could enter the world of psychology by reading *Man's Search for Meaning* by Viktor Frankl. So I took a speed-reading course and set myself a goal of reading one book a day. As you might have predicted, that turned out to be a bit of a stretch! But I was so hungry for knowledge that I read more than 700 books in seven years. I raced through them in an insatiable quest to learn everything and anything that could help me or anyone who would listen to me! In high school, I was known as Mr. Solution. If you had a question, I had an answer.

When I was seventeen years old and supporting myself by working as a janitor, I found my first moment of grace. I met Jim Rohn. A renowned personal development speaker and business philosopher, Jim was the man who helped me to see that for things to change, *I* had to change. For my life to get better, *I* had to get better. Bemoaning my past wouldn't get me to a brighter future. Complaining about my current stressful circumstances wouldn't help. Neither would hoping my luck would change or wishing on a star.

What Jim taught me was this: If you want to succeed at anything— **whether it's building a hugely profitable business, constructing a stormproof investment portfolio, or creating a healthy lifestyle that fills you with boundless energy—you need to study people who have already achieved the result you're after. In other words, success leaves clues. If a person has sustained success in any long-term ambition— whether it was losing weight, growing a business, sustaining an extraordinary relationship—then luck has nothing to do with it. They're doing something *different* than you are.** So you need to understand exactly *what* they're doing differently, and precisely *how* they've mastered the skills you'll need to replicate their success.

Jim got me to start focusing on the *few who do* in life, not just the many who talk. I began to appreciate the value of role models, those special people who can help you identify a *proven* approach instead of expending all your energy in trial and error. If there's already a paved express lane to power, why not follow it?

But remember, I was Mr. Solution! So I kept reading voraciously, kept studying the most successful people in every area I wanted to master, kept applying their time-tested strategies. Before long, I'd gathered enough answers to become a coach. I began with one-on-one sessions and built up to small seminars and then groups of several hundred people. Before long, I was working with Olympic gold medalists, billionaire businessmen, and some of the world's greatest entertainers. I had found my calling.

It was a beautiful life. I had the opportunity to share the insights and strategies I'd learned and help others connect with their inner strength, courage, and purpose. And, most important, to find out how to get quicker, faster, and more satisfying results. But the truth is, I was a different person back then than I am today. In those early years of my career, I didn't yet know how to handle the fearful part of the ancient fight-or-flight brain that exists inside us all. I'm guessing you've experienced this, too—those times when your uncertainty runs wild, spurring your mind to invent far-fetched disaster scenarios that would earn you a fortune if you wrote made-for-TV movies! I must have watched a lot of those films, because I started to develop a terrible sense of foreboding about my future.

Rationally, I could see that it was no fluke that my career had taken flight. I was working 18 or 20 hours a day on a mission to serve. But an awful thought kept worming into my brain: *What if the reason I'd been successful so quickly was that I was destined to die young?* Once I allowed myself to dwell on those irrational fears, my mind kept creating more of them. As I've taught people for years: *Where focus goes, energy flows.* So you better direct your focus!

But *this* foreboding was crazy! It wasn't just my anxiety about an untimely death. I worried that my tragic demise would be slow and agonizing. Instead of getting hit by a truck and dying instantly, I imagined myself rotting away in pain for years with cancer. I even had nightmares about it. Until one day, when my nightmares came to life and a cancer diagnosis turned my world upside down for real.

But it wasn't me who got the diagnosis.

My girlfriend at the time, Liz, burst into my apartment one day, sobbing uncontrollably. "My mom has cancer," she told me. "They think she has nine weeks to live."

It felt like a punch to the gut. It took my breath away. I loved Liz's mom, Ginny, and I couldn't believe what I was hearing. Struggling to hold back my tears, I asked, "How is this possible?" Ginny had gone to the doctor with a big bulge on her back, just below her shoulder. Now she was being told it was cancerous—and that she also had a tumor in her uterus. What's more, those doctors had decided that it wasn't even worth treating her because her cancer had progressed beyond the point of no return. All she could do was set her affairs in order and bravely face the prospect of dying in her forties.

This terrible news shook me to my core. But I was someone who could never accept pain, suffering, or defeat without searching for a solution. I knew that tens of thousands of people had beaten cancer after hearing it was incurable, and that many of them had followed nontraditional alternatives to radiation or chemotherapy. What if their success had left clues that could help Ginny?

So I went to work, reading everything about cancer I could lay my hands on. I came across a short book by a Kansas orthodontist who'd overcome pancreatic cancer and credited a nutritional program that apparently detoxified his system. At the same time, he revitalized his body with concentrated pancreatic enzymes. It was a controversial approach, and I wouldn't recommend it today because better options now exist. But at the time, Ginny had nothing to lose and no promising alternative. So she embraced this experimental approach with an unshakeable belief that it would save her.

Incredibly, within just a few days, she started to feel better. After a few weeks, as her body began to cleanse itself, she felt better still. After two and a half months, Ginny's doctor was shocked by her radical improvement. Eventually he persuaded her to undergo exploratory surgery, so he could see what was going on. When they opened her up, they discovered that a fist-sized tumor had shriveled to the size of a fingernail. The doctor was blown away. Ginny explained what she'd been doing to heal herself, but he had no interest in hearing it. He couldn't believe that her diet and her mindset could have had such a profound effect. "You don't understand," he told her in that patronizing tone. "This is just a spontaneous remission."

Today, I am happy to tell you that Ginny is alive and well in her eighties—more than forty years after being told that she had only nine weeks left to live!

That experience changed me forever. To this day, I can't explain the precise mechanisms that healed Ginny's body. But I can tell you this: **Ginny's recovery strengthened my core belief that** *there's almost always an answer*, **even in the toughest situations.** And it taught me that we need to search for those answers with an open and inquiring mind, never accepting without question that the "experts" *must* be right. Sure, there are times when the traditional "standard of care" might be the best approach. **But we all have to think for ourselves and do our own due diligence. We can't outsource the oversight of our health to anyone else, no matter how many diplomas are nailed to their office wall. We can't take it on faith that they have all the right solutions.** Likewise, we can't blindly follow the average person's example. Why *would* you, given that the average person isn't particularly healthy?

Seeing how Ginny's life was turned upside down by cancer—and then right side up again—showed me the simple truth that **nothing matters more than our health**. As you can imagine, it convinced me that taking care of my body had to be a top priority. Some people behave as if work or money is more important than health. Think about it, there are billionaires who've been diagnosed with a painful chronic or terminal disease, and who'd give up everything to restore their physical well-being.

As we'll discuss later in more detail, our lifestyle choices—especially nutrition, exercise, sleep, and mindset—play starring roles in optimizing our health. Small and simple changes in these areas can have a tremendous influence on our quality of life and our level of day-to-day energy. So I decided to go all in to adopt a healthy lifestyle that would help maximize my strength, my vitality, my capacity to grow and share, and my ability to live life to the fullest.

I started working out like a banshee. I became a vegan at a time when it wasn't exactly fashionable in America—the homeland of supersized steaks, barbecued ribs, cheeseburgers, and deep-fried chicken! It won't surprise you to hear that I occasionally took things too far. I pushed myself so hard that there were days when I found it difficult to run or even walk without back pain. But I became immensely strong and was bursting with energy. I felt for the first time that I'd truly connected to my own power, my essence, my *life force*.

YOUR SPECTACULAR BODY

"We must be willing to get rid of the life we've planned, so as to have the life that is waiting for us. The old skin has to be shed before the new one can come."

—JOSEPH CAMPBELL

When you and I are feeling energized and our bodies are functioning smoothly, we tend to take our health for granted. But if you stop and think about it for a moment, the human body is the most complex, sophisticated, and awe-inspiring piece of machinery ever invented.

Just consider the following facts:

- Your miraculous body consists of about 30 trillion human cells—and produces 330 billion new ones each day.
- Our human cells are outnumbered by *bacterial* cells in our gut. How many are there? Around 39 trillion!
- Your brain contains around an estimated 100 billion neurons, the same number of stars in the Milky Way Galaxy![3]
- What about the human eye? Well, it contains over *2 million* moving parts.
- Our thigh bones are stronger than concrete.
- Your skin sheds approximately 40,000 cells every minute, or 50 million per day, and replaces them with healthy cells without you having to do a thing.
- Red blood cells can race through our entire body in less than 20 seconds.
- Laid out end to end, your blood vessels would stretch more than 60,000 miles, or more than twice around the Earth's equator.
- Information zips across your brain's synapses at 268 miles per hour, faster than the record speed at the Indianapolis Motor Speedway.

What's more, we've been given all of this amazing equipment for free—which might explain why many people don't take such good care of it! But I was determined to make the most of what I'd been given. I *had* to perform at my peak. My mission to lead others to new heights demanded it.

As I've expanded my reach around the world, I travel incessantly. In a typical year, I visit more than 100 cities in as many as 16 different countries. Onstage, I need to hold the attention of audiences of 10,000 to 15,000 people—or even 35,000 in a stadium venue—day after day, from a four- to seven-day stretch in each of my programs. Offstage, I coach world-class winners like Serena Williams and Conor McGregor, and teams like the NBA champion Golden State Warriors and the NHL Stanley Cup winners the Washington Capitals. These phenomenal athletes expect me—like them—to operate on the outer edge of what's humanly possible. I'm not sure they'd have listened to me if I sprawled on the sofa all day, stuffing

---

3 Herculano-Houzel, "The Human Brain in Numbers: A Linearly Scaled-Up Primate Brain."

myself with cookies and potato chips! So I turned my body into a high-performance vehicle for unlimited energy.

If you're going to help create huge breakthroughs for people, the first thing you need is energy—and an extraordinary amount of it. No one can consistently take the actions necessary to break through limits or fears without a supreme level of strength and vitality. My job is to keep that happening by literally plunging into the crowd, sprinting up the stairs of the stadium, and keeping those thousands of people engaged 12 to 14 hours per day—day after day, night after night. And a big part of that is the energy that we generate together. If you've ever attended one of my events, you know what I mean. It's unbridled energy. It's energy exploding in and around you and pulsing through your mind and body. It's that feeling of being *unleashed*, where you know you can make anything possible. It launches you into a peak state of mind, a place where you're liberated to live and love and perform at a whole new level. *That's* what creates transformation.

In order to do all of this, I place insane demands on my body to generate the energy that drives these profound changes. In fact, a few years ago, an organization called the **Applied Science and Performance Institute** set out to measure how my body performs during these high-intensity events. They strapped a $65,000 contraption to me and tracked everything from my heart rate variability to the amount of lactic acid I was accumulating. They tested my blood and saliva on an hourly basis to gauge my hormonal levels throughout the day. Nine hours in, the device died, but I kept going for three more hours! They couldn't believe what they saw, so they tested me at four separate events—and each time they came up with the same results. It turned out that I jumped more than a thousand times a day—a big deal, as the researchers explained to me. **I weigh 282 pounds, and each landing multiplied the force of my body weight by four times. That's more than a thousand pounds of stress for each jump, a thousand times a day, for more than a million pounds of stress in that day. I was burning 11,300 calories per day—the equivalent of playing two and a half NBA basketball games in one day, or running three marathons.**

And then I was doing it all over again the *next* day. And the next, and the next . . .

I'm not telling you this to impress you. My point is to impress upon you

1 DAY AT UNLEASH THE POWER WITHIN FOR TONY

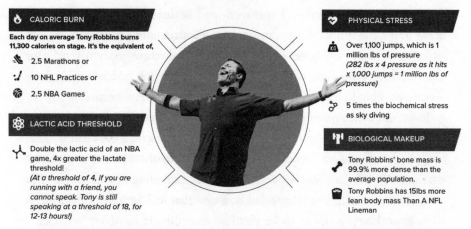

CALORIC BURN

Each day on average Tony Robbins burns 11,300 calories on stage. It's the equivalent of,

- 2.5 Marathons or
- 10 NHL Practices or
- 2.5 NBA Games

LACTIC ACID THRESHOLD

Double the lactic acid of an NBA game, 4x greater the lactate threshold!
(At a threshold of 4, if you are running with a friend, you cannot speak. Tony is still speaking at a threshold of 18, for 12-13 hours!)

PHYSICAL STRESS

Over 1,100 jumps, which is 1 million lbs of pressure
(282 lbs x 4 pressure as it hits x 1,000 jumps = 1 million lbs of pressure)

5 times the biochemical stress as sky diving

BIOLOGICAL MAKEUP

Tony Robbins' bone mass is 99.9% more dense than the average population.

Tony Robbins has 15lbs more lean body mass Than A NFL Lineman

Applied Science & Performance Institute (ASPI) has studied Stanley Cup and Super Bowl Champions, Navy Seals, Olympic Gold Medalists and published hundreds of studies on longevity. The information above is based on studying Tony Robbins across 5 events over 3 years.

just how critical it is for me to keep my body in absolute peak condition. It's the reason I've become a full-time biohacker. It's why I constantly look for new tools to strengthen and enhance my energy, vitality, and endurance.

In case you're wondering, I haven't slowed down with age, either. Today, at 62, I don't just *feel* stronger. I can measurably run faster and lift more weight than when I was 25 years old. All this, thanks to a well-designed training regimen, cutting-edge technology, a healthy diet, and the power of regenerative medicine.

Again, I'm not telling you this to brag. I'm telling you because I want you to know what's possible for you as well. **After all, my goal in writing this book is to help you unleash the pure, vibrant, turbocharged energy of your life force. What better gift could you give yourself than the ability to optimize your vitality and strength to last and even *increase* with age? What wouldn't you give to reverse the standard pattern—one that most people accept—of steady (or dramatic) decline?**

Now, I don't want to give you the wrong impression. Like you, I'm not immune from problems. Far from it! I've gone through periods when my health and even my life were in serious jeopardy, when my beliefs were tested like never before.

One of these trials by fire came when I was 31 years old, a time when I was coaching some of the most influential people on the planet and feeling on top of the world. One day, to renew my helicopter pilot license, I visited a doctor for a routine physical exam. I was so fit and health-conscious that it didn't occur to me I might have a problem. But a few days later, I arrived home late one night to find a message my assistant had taped to my door: "Your doctor keeps calling, he says you must call him—it's an emergency." Unfortunately, it was after midnight. All I could do was leave a message on voicemail.

What does your mind do in a situation like this? Well, mine went straight to: *Oh my God, after all I've done to stay healthy, is it possible I have cancer? I eat really well and train like a crazy person, but could it be the chemicals in the environment? Has all that flying exposed me to too much radiation?* When you're in a state of uncertainty, your mind sometimes goes off the rails. I decided to shut those thoughts down, to let them go and respond to reality as it came. By that stage of my life, I'd developed a core belief in the importance of a courageous mind. As the saying goes, "A coward dies a thousand deaths, a brave person only once." I would deal with whatever it was in the morning.

The next day, filled with a sense of dread I hadn't felt in years, I phoned the doctor to find out what was wrong. "You need surgery," he told me. "You have a tumor in your brain."

I was shocked and bewildered. How could he possibly know *that* from a routine physical?

The doctor, a gruff guy who would have flunked out of charm school, told me he'd performed some additional blood tests because he figured that my body contained abnormal quantities of growth hormone. (Since I was five-foot-one my sophomore year in high school, grew ten inches in one year, and am now six-foot-seven and wear a size-16 shoe, it didn't take Sherlock Holmes to make that deduction.) But then he took it one step further. He suspected that my teenaged growth spurt, when I'd shot up ten inches in one year, was the result of a tumor in the pituitary gland at the base of my brain. He told me it was a ticking time bomb inside my head.

I was due to fly the next day to the South of France to conduct one of my Date with Destiny seminars. But the doctor wanted me to skip the event and have emergency surgery instead. He obviously didn't know me well. I wasn't going to accept the first diagnosis and quickly make a decision from fear, while simultaneously canceling an event last minute and letting thousands of people down! So I flew to France, taught the seminar, and then spent a few days trying to relax in Portofino, Italy. It didn't work. My old fears of illness and mortality kept flooding back. *Was this finally it? Was I doomed to die young, after all?*

To overcome my fears, I had spent years training and conditioning my mind and body to gain a consistent sense of strength and certainty. That's the only way to prime yourself to take action. Now, out of nowhere, I'd been thrown back into the terrifying insecurity of my childhood, when nothing felt stable.

I had no idea if I'd live or die. But within a few days, I decided that I had to confront the situation head-on. So I flew home and had a brain scan. I remember emerging from the MRI machine, glancing at the bleak expression on the lab technician's face, and knowing in that moment that he'd seen something ominous. The doctor reviewed the scan and confirmed that I had a pituitary tumor. It had ballooned out of control, pushing huge amounts of growth hormone into my body and creating a condition called gigantism. The tumor had shrunk a bit on its own, and the doctor couldn't explain how or why that had happened. But there was still enough in there for him to urge me to have immediate surgery. Otherwise, he warned, the tumor could generate a disastrous overproduction of hormones and trigger heart failure or some other fatal outcome.

There was just one problem with the doctor's plan. Assuming that I actually *survived* the operation, there was still a high probability that it could wreck my endocrine system, depriving me forever of the energy that made it possible to do my life's work. For me, that was utterly unacceptable. At the very least, I'd need a second opinion before I could even contemplate such a risk. But this doctor was one of those people who are infuriated by any challenge to their authority. He refused to recommend another expert.

As I'd learned from Ginny's triumph over cancer, nobody has a monopoly on medical wisdom. I couldn't accept placing my life in a single doctor's hands without investigating my other options. I tracked down a world-renowned endocrinologist in Boston who scanned my brain again. I'll never forget his kindness and compassion—the opposite of the first doctor. He reassured me that surgery would be much too risky and that I didn't need it.

Instead, he suggested that I fly to Switzerland twice a year for injections of an experimental drug that would prevent my tumor from growing and re-duce the risk of heart problems. When I asked about its side effects, he said, "Well, to be honest, there's a severe loss of energy."

And I said, "I just can't do that. I can't fulfill my life's mission as a low-energy person." And I said, "The other doctor said I have to have surgery and now you're telling me I have to have drugs."

And this beautiful man said with a smile and a twinkle in his eyes, "Tony, you're right. The butcher wants to butcher. The baker wants to bake. The sur-geon wants to cut. And I'm an endocrinologist, so I want to give you a drug. But here's the thing: We'll just have more certainty if you take the drug."

And I responded, "But we can't be certain about all the side effects of this drug, either. There's no sign of any current issues with my heart, and I've obviously had this condition since I was a teenager. What if I just did nothing?"

And the doctor said, "Well, if you get yourself tested regularly, I guess that's an option."

Over the next three months, I met with six other doctors. One of them made a compelling case for doing nothing, other than going for regular checkups to make sure my condition hadn't deteriorated. While he agreed that my bloodstream contained enormous quantities of growth hormone, he pointed out something that everyone else had seemed to overlook: that my condition hadn't caused any negative effects. To the contrary, he said, my reservoir of growth hormone may have boosted my body's ability to recover from the extraordinary stress my work placed on it. "You've got a great gift here," the doctor told me. "I know bodybuilders who'd have to spend $1,200 a month to get what you're getting for free!"

In the end, I followed his advice and decided against surgery *and* drugs. How did that turn out? My decision may have saved my life. Six months later, the U.S. Food and Drug Administration banned the use of the medi-cation that had been recommended to me, after studies revealed it caused cancer. And three decades later, though I still have that tumor at the base of my brain, it has yet to cause any problems. It hasn't stopped me from living the most blessed and magical life I could imagine.

All of these doctors were well-meaning. All of them wanted to give me a *certainty* that I'd be okay with either drugs or surgery. **But there is a price**

for certainty when you're trying to get it from outside yourself. And I was now beginning to understand that the only true power of certainty lies within ourselves. I had to make a decision. **If I was feeling no ill effects in my life, why live in fear?** Ultimately, your health comes down to making smart decisions, developing great habits, and having a strong mindset. And remember, emotions can rule the physical body. One study showed that one five-minute angry outburst can impair your immune system for up to five hours.[4] And so: learning to master your mind is essential to an extraordinary quality of life and extraordinary amounts of energy. We'll explore more in depth the power of mindset and strategies for controlling it in the final two chapters of this book.

After a while, I simply realized that it wasn't worth feeling anxious anymore. I decided that I'd no longer live my life in fear or limit myself in any way because of some invisible threat inside my brain. Sure, I still get tested regularly to make sure that my tumor hasn't grown and that my heart is still working perfectly. But in the meantime, nothing will stop me from living fully and fearlessly until the day I die.

MAKE YOURSELF THE CEO OF YOUR OWN HEALTH

"Do not be so open-minded that your brain falls out."

—G. K. CHESTERTON

Dealing with a brain tumor reinforced my bedrock belief that you and I must take full responsibility for the most important decisions in our lives. **One of the central principles underpinning this book is that you need to function as the CEO of your own health.** We can't let anyone else determine our destiny, no matter how knowledgeable or caring they may be. **Experts should be our coaches, but not our commanders.** When it comes to your family, your faith, your finances, or your health, only you can make the critical decisions. Because in the end, you must live with the results that your decisions create.

---

4 Rein et al., "The Physiological and Psychological Effects of Compassion and Anger."

What does that mean in practical terms? **It means *taking control of edu-cating yourself about what works*, so you can make smart, informed, and independent decisions about how to protect and enhance your physical well-being.** It means *keeping a hefty dose of healthy skepticism about whatever you hear or read*, given that some of it will be misguided or harmful—or even lethal. And it means ***seeking out second opinions before making any im-portant medical decision***, since even the best doctors make mistakes—just as you and I might (very occasionally!) mess up in our own areas of exper-tise. **Where should you go for a second opinion? Obviously, it's not a random choice. You need to seek out qualified experts with a demon-strated track record for solving your specific problem.**

But I'm not asking you to take *my* word for it that one expert opinion isn't enough. A study published in 2017 analyzed the medical records of 286 pa-tients whose healthcare providers had referred them to the Mayo Clinic for a second opinion.[5] **The report found that the final diagnosis was "distinctly different" from the original diagnosis *21 percent* of the time. Yes, the second opinion contradicted the first opinion in more than *one in five* cases! What's more, for two of three patients, the final diagnosis was found to be "better defined/refined" than the first one. The first and second opinions were the same in only *12 percent* of these 286 cases![6]**

Now, let me be clear. I'm not out to undermine your faith in the medical profession. In my experience, doctors are among the most dedicated, dili-gent, and honorable people I've ever met. What could be more admirable than devoting your life to helping and healing others? But the Mayo Clinic study affirms one lesson I learned when all of my top-notch specialists dis-agreed on how to handle my tumor: *Doctors can be sincere and sincerely wrong.*

How come? For starters, our bodies are infinitely complex, and medical data can be interpreted in so many different ways. Doctors are also chal-lenged by the fact that the ground keeps shifting beneath their feet. Much of what they learned in medical school has gotten quickly outdated by the endless deluge of new research, new technology, and new treatment options.

---

5 Van Such et al., "Extent of Diagnostic Agreement Among Medical Referrals."

6 Zimmerman, "Mayo Clinic Researchers Demonstrate Value of Second Opinions."

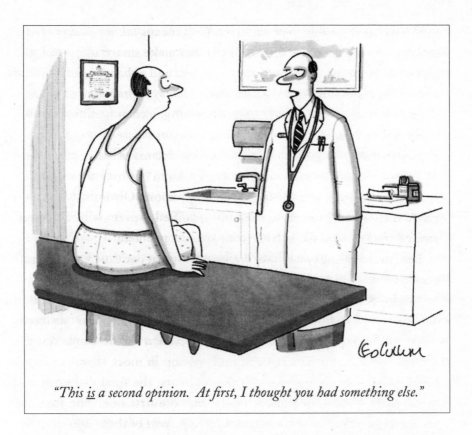

"This is a second opinion. At first, I thought you had something else."

In 2017, Harvard Medical School reported that the half-life of medical knowledge was 18 to 24 months—and predicted it was headed for 73 days by the time you're reading this! What does that mean? It means that over half of all a doctor learned in medical school is no longer valid within 18–24 months! Wow! Can you imagine how hard it must be to keep up with all those changes amid the constant pressure of caring for patients and their urgent problems?

Maybe a simple metaphor will help you appreciate what doctors go through. Picture yourself as a doctor, a person who is dedicated to saving lives with skill and empathy. You're walking along a riverside and all of a sudden you hear someone screaming! You see that they're drowning, so with no thought for your own safety, you plunge into the raging river. You grab the drowning person and swim and pull them to the riverbank. You frantically give them mouth-to-mouth resuscitation until they splutter and breathe again—you've saved that person's life! But then you hear two more people screaming from the rushing water. You're tired, but you jump in and save them both. And just as you've finished resuscitating the second one, you hear four more people screaming . . .

That's the predicament for doctors today. They're so busy saving people that they have no time or energy to go upstream to see who's throwing all those people in the river!

Atul Gawande, a surgeon at Brigham and Women's Hospital, a professor at Harvard Medical School, and a winner of a MacArthur "Genius Grant," writes candidly about the difficulties of practicing medicine in his book *Complications: A Surgeon's Notes on an Imperfect Science*. Gawande acknowledges that all doctors make "terrible mistakes," including the most respected surgeons: **"We look for medicine to be an orderly field of knowledge and procedure. But it is not. It is an imperfect science, an enterprise of constantly changing knowledge, uncertain information, fallible individuals, and at the same time lives on the line. There is science in what we do, yes, but also habit, intuition, and sometimes plain old guessing."**

> *"Over the past two decades the pharmaceutical industry has moved very far from its original high purpose of discovering and producing useful new drugs. Now [it's] primarily a marketing machine to sell new drugs of dubious benefit."*

—MARCIA ANGELL, American physician and author, 2004, first woman editor in chief of the *New England Journal of Medicine*

Finally, there's one more reason you and I need to be well informed and discerning about our healthcare. As I'm sure you've seen in the headlines, the pharmaceutical industry has its own problems. There are many great people working at drug companies, and they've developed medications that save countless lives. So please don't leap to the mistaken conclusion that I'm anti-medicine—quite the contrary. This book is filled with some of the greatest medical breakthroughs available today. Still, we can't ignore the fact that pharmaceuticals constitute a vastly lucrative business with more than its share of scandals. It can cost more than a billion dollars to research, develop, and bring to market a successful drug. So it's no surprise that a few unscrupulous people have used lies and manipulation to line their pockets at the expense of patients like you and me.

One of the more notorious health scandals in recent years involves Purdue Pharma, which touted itself as a "pioneer in developing medications for reducing pain, a principal cause of human suffering." Sounds pretty noble, doesn't it? But in reality, Purdue made huge profits by aggressively marketing OxyContin, an infamously addictive painkiller that fueled America's raging opioids epidemic. **Purdue intentionally deceived doctors on Oxy-Contin's safety record, falsely claiming that fewer than 1 percent of patients who took the drug became addicted.**[7] According to the Centers for Disease Control and Prevention, between 1999 and 2019, **nearly half a million Americans died from overdoses involving opioids.** More than 93,000 died in 2020 alone, a record high.[8]

Can you imagine that the doctors prescribing these drugs were following the pharmaceutical companies' advice? Again, physicians have no time to study every single drug that comes on the market. And can you imagine the horror of doctors trying to relieve their patients of pain, only to discover that their recommendation had been based on misinformation—and that it had led some of those patients to addiction, or even to their deaths? Meanwhile, **Purdue recently agreed to an $8.3 billion settlement to resolve a slew of criminal and civil charges, a tiny fraction of the opioid epidemic's multitrillion-dollar cost to the U.S. economy not to mention the lives that were destroyed.**[9] To add insult to injury, the company's owners, the Sackler family, agreed to their own $4.5 billion bankruptcy settlement in return for a lifetime legal shield—**but only after they made more than $12 billion in profit from OxyContin.**[10] In July 2021, Johnson & Johnson—a household name for generations—and three of the largest drug distributors—household names for generations—reached a $26 billion

---

7 Keefe, "The Sackler Family's Plans to Keep Its Billions."

8 Katz and Sanger-Katz, "'It's Huge, It's Historic, It's Unheard-Of': Drug Overdose Deaths Spike."

9 Hoffman, "Purdue Pharma Is Dissolved and Sacklers Pay $4.5 Billion to Settle Opioid Claims."

10 Sandler, "The Sacklers Made More Than $12 Billion in Profit from OxyContin Maker Purdue Pharma, New Report Says."

settlement after numerous states threatened to bring them to court for downplaying opioids' addictiveness.[11]

Plenty of other "big pharma" companies have also been embroiled in legal controversies. **Pfizer agreed to pay a then record $2.3 billion to settle federal charges of illegal and dangerous marketing of four different drugs.[12] Whistleblowers called out Questcor Pharmaceuticals and Mallinckrodt, the company that acquired it, for bribing doctors to inflate sales of a drug for an infant seizure disorder. Over 19 years, the price of the drug rose almost 97,000 percent, from $40 a vial to $39,000.** If that sounds fair, try asking your clients for a 97,000 percent price increase—or, if you work for someone else, why not ask your boss for a 97,000 percent raise?

The OxyContin scandal may be the most extreme example of a drug company putting its own financial interests before the safety of its customers. But in reality, the entire pharmaceutical industry has a powerful incentive to make us buy medications that may or may not be right for us. That's why we're bombarded with so many commercials for prescription drugs whenever we turn on the TV. Just to give you a sense of how much money goes toward coaxing us to choose a particular treatment, consider this: **In 2019 alone, more than half a billion dollars was spent on advertising in the U.S. for Humira, a blockbuster drug used to treat rheumatoid arthritis and other inflammatory conditions.**[13]

I don't know about you, but I'm always amused by how healthy and beautiful everyone looks in those TV ads for prescription drugs. They're always bursting with joy as they dance or twirl a Hula-Hoop or give a gleaming new car to their daughter! Life couldn't be better . . . until the end of the ad, when you hear about the long list of potential side effects and discover that your bladder might explode or you might stop breathing or grow an extra pair of arms!

I don't mean to sound cynical here. But the stakes are so high when

---

11 Hoffman, "Drug Distributors and J&J Reach $26 Billion Deal to End Opioid Lawsuits."

12 Rubin, "Pfizer Fined $2.3 Billion for Illegal Marketing in Off-Label Drug Case."

13 Bulik, "The Top 10 Ad Spenders for Big Pharma in 2019."

it comes to our health that we can't afford to be naïve consumers who accept without question whatever's being sold or recommended to us. That would be like buying a home based on a real estate broker's poetic listing—without looking the place over or paying for an inspector to check it out.

We need to be especially careful before taking extreme measures, whether it's a drug with potentially dire side effects or a high-risk operation. In some cases, it's worth considering less aggressive or less invasive options. **As you'll soon see, one virtue of regenerative medicine is that it's fundamentally different from the blunt-force conventional therapies most people rely on. Regenerative medicine doesn't just treat your symptoms. Its goal is to reverse or cure the underlying problem.**

I might never have learned about the power of precision medicine or many of the regenerative breakthroughs at the heart of this book if not for a terrible accident that threatened to derail my entire way of life when I was 54. I have to admit, I was acting more like a 14-year-old at the time, tearing down a mountain in Sun Valley, Idaho, on my snowboard. It went horribly wrong, and I fell with a bone-rattling force that annihilated my shoulder.

It turned out that I'd torn my rotator cuff, the set of tendons and muscles connecting the upper arm to the shoulder. Over the years, I'd dealt with lots of pain. But this hurt so brutally that I didn't know what to do with myself. On a scale of one to ten, I'd award this pain a score of 9.9! My nerves were on fire. Deep breaths even hurt. Over the next two nights, I slept a grand total of two hours.

I met with three specialists who all advised surgery. But the recovery process would be slow and arduous, and I could be sidelined for six months or even longer if things didn't go well. Plus, the long-term prognosis wasn't great. I could go for the surgery and commit to months of intensive rehab, only to have my weakened shoulder tear all over again. The doctors also warned that my arm might freeze up to the point where I'd be unable to lift it above my shoulder. How could I rip up a stage and energize tens of thousands of people with my arm frozen by my side? I'd be like a prizefighter with one arm tied behind his back!

There had to be a better answer, if only I looked hard enough to find it. So I kicked into overdrive, researching every conceivable solution. A few days later, I met an orthopedic surgeon who told me that surgery was not the best approach. And that there was a device that could immediately ease my pain and potentially help me to heal. Within 24 hours, I had someone treating me with one. It reduced my pain from a 9.9 to about a 5, which meant at least I could think coherently and finally sleep again. In our "Living Pain Free" chapter I'll tell you more about this **pulse electronic-magnetic frequency (PEMF) technology. Numerous studies have confirmed that it can speed the healing of bones by up to 50 percent.**[14] I'm confident that if you're injured or in severe pain and need some powerful relief, PEMF might be a beautiful solution for you as well.

But even though my pain was now manageable, I still wasn't my old young self again. I'd be going full tilt on stage and suddenly lose all feeling in my arm. Or I'd be halfway through the day and everything would seem fine, when the pain would suddenly hit me like a jackhammer. I was *existing*, but I wasn't *living*. And little did I know that my health crisis was about to take a turn from bad to worse.

I met with another doctor, who checked me out and delivered a devastating verdict. **He looked me in the eye and declared, "Life as you know it is over." He showed me an image of my spine and explained, "You have extreme spinal stenosis," an abnormal narrowing of the space within my spinal canal.** It wasn't a total surprise, since I'd had severe back pain for nearly a decade. But the doctor warned that my situation was so grave that one more bad hit to my body could make me a quadriplegic. Falling off my snowboard again—or one heavy jump on stage—could be catastrophic. Even going for a run would be out of the question.

After decades of relentless physical demands, it seemed like my body was starting to fall apart. My life had always been defined by my energy and mind, by my constant drive to serve people and perform for them at the very peak of my abilities. But now it looked like the whole edifice might come tumbling down at any moment.

---

14 Cadossi et al., "Pulsed Electromagnetic Field Stimulation of Bone Healing and Joint Preservation: Cellular Mechanisms of Skeletal Response;" FDA, "FDA Executive Summary Prepared for the September 8–9, 2020, Meeting of the Orthopaedic and Rehabilitation Devices Panel: Reclassification of Non-Invasive Bone Growth Stimulators."

I don't know if you've ever had an experience like this—a time when your vitality was compromised. When your energy began to slip away and you started to contemplate the possibility of continued decline. If you have, you can imagine the uncertainty and fear that I felt. But I wasn't about to surrender and accept that the damage was irreversible. I refused to believe that my fate was sealed. So I did what I've always done. I kept looking for answers.

THE MIRACLE OF REJUVENATION

"We must always change, renew, rejuvenate ourselves; otherwise, we harden."
—JOHANN WOLFGANG VON GOETHE

As luck would have it, I turned for advice to one of the smartest, most tech-savvy, and most forward-thinking people I know: my dear friend Peter Diamandis. Growing up, Peter dreamed of becoming an astronaut. But his parents wanted him to be a doctor. So, after graduating from MIT with a dual degree in molecular genetics and aerospace engineering, he earned his MD from Harvard Medical School.

In the end, though, Peter blazed his own trail, developing a dazzling breadth and depth of expertise. Among his many accomplishments, he's the founder and executive chairman of the XPRIZE Foundation, which creates competitions that inspire innovators to achieve breakthroughs in healthcare, artificial intelligence, space, and the environment. His first XPRIZE, the Ansari XPRIZE, successfully lowered the risk and cost of going to space by incentivizing the creation of a reliable, reusable, privately financed crewed spaceship that made private space travel viable. The technology was then licensed by Sir Richard Branson to found Virgin Galactic, and birth a new industry. He went on to found or cofound 24 additional companies. He cofounded a venture capital fund that invests in businesses at the forefront of health and longevity. He's also written three bestselling books and been named one of "The World's 50 Greatest Leaders" by *Fortune*. What's the common thread in Peter's passions? His deep belief is that we can harness technology to build a better, healthier, more abundant world.

Given my friend's unique background, nobody was better positioned to guide me to the most advanced medical solutions available—the leading-edge technologies that are initially accessible to the relatively small circle of people who are truly in the know. Peter operates at the epicenter of that circle. It's not just because he's a genius who understands the latest tech advances inside out. Many of the world's greatest innovators are drawn to his warmth, enthusiasm, and optimism.

When I asked for his guidance, Peter advised against rushing to have surgery, no matter how many doctors had presented it as my only viable option. **Instead, he suggested stem cell therapy. More specifically, he recommended that I speak with his dear friend, Dr. Bob Hariri.** I was surprised at first because I remembered hearing that Bob was a neurosurgeon. **"He *is* a neurosurgeon," Peter replied. "But he's also one of the world's leading experts on stem cells. There's nobody better."**

I didn't realize it back then, but this was a little like wanting to learn more about basketball and being told, "Why don't you meet my friend LeBron James? He can tell you how it's played."

Just to give you a quick snapshot: Bob Hariri, MD, PhD, is both a superstar neurosurgeon and a world-renowned biomedical scientist who pioneered the use of stem cells to treat a wide range of life-threatening diseases. Bob is a legend in the field of regenerative science because he was the first to derive exceptionally potent, healing stem cells from the human placenta—a game-changing breakthrough that we'll talk more about in the next chapter. Bob holds over 170 issued and pending patents for his discoveries. And he's also a serial entrepreneur and chairman and CEO of Celularity Inc., a clinical stage biotechnology company leading the next evolution in cellular medicine.

Bob spoke to me about the different types of stem cells and explained that they weren't all created equal. Back then, the market for stem cell therapies was like the Wild West, with many dubious treatments promoted by people who were dangerously unqualified. Bob instructed me on what to avoid and where to go for the best treatment. "You need the strongest, youngest, most powerful stem cells," he told me. "You need ten-day-old stem cells that have the force of life in them."

A few weeks later, I had my first stem cell treatment. I'll tell you the full story later because I want you to understand precisely what these regenerative therapies involve and how profoundly they can help you. But for now, I'll cut straight to the chase: **Peter and Bob set me on a road to recovery that was like nothing I could have imagined. My wrecked shoulder recovered completely in a matter of days—without surgery. My arm never froze. To this day, it works perfectly. It's like I never had that snowboarding accident.**

But something even more surprising happened—something I wouldn't have believed possible if it hadn't happened to me personally. A few days after my first treatment, I climbed out of bed one morning and realized that the searing pain I'd felt in my back for much of the previous 14 years had entirely gone away. It was a miracle. An absolute miracle.

And that, my friend, is why I'm writing this book. The healing of my own body is what brought me here today. Over the last few years, I've been on a life-changing journey. Along the way, I've experienced firsthand how this brave new world of regenerative technologies is radically altering our understanding of what's possible in terms of our health, our energy, our strength, and our longevity.

My recovery began with the stem cell therapy I've just touched upon. But I've come to realize that this technological revolution is much broader than stem cells. I want to share with you what I've learned about the many tools of transformation that are available *right now* to rewind your biological clock, rejuvenate your body, and reconnect to your life force in all its glory. I can promise you this: Once you commit to using these tools and discover for yourself their impact on your health and well-being, your life will never be the same again.

My personal experience of rejuvenation is what brought me to the Vatican. It's what led me to meet the Pope, to mix with the world's leading regenerative scientists. That said, I'm not a scientist or a doctor. Unlike Dr. Bob Hariri, I haven't spent decades toiling away in a research laboratory. I don't even know if they make lab coats big enough to fit a guy like me! So when I first considered writing this book, I asked Bob and Peter to team up with me. I'm honored that they agreed to be my coauthors and to share their unsurpassed expertise.

The three of us are blessed to be at a stage in our lives where our primary focus is on serving others. **With that in mind, we're donating 100** percent of our profits from this book to make a difference in people's lives. First, we're donating 20 million meals to Feeding America, one of the most effective organizations I know for helping those most in need. In fact, I've donated all of my profits from my last 3 books as well as provided additional donations to spark the Billion Meal Challenge. We're ahead of schedule to provide 1 billion meals by 2025, and are currently at more than 850 million meals to date. The balance of the authors' profits from this book are being donated to support some of the greatest leaders in medical research. We want to support the world's leading minds as they combat cancer, heart disease, Alzheimer's, and more. And we want to promote cutting-edge research by some of the remarkable scientists you'll meet in the chapters to come. We're excited to play a part in accelerating their efforts to save millions of lives. I want you to know that as you're reading this book, looking for answers to improve your own life, you'll be contributing not only to medical research but to feeding those most in need during these difficult economic times.

In writing this book, we've also drawn heavily on the guidance of several world-class experts who've become a part of our **Life Force Advisory Board**. They've helped to steer us to the scientists, doctors, inventors, and entrepreneurs we've chosen to spotlight.

Our advisers—to name just a few of them—include . . .

- **Dean Ornish, MD**, clinical professor of medicine at the University of California, San Francisco, and president and founder of the nonprofit Preventive Medicine Research Institute
- **David Sinclair, PhD**, a professor of genetics at Harvard Medical School and codirector of Harvard's Paul F. Glenn Center for Biology of Aging Research
- **George Church, PhD**, the legendary geneticist and molecular engineer and the Robert Winthrop professor of genetics at Harvard Medical School
- **Deepak Srivastava, MD,** president of the Gladstone Institutes and director of Gladstone's Roddenberry Stem Cell Center

- **Eric Verdin, MD**, president and CEO of the Buck Institute for Research on Aging
- **Jennifer Garrison, PhD**, assistant professor at the Buck Institute and founder of the Global Consortium for Reproductive Longevity and Equality
- **Carolyn DeLucia, MD, FACOG**—practicing OB/GYN for more than 30 years and alternative therapy expert. Pioneer at the leading edge of non-invasive sexual wellness treatments
- **Rudy Tanzi, PhD**—professor of neurology, Harvard University; director of the Genetics and Aging Research Unit at Massachusetts General Hospital; vice chair of Neurology and codirector of the McCance Center for Brain Health
- **Rhonda Patrick, PhD**—published scientist and educator, creator of FoundMyFitness. Areas of expertise include research on aging (conducted at the Salk Institute), the role of genetics and epigenetics in health status, benefits of exposing the body to hormetic stressors, and the importance of mindfulness, stress reduction, and sleep.
- **Hector Lopez, MD**, founding partner and chief medical officer, Supplement Safety Solutions, LLC, and Center for Applied Health Sciences
- **Matthew Walker, PhD**, professor of neuroscience at the University of California, Berkeley, and one of the world's leading authorities on sleep

At a meeting with some members of this illustrious group, we teased them by saying if we added up their IQs, it would total more than a million points! You'll be hearing much more from them in the chapters that follow because they're all marquee players in the world of regenerative medicine.

But the point I want to emphasize is that the material in this book is _not_ based on _my_ opinions. The answers aren't coming from me, because I'm not the expert here. **My role is to serve you by acting as your intelligent search engine. I'll help you to cut through all of the noise and introduce you to the key players, the ultimate insiders—the innovators who are actually creating the breakthroughs you need to know about.**

You can trust that they'll guide you toward some of the most effective solutions for your health.

It's much the same role that I played in *Money: Master the Game*, **the** ***New York Times* #1 bestseller that I wrote about investing.** I'm no guru on the subject, but I'm fortunate to have access to the some of the greatest investors in history. So I interviewed more than 50 giants in the field, including multibillionaires like **Ray Dalio, Warren Buffett, Paul Tudor Jones, and Carl Icahn**. I shared their most important insights, distilling them into seven simple steps to financial freedom. As I said, success leaves clues.

This time around, I'll be taking you with me to meet the masters of a very different game: the healthspan revolution. Many of their names may be new to you. But here again, they're the best of the best. **With their help, we'll introduce you to the most effective tools, technologies, and strategies to restore your energy and optimize your health.**

Many of these solutions are available today, which means you can act immediately on the information that we're about to share with you. But the field of regenerative science is advancing so rapidly that we'll also highlight some of the most important advances coming down the pike, including many transformative therapies that we expect to be available in the next one, two, or three years. In fact, in this book, I'll be taking you on a journey to meet some of the greatest experts in the world, and sharing with you more than 195 companies that are at the cutting edge of creating these innovative life-changing solutions. Many of these breakthroughs I believe in so much that I've made a personal investment in 28 of them. I want you to be clear though that neither Peter nor I intend to provide—nor are we providing—you with investment advice. Additionally, the majority of these companies are private, not publicly traded anyway, and closed for investment to the general public. Some of these innovations, already in human clinical trials, are so mind-blowing that you'd think they were decades away. In fact, they'll be here in the blink of an eye.

As a sneak preview . . .

- **Imagine a stem cell injection that can heal a damaged heart by spurring the generation of new heart muscle cells and the growth of new blood vessels.**

- Imagine an injection that can rev up your immune system to dissolve solid tumors and beat cancers long considered incurable, or prevent Alzheimer's or Parkinson's.
- Imagine 3D printers that can create an unlimited supply of desperately needed new kidneys from transplant patients' own stem cells, guaranteeing that the organs won't be rejected.
- Imagine a topical lotion that can stimulate your scalp and sprout new hair—without the traditional negative side effects.
- Imagine a onetime injection that can heal osteoarthritis by growing new, pristine cartilage in your knees or back.
- Imagine a stem cell spray gun that can heal second-degree burns without a skin graft in a matter of days or weeks verses months or years.[15]

These are just a few of the world-shaking innovations that are already available or in a fast-moving pipeline. I'm excited for you to read about these extraordinary new tools that promise virtually limitless regeneration. And I promise you an experience of awe and excitement!

---

15 Yetman, "What You Need to Know About the Stem Cell Regenerating Gun for Burns."

THE ROAD AHEAD

"When I let go of what I am, I become what I might be."
—LAO TZU

Let me ask you a question: What moved you to pick up this book? Let me guess:

- You're feeling great and want to stay that way for many years to come. You're **someone who takes full advantage of every cutting-edge opportunity to keep your energy on "high,"** avoid preventable illness, and strengthen your immune system.
- Or maybe you're an athlete seeking new ways to enhance your performance, and you want to follow in the footsteps of people like **Tiger Woods, Rafael Nadal, and Cristiano Ronaldo.** All of these champions have used regenerative medicine to recover from injury without surgery and return to peak performance in weeks instead of months.
- Or are you a person at the top of your field? You work hard and have built a life that you cherish, but lately you're **feeling run-down or burned out. Now you're ready to reignite your energy, regain your zest, and reach new heights.**
- Or perhaps, like me, you were cruising along cheerfully in the fast lane, feeling fantastic—**until suddenly you hit a pothole or a monster roadblock. You need the latest science has to offer, the least invasive solution with the best odds of a good result.**
- And **some people are longevity-seekers**, but they don't just want to live longer. They want an **extraordinary *quality* of life**.
- Finally, perhaps you're looking to extend your healthspan, to see what science and therapeutics are out there that some experts believe could add healthy decades to your life, perhaps some day in the future making 100 years old the new 60.

If you fit any of these categories—maybe more than one—then rest assured, this book is for you. Whatever age you may be, whatever stage of life you're in, whatever your physical condition, you'll find an abundance of practical solutions that will help you get to wherever you want to go.

As you can probably see by now, **this is a big book. But I hope you keep on reading, because it's also** *a book of answers* **to some of** *life's biggest challenges.* **Our objective is to help you to reach your most ambitious personal goals—and to overcome the hurdles that you or anyone you care about may face.** By the way, you may not be aware of this, but statistics show that less than 10 percent of people ever read past the first chapter of most books! Just the fact that you picked a book of this size and scope says a lot about your commitment to your own energy, vitality, and strength. Obviously, I'd like to see you read this entire book. It's got invaluable information that applies to just about every aspect of your health and vitality. The fact that you've read this far tells me that you're probably going to go for it, and for that I'm grateful, and know you will be as well! But **to help you navigate these pages, let me give you a very quick guided tour of the road ahead.** *Life Force* **is divided into five sections:**

SECTION ONE: THE LIFE FORCE REVOLUTION

This section explores the multitude of ways you can produce greater energy in your body and heal more rapidly. We'll discover why we age, and why scientists are now starting to consider that we may not need to. After this introductory chapter, we'll dive into **the raw material of life, human stem cells,** a foundational therapy for rejuvenation. Then we'll give you a peek at **the latest in preventative, predictive, personalized diagnostics tools that literally could save your life** without exaggeration. As you read you'll see this is true. **Don't miss this chapter!** We'll also show you how **simple tests for your hormonal profile** can help you map the path to regeneration—**producing more energy, strength and drive than ever before.** The section will conclude with a fresh perspective by one of the world's most respected longevity experts on the root cause of aging—and how we can follow his lead to **slow down and even turn back time on our biological clocks.** The basic mechanism unveiled by this brilliant Harvard researcher lays the foundation for many of the phenomenal tools and therapies in our subsequent chapters.

SECTION TWO: HEROES OF THE REGENERATIVE REVOLUTION

We'll look in depth at some convention-shattering technologies that are in the process of changing medicine as we know it, including a blockbuster set of tools that appears to be unmatched by anything previously known. We'll guide you to meet the heroes of this book, the maverick innovators who are driving regenerative medicine from the laboratory bench to the patient's bedside. They're people like **Martine Rothblatt, who created a whole new organ replacement industry after her daughter developed a rare terminal lung disease; Dr. Carl June, who's led the charge with CAR T-cells, the living drugs that have turned the tables on cancers of the blood and bone marrow without chemotherapy or radiation;** and the team at **Biosplice that is decipher- ing the Rosetta stone for cell-to-cell communication and appears to be on the verge of finding a cure for osteoarthritis.** In Chapter 5, "The Miracle of Organ Regeneration" you'll learn how 3D-printing technology using stem cells has already helped hundreds of patients with machine- made bladders and skin grafts—and may soon result in no one dying while awaiting a heart or kidney transplant ever again. And in **Chapter 8, "Gene Therapy & CRISPR: The Cure for Disease," we'll explore how gene therapies and gene editing techniques are fixing damaged hearts, re- storing genetically impaired vision, eliminating Alzheimer's-related anxiety—and potentially blocking the aging process itself.**

Some of these breakthrough therapies are available right now, others are still winding their way through the **FDA's intensive approval process, from Phase 1** (*is it safe?*) **to Phase 2** (*is it effective?*) **and Phase 3** (*is it ef- fective at scale and better than what's already out there?*).[16] But you do not need to wait in line for the future advancements to take action and improve your Life Force now. Here's just one example: **a noninvasive outpatient therapy that uses ultrasound to relieve the uncontrollable tremor from Parkinson's disease within a few hours** . . . and looks like it may have a real solution for opioid addiction, to boot.

---

16 FDA, "What Are the Different Types of Clinical Research?"

•

SECTION THREE: WHAT YOU CAN DO NOW

This is a must-read, because we'll be sharing with you an array of pragmatic tools to expand your physical and emotional energy. In "Your Ultimate Vitality Pharmacy," we'll introduce you to several widely available rejuvenating supplements with strong safety profiles. They range from natural "gene switches" like peptides to an inexpensive FDA-approved pill that some scientists say may protect against cancer and heart disease. We'll also share some **basic building blocks for a person's well-being: nutrition, fasting, sleep, and exercise.** We'll point you to our favorite gadgets and wearable devices, which you can use to tweak your habits, monitor your progress, and gauge what works best for your unique body. **Most important, we'll show you the tools we have found that can produce the most powerful results in the shortest period of time.**

To get down to the core fundamentals, **we'll show you a variety of diets—and more important their underlying principles—that science is showing can boost your vitality, improve your health, and increase your longevity.** We'll show how **a good night's sleep affects everything from testosterone levels to the regulation of blood sugar.** We'll discuss the importance of muscle mass in shaping your health. We'll reveal which routines can give you the most bang for the buck in improving performance, including a weekly **ten-minute workout to increase your strength and mobility. (And you'll actually have a blast doing it!) We'll even explain how to rejuvenate your appearance through cellular regeneration and other beauty-related technology, so you can** *look* **as youthful and vibrant as you** *feel,* **regardless of your biological age.** And we'll turn to **two world-class experts to unravel the complexities of women's health and help us understand the most critical factors for a woman's quality of life.**

SECTION FOUR: TACKLING THE TOP 6 KILLERS

We'll tackle the biggest health threats that most of us face and bring to you the best tools for prevention and alternative treatments. Those health challenges include:

1. **Heart Disease**
2. **Stroke**
3. **Cancer**
4. **The chronic pain that comes with inflammation and autoimmune disease**
5. **Obesity and diabetes**
6. **Alzheimer's and cognitive decline**

This section will expand on earlier chapters to explore how the latest advances in gene therapy, stem cell technology, organ transplants, and other tools are providing powerful new weapons in the wars against these mass killers. Again, you may not choose to read all the chapters in Section Four about disease. Feel free to cherry-pick what's most important to you or someone close to you.

SECTION FIVE: LONGEVITY & MINDSET

And finally, you'll discover that our concept of age—our notion of what it means to be "old" or "middle-aged"—is about to change forever. We'll look at those accelerating technologies like artificial intelligence, sensors, networks, CRISPR, and gene therapy that are enabling a longevity revolution. We'll understand why many of the world's most respected scientists believe that 80 can become the new 50, and soon 100 the new 60. Can you imagine what it will mean for you to "live young" as you age, to retain or even increase your vitality at a stage in life when decline was once the only option?

Based on his knowledge of so many different technologies coming to fruition, Peter Diamandis hopes to live far beyond the century mark, and I wouldn't bet against him! Still, we all know that living longer can be a mixed blessing. For a person who's sick, suffering, and miserable, the idea of extending life by several decades may sound more like a punishment than a prize. **The greatest gift is the ability to rejuvenate our body—to stay joyfully active, productive, fully functional, fulfilled, pain free, and brimming with energy into our seventies, eighties, nineties, and** beyond. In other words, what I'm aiming for—and what I wish for you—isn't just *quantity* of life, but *quality* of life. I want *more* than a long *lifespan*; I want a long *healthspan* as well.

What's the secret to enriching the quality of your life? Though physical wellness is priceless, nothing matters more than our mindset and the power of our mind and emotions to heal every facet of our being. Our final two chapters will teach you about the amazing power of placebos, how our mind can heal our bodies, and the most important decisions that you can make to change the quality of your life.

Please, whatever you do, make sure to read the two final chapters, as they may be some of the most important ones you'll read in this entire book. Why? Because whatever we do with our bodies, if we don't manage our minds and emotions, we'll never experience the quality of life we truly desire and deserve. They will show you the power of the mind to heal, and in addition, guide you to live in a beautiful state that elevates your mind, body, and spirit, enabling you to connect more powerfully than ever before with your own life force. By liberating yourself from fear, you'll be free to live more, love more, achieve more, and share more—to experience at a higher level the astounding miracle of being alive.

So why not take a moment now to create a game plan. Set a goal for yourself. Maybe you'll read a chapter a day, or two in a week so you'll have completed this book in roughly 12 weeks. Or if you are quite passionate about the subject like I am, maybe you'll consume the book over a long weekend. What I can promise you is at the end of this journey, you'll know not just more about the latest breakthroughs and technology to increase your strength, vitality, and power but also how to combat disease and actually prevent it. Having those insights will not only empower you for yourself, but your family or anyone else you love. In addition, all the chapters moving forward also have a small summary at the top so you know what to expect, and what promises are in store.

Does this sound like a road worth traveling? I promise you an experience of awe and inspiration as together we uncover some of the most powerful tools for transforming our lives. Let the journey begin . . .

CHAPTER 2

THE POWER OF STEM CELLS

Harnessing Nature's Repair Kit

"The regenerative medicine revolution is upon us. Like iron and steel to the industrial revolution, like the microchip to the tech revolution, stem cells will be the driving force of this next revolution."

—CADE HILDRETH, founder of BioInformant, a stem cell industry research firm

In this chapter, you'll learn about **stem cells, the basic building blocks of every tissue and organ in the body. Most of all, we'll share with you the compelling clinical results they are being generated on a daily basis. The early results are in, and they are nothing short of spectacular. In this chapter, you'll learn how:**

- Athletes like **Tiger Woods, Rafael Nadal, and Cristiano Ronaldo** have used stem cells to **recover** from torn ligaments and degenerative back pain—**without surgery, and often within weeks rather than months**[1]
- **Five patients with age-related macular degeneration**—a progressive condition that commonly leads to blindness—**stabilized their eyesight**[2]
- A young man in California **regained the use of his hands and arms after a car crash had left him paralyzed from the neck down**—and now plans to walk again[3]

---

1 O'Neil, "No More Knife: The Stem-Cell Shortcut to Injury Recovery."

2 Akst, "Donor-Derived iPS Cells Show Promise for Treating Eye Disease."

3 McCormack, "Stem Cell Treatment for Spinal Cord Injury Offers Improved Chance of Independent Life for Patients."

- A four-year-old boy overcame the odds and beat leukemia with the help of stem cells from his newborn sister
- A teenager put the lifelong agony of sickle cell anemia behind her
- A 26-year-old woman who'd been immobilized by multiple sclerosis is now out on the ski slopes!

All told, well over a million people have seen their lives transformed—or even rescued—by stem cells.[4] **This chapter is special to me because I am one of them.** To discover more about these amazing breakthroughs, stay with me. What you'll learn might change your life, too.

"In the beginning there is the stem cell; it is the origin of an organism's life."

—DR. STEWART SELL, an immunologist who has studied
the link between stem cells and cancer for 50 years

I **was still in searing nerve pain from my torn rotator cuff when I first met Dr. Bob Hariri, the surgeon-scientist-entrepreneur who's one of the early pioneers in stem cell biology.** For some reason I'd imagined a skinny, older, balding guy in a lab coat. Bob was the best at what he did, and I assumed he'd be reserved and maybe a little arrogant. Was I ever wrong! In walked this muscular, charismatic guy with a full head of hair and the most unbelievably warm and humble manner. Pulling no punches, Bob proceeded to give me the short-form education of a lifetime, and right away I knew we'd be great friends. For twenty years, he'd been on a crusade to bring the best and safest stem cell therapies to the U.S. mass market—to transform reactive sick care into proactive, precision healthcare. Dr. Bob is the rare individual who's decided to change the world. And here's the kicker: He's got the intelligence, the savvy, the experience, and the bulldog tenacity to pull it off.

I **know you've heard about stem cells, the precious birthright given to each and every one of us.** They have two unique superpowers. **Unlike other cells, they can divide and renew themselves for a lifetime. What's more, like a cellular skeleton key, they can unlock an almost limitless**

---

4 Charlotte Lozier Institute, "Fact Sheet: Adult Stem Cell Research and Transplants."

array of healing powers. They can differentiate into whatever type of cell our body needs. They can repair or replace more specialized tissues in our skin, bone, muscle, blood, retinas, liver, heart, and brain. On top of everything else, **stem cells can strengthen our immune system to help keep us healthy and strong.**[5]

In a nutshell, stem cells are the body's repair kit. They deliver the raw material—the molecular signals and growth factors—that enable us to stave off disease, bounce back from injury, and live our lives with optimal energy and at peak performance.

Heading into my talk with Dr. Bob, I'd done my due diligence. **I knew that the U.S. Food and Drug Administration, the strictest medical regulatory body in the world, had overseen the use of stem cells for more than 80 diseases of the blood and immune system, including leukemias and lymphomas. I knew that more than a million people had undergone stem cell transplants worldwide, with disease-free survival rates as high as 90-plus percent.** Hundreds of thousands more have made it safely through clinical trials for autoimmune diseases, Alzheimer's, Parkinson's, and many other chronic conditions.

I knew firsthand of several people with joint problems who swore by their "off label" stem cell treatments. I found several small studies that suggested the benefits were real. **But when I went to three different specialists to try and deal with the massive pain that my torn rotator cuff was causing, all I heard was a chorus of negativity.**

"Stem cells aren't proven," they told me.

Stem cells hadn't been approved for what ailed me, they insisted.

"It's not worth the risk," one said. "You've got a serious condition—you need immediate surgery, not pie-in-the-sky promises!"

Maybe you've run into similar remarks from your own doctors. It's what happens to patients who start looking at alternatives to the official "standard of care." I heard those specialists out; they were smart and accomplished, and I'm sure they wanted the best for me. But I couldn't escape the nagging intuition that my solution wouldn't be found on an operating

5 *ScienceDaily*, "Blood Stem Cells Boost Immunity by Keeping a Record of Previous Infections."

table. **In an average year, I'm up on stage in 115 cities in 12 to 16 countries, some of them multiple times. I take my commitments seriously. Months of downtime rehabbing from surgery just wasn't going to work for me.**

To get the help I needed, I had to travel to another country—to a place where my body could heal itself with some natural encouragement. I'll admit that I wasn't crazy about my stem cell options inside the U.S., where clinics extract *autologous* cells (a big word for cells from your own body) out of a patient's own adipose (fat) tissue or bone marrow. That's a painful, invasive procedure—and what's worse, the results are unreliable. At best, I would be putting my old stem cells back to work and hoping they'd get the job done with a wish and a prayer. After weeks of investigation, I thought I'd hit a dead end. I was in a bad way, hurting and discouraged—until I met Dr. Bob Hariri.

Cutting straight to the chase, Bob told me that autologous, fat-derived stem cells had significant clinical limitations. **As he explained it, our tissues and organs go through a continuous process of renovation and renewal, a process naturally driven by our stem cells. Here's the catch: From the moment we're born, our stem cell reservoir starts drying up. It's a process called "stem cell exhaustion," and it's believed to be one of the main causes of aging. As we get older, some of our stem cells get used up. Most of them stick around but lose the ability to repair or replace our damaged tissues.**

As we reach 25 or 30, the rate of decay begins to accelerate. By age 80, we might have *one thousandth* the number of stem cells we had as an infant—and the few we have left are barely wheezing along. Our bodies—our fine-tuned, natural regenerative machines—start running into problems they can no longer fix.

Bob's a gifted communicator, and he laid it out to me: **"Picture your body as a beautiful mansion.** When it was first built, **it came with a big staff of maintenance and repair people who knew just what to do when anything went wrong. They'd fix leaks in the pipes or shorts in the wiring before small problems became big ones**—you wouldn't even have to ask. **Then the years pass, and your mansion gets older. The staff is dying off, or they're exhausted, or senile. They can't keep up with the**

holes in the roof anymore, or the mold in the master bedroom. Worse yet, the materials they need for repairs start to run out, and the ones they've got left aren't as good as the originals. **At some point the mansion falls apart."**

At the time I was 56, and I took his point: My aging resident stem cells might not be up to the job of healing my shoulder. In a perfect world, Bob said, we'd be calling in the cavalry from **the most abundant source of fresh stem cells: the placenta, after a healthy birth**.

The placenta is the organ that protects fetuses from harm and provides the oxygen, nutrients, and growth factors they need to flourish—or what Peter calls "nature's own 3D printer that manufactures the baby." As Bob will tell you, **"Human beings are at their biological best at birth—it goes downhill from there." Frozen at age zero, placental cells are in top condition. Their DNA is uncorrupted by viruses or UV rays, untainted by alcohol or tobacco or the cosmic radiation that penetrates planes at high altitude. They're as close to a pure natural commodity as it gets. Best of all, they come from the natural afterbirth of a healthy newborn, which makes them both plentiful and free of ethical issues in their use.**

During Bob's surgical training at Cornell, he was intrigued by fetal surgery performed in utero on an unborn patient with spina bifida, a disease where the backbone fails to completely close, damaging the spinal cord and leading to disabling birth defects. The surgeon opened the pregnant mother's uterus, pulled out the fetus, sewed up its back to cover its spine, and returned it to the uterus. Months later, after the birth, Dr. Bob was astonished to find a thriving infant *without the faintest trace of a scar*. It was as though the surgery had never happened. And Bob realized: *If we could harness this regenerative power, we might be literally able to rebuild ourselves.*

Did you know that our species has X-Man potential that has yet to be fully explored? In a paper cowritten with stem cell godfather Arnold Caplan of Case Western Reserve University, **Bob noted that infants and even some young children can regrow severed fingertips as long as the wound isn't stitched up. They channel their "inner salamander" to regenerate the lost tissue!**

And how about this for a bonus? **The placenta also acts as a defense** system to protect the developing fetus from a wide range of threats. **The organ contains supercharged, anticancer immune cells . . . which may be one big reason that it's virtually unheard of for pregnant mothers with cancer to pass it on to their babies.**

Are you convinced yet? I sure was. But then Dr. Bob gave me the bad news: Despite their apparent safe and effective track record wherever their use was permitted, placenta-derived cells weren't as yet approved as an orthopedic therapy in the United States. As Bob explained it, the FDA has the enormous responsibility to guide and ensure the safe use of these therapies, and there was still a lot of work to be done. **My remedy seemed so close and yet so far. It was really frustrating.**

Fortunately for me, Bob's a bulldog. He solves problems for breakfast. He knew of a clinic in Panama that had permission to treat patients with the next best thing to placental cells: high-quality stem cells from umbilical cords. **"This isn't fetal tissue**, it's nothing like that," he emphasized. For decades, he told me, **babies' umbilical cords and placentas were simply thrown away after birth—even though they were "a lot more powerful than your own aging stem cells."** Dr. Bob shared with me story after story of clients with all sorts of dramatically positive results after treatment with these pristine stem cells.

I put on my consumer hat and asked the next obvious question: How much did it cost? I reached out to the Panama clinic and learned that treatments could range from $10,000 up to $25,000. Knees or ankles or elbows could often be treated for as little as $5,000, but my rotator cuff was a lot more involved.

Though I trusted Bob explicitly, I had a moment of sticker shock: "Up to twenty-five thousand dollars, are you kidding me?"

But as Bob reminded me, shoulder surgery can cost that much or more, and that was before you factor in the expense of months of rehab and recovery time. And even after the surgery, there's was no guarantee I'd get back to where I was before I got hurt.

Still, I hesitated. **I had no way of knowing then that this treatment would be the biggest bargain of my life.** At the time, my nerve pain was nearly unbearable. If I moved my shoulder just a tiny bit at the wrong angle, it was like an electric shock. It literally took my breath away, the pain was so

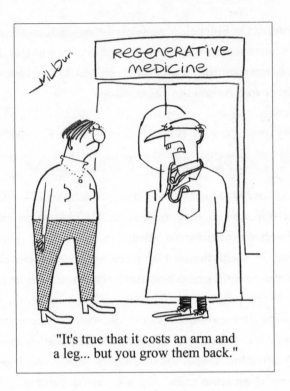

"It's true that it costs an arm and a leg... but you grow them back."

strong. My career was on the line; I couldn't afford a mistake. Why should I listen to Bob and head to Central America when all these well-known specialists were steering me in the opposite direction?

Then I did what I do in these situations. **I evaluate the risk-reward proposition.** If stem cells didn't work, what would be my worst-case scenario? I could still go in for the surgery. But if the stem cells worked, I could be out of pain immediately and have a fully functional shoulder with a much shorter recovery time. So why not give them a shot? **I don't know about you, but if my choice is between a needle and a knife, you can give me the needle every time!**

Most of all, I trusted Dr. Bob, a working-class kid from Queens who found his calling to become one of the world's top neurosurgeon-scientists, a matchless innovator in microsurgery, and then a father of regenerative medicine. **He's someone who defied the conventional wisdom to find an alternative road to rejuvenation. It wasn't paved with toxic chemicals, but with living cells, the original building blocks of life.**

Over the years, Dr. Bob has saved so many lives. But how he got to where he is today is a fascinating saga. It shows how any of us can find our life's answers if we stay true to what drives us—in Bob's case, his overwhelming desire to help people, to heal their pain, and to transform the field of regenerative medicine.

THE POWER OF YOUNG BLOOD

Dr. Bob's glorious obsession with the power of stem cells began in the early 1980s, nearly 40 years ago, when he was an MD/PhD student in New York, at Cornell. For his dissertation, he wanted to do something that could truly make a difference. **So he focused on a major cause of heart disease and heart attacks, the world's number-one killer:** the thickening of the arteries known as **atherosclerosis**.

According to the conventional wisdom of the day, atherosclerosis was caused by metabolic problems like high blood pressure and cholesterol. But Bob suspected that it might instead be driven by age-related inflammation. After teaching himself microsurgery, he did something that would alter the history of our understanding of stem cells. In essence, he swapped out microscopic blood vessels from young mice and put them into older mice, and vice versa.

What happened next was astounding. First, the older mice appeared to get younger. Their hair became thicker and darker. Their muscles got stronger. They zipped through their mazes much faster. Meanwhile, just the opposite happened to the young mice who'd received the older mice's blood vessels. They seemed more lethargic. They went downhill—they started breaking down.

Bob wanted to see if there might be **factors in "young blood"** that could **help the older animals heal**. So he made an incision in the transplanted tissue in both groups to gauge how fast the damage would be repaired.

Once again, he observed something amazing. The injured tissues from the older mice healed quickly inside the younger animals—at a miraculous rate. In fact, they healed even *faster* than the young blood vessels he'd put into the older mice. **Dr. Bob had made an extraordinary discovery. He'd accomplished a feat of rejuvenation that most had thought impossible.**

Though it would be years before Bob and others would demonstrate that our stem cells are depleted and weaker with age, the seed had been planted. **Inflammation, Bob realized, was "the slow, sweep second hand of the clock of aging.** It's always going around, always adding time. Your state of inflammation circulates the factors that erode your organs and tissues, which damages your reservoir of stem cells."

From that point forward, Bob said, "My thesis became that aging was really a stem cell problem." What's more, the mice experiments showed that you could turn back time within an organism—that time could be *subtracted* **as well as added. Stem cells had the power to reduce inflammation, heal tissues, restore organs, and bring back youthful functionality. What was the upshot? It meant that aging was reversible!**

That's when Bob realized that stem cells would inevitably become a disruptive health technology across a wide range of aliments. All that was missing, he said, was a product "that a doctor could deliver like a pharmaceutical or any other therapeutic." But Bob also knew the field would never flourish as long as it relied on embryonic or fetal stem cells. And he thought, *There has to be a better mousetrap.*

THE POWER OF THE PLACENTA

"The placenta is a supply depot for stem cells."
—DR. BOB HARIRI

A few years later, he found it. When Bob hustled in from work to see the first-trimester ultrasound of his daughter Alex, she was the size of a peanut—perfectly normal. **What surprised Bob was the placenta. It seemed gigantic—much bigger than he'd expected, and way out of proportion to the unborn child.** Like all former med students, Bob had been taught that the placenta was a vascular interface between mother and developing fetus, a dense collection of blood vessels for channeling vital nutrients and oxygen—no more and no less. But if that's all there was to it, he wondered, wouldn't the placenta develop in lockstep with the fetus it was nourishing? **What possible reason could there be for the placenta to get so big so soon?**

Bob probably wasn't the first medical scientist to notice this anomaly, but he was probably the first one to obsessively investigate it—and to understand the placenta's biological value. He theorized that these organs had been ignored because they "come out looking horribly alien and bloody. Maybe being a trauma surgeon and not the least bit squeamish made it easier for me to appreciate them."

Bob was trained as an engineer before he became a doctor. Engineers know that form follows function. Ergo: **The placenta had to be *more* than an interface. Bob thought it must somehow govern development, controlling the baby's growth rate. But if so, why? And how?**

His engineer's brain kept gnawing at the problem. One day he fished a placenta out of a medical waste bin and brought it back to his lab: "People thought I was a lunatic." When he perfused it with fluid and began taking it apart, "it didn't look like a vascular interface. *It looked like a bioreactor.* It's a very lobular organ with dense areas of tissues and huge numbers of cells, and those cells are dividing and propagating and differentiating, and **they're making their way from the bloodstream of the placenta to the bloodstream of the fetus.**"

That's when "it dawned on me," Bob said, "that maybe **the placenta was a supply depot for fetal stem cells**. And I was offended that people were throwing these fantastic organs away."

The rest is history. **Bob left Cornell and founded Lifebank USA, which used patented technology to harvest and test and preserve cord blood and placental stem cells in nitrogen-cooled freezers. The service was offered to new parents who wanted to "deposit" the stem cells of their newborn, preserving the child's original, uncorrupted DNA and their pluripotent stem cells. What's the point of this? Those stem cells may be used in the future to regrow organs or repair damage. Talk about a rainy-day account!**

Over the next 20 years, Bob threw himself into stem cell science. His research team—anchored by Xiaokui Zhang, PhD, from prestigious Rockefeller University, and Qian Ye, PhD, from Memorial Sloan Kettering—confirmed that the placenta manufactured huge numbers of *pluripotent* stem cells. What does pluripotent mean? These are cells that can develop into almost any tissue or organ: skin or brain, heart or bones, lungs or pancreas or bladder. By contrast, cord blood stem cells—extracted from umbilical cord blood—can differentiate only into different types of blood cells.

In their undifferentiated state, **placental pluripotent cells contain a complete set of the information that's housed in our DNA—and in out-of-the-box condition, like the master installation disk inside a vintage laptop.**

As Bob explains, "You used to run your computer off your installer disk, right? You installed the software and then you put the disk away. You protected it from anything that would corrupt the software—like sources of electromagnetic radiation—just in case you needed it down the road. And **if the software in your computer started to go bad, you could just erase it and reinstall it. And it was like new again.**

"With placental stem cells, I thought I could protect the biological software in the DNA by putting it into a deep freeze. So when somebody needs it, we can give them their stem cells with their full, uncorrupted genome, the blueprint for all their proteins and enzymes and so on. That was my theory."

Once babies are born and their afterbirth tissue is discarded, there's no retrieving those flawless stem cells, our pitch-perfect installer disks.

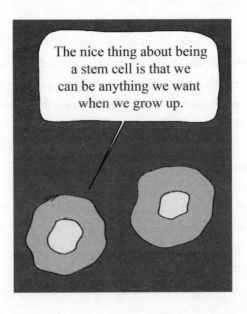

Bob will never forget a couple who'd been discouraged by their family doctor from banking their firstborn's cord blood. When their second child developed leukemia and desperately needed a stem cell transplant, the couple came back to him in tears.[23] A potential cure had slipped through their fingers.

Peter Diamandis has banked the placentas for his twin boys with Lifebank USA. I've done the same for my baby daughter. And we've invested in this organization to make this the norm. As Bob says, "Science is always evolving, with tremendous applications in store. If your baby was born with a spare set of lungs or kidneys, why would you throw them out at birth?"

Unlike autologous stem cells from our own fat tissue or bone marrow, the use of placental stem cells involves zero risk or discomfort for donors. They can be standardized and made available on short notice like any off-the-shelf medicine. Service-based expenses, the line items that make other therapies so exorbitant, are eliminated. And once stem cell products are manufactured at scale, they'll be affordable across the board.

With roughly 140 million births per year across the globe, placenta-derived stem cells could usher in a future of democratized regenerative and precision medicine. They could be made available to *everyone,* **regardless of wealth or income. A single placenta supplies more than 100,000 therapeutic doses, exponentially more than umbilical cords or any other source.**[24]

Bob took this information and built a startup called Anthrogenesis. Then he merged it with **Celgene**, the world's largest biotechnology company. Over the next seven years, as Bob ran Celgene's cellular therapeutics division, he uncovered more about cellular medicine's potential **to treat diabetes, Crohn's disease, skin wounds and burns, even the malignant solid tumors that have vexed the most gifted minds in science! In 2017, Bob teamed up with Peter Diamandis to spin off a new enterprise, Celularity. I also invested in the company, which is now a publicly traded company on NASDAQ. This "biorefinery" is setting the bar for an array of off-the-shelf therapies, from pluripotent stem cells to modified T cells and natural killer (NK) cells.**

Bob described how "Celularity is already beginning to change the game by treating leukemias and other blood cancers with placenta-derived natural killer cells." Once FDA approval is in place, the company will have the capacity to deliver millions of treatments for a myriad of other cancers. **What a crazy turnaround for the placenta, from medical trash into healing liquid gold!**

As for embryonic stem cells, Bob considers them unsuitable for broad clinical applications. Ethical questions aside, **he believes that placental cells are flat-out superior for the development of medicines**: "A lot of fertilized eggs can make it to a blastocyst-stage embryo but not be good enough to make it through a full-term pregnancy. **When you take a close look at embryonic stem cell lines, a very large number—as many as 80 percent—have gross chromosomal abnormalities. These defects would ordinarily stop a pregnancy from going all the way to full term, which is what happens when a woman has a 'missed' period.** Off the bat, that's a quality control nightmare for embryonic stem cells."

And Bob went on: "I'd argue that **stem cells from a placenta, from a healthy newborn, come with a *Good Housekeeping* seal: 'Approved by Mother Nature.'"**

Ten years after he started working with placenta-derived stem cells, Bob found his proof of concept for a new platform to develop regenerative therapeutics. **Quentin Murray, a four-year-old boy from New Orleans, was diagnosed with acute lymphoblastic leukemia.** With his bone marrow glutting his system with immature white blood cells, **Quentin's chances of survival were pegged at under 30 percent.**

As luck would have it, the boy's mother was five months pregnant with her second child, a girl. When Jory was born, her doctors rushed a blood sample to Celgene for analysis. **Bob's hope was to treat Quentin with a two-pronged approach: "The cord blood cells would rebuild his bone marrow. Plus I believed the placental cells would boost the potency of the cord blood cells and possibly have an anti-tumor effect."**

Everyone held their breath. The odds of a cord blood match between boy-girl siblings was about 25 percent—"a genetic crapshoot," Bob says. This time it worked. Jory's placenta and cord blood were shipped to Lifebank USA for cryopreservation. **In March 2008, after the FDA approved the procedure as a special "compassionate use," Quentin became the first U.S. patient to receive a donor transplant consisting of cord blood and placental cells.**

The young patient came through with flying colors. In fact, Quentin rallied so quickly that the hospital discharged him a week earlier than the typical cord blood transplant recipient.[25] Ten years later, he shared his experience at the Vatican conference. It was one of the most moving and powerful stories that was shared that week.

Quentin is still in remission today, an active teenager who loves playing the trombone and video games. Little sister Jory takes credit for everything he does. After all, he wouldn't be around without her—and the stem cells she gave him!

STEM CELLS NATURE'S REGENERATIVE ENGINE

On my first day in Panama, I had my first painless half-hour IV stem cell infusion and three injections into my rotator cuff, and I felt okay. After the second day's treatment, I had what's often called a "cytokine response." I felt chills and shaking, but I wasn't scared. They told me it was normal: "Your body's healing, just get some rest." The shaking passed after about twenty minutes. The next morning, before my final treatment, I woke up . . . and something miraculous happened. I stood up . . . and for the first time in 14 years, I felt . . . *nothing*! No pain. No stiffness in my spine . . . no stabbing in my suddenly flexible shoulder . . . not so much as a twinge!

And here was the most amazing part. After so many years of agony from my spinal stenosis, now I was standing straight and strong without an ounce of pain in my back. It felt supple and free, better than it had in decades. You know that expression, *I felt like a brand-new person*? Without exaggeration, that new person was me.

Six years later, my shoulder is still perfect, with full range of motion. I don't baby it; to be honest, I don't even really think about it. I took the road less traveled on and never looked back. My body healed itself with nature's creators of *sheer life force*: with stem cells.

When I first got back home, nobody could believe it, not even my trainer. "How could you possibly heal that shoulder that quickly, without surgery?" he said. "This is mind-blowing!"

Not long after, I saw a dear friend of mine, an entrepreneur and movie producer who'd also torn his rotator cuff. I informed him of the power of stem cells, and he was intrigued. But he went to some of the best surgeons in Los Angeles, the ones who treat star athletes, and they told him what my specialists had told me: "Stem cells will never work—it's a pipe dream."

So my friend went in for surgery. I felt so sad and frustrated watching him endure that painful experience and all the subsequent time it took for his rehab. Since then, I've had better luck persuading other people to get a second opinion and give stem cells a try. And I've been delighted to witness miraculous healing for them as well.

In my case, I also received an unexpected dividend from the treatment. For about a year I'd worked with **Tim Royer, PhD, one of the world's top neuropsychologists, someone who's consulted by top NFL teams before they choose their next quarterback in the draft**. He measures athletes' current brain capacity and projects what they might accomplish if that capacity was enhanced. **He's helped me maximize my own capacity to stay "in the zone" for peak performance at my events, in business, and in life.**

Dr. Royer has archived a history of my EEG brain waves. After I returned from Panama, he tested me again and he said, "This is crazy! Your brain is able to do things I've been trying to get it to do over months of training—and it's doing it instantly and easily! What have you done?"

I shared with him my experience with stem cells, and he said, "I have to find out more about this." He called Dr. Bob Hariri and said, "I've got to talk to you about Tony. I don't know what he's been doing, but his quantitative performance has *dramatically* improved. His brain looks twenty years younger!"

Long story short, regenerative medicine changed my life—and maybe it can change yours as well. My experience isn't unusual. Dozens of world-class athletes—including **Tiger Woods, Rafael Nadal, Alex Rodriguez, and the late Kobe Bryant**—have turned to stem cells for pain and injuries that threatened to ground them.

Golfing legend Jack Nicklaus, dogged by chronic back pain since he was a teenager, chose a stem cell treatment in Germany over spinal fusion surgery. He took the stage at the Vatican conference that I told you about in our first chapter. The therapy went so well, he reported,

that he was going back for a second helping for his cranky shoulder. "I can now hit a tennis ball and a golf ball without hurting," he said, sounding awfully gleeful for a 78-year-old. "I've become a believer." I've heard similar reports from everyday runners and gym enthusiasts and corporate-league ballers—from people just like you!

After my miraculous healing experience in Panama, and the amazing changes in my spine and shoulder, I became obsessed about showing other people what stem cells could do. But I knew something was still missing from the picture: broad availability. And so I asked Bob, "How are you going to get all of this out to the general public, so they can have access to these incredible technologies?"

A few months later, Bob came back with an answer. He envisioned a place where we could work with all sorts of people to get to understand and meet their needs: athletes and biohackers laser-focused on performance, ordinary people craving more energy, or anyone seeking to ward off a big health challenge—or to find nontraditional options for treatment if that challenge has already arrived. He and Peter decided to form a new company called **Fountain Life. They brought together advanced diagnostics (MRIs, CTs, genomics) alongside their state-of-the-art therapeutic tools from Celularity with the leadership of Dr. William Kapp, a renowned orthopedic surgeon with master's degrees in immunology and genetics. Dr. Kapp has an extraordinary passion for healing people and a rare capacity to target the real source of any problem.** (Some people call this *common sense*, which you and I know is anything but common!) **After building nine hospitals from scratch, he decided he was done with the sick care business and was ready to perform more proactive, predictive, personalized healthcare.**

Together the partners asked me to join them as a cofounder. Our new venture has opened six Fountain Life centers across the U.S., and is on track to expand up to nine in the U.S. and three overseas by the end of 2023.

Think of Fountain Life as your personal health coach, identifying the most advanced and effective treatments available today and delivering them to its members. While you'll still be the CEO of your own health, Fountain Life can assist you in maximizing your strength, energy, and quality of life. **The company's unique fitness centers incorporate a patented, AI-driven, 30-minute workout to help you build muscle mass, an essential component of vitality and extended healthspan. Fountain Life's clients range from billionaire businesspeople to soccer moms to the Pittsburgh Steelers.**

You say you don't live near a Fountain Life center? I've got good news for you: You don't need to wait to join the regenerative medicine revolution. We've created a new app—*FountainOS*—that can assess your true state of health, gain access to an AI-driven suite of diagnostics and help steer your healthspan journey. Your doctor can even use it to coordinate some of the most advanced tests for you. You'll find out more about this in our third chapter, on diagnostics. **In the meantime, you can download the free FountainOS app at www.LifeForce.com, or simply take your phone and scan the QR code below.**

Why did I get involved with Fountain Life? Because I'd experienced firsthand the tremendous benefits of advanced diagnostics and cell therapy and wanted others to share it. Plus I wanted to stay on the cutting edge for my own sake and my family's, as well. Most of all, I shared my cofounders' vision to scale up delivery of these marvelous therapies and make them accessible to millions of people.

Peter, Bob, Bill Kapp, and I are on a mission to democratize regenerative medicine and make it widely available. We're leveraging the impact of many new breakthrough treatments, as well as *allogeneic* stem

cells—a ten-dollar word that basically means they come from someone else, not from you. Over time, we're determined to find a way to slash the cost of pharmaceutical-quality, off-the-shelf cellular medicines and treatments by 90 percent or more. That would bring us down to two to three thousand dollars to treat a typical case of osteoarthritis.

It boils down to this: Bob had a beautiful, audacious dream, and I wanted to be part of it. He imagines a world where we'll all be able to recharge our natural regenerative engine to manage and contain the causes of premature death and chronic illness. **He wants athletes to be able to perform at a higher level, and ordinary people to have an *extraordinary* energy level and quality of life.**

It's a wildly ambitious vision, no doubt about it. But that's something I love about Bob, Peter, and Bill, and it's what makes me feel most alive. We go all in on everything we do. (On top of everything else, we're all pilots. Years ago, Bob and Peter founded the Rocket Racing League, the world's first civilian use of custom-built, rocket-propelled airplanes—just for fun!) **In any voyage that demands on-point navigation and rapid acceleration, I want Bob and Peter and Bill on my side.**

Besides, I've got a passion for hanging out with geniuses. In my experience, something rubs off when you're around people this brilliant. Proximity is power!

So now, before diving into the bigger picture of stem cells and their enormous promise, allow me to let you hear directly from Dr. Bob Hariri, in his own words. Bob, you're on!

*   *   *

Thanks, Tony . . . I want to give some context to the story Tony just shared with you. Tony Robbins is an extreme athlete. With a six-foot-seven-inch, 280-pound body, **he takes on physiological demands that are unprecedented for a 20- or 30-year-old, much less someone who's 62. You can't limit a physical specimen who goes on stage and does things other human beings cannot match.**

After Tony tore his rotator cuff and was diagnosed with spinal stenosis, I knew that the conventional therapies for degenerative joint disease had a low probability of getting him back to the level his lifestyle demands. **And**

let's be real, once you replace a joint, you've crossed the Rubicon. It's irreversible. So for Tony, stem cell therapy turned out to be a reasonable choice. If it failed, he could always go back to surgery.

But it didn't fail, and now we have one of the most trusted voices in the world who put himself on the line to learn how stem cells actually worked. Because Tony experienced the results in his own body, he can speak with real authority. Like few others, he's put in the time and effort to understand the experts' landscape.

When I formed Celularity, it was the product of two decades of efforts to develop cellular medicines and deliver them with quality and affordability and at scale for a wide range of clinical applications. That includes **autoimmune disease, one of the ten leading causes of death for young and middle-aged women.**[6]

In cancer immunotherapy, we're aiming to "disrupt the disruptors." Our objective is to make what are now six-figure therapies affordable and insurable for people of average means. Within the next ten years or so, I can envision a time where cell therapy costs no more than today's biologics for inflammatory disease or cancer—and with far greater safety and effectiveness.

Around the turn of this century, we looked in the wastebasket and started isolating unique stem cells from discarded postpartum placentas. Now the time has come to take the next step, for people to recognize cell therapy as a practical option for their health problems. That's the challenge straight ahead of us.

Tony, Peter, and I, along with our partner, Dr. William Kapp, see the future for cellular medicine as virtually limitless, from curing your cancer to repairing your joints or your heart or your brain. We already know how powerful these tools are. People are beginning to get comfortable with the fact that they're really safe. **The four of us are in a hurry, because there's a moral imperative to accelerate these advances and make them available to *everyone*. (Plus we're not getting any younger!)**

---

6 Ericson, "A Multi-Center Study to Evaluate the Safety and Efficacy of Intravenous Infusion of Human Placenta-Derived Cells (PDA001) for the Treatment of Adults with Moderate-to-Severe Crohn's Disease."

I hope we'll have the chance to serve you or someone you love—either to prevent a serious problem or to be there at a time when you need help the most. Thank you.

*   *   *

Thank you, Bob. . . . Now let me ask you a simple question. Have you ever bought a car or an outfit and suddenly you see it everywhere? Once we know something's important, there's a part of our brain that becomes hyperperceptive to spot it wherever it emerges. Once I began following stem cell breakthroughs in the media and medical journals, it felt like something new was exploding every month. It dawned on me that **stem cells are the backbone of today's regenerative medicine revolution, the stuff of everyday miracles. To get your full attention, we've collected just a handful of the many riveting developments that are transforming medicine as we speak. Here are eight examples that will blow your mind:**

1. At Stanford, researchers were startled when seven stroke victims showed *dramatic* improvement in motor function after having stem cells injected directly into their brains. Even more amazing, **all of them were treated more than six months *after* their strokes, the point where damage is usually considered permanent. A 71-year-old wheelchairbound man could suddenly walk again. In another case, *more than two years* post-stroke, a 39-year-old woman improved so much that she regained the confidence to marry her boyfriend—and get pregnant!**

2. After his car fishtailed into a telephone pole, 20-year-old Kris Boesen was paralyzed from the neck down. Kris had what they call a "chronic and complete" spinal cord injury—a total loss of both sensation and muscle function. Then he entered a long-shot stem cell trial at the Neurorestoration Center at the University of Southern California. **Within two weeks, Kris had regained feeling and strength in his arms and hands. After three months, he was wearing out his smartphone, feeding himself breakfast, hugging his parents, even working out with weights.** Before his treatment, Kris says, **"I was just existing. Now I'm able to live my life."** His next goal is to walk again, which isn't as far-fetched as you might think. **In a study at Rutgers, 15 of 20 patients with similar injuries were walking 11 yards after treatment with cord stem cells and intensive physical therapy.**

3. I read about **Jennifer Molson**, just 26, who'd lost feeling from the chest down from a brutally progressive case of multiple sclerosis. After joining an experimental trial in Ottawa, Canada, **she received a bone marrow stem cell transplant plus chemotherapy. Now she's skiing and kayaking like a champ! Seventy percent of her study's cohort stabilized their condition, with no further deterioration. They're the first MS patients to find an effective treatment without conventional drugs.** "I got a second chance at life," Jennifer says.

4. Meanwhile, **in London, stem cells from an HIV-resistant donor were implanted into a man with HIV and Hodgkin's lymphoma—and pushed** *both* **conditions into remission. He became the second person to "beat" HIV with cellular medicine.** While anti-retroviral therapies are highly effective in treating HIV, stem cells could point the way toward the first real cure.

5. **After a 57-year-old cardiologist had a massive hemorrhagic stroke that paralyzed the whole right side of his body, the FDA gave Bob Hariri's team at Celularity special permission to treat him with placental stem cells.** The man sat for an hour with his family, watching TV and joking around, barely noticing the IV infusion. **Less than three weeks later, he was standing on his own. He'd regained more than 50 percent of the function in his right arm. After a few more treatments, he was strong enough to return to work.** Was it the cell therapy or a natural course of recovery? We don't yet know for sure. "But what's indisputable," Bob said, "is that the treatment was well tolerated, and that it's opened the door to ongoing studies."

6. Dr. Chadwick C. Prodromos MD is a Princeton-educated, Johns Hopkins and Harvard– trained Orthopaedic surgeon internationally renowned for his pioneering work on ACL reconstruction and editor of the textbook on the subject for Orthopaedic surgeons. His passion for preserving rather than replacing joints led him to becoming a world leader in the use of stem cells to avoid joint replacement for osteoarthritis. Due to FDA limitations in the United States, he opened a center in beautiful Antiqua, because the prime minister, Gaston Browne, has declared his goal is to make the beautiful destination the stem cell capital of the world. Now in this environment, he's able to use cultured cells and is able to avoid joint replacement in most severely arthritic patients he sees, while also never using destructive cortisone and stopping all pain-killing and anti-inflammatory medicines. With well over a million joint replacements performed annually in the USA, the public health implications are staggering.

7. Researchers at Osaka University in Japan are farming patches of adult skin for *induced pluripotent stem cells* that can grow into parts of the human eyeball, from retinas to lenses. The team treated one woman who had nearly lost her sight from a diseased cornea, the transparent sheet at the front of the eye. The damage was supposed to be "permanent." A month later, the woman's vision had significantly cleared.

8. And finally, here's a story that moved me to tears. **Helen Obando**, a 16-year-old from Massachusetts, had suffered all her life from **sickle cell anemia, the inherited blood disorder that causes agonizing pain plus heart disease and stroke in children as young as three.** For too long, doctors had nothing close to a cure. **But after an infusion of her own genetically modified stem cells, Helen's bone marrow began producing normally shaped red blood cells. Over the months that followed, Helen's symptoms faded away. She joined her school's dance group, her great passion in life. At her six-month checkup at Boston Children's Hospital, her hemoglobin count was nearly normal. The sickle cell scourge was gone.** Here's what I found on Helen's Facebook page: **"This year has been one of the toughest years for me."** But now, she went on, she's about **"to start a new life and I'm going to live it the best I've ever lived life."** Who could say it any better than that?

A stem cell spray gun can heal severe burn injuries to the largest organ in your body: your skin. ReCell's regenerating gun essentially works like a

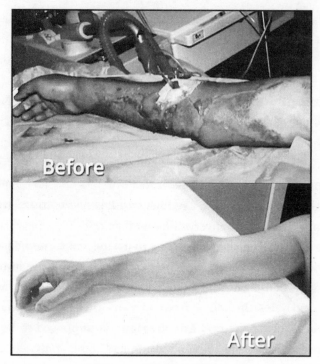

Same arm after stem cell regenerating gun treatment.

paint gun—except that it sprays your own skin cells on the damaged patch of skin. With minimal scarring or risk of infection, this procedure is now an experimental alternative to skin grafts for second-degree burns, and has the potential to treat third-degree burns—the most severe ones—as well.[7] Go to www.youtube.com/watch?v=eXO_ApjKPaI to see the difference!

I could give you dozens more of these stories without even scratching the surface. There are thousands of ongoing clinical trials with stem cells—for Parkinson's and Alzheimer's, heart disease and liver ailments, type 2 diabetes and type 1. If something in your body is "broke," the odds are better than decent that a scientist somewhere believes stem cells can fix it.

Paul Root Wolpe is a bioethicist at Emory University, someone

---

7 Yetman, "What You Need to Know About the Stem Cell Regenerating Gun for Burns."

whose job is to be a skeptic. He never hesitates to slam what he calls the "fetishization of progress," the unquestioning worship of some bright and shiny new idea. Yet even Wolpe recently tweeted that **stem cell research "is turning a corner and beginning to offer the kinds of cures advocates envisioned."**

Sounds like a win-win for everybody, doesn't it? Could stem cells, exosomes, and other cellular therapies be the express lane to a healthier future for humanity? All that's slowing progress on these phenomenal therapies products is the gridlock that often slows approval by the U.S. Food and Drug Administration. Don't get me wrong, the regulators have a tough job. Dynamic living cells are very different than traditional pharmaceuticals. The FDA is hamstrung by outmoded tools and guidelines. They're also walking a knife's edge between protecting the public and fostering innovation. And I'm sure they were troubled by headlines like these:

"YOUTUBE TESTIMONIALS LURE PATIENTS
TO SHADY STEM-CELL CLINICS"—*WIRED*

"STEM CELL TREATMENTS FLOURISH WITH LITTLE
EVIDENCE THAT THEY WORK"—*NEW YORK TIMES*

"THE BIRTH-TISSUE PROFITEERS"—*NEW YORKER*

We all know the press can sometimes go overboard with negativity. But I'm not here to shoot the messenger. The fact is, the stem cell industry has had some real problems. More than a thousand loosely regulated clinics have set up shop in the U.S., and God knows how many more overseas—**it's the Wild West out there**. Some are legit operations, managed by experienced medical professionals. They do their best to follow basic standards for protocols and hygiene. But even some of these facilities fall short on patient follow-up, quality control, and dose-to-dose standardization. Even the best of them can at times over-promise and under-deliver.

But it gets worse—a *lot* worse. A few rogue operations navigate *just* inside the FDA's line, or count on not getting caught when they cross it. They'll promise to cure Grandpa's dementia or young Johnny's autism or cerebral palsy. They'll claim that they'll make the blind see and the lame walk—all without adequate investigation or a track record of results to demonstrate real impact. Often they'll tell people they're being recruited for an important research "study," knowing there are plenty of desperate patients ready to pay up front to play.

There are places where semi-trained technicians whip up a stew of cells, often drawn from the patient's belly fat, and reinject them in what may be a nonsterile environment. You wouldn't expect your child's pediatrician to make his own penicillin, right? Yet many stem cell clinicians are asking you to trust them to do pretty much the same thing.

Most of these scenarios aren't tragic. The only harm done is to the customer's bank account, the $5,000 or $30,000 or $50,000 fee for a failed procedure that had next to no chance in the first place. **But in a small handful of cases that have drawn a ton of publicity, the outcome can be a nightmare. In San Diego, California, a clinic mixed stem cells with smallpox vaccine for an unproven and dangerous cancer treatment. In Florida, three elderly women with macular degeneration went blind after being injected with stem cells derived from fat tissue, in *both* eyes at once, a gross violation of surgical protocol.** In addition, preclinical studies have linked human embryonic stem cells to benign tumors called *teratomas* in mice.

Scary stuff, no question. But as Dr. Bob shared with me from his decades of clinical experience, "Cellular medicine is safe and well tolerated when it conforms to the FDA's Current Good Manufacturing Practices (CGMP) and when it's administered as an approved IND," or Investigational New Drug. **"As compared to traditional chemical drugs and biologic agents,"** Bob adds, **"cellular medicine has an excellent safety track record in lab and clinic alike."**

The Florida disaster was a case of egregious negligence. After they injected improperly manufactured cells with substandard quality control, it's believed that a chemical contaminant wound up damaging the women's retinas—a runaway train of unintended consequences. But as Bob makes clear, while it's theoretically possible for stem cells to trigger growth of the wrong tissue in the wrong place, these cases are *extremely* rare—and with stringent clinical standards and quality controls, any risks can be minimized.

You don't have to take my word for this. As Dr. Bob points out, **the**

FDA holds companies to highly rigorous testing and quality standards. There is absolutely *no* data to suggest that stem cells from the placenta or bone marrow are an "ignition source" for malignancies. "Healthy stem cells from the right source don't appear to increase the risk of cancer," Bob says. **"In fact, we believe that stem cell therapy may boost our immune system and *lower* the risk of cancer."**

Why are stem cells so safe? The short answer is that they don't stay in the body very long. The treatment is not some magical one-off that lasts a lifetime. While I've had no problems with my shoulder since my treatment in Panama, I appreciate the energy boosts—and my body's enhanced ability to rejuvenate—from stem cells. So I've given myself the benefit of regular tune-ups, a simple stem cell infusion once or twice a year.

Thanks to research by groundbreaking scientists like Dr. Bob Hariri and Dr. Arnold Caplan, we know that most imported stem cells clear out of the body within a few days, leaving behind a small reserve for a few months at most. They make their biggest impact by secreting squads of signaling molecules to energize our *existing* cells. These bioactive molecules are the stem cells' secret sauce. They block premature cell death and scar tissue. They stimulate the growth of fresh blood vessels and help to normalize our autoimmune response. Bottom line? Stem cell secretions restore our "old" cells to a younger, higher-functioning state.

And as Dr. Caplan has noted, allogeneic stem cells—healthy stem cells taken from a donor—"have been introduced into thirty thousand to fifty thousand people worldwide, and we don't know of any adverse events." Does that sound like a compelling proposition to you? It certainly was enough for me to move forward with my life-changing stem cell intervention.

But let us be clear: There's no free lunch in medicine. It's like the stock market, where the most successful traders are the ones who look for *asymmetric* risk-reward. They want the smallest possible risk with the greatest potential upside. This is exactly how you should weigh your decisions on anything you learn from any experts any where in the world, and including what you read in this book. It's an essential part of our journey to an expanded quality of life and healthspan. As the FDA points out, **"All medical treatments have benefits and risks."**[8] That's another way of saying that no treatment is completely risk-free.

Back surgery is a dramatic case in point. In a study of data from the Ohio Bureau of Workers' Compensation, more than 700 patients were diagnosed with herniated discs or similar conditions. **Of the group undergoing spinal fusion surgery, only 26 percent improved enough to be able to return to work—as compared to *67 percent* who improved enough without getting the surgery.**[9]

Believe it or not, aspirin has tons of risk, from allergic reactions to gastrointestinal bleeding to strokes.[10] So does your over-the-counter decongestant. And don't get Bob or some of the other medical scientists started about statins.

Until very recently, the stem cell field was polarized between two flawed models. Elite institutions like Stanford managed boutique clinical trials with maybe a few dozen subjects and per-patient expenses running into six figures. That's great for pure science, but it's an unsustainable business model. On the other extreme were the neighborhood stem cell clinics, whose interest in follow-up pretty much ends the moment they swipe your credit card. When people are over-promising and under-delivering, the last thing they want to do is tell you how they're actually performing. **Do you want to know the real tragedy of the stem cell industry? It's all the lost data from literally millions of stem cell patients, the so-called "tourists" passing through these clinics' revolving doors, never to be heard from again.**

With such a huge opportunity to help so many people, our new healthspan enterprise, Fountain Life, has set out to create an unassailable standard for healthspan optimization—from scratch. Our mission rests on three pillars:

---

8 FDA, "FDA Warns About Stem Cell Therapies."

9 Nguyen et al., "Long-Term Outcomes of Lumbar Fusion Among Workers' Compensation Subjects: A Historical Cohort Study."

10 Jiang He et al., "Aspirin and Risk of Hemorrhagic Stroke: A Meta-Analysis of Randomized Controlled Trials."

- **The first is diagnostics.** By leveraging the latest technology, you'll see what's happening inside your body while any problem is still manageable, *before* it becomes a major challenge. (More on this in our next chapter.)
- **The second pillar is all about performance.** Whether you're a professional athlete, an everyday workout fiend, or a weekend warrior, Fountain Life can guide you toward a practical plan to become your best self in body and mind, with maximum vitality!
- **The third pillar is the latest in regenerative treatments,** personalized to your diagnostics and performance goals and how they fit together. These include accessing stem cell therapies, NAD+ precursor supplementation, hormone treatments, placental exosomes,[11] and more.

One of the transformational goals of Fountain Life is to bring regenerative medicine, also known as precision medicine, into the mainstream. How will they do that? Our plan at Fountain Life is to collect data on stem cell therapies under an FDA-approved Investigational New Drug (IND) trial. We will collect data for review and validation from an Institutional Review Board (IRB) for submission to the FDA as part of the approval process for new biological therapies.

The time is ripe. The FDA is committed to fast-tracking legitimate cellular therapies through the 21st Century Cures Act. The agency is determined to speed approval timelines for serious or life-threatening conditions: cystic fibrosis, Duchenne muscular dystrophy, Lou Gehrig's disease, and many more. Peter, Bob, Dr. Kapp, and I are eager to do whatever we can to make this new era happen—to speed the trajectory of regenerative medicine for everyone who needs it.

---

11 Exosomes are composed of tiny extracellular sacs that deliver growth factors and other rejuvenating molecules from stem cells to surrounding tissues that need them most. You'll learn more about them in Chapters 10 and 11.

IF YOU WANT TO FIND TREASURE, YOU NEED A MAP

"We have to take stem cells from bench to business to bedside."

—ARNOLD CAPLAN, stem cell science icon

By the end of this decade, Peter Diamandis predicts that stem cell treatments will cost "less than the price of a laptop today." For relatively small interventions for knees and elbows, prices are already dropping to that level. Eventually these treatments will be available at your private doctor's office, with most of the price covered by private insurance or Medicare. If that sounds unlikely, consider the history of HIV/AIDS. Not so long ago it was a death sentence. **Now it's routinely managed as a chronic illness—a development that has saved millions of lives.**

Thirty years after his life changed course with a glimpse of his daughter's ultrasound, Bob is still dreaming big dreams. He's convinced that we're "about to harness the power of the living cell to treat all the chief causes of mortality: degenerative disease, cancer, autoimmune disease."

Bob has never steered me wrong, and I have no doubt that we're on the cusp of a thrilling new era in regenerative medicine. But one thing kept nagging at me. How could people across this country and the world—people like *you*, the readers of this book—take full advantage of these life-enhancing therapies? How could they find out what they needed—and when they needed it? And how could they best protect themselves from the ravages of aging?

Bob and Peter made it clear to me that the first step in avoiding a severe health problem was early diagnosis and prevention. In fact, according to Dr. Bob, experts say that it pays to begin stem cell treatments *before* a crisis strikes—say, by age 45 or 50. **You want to kill the monster when it's small, not wait until it grows into Godzilla. That's why I invested with Peter and Bob some years ago in a company called Human Longevity Inc. (HLI), where my friends had partnered with hall-of-fame biotechnologist Craig Venter to advance the field of medical diagnostics and why I invested in Celularity Inc as well.**

In the next chapter, we'll show you some tests you can do yourself—not only to perform at your best, but **to flag early warning signs of heart** disease, cancer, and Alzheimer's. We'll also steer you to what you can do right now to boost the quality of your health by checking the toxic metals you've accumulated from your environment. These poisons can affect your memory, your mental clarity, and your overall level of energy. Most important, we'll share how you can optimize your hormones. As we age into our 40s and 50s, sometimes even our 30s, we can see significant drops in our vitality, physical strength, and sexual drives. The good news is that these dips are reversible.

We all know that if you want to find the treasure, you need a map. To get to where you want to go, you must first know where you are. And when it comes to your health, you need the best possible data to tell you where you stand and where you're headed—and what you need to change if you don't like the answers. **The breakthrough technologies we're about to share with you can lead to lifesaving early treatments, or (knock on wood) give you priceless peace of mind. To learn more about them, let's move on to the next chapter and learn how the newest science on diagnostics and prevention can free you from some of the biggest health fears and show you the precise needs of your body in order to expand your health, vitality, and strength. Let's learn the power of diagnostics. . . .**

CHAPTER 3

DIAGNOSTIC POWER: BREAKTHROUGHS THAT CAN SAVE YOUR LIFE

Advances in Testing Can Help Detect Disease Earlier, Which Leads to Earlier Treatment and Vastly Better Outcomes

"If you can't measure it, you can't improve it."
—PETER DRUCKER

When you embark on a journey, you need a plan. You need to know where you're starting from, where you're going, and how you're going to get there. You need a map. You have to establish where you are and where you want to be. Whether it's a journey to an actual place or a journey to better health and vitality, knowing your starting point is essential to achieving your goals. Are you a couch potato who wants to run a marathon? Are you craving more energy so you can crush it in your business? Are you a mom juggling your kid's carpool and work who needs more stamina to fit everything in? Or are you a professional athlete looking to take yourself to the next level? Knowing your baseline will help you get to the finish line.

In this chapter, I'm going to share with you the newest technology—**five tests** that are critical to help you assess the state of your health. The first three deal with the most feared and formidable killers in our society: **heart disease, cancer, and Alzheimer's. The other two can help you attain peak vitality at any age, whether you're in your early thirties or**

mid-eighties, by helping your body purge metal toxins and your hormones maximize your capacity as opposed to slowing you down.

As humans, we're hardwired to be optimists about the state of our bodies. We assume we're relatively healthy, that the 30 trillion cells in our bodies are behaving just as they should, that our organs, tissues, hormones, and neural signals are going about the critical business of keeping us alive and well. Yet we've all heard about that friend who seemed trim and fit yet died of a stroke on the tennis court or went to the emergency room with stomach pain only to find out that they had late-stage cancer.

So how do we make sure we stay in top physical form so we can live our lives to the fullest? How do we ensure there's nothing wrong with our bodies that requires immediate attention? And if there is something awry, how can we get an early warning so that we have the best chance to fix it?

Most people assume their annual physical can sniff out any problems. Here's the challenge: As well-trained and skilled as doctors are, the physical they perform is really not set up to dive deep and catch complex conditions. **With all due respect, tapping your knee, peering into your ears, and listening to your heart started in 1920 . . . it's certainly better than nothing, but it's kind of analogous to opting for a clunky early model computer that weighs 50 pounds over today's sleek MacBook Air that tips the scales at 2.8 pounds and has lightning-quick processing speed. Kind of like choosing to drive a Model T when there's a Bugatti, keys in the ignition, around the corner.** I'm excited to tell you about what you can think of as the medical equivalent of the MacBook Air or the Bugatti— some amazing new diagnostic technology, some revolutionary tests that are transforming our ability to preserve our health and vitality.

What if you're the kind of person who's scared to find out what might be happening beneath your skin? If you prefer not to know, read on! You may change your mind when you discover this quick overview of these powerful new diagnostic tools. These diagnostics can help you understand what's going on inside your body with *precision* and alert you to any issues early enough so you can take quick and decisive action while the problem is small and easy to solve. You can think of these diagnostic tools as your check-engine light. You'll hear about them here, in this book, long before you might encounter them at most doctor's offices.

How can I be so sure? Well, a 2003 report from the Institute of Medicine in Washington, D.C., estimated that the time between discovery to adoption in clinical care can average seventeen years! We don't have time for that. If there's one thing I want to get across to you in this book, it's that **knowledge really is power when it comes to your health**. If you detect medical problems **at their earliest stages, they're easier to address and the problem can often be eliminated altogether**.

So let's take a quick look at the key diagnostic tests that are available now to detect disease early and solve problems when they're most treatable. To understand the importance of these tests, let's take one second to look at the statistics on three of the top killers—heart disease, cancer, and Alzheimer's.

- As of September 2021, 4.55 million people worldwide had died of COVID-19. But **the tragic death toll from this pandemic pales next to an even more formidable killer: cardiovascular disease.**

  In fact, each year, 18 million people succumb to cardiovascular disease, including one American every thirty-seven seconds. But now a combination of artificial intelligence and imaging technology can help determine who's at risk years before a heart attack or stroke could occur and—most important—show you what you can do to prevent it.

- Cancer is another fiend, causing 9.5 million deaths worldwide each year. Cancer is so commonplace that nearly 40 percent of Americans are expected to receive a diagnosis at some point. But now a new powerful blood test can detect more than 50 different types of cancer at their earliest stages, when they're easiest to treat.

- Alzheimer's disease may be the most feared of all—and for good reason. One of every three seniors dies with a diagnosis of Alzheimer's or another type of dementia. But now artificial intelligence can determine if your brain is showing signs of Alzheimer's—or if you're in the clear. And early diagnosis is the first step for a cadre of therapeutics being developed that we will discuss in Chapter 22, "Alzheimer's: Eradicating the Beast."

The tests we just mentioned help detect disease, but it's equally important to keep things running smoothly, to measure performance levels just like you use the gauges on a car's dashboard to get a sense of how the engine is functioning. Are all the fluids topped off? Are the brake pads in good condition? Similarly, there are **two elements that massively impact our quality of life yet are not routinely measured: levels of hormones and heavy metals.** Suboptimal hormone levels represent the greatest solvable cause of reduced performance, lack of energy, and even brain fog. Heavy metals can silently build up to toxic levels in your body and have a similar impact. But quick and easy blood tests can help you find out where you stand and what you need to do to restore your body to peak condition.

- **Hormonal balance is critical if you're going to experience optimal energy and sexual vitality.** As we age, our hormone levels decline, but did you know that testosterone and estrogen are both critical for heart health? Yep, they keep your arteries clean. **While we tend to think of hormone replacement therapy (HRT) as the only solution for plummeting hormone levels—especially for women as they go through menopause—modern science is discovering that hormone optimization can also help solve problems before they get out of control. Let me give you one example.** Consider that optimal testosterone levels for a male can range widely from 250 to around 1,000 ng/dl (nanograms per deciliter). **Here's the problem: No one will tell you to seek out hormone replacement if you're slightly above the base level of 250, but some men feel tired, listless, and lose their drive unless their levels are between 700 and 900 or higher.**
- **Tests to measure hormone levels and their impact on your life are essential to maintain strength along with optimal levels of mental and physical performance.**
- In addition, consider the fact that our environment, including the very food we eat, is brimming with toxic metals like cadmium, lead, and mercury. For example, I thought I was doing the right thing for my body by eating lots of fish, a healthy form of protein, but I had no idea that the fish I favored—tuna and swordfish—were full of mercury.

- **It was only after I started losing my memory and feeling unbelievably exhausted that I got a simple blood test that revealed I had an
outrageously high level of mercury poisoning. Most people don't
even consider that a dangerously high concentration of metals
might be causing their lack of energy, gastrointestinal problems,
and brain fog. But this threatening level is much more common
than you might imagine. In fact, when I suggest that people get
tested, nearly a third eventually tell me that they had some form
of toxic metal accumulation.** I want to make sure you know about **this
test, which can alert you to dangerous concentrations of metals in
your body. And most important, show you what to do to cleanse and
restore your natural vitality and life force.**

These **new diagnostic tests available today mean that you don't need to
sit back and wait for disease to strike or performance to decline. You
can be proactive.** But there are two kinds of people in this world: those
who want to arm themselves with information and those who find knowledge scary.

I have to admit, I used to fall into the second category. What if they
find something small and overreact, making a mountain out of a medical
molehill? But as I became more educated and aware of the importance of
early detection, I wound up discovering issues that would have been so
much easier to address had I only known about them earlier. **I became an
information warrior. I'm someone who feels that the more I know, the
better equipped I am to make the very best decisions based on hard
evidence, not speculation.**

It's vital to educate yourself. Sticking your head in the sand isn't the
answer. **Ignoring a problem, or not even being aware of it in the first
place, doesn't mean it doesn't exist. Ask yourself: Would you rather
know about an issue early on, when treatment is effective, easy, and
cheap? Or much later on when you have few options for effective
treatments? You have the power to take matters into your own hands
and ward off or lessen the impact of these diseases while increasing
your healthspan.** How? By being curious and informed!

In upcoming chapters, you'll learn about the stem cell revolution,

ultrasound treatments, 3D-printed organs, and gene therapies that can restore sight to the blind and cure inherited diseases. These innovations and many others you'll hear about are incredibly exciting. But before we get to them, you've got to have a baseline understanding of your health. And these new diagnostic tests are designed to give you just that: clarity and truth about your normal baseline and how it can be improved. We're talking about the essence of quality of life—vitality, energy, zest, and the ability to enjoy life when you're in your 30s, 40s, 50s, 60s, 70s, 80s, and beyond.

Fortunately, these new diagnostics are easy to access and relatively inexpensive compared to the costs and inconvenience incurred if you detect disease once it's significantly progressed. If there's one thing that's unassailable when it comes to your health, it's that ignorance is not bliss. Ignorance is pain. Ignorance is disease. And ignorance can lead to unnecessary, avoidable procedures and even death. So are you open to finding out the latest tools available to protect yourself, help maximize your potential, and get the most out of your life? Let's start with ways you can fight back against the number one killer: heart disease.

DETECTING HEART DISEASE

"An ounce of prevention is worth a pound of cure."
—BENJAMIN FRANKLIN

As I was in the late stages of writing this book, I got a call from Dr. Bill Kapp, the CEO of Fountain Life, the extraordinary diagnostics and performance company I cofounded along with my coauthors, Peter and Bob. Bill, an orthopedic surgeon by training with a master's in immunology and genetics, is on a mission to revamp medicine from "sick care" to "well care" by being proactive and finding disease before it spreads. He was excited to tell me about one of the greatest breakthroughs in cardiovascular disease in recent memory: the use of artificial intelligence to read a heart scan and differentiate between safe and dangerous plaque. If there's a heart attack looming in your future three, five, ten years down the road, this new AI-guided approach to CCTA—coronary CT angiography—called Cleerly can detect the warning signs so that you can take action to prevent it. Fountain Life is one of the first organizations to get access to this incredible technology, and Dr. Kapp was bubbling over with enthusiasm. "Tony, you have to come do this scan," he told me.

For me, it was a no-brainer. I'm all about prevention as the key to longevity. As soon as Dr. Kapp told me about this new scan, my thoughts turned to my father-in-law. Dad is one of the most hardworking human beings you can imagine, a self-educated business owner—he's been in the lumber industry his whole life—and a man with boundless integrity. Yet as he began to approach 80 years old, I noticed a difference in him. His attitude has changed and his energy has, too. He's had some health issues, which is hardly surprising at his age, and he's worried about a potential heart attack or stroke. As with so many people as they grow older, fear and uncertainty can start to creep in. I know when I turned 60, I even had a few thoughts about my own mortality, wondering: *How many years have I got left?*

Dad and I hopped on the plane together. When we arrived at the Fountain Life center in Naples, Florida, Dr. Kapp showed us charts and graphics that illustrated exactly how AI can take a regular CT scan and amplify it so you can actually look through every artery and distinguish between calcified cholesterol plaques, which are stable, unlikely to rupture and therefore safe, and noncalcified, or soft, unstable, plaques which can mean bad news. You get a score that indicates exactly where you stand so you can know what changes you should make in terms of diet, exercise, and medication to decrease your risk of heart disease. It's truly mindblowing: Cardiovascular science has never had any test this accurate.

Dad and I are both of an age where we're likely to have some of that soft plaque, but knowing the extent allows us to take advantage of strategies to clean it up and make our hearts as strong as ever. As it turned out, my lumberjack father-in-law came out clean as a freaking whistle. When he looked at the scans and was told by the doctor that he had just the tiniest amount of soft plaque, which can be easily reversed, a change came over him. To say that a spring came back into his step is cliché, but that's exactly what I watched happen. My results were great, too. In fact, I'm in better shape than I was three years ago, which is something I found out after Dr. Kapp compared my current CT scan to my previous scans that had now been analyzed with AI. **Technology is truly amazing! It holds the key to optimizing our health and well-being.**

This **AI-guided approach to CCTA** completely reshaped Dad's mindset—and mine, too. **It was incredibly reassuring and invigorating for us to see these great results, and it gave us confidence that we should continue with our current diet and fitness regimens, no medical interventions needed.** But there was an added bonus. Dad had started to have real hip issues, which can make you feel old when you're in pain all the time. Fortunately, Fountain Life does not just perform a battery of diagnostic tests; they provide some of the most cutting-edge revitalization and regenerative therapies available today. One of them is a ten-minute procedure that we'll cover in more detail in Chapter 11, "Living Pain Free." It consists of a doctor using ulatrasound to identify hardened connective tissue and trapped nerves, and then giving a few injections of saline and placental matrix—the latest cutting-edge biologic isolated from the placenta—which releases trapped nerves and rejuvenates the soft tissues of the body. After just ten minutes, Dad was walking as smooth as silk!

I'll never forget getting back on the plane that night and Dad looking at me and saying, "You know, Tony, these people have shown me what's possible. I'm moving completely differently, with no surgery, my heart is in great shape. I don't know if I buy into living to be a hundred and ten or a hundred and twenty, but I could live to be a hundred. That's twenty more years! That's as long as you've been married to my daughter. That's like another lifetime!"

The joy I felt seeing Dad have a compelling future once again, no matter how long he lived, and knowing he'd be experiencing a greater quality of life was incredibly gratifying. **That compelling future, and the energy boost that comes with having certainty and peace of mind from taking charge of your health, is exactly why I wrote this chapter.**

Peter Diamandis describes a similar feeling after he goes through his annual battery of diagnostic testing, the same tests described in this chapter—and the same tests that are also accessible to you. **"I call this process 'digitally uploading myself,'"** says Peter. "It's incredible! You get more than 150 gigabytes of medical data analyzed by AI and interpreted by a doctor. **I don't wonder how my body is doing, I know exactly how my**

body is doing. If there's a small challenge, I can handle it immediately. In my most recent test, I found out that I was measurably in the best health that I've been in in the last five years! It made me feel elated and incredibly empowered."

The CCTA test that **Dad and I had can reveal years in advance that a heart attack is likely and, more important, what to do right now to prevent it from ever happening. Thanks to artificial intelligence, we can find problems when they're small and handle them before they grow and become insurmountable. And as we'll see later in the book, what is now humanity's number one killer—heart disease—is becoming increasingly treatable. But remember that therapies are most effective when deployed early!**

One of the greatest benefits of utilizing these CCTA scans created by a New York–based company called Cleerly is that their sophisticated technology deciphers scans and makes them far more accurate and useful. **Incredibly, Cleerly can distinguish between safe and dangerous plaque** *before* **a heart attack ever occurs.** Often, doctors doing their best to read a traditional CT scan have difficulty telling the difference in some cases. In fact, **Cleerly CEO and founder James Min, a cardiologist, published data in 2019 that found a full two-thirds of patients sent for an invasive catheterization procedure to measure blood flow didn't even actually have heart disease![1] Cleerly slashes the number of unnecessary cardiac procedures by determining whether they're necessary in the first place**.

If I had had this test earlier, doctors would have been able to distinguish between my hard and soft plaque, and I would have had answers three years sooner, and with a lot less concern! I'm grateful to my concierge doctor, Dr. G from New York who specializes in cardiovascular disease and brought the CCTA technology to our team. Plus, applying AI to CCTA scans provides results in just a few minutes compared to what can be hours with manual analysis.

Another thing that's so great about Cleerly is that it's not targeted to

---

1   Chang et al., "Selective Referral Using CCTA Versus Direct Referral for
    Individuals Referred to Invasive Coronary Angiography for Suspected CAD."

specialists. Instead, it's intended for primary care physicians as a way to help them better interpret imaging, enabling them to help guide patients along the path to better health without having to refer them out to specialists.

That's exactly how things played out with one Fountain Life patient, a real estate investor in his late fifties who appeared to be the picture of health. He had successfully lost over thirty pounds, lowered his blood pressure and cholesterol, made better food choices, and stabilized his hormone levels. Over time, he became a new man. He exercised every day. He ate well. **But when he applied for life insurance, his calcium score of 1,000 was like a giant red flag being waved in front of a bull. The insurance company flat-out turned him down.**

But you know what happened next? **The Cleerly test showed that the insurance company was dead wrong. The patient had no signs of any dangerous soft and unstable lesions.** Fountain Life wrote a letter to the insurance company explaining that the Cleerly analysis offers a new way to look at heart disease that's much more precise and accurate. Now, we all know that insurance companies really don't like changing their minds, but they did in this instance. **The man got the life insurance he needed, and the insurance company got introduced to a completely new, much more accurate way of assessing heart health. But more important, the patient was relieved of the fear and the uncertainty of wondering when a heart attack might occur.** In fact, it transformed and impressed him so much that he became a financial backer of Fountain Life, investing $1 million in the company.

That's essentially the same thing that Dad experienced. He had been told by other doctors that he might need invasive testing, might even need some stents, but Cleerly discovered that most of his plaque was stable and nothing to worry about. Stable plaque doesn't trigger heart attacks. The tiny amount that was unstable could be converted to stable plaque with the help of some newer medications. **Dad had been worried about his heart health for months, but Cleerly's unequivocal results gave him a new lease on life. And it could do the same for you and your loved ones.**

If you would like to access these CCTA scans for yourself or a family member, you should know that this tool and other sophisticated

technology are now being made widely available. We are sharing examples from Fountain Life for each of these tests because I know they're available there, but I don't want you to get the impression that you can't find them elsewhere. The caveat? Only doctors who are on the cutting edge will know about these tests. If you're having trouble finding someone in one place who knows about all of them, we've created a way for your doctor or for you personally to get access through our FountainOS app. In essence it's a one-stop shop for accessing all the latest diagnostic tests. Again, some of these can be done from your home, or they can be ordered by your doctor. So please bear in mind that while I'm passionate about Fountain Life, if you don't live near one of our centers, you can still tap into these tools thanks to this app, which will help you or your doctor easily do so in minutes.

DIAGNOSING CANCER EARLY

"Awareness is key. In the absence of information, none of us know what is happening and what could be jeopardizing our health."

—ERIN BROCKOVICH

Just saying the word "cancer" strikes fear into the hearts of so many people.

In 2020, the American Cancer Society predicted that the disease would claim the lives of more than 600,000 people. That's 1600 people a day in this country alone. The good news? Deaths from cancer are actually falling. In fact, from 2014 to 2018, the overall cancer death rates decreased by about 2.1 percent per year for women and 2.3 percent per year for men. Since 1991, when deaths from cancer were at their peak rates, nearly 3 million deaths have been avoided.[2] Equally good news is coming from the wide range of cancer-related treatments that you'll read about in Chapters 8 and 19. As you already know, the number one thing you can do to fight and survive cancer is to find it early.

So things were already headed in the right direction even before the revolutionary GRAIL test came along. In the cancer chapter later

---

2 Islami et al., "Annual Report to the Nation on the Status of Cancer."

in this book, Chapter 19, **I'll tell you every detail of the dramatic story that underpins the development of this game-changing blood test that can identify cancer long before symptoms pop up, in its earliest stages before discomfort brings you to your doctor. But suffice it to say that GRAIL has a very clear goal: reshaping the landscape of cancer diagnostics.** GRAIL arrived on the scene in the spring of 2021, and Fountain Life is one of the first places to offer this incredible test, which is part of its baseline testing for all members. Before GRAIL, it was possible to screen for just a few types of cancer, like breast, colon, cervical, prostate, and lung cancers. **Prior to the GRAIL, we've been able to detect only 20 percent of cancers, which means that four of five cancers went undetected until they had grown and started causing trouble! Now as GRAIL is hitting the market, it has the potential to completely overhaul the field of cancer diagnostics.**

While GRAIL can search for more than 50 different types of cancer with a simple blood test, like any test it isn't perfect. It can't detect every cancer type, especially brain or kidney cancer. But that's where the use of full-body MRI comes in. MRI (magnetic resonance imaging) is a powerful type of imaging that uses magnets, not radiation, to form high-resolution internal images of your body, imagery that can find early solid cancer cancers wherever they are lurking. **Together, GRAIL and MRI full-body imaging can detect a complete spectrum of cancer at very early stages. And you know what that means, right? Early detection equals early treatment, less invasive treatments, and better survival rates overall.**

Ponder this mind-blowing statistic from Dr. Bill Kapp: Using the modern diagnostic tools described in this chapter, some 14 percent of individuals tested will find that they have an actionable disease, meaning that **one in seven people walking down the street have a critical health condition they don't know about, but could diagnose and treat if they only had the tools!**

Some general practitioners may question the wisdom of doing so much testing. "If you keep looking," they could point out, "you're going to find something." That's the whole idea! "We are all aging, and we are all experiencing wear and tear," says Dr. Kapp. **"Our mission is to keep you in optimal health, and to find something before it gets you."**

In other words, using technology such as routine full-body MRI to detect cancer or other problems, such as aneurysms, is the pinnacle of preventive medicine. It's the ultimate checkup. Here's why this is so critically important, especially as it relates to cancer: **When cancer is detected at Stage 4, the most advanced stage, the outlook is very grim. Compare that to finding cancer at Stage 1, the earliest stage, when survival rates are extraordinarily higher.** In fact, a massive study of more than 100,000 patients examined early detection of cancer. <u>**That study has determined that there's an 89 percent chance of survival for early stage detection compared to a 21 percent chance of survival with late-stage detection.**</u>[3] Basically, the chances of a full recovery at Stage 1 are much, much better than they are at Stage 4. So you can see how the chance of recovery really hinges on early detection.

To illustrate just how game-changing it can be, **let me share with you a story about a 60-year-old man who came to Fountain Life at the urging of his wife, who had heard about the advanced diagnostics offered to members at the clinic.** This man, who works in the tech industry, had just had a physical. He tried to dodge his wife's pleas, telling her, "I'm fine. I'm great. My doctor says I'm healthy as a horse. I don't need any testing." But she didn't give up—and he's now thanking her for that.

To make her happy, **this man grudgingly came to Fountain Life for a complete workup. A full-body MRI revealed something shocking: Stage 1 bladder cancer.** His primary care doctor had done nothing wrong; he hadn't overlooked anything. In fact, **this early stage bladder cancer wouldn't have been picked up by any means other than the MRI, which isn't standard operating procedure for an annual physical**. Consider that this man's urinalysis was negative, and there was no blood in his urine. In essence, there was no reason to suspect a cancer was quietly growing inside him. **But because he listened to his wife, he discovered the problem early and jumped on treatment.**

Now, the treatment for bladder cancer can be brutal; if the cancer burrows deep into the bladder, you often have to remove the entire bladder and end up with a pouch on your side for the rest of your life where your urine collects.

---

3 Howlader et al., "SEER Cancer Statistics Review, 1975–2018."

But early stage bladder cancer can be treated very easily with an outpatient procedure. And that's exactly what happened. "It was a complete cure and now he's just in for routine follow-ups," says Dr. Kapp.

What's particularly unique about this situation is that this man's primary care physician is a concierge doctor, exactly the kind of doctor devoted to personalized care whom you might expect to do the sort of deep dive that would have turned this up. **Yet routine MRI imaging is not part of classic concierge wellness care—or most other preventive care.** "This guy is thinking that he's getting the best care," says Dr. Kapp. "But I keep telling people, 'Concierge care is great, but it usually means you're at the front of the line for traditional care.'"

According to the National Cancer Institute, there's an 89 percent chance of survival for early stage detection compared to a 21 percent chance of survival with late-stage detection.

The plain truth is that traditional care is not cutting-edge. It doesn't routinely leverage the latest and greatest innovations. We all deserve better. **We all deserve the most innovative technology to detect cancer at its earliest stages so we can live better, longer, healthier lives.** Again, if you'd like to be able to get this test, there are many full-body MRI centers around the world, but you or your doctor can also access them directly through the FountainOS app.

DETECTING EARLY ALZHEIMER'S AND DEMENTIA

"Dementia is our most-feared illness, more than heart disease or cancer."

—DR. DAVID PERLMUTTER, neurologist and
five-time *NY Times* bestselling author

I have an unbelievable figure to share with you about aging and dementia: At any given point in time, would you believe that 6 million Americans are living with Alzheimer's disease or mild cognitive impairment,

which can be a precursor to the disease? The death rate is skyrocketing: In fact, deaths from Alzheimer's increased by 145 percent in the nearly two decades between 2000 and 2019, even as deaths from another top killer—heart disease—decreased by 7 percent. The National Institute of Health estimates numbers will more than double to 15 million by 2060 as the population ages.[4]

Heart disease and stroke are scary. Cancer is scary. But Alzheimer's? That just may be the scariest of all end-of-life diseases because of how it steals our memories, our connections with loved ones, and our independence, taking a huge toll on those we love. Anyone who has loved someone with Alzheimer's or dementia knows how brutal and dehumanizing the end can be.

Dr. Kapp has seen the fear that Alzheimer's strikes in the hearts of people, including one of his friends who is an accomplished attorney, and in his early 50s was a semi-pro golfer who evaluated golf courses for a popular golf magazine. His parents were both athletes as well. He grew up playing sports and staying active along with his parents. **As they grew older, his father developed Alzheimer's disease, followed quickly by his mother. They were both placed in the same Alzheimer's dementia facility, and Dr. Kapp's friend feared that it was his fate to follow in their footsteps.**

Over the course of a decade, he watched his parents decline and witnessed their deaths, one after the other, absolutely distraught over their fate, and his fear was that he was going to wind up in the same position and be a burden on his family down the road. **Rather than wonder about what lay ahead, he decided to take advantage of technology available at Fountain Life to perform sophisticated AI mapping of an MRI image of his brain. This technology, from a company called Combinostics, uses AI to analyze brain tissue.** It measures 132 areas of the brain and applies AI to determine whether you show signs of an Alzheimer's brain or a pre-Alzheimer's brain, as well as Parkinson's disease. At the same time, it can also measure the volume of various parts of your brain, whether they are increasing or decreasing and whether you have any vascular disease in your brain. **All these data points taken together provide an in-depth**

4 Brookmeyer et al., "Forecasting the Prevalence of Preclinical and Clinical Alzheimer's Disease in the United States."

look at your brain that reveals abnormalities or patterns of disease that indicate various types of neurological decline, including dementia and Alzheimer's.

In addition to the Combinostics testing, Dr. Kapp's patient was so worried that he also did the genetic testing to assess if he was genetically susceptible to Alzheimer's. He was very nervous, as you might imagine, but once Dr. Kapp gave him all his results, he was overjoyed. Fortunately for him, he tested negative on all counts. Immediately, it was just like a huge, overpowering weight had been lifted from his shoulders. His whole outlook shifted, just because he was brave enough to take advantage of the incredible technological tools we now have available to detect disease at early stages.

You may be wondering, what if testing provides evidence that you might in fact develop Alzheimer's? As we shall see in Chapter 22, "Alzheimer's: Eradicating the Beast," what was once a disease that meant certain death now has a number of impressive therapies in Phase 3 clinical trials, as well as recently approved treatments that appear to significantly slow the progress of the disease. At the risk of sounding like a broken record, the earlier you start treatment, the better it works and the longer you remain symptom-free.

Let me share another story, about a well-off woman in her 70s who was married to a former CEO a large financial services company. She was brought to Fountain Life by her family, who were preparing to move her into a nursing home for Alzheimer's patients. Her family members had heard about the Combinostics technology and decided it couldn't hurt to run the test, just to confirm her diagnosis. Well, the AI-interpreted scans showed that she had fifty white matter lesions on her brain. While this was concerning, it wasn't Alzheimer's; instead, it was Lyme disease! Yep, you read that right: She didn't have Alzheimer's; she had a treatable tick-borne disease. This woman was from a small town in the northeast known to have ticks, yet she had never been tested for Lyme disease. The woman was prescribed antibiotics for thirty days and completely recovered. Having access to the must cutting-edge technology kept her out of a nursing home, and that changed the trajectory of her entire life. It was like a rebirth.

The attorney whose parents had died of Alzheimer's experienced a similar feeling. How did he celebrate? Well, shortly after getting his results, he went out and ran an Ironman Triathlon. **"Not that he was in bad shape to begin with, but he has a renewed lease on life because now he knows that his probability of dying of Alzheimer's is extremely low, if at all,"** says Dr. Kapp. His new goal? To optimize his health in every phase.

Peter, Bob, and I share that goal and it is the reason we wrote this book. And we believe that should be everyone's goal.

THE POWER OF BLOOD TESTS

"Everything in life . . . has to have balance."
—DONNA KARAN

One of the most valuable tools in today's diagnostics arsenal is the wide range of modern-day blood tests available through companies such as Quest Diagnostics and Labcorp. These companies have developed low-cost and accurate means to analyze and report on over 50 different blood biomarkers to help you and your physician evaluate whether or not your body is operating within normal parameters. What are these blood tests analyzing? Everything from your vitamin nutrient levels, your insulin and glucose markers, and your cholesterol, to inflammatory markers, hormone levels, and whether you have heavy metals in your system.

Let's talk about hormones first. It's a fact of life: As you get older, your hormone levels start to fluctuate and decrease. Typically between the ages of 40 and 50—sometimes as early as the mid-30s—the amount of hormones coursing through your body starts to drop off. For some individuals the levels rapidly drop off a cliff, and for some that begins as early as 35. That matters because hormones are a primary driver of energy, vitality, strength, beauty, power, and focus. When hormones plummet, these characteristics do, too. You'll learn more about this in the next chapter, but it's important to understand that evolution never designed the human body to live past the age of 40; in fact, just **200 years ago the typical lifespan was just 35 years**! From an evolutionary standpoint, once you'd reproduced and had your kids, you weren't needed. After that age, it didn't matter whether you stuck around or not, and human evolution is sloooow, so it hasn't done a great job of keeping hormones at peak performance levels for those of us now living into our 60s, 70s, 80s, and beyond.

One of the most overlooked aspects of a traditional physical health checkup is a person's hormonal profile. More attention is paid to blood sugar, cholesterol, hemoglobin, and kidney function than to perhaps the most critical part of anyone's health profile: sex hormones. **Sex hormones are the messengers that not only govern sexual health but also play a critical role in many physiologic functions, including blood sugar regulation, inflammation, neurological status, cardiac health, muscle health, and bone metabolism.**

It is no secret that general health begins to trend downward for many people at about age 50, just as hormonal decline become more intense for both sexes. Of course, due to menopause, women experience this decline even faster than men; hormonal imbalance in women can lead to unwanted weight loss or gain, depending upon fluctuations within their body. In Chapter 10, "Your Ultimate Vitality Pharmacy," we'll take a deep dive into what is traditionally called hormone replacement therapy (HRT), but what one of our advisers, Dr. Hector Lopez, calls hormone optimization therapy (HOT), an approach that looks more holistically at your full clinical picture. Hormones can have such major impacts on health that these simple tests should be performed every six months for those in the affected age group. Remember: Optimal hormonal balance is critical to healthy lifespan!

You don't have to accept declining hormone levels as a fact of life! **Hormones can be supplemented to optimal levels with life-changing outcomes. For men, testosterone is the most important factor in health and well-being.** Not only does it govern traditional male characteristics, but it's a major neuroregulatory hormone. Take, for example, one of Dr. Kapp's patients—a 35-year-old man with a history of traumatic brain injury who had been gaining weight, experiencing profound depression, and couldn't seem to hold down a job. Multiple doctors had diagnosed him with depression, but the prescribed antidepressants were having little effect. By the time he came to see Dr. Kapp at Fountain Life, he was at the end of his rope and on the fast track to divorce. **Testing his hormones immediately revealed** that his testosterone level was 97 when it should have been 700! Replacing his testosterone led to him quickly coming off his antidepressants, losing weight, landing a stable job, and revitalizing his marriage.

Women have their own unique hormonal needs. **For women, the most important hormone is estrogen, which—along with progesterone— gives them their traditional female characteristics.** Fortunately for women, OB-GYNs are more attuned to hormonal health, so their hormonal profile tends to be assessed more often. However, **it's not unusual for them to miss effective hormonal treatment, particularly after menopause**.

That was certainly the case with a 70-year-old woman who came to Fountain Life for testing. When she went through menopause in her late forties, her OB-GYN had told her not to take hormone replacement due to the risk of breast cancer. Unfortunately, **a scan of her coronary arteries using the AI-interpreted CCTA test we talked about earlier in this chapter—the one that Dad and I had—revealed severe coronary artery disease with a lot of unstable plaque. Dr. Kapp stressed that this could have been avoided had she simply been put on bioidentical hormones twenty years ago.** I share all this with you not to scare you but to educate you. With the right information, you will be empowered to ask the right questions so you can access the right hormone testing and optimize your health—and your life.

Women's health is so important, and there are so many myths as a result of outdated studies, that we have an entire chapter in Section Three dedicated to it, featuring two extraordinarily respected doctors—**Jennifer Garrison**, PhD, assistant professor at the Buck Institute in Marin County, California, and a member of our book's advisory board, and **Dr. Carolyn Delucia**, a pioneer of noninvasive sexual wellness treatments and a practicing OB/GYN for nearly thirty years.

I know this is a lot to absorb. But the bottom line is that not only do you have the power to help prevent disease from taking root in your body, but you also have the power to maximize your health and vitality, through a handful of tests that promote both healthspan and lifespan. **In the next chapter, you're going to meet the scientists who are actually reversing the aging process, slowing it down with the goal of stopping it.** We're going to introduce you to an extraordinary scientist at Harvard who is

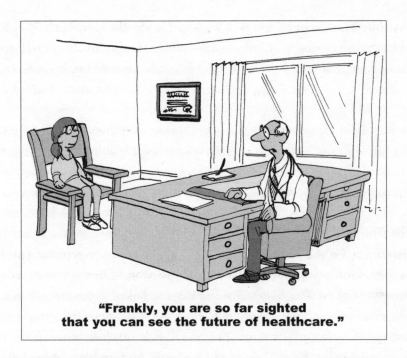

"Frankly, you are so far sighted that you can see the future of healthcare."

cracking the code of aging, as well as other researchers who realize that age is just a number, a social construct that doesn't need to define you. Instead, with renewed energy, vitality, and strength, we'll tell you how you can define age.

Hormone Testing

If you feel like you've lost some of your drive or passion or lack some of the energy you used to channel five or ten years ago, hormones might be to blame. The great news is that it's easy to find out through simple blood tests.

Men and women have many of the same hormones, albeit in different ratios. Achieving the right hormonal balance can help optimize your health, so it's critical to seek out a doctor who is well versed in the treatment of hormonal regulation. Make sure your doctor uses only carefully sourced bioidentical hormones for treatment and monitors your health for any potential side effects.

- A basic assessment of male hormonal health should include: total testosterone, free testosterone, dihydrotestosterone (DHT), estradiol (E2), sex hormone binding globulin (SHBG), and dehydroepiandrosterone (DHEA).

- A basic assessment of female hormonal health should include: estradiol (E2), progesterone, testosterone, free testosterone, SHBG, and DHEA, at a minimum. It would also be helpful to assess other estrogen metabolites as well.

Once again, these are tests that can be done in your home in coordination with telemedicine doctors. There are many organizations that do this, or if you want to work with our organization, you're welcome to reach out through our app.

The Importance of Heavy Metal Testing

Since we're on the subject of testing, I also want to encourage you to get tested for heavy metals, given a surprising experience I had several years ago. At that time, as described earlier, I had torn my rotator cuff in my right shoulder and done a series of tests on my body, including a blood test to screen for toxic metals. Afterward, the doctor asked me to call him. **To my astonishment, he told me that I had such high levels of mercury in my system that I was at risk of going into cardiac arrest.** "Mr. Robbins, we measure mercury on a scale of zero to five," he said. "If you're a three, four, or five, you're in danger and have got to get it out of your nervous system. The most I've ever measured in a human is seventy-five. You're one hundred and twenty-three."

I was dumbfounded. **Then the doctor asked if I'd had any problems lately with losing my memory. "Yes," I said. "It's been happening on stage." I hadn't even told my wife about it because I didn't want to worry her. The doctor told me, "A lot of people are misdiagnosed with dementia when really it's mercury poisoning."** Then he asked if I'd also been feeling unusually tired. I replied, "I don't think I've ever felt more exhausted in my life. I thought it was just my crazy schedule." Well, it turned out that **exhaustion is another symptom of mercury poisoning, which disrupts the mitochondria in your cells and leaves you feeling utterly depleted**.

How did this happen? I'd been incredibly conscientious about my diet. I use food purely as fuel, not entertainment, so I ate lots of big salads and fish every day. **Tuna and swordfish were my favorites, and I ate them** virtually every day. **What I hadn't realized is that tuna and swordfish live unusually long lives and consume lots of smaller fish, so they accumulate exceptionally high levels of mercury. They were essentially poisoning me.** I also found out that genetically, I don't methylate well, which simply means that my body does not easily repair my DNA or regulate my hormones, and compounded the problem. **Why am I telling you this? Because it's really important for you to get a toxic metals test. It's no big deal—just a simple blood test.** The company that detected my mercury poisoning is called **Quicksilver Scientific**. Thankfully, its founder and CEO, **Christopher Shade, PhD**, put me on a protocol that gradually detoxified my body. **If I hadn't been tested and gone on this mercury detox program, I probably wouldn't be alive today. In fact, I'd say roughly one in three people whom I recommend for testing have some form of toxic metal accumulation. You need to get it out of your system, so take it from me and get the simple blood test.**

Now again, all of this may sound a bit overwhelming, but in reality, **you could do all these tests—the CCTA test for heart disease, the MRI and GRAIL test for cancer, and the blood tests for metals and hormones in a few hours.** The metals test and the hormone test can even be done from home. Or you might say, I'm only concerned about heart disease, let me just do the CCTA test. As we'll show you, your doctor can also arrange for you to do this test on their own, or through the FountainOS app. So it's not a lot of time, but it can really change the quality of your life, or even save your life or the life of someone you love.

A QUICK BONUS: 5 MORE SIMPLE TESTS THAT CAN HAVE A DRAMATIC IMPACT ON YOUR LIFE

Precision medicine has come up with a whole new set of diagnostic capabilities that can radically alter the course of your health. **Let me quickly share with you five additional tests that I and many of Fountain Life's clients do regularly. They take less than ten minutes total. Some can even be done from the comfort of your own home**; you just have to send them in for analysis.

1. <u>**Bone density**</u> **is critically important for long-term health and well-being. One in two women today over 50 will fracture a bone due to osteoporosis. There's a simple, noninvasive test that** measures your bone mineral density, bone strength, and percentage of total body fat and lean muscle mass, providing data necessary to determine whether osteoporosis treatment is recommended to prevent fractures. **Many athletes do this test, and I've done it as well. It takes as little as three minutes, with minimal radiation involved. It's called the dual X-ray absorptiometry (DEXA) bone density + metabolic scan and is the most advanced test for measuring osteoporosis.**

2. <u>**The power of DNA Analysis. Complete DNA analysis**</u>**, sequencing your genome and having the results analyzed by the right AI algorithms,** can provide insights into your genetic risks for many health conditions and your carrier status, which refers to traits that can be passed on to future generations. Through a simple swab of your cheek, you can know in advance what reactions you'll have to certain medications, understand if you have a higher or lower proclivity to certain cancers of other diseases, and also gain insight into your physical traits and things such as food intolerance that can help guide lifestyle decisions. Plus today, there are companies aggregating all of the newest genomic discoveries and correlations, and **they will send you (and your doctor) a news bulletin if there is something newly discovered about a gene you carry. How amazing is that?**

3. <u>**Microbiome Analysis.**</u> **You may know that you have even more microorganisms (your microbiome) living in your body than cells.** The newest breakthrough in mapping your microbiome, called **GI-map microbial assay plus,** is an innovative clinical tool that measures gastrointestinal microbiota DNA from a single stool sample using state-of-the-art technology. Knowing what's going on inside your GI tract is invaluable. Better yet, this test can be done in the comfort of your home. **If you're having challenges in your gut, or suffering from lack of energy, it's highly likely your microbiome is playing a role. This analysis tells you what's going on and provides you with solutions.**

4. **<u>Vital Health Skin Analysis.</u> AI facial imaging + analysis** uses artificial intelligence to evaluate the health and age of your skin. Computer imaging also enables Fountain Life specialists to simulate the effects that sun damage and aging will have on your skin's appearance up to the age of 80. These results help our team develop a customized skin rejuvenation and anti-aging plan to treat and prevent future skin damage. You'll find many of the solutions in Chapter 15, in our chapter on beauty, later in the book.

5. **<u>What's your TruAge?</u>** As you'll discover later in this book, **you have a chronological age and a biological age**. Some of us age faster than our chronological age, and some slower. Wouldn't you like to know where you stand? This simple test is the #1 biomarker for healthspan and lifespan. It measures epigenetic markers in your DNA to determine your effective biological age and also provides a full suite of aging-related metrics, including telomere length measurements (the length of the little protective caps on the ends of your chromosomes) and your current pace of aging. **I took this test last year, at the chronological age of 61, but my body was just 51 years old—very encouraging!**

SO WHAT ARE THE NEXT STEPS?

I hope that I've gotten you as excited as I am about the power of these new technologies to help us anticipate challenges, experience peace of mind, and maximize our physical energy and potential. Again, while we're very proud of what we do at Fountain Life and of our team for bringing the most cutting-edge tools and regenerative therapeutic breakthroughs to our clients, **these tests can be accessed by your physician on their own or through our app.** We designed it so that anyone using the app can access 90 percent of the same technologies offered in a Fountain Life center—even if you don't live near one.

However, if you are lucky enough to live near a Fountain Life center, we welcome you to stop by and check it out. As of publication, there are six centers, in Florida, New York, and Pennsylvania, with additional centers planned by the end of 2023 in Dallas, Chicago, Los Angeles, Dubai, India, and Toronto.

And if you're a resident of San Diego or San Francisco, you may want to visit our sister organization, the Health Nucleus, which is part of Human Longevity Inc. (HLI). HLI was cofounded by Peter and Bob, alongside genomics pioneer Craig Venter. I'm a client and an investor as well. At the Health Nucleus, you can access many of the same technologies. Again, you're not limited to going to Fountain Life for these tests. They are available through a variety of practitioners; your doctor may already have access to them.

In fact, these days, there are so many digital tools designed to help you optimize your health that you can do much of it from your home. Today there is everything from a credit card–sized device called UHealth that can measure your heart rate, to Tyto, a palm-sized handheld exam kit and app that lets you perform your own guided medical exam that your physician can see remotely in real time. Have a sore throat? Tyto's camera can look clearly into the back of your throat. You can read about these technologies and many more in the reference section at the end of the book.

Our goal in this book is to give you the tools to be the CEO of your own health, supported by experts including clinicians and nutritionists. The real goal is to have the average person gain access to more information about their health than a traditional physician would even have access to.

One of the greatest advantages is to have an ongoing snapshot of your health with all of your records and progress recorded. It's nice to be able to compare your physiological age to your chronological age. We even use sport gait technology to detect changes in your gait that can indicate neurological problems including concussion, Parkinson's, and Alzheimer's, just by having you walking ten steps forward and back with your phone!

So let's move forward and discover all of the ways that you can reverse your physiological age, reduce your risk of chronic disease, and extend your healthspan.

So what should you do? Give yourself the peace of mind of knowing where you stand on the big three—heart disease, cancer, and Alzheimer's—and also increase your energy, drive, and vitality through hormone optimization via a simple blood test. If you want, do it right now, and set yourself up to get the answers that you need.

I hope this chapter has awakened you to just how far technology has come and convinced you not to wait until there's a challenge. I was actually finishing this chapter when my wife called me after traveling to LA to visit with a dear friend of ours to introduce her to our four-month-old baby girl. Toward the end of the visit, she could feel a difference in our friend. When pressed, our friend revealed that her beloved husband of 40 years had just been diagnosed with a brain tumor and told that he has six months to live. We both cried because we love this couple so much, but it's also the very reason I wrote this chapter and am writing this book. Again, remember, prevention and capturing a challenge early is everything!

Just remember, like a race car, many of us are trying to live our lives so fully that we push ourselves without checking in on how our engine is doing. But even race car drivers have all kinds of gauges to tell them what's going on inside the engine.

Please give yourself the gift of knowing what's going on under the hood and getting those you love to know where they stand. And one last time, a as a ridiculously repetitive reminder—problems are easy to solve if you catch them when they're small! Don't wait until they become a challenge so big that they override your ability to take action.

Now let's turn to our next chapter, a powerful one about a disease that every single one of us, no matter how fit or strong or healthy, must face. It's what scientists are now calling "the disease of aging." Believe it or not there is now new hope that we can live longer and better, so let's see how a Harvard longevity scientist is beginning to turn back our biological clock. . . .

FOUNTAIN HEALTH INSURANCE

If you are the owner of a company and self-insure your employees, (63 percent of companies today do), you may be interested in knowing about an insurance plan that includes all of these latest diagnostic tests for your employees. To learn more, refer to the Fountain Health Insurance Breakout Box in the back of this book on page 662.

CHAPTER 4

TURNING BACK TIME: WILL AGING SOON BE CURABLE?

The Incredible Story of the Power of Your Epigenome, Sirtuins, and Mitochondria

"What if we could be younger longer? Not years longer but decades longer. What if those final years didn't look so terribly different than . . . the years that came before them? And what if by saving ourselves, we could also save the world?"

—DAVID SINCLAIR, *Lifespan: Why We Age—and Why We Don't Have To*

For the first time in human history, scientists are cracking the code to understanding why we age, and what can be done about it. **In this chapter you'll learn:**

1. What one of the leading longevity experts from Harvard does to boost his energy and keep his biological age twenty years younger than his chronological age.
2. What is meant by the "information theory of aging" and how this theory opens the possibility of slowing, stopping, or even reversing the aging process.
3. Why your DNA, your genome, is NOT your destiny, and how your epigenome can be modified to stave off degenerative disease and change the quality of your life.
4. The role of your mitochondria, the powerhouse of your cells, which deliver high levels of *cellular energy* to power your body, mind, and psyche.

5. The intricate dance of your sirtuin genes that serve to both repair your DNA and regulate your genome, and could be the key to age reversal.

6. How a recent discovery rocked the longevity world, demonstrating that a gene therapy treatment was able to "turn back time" in mice— effectively reverse their age, restoring eyesight and regrowing their optic nerve.

People often say that age is just a number—but for David Sinclair, it's two numbers. He's 53 going on 33. If that sounds confusing, stay with me, because the explanation could change your life, or at least your expectations for your *healthspan*—the number of years you stay healthy and active and fully functional on this earth.

David Sinclair, PhD, is one of the world's top authorities on rejuvenation. He's a tenured professor of genetics at Harvard Medical School. He runs two state-of-the-art labs on the biological mechanisms of aging, one at Harvard and the other in his native Australia. He's founded nearly a dozen biotech startups, written a *New York Times* bestseller, and patented 35 inventions. He's the chairman of Life Biosciences, the mother ship for a family of research and drug development companies that are engaged in hand-to-hand combat with aging on every front. In case you're not impressed yet, **he made *Time* magazine's list of "The 100 Most Influential People" in the world**.

Pretty remarkable, wouldn't you agree? But a few years back, when Peter Diamandis first told me I *had* to meet this "leader in the field of longevity," I'll admit I wasn't so excited. "Wait a second, Peter," I said. **"I don't need to live forever. What impact would this have on my life *right now*? What I'm interested in is increasing our energy and strength and flexibility and vitality—our quality of life *today*, not just some time in the future."**

But Peter was persistent. He told me about Sinclair's huge breakthrough, a groundbreaking study to turn back our biological clock. **And he explained to me the scientist's mind-blowing "Information Theory of Aging."** According to Sinclair, **most chronic or degenerative diseases—the ones that hijack our energy and degrade our health—aren't hardwired into our genes**. In reality, **they're the result of bad "information" that makes our genes turn "on" or "off" at the wrong times or in the wrong places**

in the body. It's like corrupted code on a computer hard drive, only on a molecular level.

Since 1995, when he joined Leonard Guarente's vanguard lab at MIT and codiscovered a cause of aging in yeast cells, Sinclair has wrestled with the riddle of why we physically decline over time. *Lifespan*, his first book, was the culmination of decades of moving two steps forward and one step back, of endless experiments with worms and flies and mice and monkeys.

And the upshot of all this relentless research? Sinclair concluded that the nine classic "hallmarks" of aging—from exhausted stem cells to tangled proteins to a rundown metabolism—didn't actually *cause* the process. **Instead, they were the *result* of DNA damage and improper regulation of genes. He found the same mechanism operating "in every organism in the universe," from yeast and bacteria to *Homo sapiens*: "Aging, quite simply, is a loss of information." That's another way of saying that aging is *entropy*, the disorder that results from missing or corrupted data.** It's like a computer program that has damaged lines of code and also has forgotten where the computer code is located! Your cells' ability to do what they're supposed to do just isn't up to snuff.

Can I give you the headline? Environment and lifestyle choices really *matter*—even more than people once thought.

David Sinclair is a card-carrying contrarian, a master of disruption. He's that unicorn of unicorns—**a truly original thinker, the rarest creature on this Earth**. He has doubled down on three revolutionary ideas:

- **Principle #1: Aging is a disease, which means it's not inevitable—or acceptable.**
- **Principle #2: Aging is a *single* malady with many manifestations, from heart disease to cancer to diabetes to autoimmune disorders.**
- **Principle #3: Aging is treatable and even reversible.**

Take a moment to digest those three sentences. Think about their implications. Consider the possible payoff as Silicon Valley pours in tens of billions of dollars and countless petabytes of AI to take on degenerative disease and restore our life force. To be clear, not all scientists agree with Sinclair on every point. He's working in a very young field, where arguments are passionate and consensus is still emerging. But if his **Information Theory** is onto something (and a number of Nobel-level brainiacs believe that it is), the insights we'll be sharing in this chapter could change *everything* for you and those you love. **They could open the door to a *new* you. To be healthy and vital and strong at nearly any age!**

I'm proud to have David Sinclair on our Life Force Advisory Board. I feel privileged to support his amazing, transformational, pragmatic research to lift the quality of life for human beings across this planet. And I'm honored to introduce him to you in this chapter. Read on, and prepared to be surprised, encouraged, and inspired!

DAVID SINCLAIR'S REJUVENATION RECIPE

As you can imagine, Sinclair has enough on his plate to exhaust two or three normal people. But when you meet him, his dynamic energy is sparkling, commanding, unquenchable. He has a boyish face, a quicksilver intellect, and a mischievous sense of humor. In a very real sense, he's the embodiment of youth. How so? **Well, Sinclair's *chronological age*—the one on his birth certificate—is 53. But his *biological age*—from biomarkers in his blood that tell the tale—is around two decades younger. And for the record, it's our biological age that matters. It's the number that best predicts our prospects for living another thirty or fifty vibrant years or more.**[1] **Science shows that we *don't* all age at the same tempo.** Take a look at my friend **Tom Brady**, a man who just won his seventh Super Bowl at the tender age of 43. Tom now has more Super Bowl victories than any NFL team! If you're looking to sustain that kind of peak performance in whatever competition you're in, whether in business or life, then read on.

So how did Sinclair do it? How did he pull off this nifty trick to become as healthy as a typical person nearly twenty years his junior? Did he just get lucky and win the genetic lottery? Or is there something he knows and *does* that you and I need to understand, so we can follow his example?

---

1 We'll be getting to this in more detail later in the chapter, but Sinclair's biological age was computed by a method similar to the gold-standard "epigenetic clock" devised by Steve Horvath, the UCL Ageneticist.

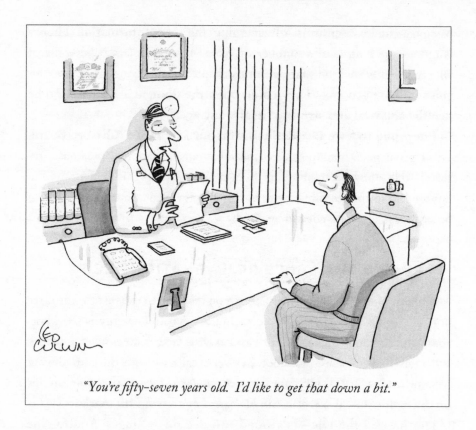

"You're fifty-seven years old. I'd like to get that down a bit."

As it turns out, Sinclair has leveraged his encyclopedic knowledge of longevity science to make some high-impact lifestyle choices and vastly improve his prospects of a long and healthy life. First of all, he's smart about what he eats; he's especially careful to limit his red meat and avoids almost all sugar. Second, he confines himself to one meal per day (dinner)— a form of caloric restriction that many have found to be one of the smartest, healthiest moves you can make. Third, he moderates his intake of alcohol. Fourth, he strives to get eight hours of sleep per night. Fifth, he exercises at least three days per week.

As we will discuss in Section Three, the lifestyle changes that can affect your life, **simple moves like these, have an outsized impact on your health, energy, vigor, and longevity**. Best of all, they're easy to understand—and to replicate. You don't have to be a Harvard longevity guru to decide that it's probably unwise to gorge on sugar!

But the truth is, Sinclair's lifestyle is healthy but not all *that*

exceptional. Though he's a big believer in the benefits of exercise, he will freely admit that he's not exactly a hardcore gym rat. What's more, he wasn't exactly blessed with fabulous genes. His family tree has lots of diabetes and more than its share of early deaths and disabilities.

So what is Sinclair's secret? In part, at least, it's a small handful of vitality supplements and simple medications taken most days for the last five years.

Sinclair's blood sugar and inflammation markers used to be high but have dropped to healthy levels. **His 83-year-old father, Andrew, takes these rejuvenation supplements as well—which may help to explain why he's no longer saddled with aches or pains or memory deficits. Bursting with energy, Andrew walks three to four miles a day, outlifts his son at the gym, and spends his spare time mountaineering and hiking through the Serengeti in Africa. "Compared to ten years ago, he's a different person,"** says Sinclair. "Physically and mentally, he's more active in both regards."

In case you're wondering, Sinclair's regimen isn't anything especially exotic. **He takes a vitamin cocktail, D3 and K2**, a simple, life-changing breakthrough that too few people know about. **D3** has been scientifically proven to strengthen our bones, balance our hormones, and fortify our immune systems—a critical benefit as we age and our immune response weakens. According to a study at the Mayo Clinic, **recent studies have found that people with vitamin D deficiencies were far more likely to test positive for the virus that causes COVID-19—and to experience acute respiratory failure or death after they were infected.**[2] In Scotland, the government went so far as to give free vitamin D supplements to vulnerable populations who'd been isolating indoors and getting limited sunlight.

Meanwhile, **vitamin K2** actually keeps our arteries from clogging with calcium plaques, a leading cause of heart attacks. (And if you want to detect asymptomatic heart disease *before* it causes a big problem, and you've read our previous chapter, you already know about a new, noninvasive coronary CT scan developed by a startup named Cleerly, which uses AI to predict the risk of any potential blockages.)

---

2 Marshall, "Can Vitamin D Protect Against the Coronavirus Disease 2019 (COVID-19)?"

In addition, Sinclair spoons a gram of *resveratrol* into his morning yogurt (for maximal absorption)—it's a potent antioxidant, found in grapes and red wine, that may protect our brain and heart. As you may know, resveratrol was all the rage for a period of time, until some studies showed that without fat, resveratrol absorption was five to ten times lower. According to Sinclair, consumption with yogurt (or another fat source) is critical. He takes a gram of *metformin*, **the pennies-per-dose first-line treatment for type 2 diabetes that could have a far-reaching impact—even if you're not diabetic. By boosting our sensitivity to insulin and thereby lowering our blood glucose,** Sinclair believes that this garden-variety wonder drug is a healthspan gold mine. **We'll tell you more about metformin in Chapter 10, "Your Ultimate Vitality Pharmacy," and about a recent study that indicates that it may protect against everything from cancer to heart disease to dementia.**[3]

Last but not least, Sinclair takes one gram of an over-the-counter supplement called NMN (nicotinamide mononucleotide), which we'll return to shortly and again in more detail in Chapter 10. Naturally generated by the body, this compound gets converted into a molecule called **NAD+, which plays a central role in regulating and energizing our cells. The problem is that we make less and less NAD+ as we get older**—which is where supplementing with NMN comes in. **If you search on Google or Amazon, you'll find at least a dozen different brands selling what they claim to be NMN, with prices ranging from $24 to $95 for 60 tablets. The challenge is that a lot of these supplements do not in fact contain actual NMN when tested in the lab. And in many cases, what they contain isn't a stable form of the molecule and can degrade in under 60 days. In Chapter 10 we'll share with you what we believe to be safe options for you to consider.** You can buy something similar online for $50 a month, probably less than what you're paying for Wi-Fi,[4] but you need to be careful about your source. Sinclair is banking on early studies

3 Campbell et al., "Metformin Use Associated with Reduced Risk of Dementia in Patients with Diabetes: A Systematic Review and Meta-Analysis."

4 Citroner, "Diabetes Drug Metformin May Help Reverse Serious Heart Condition"; Saraei et al., "The Beneficial Effects of Metformin on Cancer Prevention and Therapy: A Comprehensive Review of Recent Advances."

that say the pill is safe. Besides his father, his brother also takes it; so do the family's dogs.

But before you pull out your credit card, let me add a caveat. Various NAD+ precursors have delivered remarkable payoffs for animals' health-span. But we can't yet be sure of their benefits—or risks—for human beings. Sinclair himself cautions that no one magic molecule can solve all of our ills. And he knows better than almost anyone that anecdotal evidence is no sub-stitute for rigorous, controlled, double-blind clinical trials.

Still . . . **according to some of the most respected scientists in the world, the rewards could be astounding. If Sinclair's hypothesis proves out, his chosen supplements—or something like them—could actually slow the ravages of time and change the course of human history. We might stop aging in its tracks, or even recover the energy we took for granted as twentysomethings. The implications are epic.** As Sinclair wrote in his runaway bestselling book, *Lifespan*: "What if we didn't have to worry that the clock was ticking? And what if I told you that soon—very soon, in fact—we won't?"

It's an extreme proposition, no question. I'll understand if you find it hard to swallow, no pun intended. But as you'll soon discover, the future painted by *Lifespan* isn't some far-fetched fantasy. **We're quickly reaching a tipping point in knowledge and technology. We're at the brink of big-time advances that could dramatically expand our energy and extend our healthspan *and* our lifespan.** The science is around the corner—**in many cases, it's a practical reality right now**. Sinclair's rejuvenation supplement cocktail is just one of a multitude of technologies with massive potential to propel us into a shining new world of longer, healthier, more dynamic and productive lives.

KLOTHO: A GENE THAT CAN BE UNLOCKED TO INCREASE LIFESPAN

Here's another potent rejuvenator coming your way: a naturally occurring human enzyme called klotho. According to a San Diego–based company called Klotho Therapeutics, higher levels of the human

Klotho gene can be linked to with dramatically higher survival rates in older people.[5] Though preclinical animal data is no guarantee, what we know so far is intriguing. **When a mouse's klotho gene was "knocked out," its lifespan was shortened by 80 percent. But when the gene was manipulated to "turn on" at a higher level, the mouse lived** *30 percent longer* **than normal mice . . . a longevity bonus equivalent to more than twenty human years.** And since the identical protein is found across the animal kingdom, scientists believe there's reason to be optimistic that people will benefit, as well.

As Klotho Therapeutics CEO and founder Jim Plante explained to us, the klotho story is much like the tale of NAD+. **As our bodies age, we develop deficiencies of this critical anti-inflammatory.** His company has developed a small-molecule pill that promises to "unlock" the klotho gene, restore its "information" to youthful levels, and stop degenerative illness in its tracks. Their first human clinical trial will be aimed at acute diseases of the kidney, where klotho concentrations are highest. But they're also planning to tackle cancer, heart disease, diabetes, and frailty. **And since klotho penetrates the blood-brain barrier, they're optimistic that it could help prevent dementia. It's already established that a healthy amount of klotho is associated with larger brain volume and enhanced memory and other cognitive functions.**[6]

Before we get back to NAD+, I want to discuss something more fundamental. Let's focus for a moment on what scientists like to call **"first principles,"** the precepts that can guide us to solve the most basic puzzles of existence. If the quality of our lives and the state of our health is defined by our energy, our vitality or life force . . . **then what could be more fundamental than this critical question:** *What generates our body's energy?*

---

5 Semba et al., "Plasma Klotho and Mortality Risk in Older Community-Dwelling Adults."

6 Kurtzman, "Brain Region Vulnerable to Aging Is Larger in Those With Longevity Gene Variant."

What powers the 30 trillion cells in our body? **Even more important, how and why do we lose energy over time? Why are so many young people falling prey to illnesses usually associated with the aged, like diabetes, cancer, and heart disease? And *most* important: How can we restore our life force to its youthful peak and sustain our energy throughout a long and exuberant life, into a ripe and active old age?**

Here's a clue: The most powerful answers can be found in the smallest elements of life.

MEET YOUR MITOCHONDRIA: YOUR ENERGY GENERATORS

"What the Indians call prana and the Chinese call ch'i, Christians refer to as grace or the Holy Spirit, and secularists might call vitality or simply life-force. . . . Every cell in your body must have a fresh supply of energy each day in order to thrive."

—CAROLINE MYSS, *Why People Don't Heal and How They Can*

For some time I've understood that **our quality of life is determined by our emotions.** If you've got a billion dollars and you're angry all the time, your life is anger. If you've got beautiful children and you're worried all the time, your life is worry. **But emotions don't exist in isolation. They're heavily influenced by your physiology, most of all by your *energy*. Low energy tends to bring negative emotions.** How do you feel after a night or two of poor sleep? That's a low-energy state. The flip side is that high energy sparks *positive* emotions. Think of how you feel when you're rested and calm—a lot more hopeful and confident, am I right?

Here's the crux of the matter: Your energy is determined by the universe inside you: your 30 trillion or so living cells, the fundamental units of every tissue and organ and system in your body. To put two and two together, *our quality of life is the quality of life of our cells*—it's where the rubber meets the road. **When our cells are healthy and strong, we are fully *alive*.** When our cells are in equilibrium, or what scientists call *homeostasis*, our emotional life will be balanced as well. And as you'll see, **we need high levels of *cellular energy* to thrive in body, mind, and psyche.**

We all know people who seem to have "fast" or "slow" metabolisms. In fact, our bodies are motored by *multiple* metabolic pathways. By changing one chemical into another, they regulate everything from our hormones to our sleep cycle to our immune system. But the metabolism most of us think of first—and the critical one for this chapter—is *glucose metabolism*, **the chemical reactions that convert carbohydrates and sugars into energy. This happens inside our *mitochondria*, the cell's tiny blast furnaces that keep us humming through our days. They are nothing less than our life force generators!** Peter Diamandis has twin ten-year-old boys. They spill over with high spirits—they're turbocharged! Their mitochondria fire at full blast all the time. **As one National Institutes of Health–funded study noted, "Perhaps no structure [mitochondria] is so intimately and simultaneously connected to both the energy of youth and the decline of the old."**[7]

Mitochondria create the fuel that powers each and every cell in our bodies. They live in the cytoplasm, the salty sea between a cell's outer membrane and its nucleus. **Their biggest job is to import nutrients, break them down, and turn them into complex molecules called ATP,** *the cells' battery packs*.

We need ATP to flex a muscle, to feel heat or cold, to digest nutrients, to eliminate wastes like carbon dioxide—basically, for our body to do anything! The higher the animal on the evolutionary scale, the more energy—and hence the more ATP—it needs to survive. If your mitochondria are lying down on the job, there's no ATP—and **without ATP, there's no life! Our species can last three weeks without food. We can go three days or so without water. But as little as three minutes without oxygen can damage the brain—because oxygen is needed to "burn" the glucose in our mitochondria and produce ATP.** (Another "fun" fact: Cyanide is so lethal because it targets the mitochondria and blocks them from using oxygen or manufacturing ATP. A tiny amount—less than a drop—can kill a medium-sized person in 30 seconds flat!)

For David Sinclair, the mitochondria are the cells' Da Vinci Code, the place where the secrets of life and vitality and decay and death are

---

7 Sun et al., "The Mitochondrial Basis of Aging."

most likely to be found, if only we can decipher them. In his team's ongoing research into what promotes healthspan and longevity, "we go in unbiased," he says. "We ask the cells and the animals to tell us what's important in aging, and we keep getting dragged back to the mitochondria."

AGE: THE ROOT CAUSE OF ALL DISEASE

"Old age isn't a battle; old age is a massacre."

—PHILIP ROTH, legendary U.S. novelist

Whether we're 20 or 40 or 60, we're getting older each moment, every day. And it's not just you and me. As people live progressively longer, the entire world is aging—and the trend is accelerating. In 1800, the world's average life expectancy was only about 30 years. By 2019, thanks to antibiotics and vaccines and better hygiene, plus a sharp drop in child mortality, the worldwide average had zoomed up to 73— and a lot longer than that in Western nations like the United States with strong healthcare and modern sanitation systems.

By 2050, the segment of the world's population over 60 (my new cohort) will be nearly twice what it is today—more than 2 billion people, nearly one of five souls on Earth. Fortunately, I can tell you that our longer lives will also be more active, more dynamic, and flat-out *healthier* than ever before if we align with many of the principles shared by the experts in the pages to follow.

Even with a recent statistical dip from opioid overdoses, suicide, and chronic liver problems (the so-called diseases of despair that took a deeper hold with COVID-19 lockdowns), **the typical person in the United States now lives to age 79. Once we make it to 65, statistics show that we can look forward to another 19 years, on average. A healthy 80-year-old, free of terminal illness, has a good shot at lasting another decade or more, to 90 years-plus.**

But while our quantity of life has risen significantly, our collective *quality* of life is—for the moment—stuck in neutral. Though we've made huge strides against viral and bacterial infections, more than 1.7 million Americans a year die from chronic diseases. **Overall, more**

than two of three deaths come from one or more of the Big Six: heart disease, cancer, stroke, chronic obstructive pulmonary disease, diabetes, and Alzheimer's. We'll be addressing all of them—and the latest breakthrough treatments and prevention tools—in Section Four of this book.

Here's a question: What's the biggest risk factor for these devastating conditions? Smoking? Too many nightcaps? Big Gulps with a double helping of McDonald's fries?

The answer is, none of the above.

The biggest risk factor *by far* is aging. While smoking increases your cancer risk fivefold, according to Sinclair, *aging raises it fivehundred-fold.* (It makes sense when you think about it. How many 12-year-olds do you know with hardened arteries or lung cancer?) Aging itself is the mother of virtually *all* diseases—including most infectious diseases. While nursing homes reported only 4 percent of coronavirus cases in the U.S. (as of mid-2021), they accounted for 31 percent of total deaths.[8] According to the Centers for Disease Control and Prevention, the 85-and-up demographic was *630 times* more likely to die of COVID than people in their 20s, many of whom had the virus with no symptoms at all. Why the huge difference? The older people had lethal underlying conditions like heart disease or diabetes, or what doctors call "comorbidities"—the illnesses linked overwhelmingly to aging.

More and more top scientists now agree with Sinclair on this point, though the medical establishment is still playing catch-up. In 2018, the World Health Organization finally included "aging-related disease" in its international coding manual, a grudging step in the right direction. And get this: The National Institute on Aging—America's only federal research center for preventative healthcare, instead of reactive sick-care—receives just 7.5 percent of total funding from the National Institutes of Health.[9]

"If we put as much money into aging as diseases," Sinclair argues, "we would have many [approved] medicines by now." We'll know we have turned

---

8 Conlen et al., "Nearly One-Third of U.S. Coronavirus Deaths Are Linked to Nursing Homes"

9 Peterson, "Final FY21 Appropriations: National Institutes of Health."

the corner, Sinclair says, when anti-aging drugs are prescribed as freely as statins are today.

SO, WHAT IS AGING?

"Without energy, life would be extinguished instantaneously, and the cellular fabric would collapse."

—ALBERT SZENT-GYÖRGYI, Nobel Prize–winning biochemist

But what exactly do we mean by "aging"? As it turns out, gray hair and forgetfulness and cataracts and hearing loss are just the obvious downstream ramifications. The aging syndrome itself takes root early on, in our mid-twenties, and operates invisibly for a long time. It's like Jaws, the killer shark, skimming silently beneath the surface—until one day it strikes.

By middle age, our cells have grown larger and fattier. Their membranes are less permeable, making it harder to pull oxygen in or push waste products out. They divide more slowly, thinning out our tiny blood vessels and shrinking our muscles. And they get stiffer, bad news for our joints and circulation and airways.

Just as the knee bone connects to the thigh bone, **tissue changes lead to organ changes—especially in our heart, lungs, and kidneys, which gradually lose functionality**. Early on, we may not notice that we've passed our peak; like a well-built office tower, our organs are designed with spectacular redundancy. **A 20-year-old heart can pump ten times as much blood as the body needs. But around the time we hit 30, we're losing some of that reserve each year.**[10] (There's a reason people stop racing their children in middle age!) **Our hormone and stem cell levels also drop off a cliff between the ages of 30 and 40. Why? Because we weren't designed by evolution to live past 35.** Once we procreated and kept the species going, our job here was considered done. The all-too-typical results? All the dreaded features of aging, from chronic disease and dementia to "geriatric syndromes" like frailty and falls.

---

10 Mandal, "Heart Rate Reserve."

Aging is also an enormously complex problem, with countless moving parts. So it's a tall order to get to the bottom of it. "Aging is not one thing going wrong," says **Leonard Guarente, PhD**, the longevity research pioneer who gave Sinclair his start in the field. "It's many things that go wrong at the same time [and] reinforce each other in their decline." **Or as Tad Friend memorably observed in the *New Yorker*: "Solving aging is not just a whodunnit but a howdunnit and wheredunnit and a why-oh-whydunnit."**

Fair enough. But the book you hold in your hands is all about actual proven solutions that you can use today, as well as futuristic tools quickly coming down the pike. There are some really smart scientific detectives hunting for clues, getting closer each day to the source of our physical troubles. It goes without saying that David Sinclair is one of the top sleuths around. He's come up with an idea that is bold, provocative, and elegant, all at once. Are you ready? **Sinclair is convinced that aging results from lost or distorted *information*. He believes that the source of our later-in-life woes is a breakdown in cellular communication and regulation**—no more, no less.

Our genetic code is a miraculous thing. Our original "information" is the instruction book that grows a microscopic romance between sperm and egg into an eight-pound newborn with billions of cells—all in the space of nine months! This manual, our genome, directs the body's genetically identical stem cells to morph into nerve cells or heart cells or muscle cells or skin cells. In most cases, everything comes out working perfectly. All of a baby's systems are *go*, like a brand-new Tesla under warranty.

But over time, bad things happen. We're bombarded by radiation, stress, and environmental toxins. We suffer from crappy diets and not enough real exercise. Our physical and emotional fitness get sorely neglected. There's a reason why the U.S. cancer rate stays stubbornly high, in spite of all we've learned about prevention . . . or why childhood diabetes keeps rising every year.

But here's our promise: We can stay disease-free for nearly all our lives. We can write a new ending to our biological stories—and a new middle, too.

If Sinclair's Information Theory of Aging is on the money, and we're able to reboot our genome and correct those master instructions to their pristine state, the time may not be so distant when we'll sustain our youth throughout our life! We'll stop getting "older" in any sense that matters. **Biologically speaking, we'll get *better*. More zestful and powerful. More tireless and energetic. More robust and *alive*!**

THE HOLY GRAIL

"What we've got here . . . is failure to communicate."

—CAPTAIN, the warden in *Cool Hand Luke*

Let's start with a bit of background. There are **three words** I want to help you understand. They sound scientific, but go a long way in understanding the process of aging, and most important, changing the level of energy you experience even today. Those three terms are *genome, epigenome,* **and** *sirtuins*.

<u>What's your genome?</u> Every cell in your body has an identical instruction set of 3.2 billion letters from your mother and 3.2 billion letters from your father. **These letters make up your DNA and are known as your genome.** Your genome codes for some 30,000 proteins that are the enzymes and building blocks of life. **The proteins your genome codes for at birth are the very same they code for when you are 80 years old!**

So, if it's true that your genome doesn't change over the span of your lifetime, and you have basically the same genome at 80 that you had when you were 20, why don't you look the same as when you were 20?

<u>That's where your epigenome comes in.</u> Your epigenome (where the prefix "epi" means above) is the cellular software that controls your DNA, your genome. It tells each cell what genes it should turn on and what genes it should turn off. This is how cells with identical DNA can have very different functions, why one cell becomes muscle, and another forms a neuron. **While your genome is a set of instructions, like keys on a piano that each make a note, your epigenome is like the piano player who decides which keys should be played at what exact time during a concerto.** Biologically, the epigenome is made up of chemical compounds and proteins

that attach to DNA and direct which of your 30,000 genes are turned on or turned off, throughout your life.

When it comes to our healthspan, lifespan, and how our body and mind function each day, our genes and DNA are *not* our destiny. The epigenome, which controls gene expression, is *the* main mechanism that decides our destiny. Let me say this again, because so many people are hypnotized into believing the opposite: ***Our genes are not our destiny.*** Don't take it from me. Listen to what David Sinclair told us: **"If you look at twin studies, at thousands of people, you come to the conclusion that only 20 percent of our health in old age and our lifespan is genetically determined, which is a stunning thing."**

What accounts for the other 80 percent? *The epigenome.* **Among biologists and geneticists, the issue is no longer in serious dispute: <u>The epigenetic joystick that controls *how* the genome functions is more powerful than the genetic code itself</u>. Importantly, several lifestyle factors have been identified that are believed to powerfully modify epigenetic patterns, such as diet, obesity, physical activity, tobacco smoking, alcohol consumption, environmental pollutants, psychological stress, and working on night shifts.**

At this point, we've spoken about how **aging is the misregulation of your epigenome—having the wrong genes turned on or off as we get older.** Errors in our epigenome accumulate over our life. Throughout life, as we age, our cellular DNA is constantly challenged by damage-inducing factors such as smoke, radiation, and toxins in the environment. **This is where our third ingredient of why we age, sirtuins, plays a critical role.**

<u>Sirtuins (pronounced SIR-TO-INS) are a set of seven regulatory genes that have two different and competing functions in your cells.</u> First, they **govern the epigenome, "turning the right genes on at the right time and in the right cell, boosting mitochondrial activity, reducing inflammation, and protecting telomeres."** And second, they have another **critical function in directing DNA repair.**

As we age, the need for DNA repair increases because of accumulated damage. Makes sense, right? At age 20 we've only had a little exposure to environmental toxins, but by age 60, we have had three times the exposure, and because DNA damage accumulates, the need for repair is constantly increasing. As such, our sirtuins become overtaxed, frantically responding to one fire alarm after the next. As they get spread too thin, they get distracted from their second critical job of regulating the epigenome, deciding which genes should be turned on and which should be off.

The double-hit result? As we age and accumulate more and more DNA damage, our ability to repair the damage at the same time becomes more and more challenging. **From entire organ systems down to individual cells, our bodies become dysregulated.** Epigenetic noise accumulates. Genes that have no business being on are steadily switched on and vice versa. **It's epigenetic mayhem!**

In a nutshell, that's the dynamic of aging on a molecular level: the tension between gene regulation and gene repair, and how we pay the price when our sirtuins become overwhelmed.

This leads us to another important question, for which the answer can combat the disease of human aging: **How can we revive and supercharge our sirtuins?**

How to Help Sirtuins? Answer? NAD+

Thanks in large part to Sinclair, we now know that our sirtuins can't do much of *anything*—**including fixing our DNA—without a heaping helping of NAD+, a molecule that is critical to power the entire sirtuins system. So it's sobering to learn that we lose about half of our NAD+ by our 50s . . . right around the time when we need it more than ever to function at peak efficiency.** **Not only do our sirtuins have more and more work to do as we age, but they don't have enough NAD+ fuel to do their job!**

Does this sound like a grim story to you? In fact, it's just the opposite. First, as we shall see in Section three in Chapter 10, "Your Ultimate Vitality Pharmacy," there is something you can do to aid your sirtuins and boost your NAD+ levels. Second, if you've stayed with me this far, you should be ecstatic about this recent shift in scientific thinking. Because unlike mutations in our genome, epigenetic aging is predictable, reproducible—and, based on recent clinical trials, possibly *reversible*.

Think about it, without exaggeration Sinclair is talking about the Holy Grail—the fountain of youth! **Once we figure out how to restore our**

epigenome to an earlier age, everything changes. "Incurable" maladies— from diabetes to Parkinson's to macular degeneration—will become *bugs* in the aging process instead of standard features. They'll be fixable or even preventable. **Once we crack that code, humanity will be liberated from age-related disease. "Imagine you have a treatment for heart disease,"** **Sinclair says, "but as a side effect you'd also be protected against Al-** **zheimer's, cancer, and frailty."**

Now, let's pause for a moment and take stock. Because I have to admit, we've plunged you into the deep end of this scientific pool. It's a lot to di-gest in one fell swoop. So, take a deep breath. Stretch your limbs. Grab a cou-ple of glazed donuts (no, forget that). And now that you're feeling refreshed, let me tell you what all of this adds up to. It's as profoundly important as it is simple and straightforward. Here, in short, is the big message of this chapter:

Aging isn't scripted into our biological program. Unlike death and **taxes, it's not inevitable.**

And if you want more evidence, let me introduce you to some four- **legged friends of ours.**

NMN AND MUSCULAR MICE

It's now generally accepted that the shrinkage and death of our micro-capillaries, our smallest blood vessels, is a primary aspect of aging. As blood flow diminishes, tissues and organs get less oxygen. Waste products build up. Wounds heal more slowly. We lose bone (osteoporosis) and most of all muscle mass. **This helps to explain why physical performance** **peaks in most people in our twenties, and why professional athletes** **generally get forced off the field by age forty.**

We know that regular workouts can help stave off this decay. **Exercised** **muscles release growth-stimulating proteins that tell our endothelial** **cells (the cells lining our blood vessels) to form new capillaries.** But without enough active sirtuins in the neighborhood, says Sinclair, "it's as if these cells had grown deaf to the signals that muscles sent their way."[11] Once again, critical information is lost.

---

11 Pesheva, "Rewinding the Clock."

In his quest to better understand what was happening, Sinclair conducted a remarkable experiment. **His team at Harvard gave NMN (nicotinamide mononucleotide), the precursor molecule that is converted into NAD+ inside our cells, to twenty-month-old mice (equivalent to a human in their late 60s or early 70s).** And do you know what happened? **The animals were revitalized. They formed new and more densely networked blood vessels. Their mitochondria revived as well. And with more blood flow and oxygen, their muscles got larger and stronger.** The transformation was quite amazing. Within two months, the revitalized animals were running 60 percent farther than an untreated control group. **They'd become as vigorous as mice half their age. By every measurement that mattered, they were young again! This is why Sinclair and his dad take a gram of NMN every morning as a supplement.**

AN NAD+ BOOSTER BEING TESTED BY THE US SPECIAL FORCES

When it comes to boosting NAD+, there may be a new game in town in the next two or three years and it goes by the code name MIB-626. MIB-626 is a proprietary, synthetically manufactured molecule that is similar to, but not identical to NMN. It's being developed and tested by a company called Metrobiotech that Peter and I have invested in. Historically, when measured, the most NMN has been able to boost NAD+ levels intracellularly has been 40 percent, but recent studies in humans show that fourteen days of dosing with MIB-626 can raise NAD+ levels by as much as 200 to 300 percent!

"We've discovered a way to reverse vascular aging by boosting the presence of naturally occurring molecules in the body that augment the physiological response to exercise," said senior study investigator David Sinclair.

When evaluated in mice, researchers fed 400 mg/kg of NMN per day to 20-month-old mice, an age comparable to 70 years in people. After two months, the **mice had increased muscular blood flow,** enhanced physical performance and endurance, and the old mice became as fit and strong as young mice. A teenage mouse will run about one kilometer straight on a treadmill. You give this compound to an adult mouse (age 70 equivalent), which is not as muscular, for thirty days, it can run between two and three kilometers.

Rather than go the supplement route (which does not require FDA trials), Metrobiotech is pursuing FDA approvals, and is in early Phase 1 and Phase 2 trials using MIB-626 for a wide variety of indications, ranging from increased muscle endurance and neurogeneration, to treating COVID-related kidney failure and even heart failure.

Perhaps most interesting, in July of 2021 it was leaked that the U.S. Special Operations Command (SOCOM) has "completed preclinical safety and dosing studies in anticipation of follow-on performance testing" using Metrobiotech's MIB-626 molecule. "If the preclinical studies and clinical trials bear out, the resulting benefits include improved human performance, such as increased endurance and faster recovery from injury," said Navy Commander Timothy A. Hawkins, a spokesperson for SOCOM,

If all goes well with clinical trials, it's hoped that MIB-626 will gain regulatory approval as a new drug, available to all of us by the end of 2023.

EPIGENETIC TIME MACHINE

"Our study shows that aging may not have to proceed in one single direction . . . with careful modulation, aging might be reversed."

—JUAN CARLOS IZPISUA BELMONTE,
groundbreaking stem cell biologist, Salk Institute

Sinclair is most excited these days about the potential of cellular reprogramming to alter our epigenome and keep us healthier longer. In 2006, a Japanese researcher named Shinya Yamanaka made a thunderclap, Nobel Prize–winning discovery that changed the course of medicine and human biology. He showed that a set of four genes could transform garden-variety adult cells into age-zero stem cells. **These manipulated stem cells—known by scientists as *induced pluripotent stem cells*—had the magical ability to repair or replace injured tissue anywhere in the body. By pushing cells back in time, decades of epigenetic scuffs could be wiped away.**

Ten years later, the Salk Institute's Juan Carlos Izpisua Belmonte turned on all four "Yamanaka factors" in prematurely aged mice. Belmonte's first approach created dramatic results, but some of the mice died. He then modified his approach and successfully drove their cells into "molecular rejuvenation." That's right. **Izpisua Belmonte achieved the astonishing feat of refreshing the animals' waning mitochondria—and thereby *increased the mice's lifespan by 30 percent*.**[12] "It was a crazy experiment," says Sinclair, "and he'll probably get a Nobel Prize for it." In fact, Sinclair predicts that this work will go down as one of the touchstone papers of the twenty-first century.

In 2019, Sinclair's Harvard lab, standing on the shoulders of Izpisua Belmonte and the entire sirtuin field, **turned on three of the four Yamanaka factors in mice blinded by age-related glaucoma. In adult mammals, cells in the central nervous system—which includes the optic nerve— aren't known to regenerate. Once vision has been lost to glaucoma, there's never been a way to get it back . . . but maybe now there will be. Sinclair's REVIVER mice (*RecoVery of Information Via Epigenetic Reprogramming*) had their sight restored, "the first treatment to reverse vision loss in a glaucoma model."**[13] **Even better, none of the mice died.**

Then Sinclair's team moved to the acid test of his Information Theory of Aging. Using the gold-standard **"epigenetic clock"** invented by **UCLA's Steve Horvath**, they measured a chemical change called **"methylation"** along the mouse genome. **Horvath compares methylation to rust on a**

---

12 Ocampo et al., "In Vivo Amelioration of Age-Associated Hallmarks by Partial Reprogramming."

13 Mendelsohn and Larrick, "Epigenetic Age Reversal by Cell-Extrinsic and Cell-Intrinsic Means."

car: The more you've got, the older you are biologically and the fewer years you likely have left.

So what did Sinclair find? After the three Yamanaka factors were turned on, his REVIVER mice showed *less* methylation. **They actually got younger and could actually see; the glaucoma was *gone*! Demethylation made the old neurons behave like frisky young nerve cells.** Sinclair called Horvath and said, "Guess what, Steve—your clock isn't just a clock. It actually controls time!" (If you're curious to know your own level of methylation and your epigenetic biological age, Sinclair's team will soon be marketing a test based on a quick and painless cheek swab. It promises a turnaround time of just a few days and has a real cost of only a dollar.)

To be clear, many a promising therapy has crashed and burned in the gulf between animal studies and human clinical trials. Even so, the REVIVER results thrilled the scientific world. Maybe we *could* return our epigenome to its youthful state. If so, the implications are breathtaking! **Once we can safely reprogram our biological clocks and wind them back, what's to stop us from returning patients to the point *before* they suffered a stroke, severed their spine, or formed their first pancreatic cancer cell? "The body would heal," says Sinclair, "as though it was very young, even neonatal."** All we'll need to do is take is a ride in the epigenetic time machine!

> *"Tackling aging isn't a selfish act. It's probably the most generous act I could give the planet."*
>
> —DAVID SINCLAIR

While the road to a healthy epigenome and hearty mitochondria may ultimately be paved by supplements like NMN, lifestyle also plays a starring role. The older we get, the more important our personal habits become. As we'll discuss in later chapters, calorie restriction—a condition mimicked by NAD+—is a critical piece of the puzzle. So is regular exercise.

"This is why I actually now bother to worry about my health," says Sinclair. "I thought we could affect it only slightly, but no. **We really *do* have**

our longevity in our hands." I hope you take that to heart, because it might just be the single most important lesson in this entire book.

The last thing he'd want to do, Sinclair says, "is keep people sicker for longer." His goal isn't just to help you and me to live into our nineties and beyond, but to arrive there vibrant and intact, ready to rock and roll. That's what we mean by expanding our healthspan—to keep feeling young until our very last days! In preclinical trials, Sinclair reports, mice given NMN (that NAD+ precursor) "don't get heart disease, cancer, Alzheimer's, until sometimes 20 percent later in their life. And so that's 20 percent longer youth, not just 20 percent longer life."

When super-old mice finally *do* get struck down by chronic disease, they don't linger on in misery. On the contrary, they die more abruptly. These findings are in line with research by Nir Barzilai, chief medical adviser at Life Biosciences. In a study of 700 people past their 100th birthday, he found an unexpected phenomenon: "At the end of their life, they are sick for a very short time."[14]

A "longevity dividend" translates to fewer and shorter hospital stays and far smaller medical bills. **Over their last two years of life, according to the Centers for Disease Control, centenarians rack up just *one-third* of the healthcare expenses of people who die younger.**[15] If we could push back the typical onset of chronic disease—say from people's 60s to their 90s—**the U.S. alone would save billions of dollars a year.**[16] **Most important of all, millions upon millions of people would lead healthier, happier, more socially useful lives.**

Early in his career, when David Sinclair called himself "a science rebel," his zeal rubbed the establishment the wrong way. Even today, he tells us, his team is still working "against the flow, because we think differently here about problems. What we discover is counterintuitive. And sometimes it takes twenty years for us to get to the answers of the questions we're asking."

---

14 Bluestein, "What if Aging Could be Slowed and Health Spans Extended? A Q+A with Nir Barzilai, M.D."

15 Lade, "Reaching 100: Survivors of the Century."

16 *The Science of Success Podcast,* "How to Stop and Reverse Aging with Dr. David Sinclair."

Maybe you've heard of the great insight about **the three stages of all truths**? Here's how it goes:

1. First they are ridiculed.
2. Then they are ferociously opposed.
3. And then finally they are accepted as self-evident.

In the next section of this book, you will meet a series of genius scientists who have created extraordinary breakthroughs by following this very path. In fact, you might start out reading these chapters as one of the doubters yourself. *There's no way*, you may say to yourself. Or: *How can this be possible?* But I would encourage you to stay the course and read on. Because the results are real.

In many ways, Sinclair has a lot in common with our first set of heroes. We've all heard about people who die on the waiting list for organ transplants. But it doesn't have to be that way, thanks to pioneer scientists who are rewriting the story. Let's turn now to breakthrough science that might sound like science fiction but is being done successfully today, as we speak: the regeneration of new replacement organs.

Turn the page now—and fasten your seatbelt!

HEROES OF THE REGENERATIVE MEDICINE REVOLUTION

Learn five of the most powerful tools for the healing, transformation, and regeneration of the human body, and hear the inspiring stories of the heroes who have created them. These tools and discoveries are the basis of so many treatments you'll read in this book, including . . .

- The miracle of organ regeneration

- The mighty CAR T-cell: A breakthrough cure for Leukemia

- Incisionless brain surgery: The impact of focused ultrasound to heal Parkinson's symptoms and even opioid addiction

- Gene therapy and the power of CRISPR; a potential cure for disease.

- The Wondrous Wnt pathway: The Ultimate Fountain of Youth? Learn about a breakthrough molecule in Phase 3 trials that could literally regrow all your tendons in less than 12 months, eliminating osteoarthritis. Also learn about some of the newest cancer treatment alternatives to traditional chemotherapy, radiation, and surgery.

CHAPTER 5

THE MIRACLE OF ORGAN REGENERATION

"If we keep cars and planes and buildings going forever with continuous maintenance and an unlimited store of parts, why can't we create an unlimited supply of transplantable organs to keep people living indefinitely?"

—MARTINE ROTHBLATT, creator of SiriusXM
Radio and CEO of United Therapeutics

The decade ahead will be known for many dramatic health advances, but few will be more astonishing or impactful than this one: We may each soon have access to a set of backup organs. Today the transplant waiting time can be years, which for many people might as well be never. But what if people didn't need to wait for someone to die before they could get a healthy kidney or heart or liver? In this chapter, you'll learn how five brilliant scientists and entrepreneurs are taking on this gargantuan challenge as we speak. Here are just a few of their stunning advances:

- "Dead" and damaged lungs can now be restored and preserved in good condition for up to twenty-two hours, enough time for them to be flown out for transplantation—with a 100 percent success rate.
- Another stem cell–based platform—3D-printed organs, a twenty-year-old technology—is fast advancing from skin and bladders to solid organs like hearts, kidneys, and lungs. The ultimate payoff, projected before the end of this decade, will be an unlimited supply of safe and affordable

on-demand transplants, with the finished product available within a
month of the order being placed.

- "Humanized," genetically modified pigs could provide more than enough
  off-the-shelf organs for everyone on the transplant lists—with no risk of
  viral contamination or a life-threatening immune response. The transplants might even be stronger and more resilient than our original organs!
- Yet another organ regeneration platform is rebuilding lungs from scratch
  by combining a pig collagen scaffold with the future recipient's own stem
  cells. With perfect DNA matching between the patient and the regenerated tissue, there's no chance of rejection—and no need for lifetime immunosuppressant drugs.
- Our lymph nodes can be turned into bioreactors to manufacture "mini-
  organs" to support or replace diseased originals.
- On-demand "cyborg kidneys"—synthetic scaffolds infused with stem
  cells—can generate normal urine and are targeted to be tested in human
  patients by 2023.
- Plus, as you read this, you'll learn principles that have guided these
  inspirational scientists to create breakthroughs in areas where the task
  seemed impossible. As you read, notice the patterns they use to create
  these breakthroughs because you can model their beliefs and actions to
  solve your own challenges or to achieve goals that might initially seem
  impossible.

**I know this all sounds like science fiction, but Dr. Anthony Atala
of Wake Forest University has been using stem cells to grow 3D-
printed human bladders for almost twenty years now, and there are
people today whose lives have been saved and transformed through
his work.**[1] Most of what you will read about in this chapter will be coming to the public between the end of 2022 and 2025. So let's begin the
journey. . . .

Of all the brilliant people breaking through this frontier, one stands
out: **Martine Rothblatt, the chairman, CEO, and founder of United**

---

1 Atrium Health Wake Forest Baptist press release, "Wake Forest Physician
   Reports First Human Recipients of Laboratory-Grown Organs."

Therapeutics, or UT. The quality and scope of Martine's thinking, the depth of her curiosity, the passion of her execution—**she just gets to a different level than anyone else**. She's become a friend of mine, and has been a close friend of Peter Diamandis for more than thirty years. When Peter and I recently caught up with her for an interview, what I learned left me in awe. Read on, and I'm betting you'll feel the same way.

United Therapeutics is changing the game with a multitude of options for life-and-death organ transplants. For anybody else, that alone would be an impressive life's work. But for Martine, it's just the latest in a long series of odds-defying quests. Years ago, she envisioned a way to connect the whole world to the best in news and music, no matter how remote a listener might be. The result? Satellite radio, now known as **SiriusXM**. Next, as a lawyer with no pharmaceutical background, Martine drove the discovery of "orphan" drugs to save the life of her own daughter and thousands of others with once terminal diseases. She is an author, a lawyer, a helicopter pilot, and a green revolutionary. **She has the brain of an engineer and the soul of a philosopher—and what could be more beautiful than that?** After living the first half of her life as a male, Martine became the highest-paid female CEO in the United States and the first openly transgender CEO of a public company. To paraphrase *Star Trek*'s old tag line, she goes where no one has gone before.

Let me share with you a bit of Martine's amazing personal story . . . and then I'll explain in more depth the breakthroughs she's making in the field of organ transplants. Why learn more about her? Here's why: There are times when all of us face seemingly insurmountable challenges. Most of us accept these challenges as part of life and do our best to manage our problems or suffering. **But then there are people who create solutions and bring them to the world, to help others. Martine is one of those.** As you read the following pages, I'd ask you to think about the principles she follows to attack and solve the toughest problems. Because, as already noted, these same principles will work for you in any area of your life—including your health.

You don't have to take my word for this. *Forbes* put Martine on their list of **"100 Greatest Living Business Minds," right next to Bezos, Buffett, and Bono.** As *Inc.* magazine exclaimed: "She is breaking glass windows all over the place!"[2] Or as legendary futurist Ray Kurzweil put it, Martine has "a perfect track record"[3] in turning her visions into reality.

It's extremely rare to find someone so consistently inspirational across such a wide swath of human endeavor. When I do, I want to figure out what makes them tick. **Here are two things I can tell you about Martine. First, she knows no fear**—least of all about being wrong. **"The person who makes no mistakes is making the biggest mistake,"** she says, "because they're just standing still and doing nothing." **Second, she's a serial obsessive. And everybody loves it when Martine gets obsessed, because it means that life on this earth is about to change for the better.** As she told me at the Vatican, "The world's biggest problems are the biggest opportunities."

Going back to the time when Martine was still Martin Rothblatt, she was already the emperor of moonshots, or what Peter Diamandis calls "massively transformative purposes." From a very young age, she realized that it wasn't crazy to think you could do something that had never been done before. As I've always taught, **if you want new answers, you've got to ask new questions**—and to ask them with the certainty that they *need* to be answered. Martine embodies that principle to a T. At every step she's been dismissed by those "in the know." But she shows us that no matter what anybody tells you, no matter how many roadblocks get thrown in your path, **you keep digging until you reach your destination. You go full tilt. You liquidate doubt. You do not waver.**

Better than just about anyone I've ever met, Martine rejects what I call "the tyranny of how." When most people have a dream or goal, they get excited until they start to confront *how* they're going to achieve it. Since they don't yet know *how*, they get demoralized. They lose the sense of certainty that breakthroughs require. Soon they stop trying—they give up. But Martine never gets discouraged by logistics. **When something that matters is on the line, she** *decides* **that she'll find the solution,** even if all the

---

2 Daum, "Celebrate These LGBTQ Business Leaders Who Are Changing the World."

3 Tucker, "Martine Rothblatt: She Founded SiriusXM, a Religion, and a Biotech. For Starters."

engineering details and logistics aren't quite ready for prime time. Does that make sense to you, too? I hope so. Because no matter what your ambition may be, it's that kind of resolve and absolute persistence that fuels success.

What is Martine obsessed about these days? What's driving her every living, breathing moment? Try this one on for size: **a world of "organs on demand," where no one will ever need to die for the lack of a working lung, liver, kidney or heart**. Martine's certainty never wavers. "**Persistence is omnipotence**," she says. "**If you don't give up, you *will* succeed**."

Organ regeneration is a fascinating field—it's literally sci-fi in the flesh. But before we dive into it, I want to tell you a little more about the person whose unflinching determination is making it happen today, in real time.

"Truth and technology will triumph over bullshit and bureaucracy."

—RENE ANSELMO, founder of PanAmSat, the first privately held international satellite communications enterprise in the U.S.

Martine grew up feasting on the science fiction of Arthur C. Clarke, the godfather of satellite communications. In the 1970s, as an adventurous 19-year-old taking a break from college, she traveled to the Seychelles, islands off East Africa where NASA had installed a tracking station for deep space missions. After climbing a mountain for a peek at the gigantic dish, she had a full-blown epiphany: "It was like we stepped into the future."[4] She began "going to bed each night saying if it's the last thing I'm going to do in my entire life, I'm going to connect the world with satellites."

Flash forward a few years. Martine had her law and MBA degrees from UCLA, with a focus on space law and finance. She joined Gerard K. O'Neill, the visionary Princeton physics professor, as CEO of Geostar, a vehicular tracking system—an early version of today's GPS. Martine's big idea was that the same signals that tracked trucks and planes could also transmit sound. She'd spent too many hours on country back roads searching in vain for a jazz station. Or—even more frustrating—having one fade into a dead zone just as one of her favorite artists came on. Then it came to her: Why couldn't satellites be used to broadcast radio? Why couldn't

---

4 Miller, "The Trans-Everything CEO."

listeners the world over get access to hundreds of crystal-clear channels—from anywhere they could see the sky? Why shouldn't people in Omaha or Reno get the same programming we take for granted in New York or D.C. or San Francisco?

Martine is an engineer at heart: "If you can't make it or build it, I'm not that interested in it." She did the math and knew her idea could work. As satellites kept getting bigger and more powerful, they'd be able to beam a signal to "a flat little plate embedded into the roof of an automobile."[5] **That was the genesis of Sirius Satellite Radio, now SiriusXM. In our interview, Martine made it clear how this vision met her three criteria for a legitimate moonshot:**

1. **The goal—in this case, a global satellite radio service—could realistically be accomplished within a decade;**
2. **It had the potential to transform society: "My idea was to broadcast dozens of channels of content people can't get any other way into every city and town in North America—to 10x blow the limit away!"**
3. **It was something that "probably 99 percent of the population thought was impossible."**

It wasn't easy—it never is, when you're doing something original. Martine ran up against doubters at every turn. First there were the experts who insisted that satellite radio signals could never reach a small planar antenna from more than 20,000 miles from Earth's surface[6]—not if they had to pass through trees or get around tall buildings. (Remember, this was before cell phones or a commercial internet.) Then there were the skeptics who said the Federal Communications Commission would never assign its valuable frequencies to an unproven satellite system. (That included the National Association of Broadcasters, the terrestrial radio lobby. They were terrified of new competition and wanted to monopolize the frequencies for their electronic news-gathering trucks.) But Sirius aced the technology. In 1997, seven years after Martine founded the company, it

---

5 Rothblatt, "My Daughter, My Wife, Our Robot, and the Quest for Immortality."

6 RF Wireless World, "Satellite Orbit Types."

received its FCC license. Still, the naysayers weren't done. **There wasn't any market for subscription radio, they said. Who would pay for music and news and sports when they could get AM or FM for free?**

But as it turned out, *lots* of people were ready to pay, especially after Howard Stern brought his show into the fold. **Today, SiriusXM counts more than 30 million subscribers.**[7] As Martine shared with me at one of my Business Mastery seminars, she's met hundreds of people from all walks of life, from all corners of the country, who say that her brainchild "helps them get through each and every day." She's been hugged by women in the most isolated places who can now connect to heartwarming talk media and a smorgasbord of musical genres. Thanks to over-the-air academic course work, her pioneering technology enabled young people in India to get accepted to top universities. (She extended SiriusXM to Africa and Asia via related companies and additional satellites.) Martine is always gratified to hear these stories. But she wasn't surprised by SiriusXM's success, because she knew how much power and momentum a moonshot can generate. As she told me, **"You can construct the reality you desire when you have your massively transformative purpose. You know you're going to win before you actually win."**

> *"The beautiful thing about the human mind is it's like a quantum computer. It can take in so much information and then just collapse into a solution right away."*
>
> —MARTINE ROTHBLATT

Sirius was still getting off the ground when its creator launched another transformation—a personal one. Because Martine wasn't yet Martine. She was still Martin Rothblatt, though she'd long felt at odds with her label as a male. She'd bottled up her female side: "I was super-sensitive to not wanting to be laughed at, not wanting to be bullied, not wanting to lose all my friends." Only Bina, her wife and soul mate, knew the truth. Before changing her name and gender, Martine consulted each of their four children. She gave each of them a veto; if they didn't want her to make the transition, she

---

7 SiriusXM press release, 2020.

wouldn't go through with it. All four supported her choice. Jenesis, just seven years old, pierced to the heart of it: **"I love my dad and *she* loves me."**

It was around that time that Martine and Bina noticed something not right with their youngest child. On a family ski trip in Telluride, Colorado, **Jenesis's energy flagged and her lips kept turning blue.** Back home, she had to be carried upstairs to her bedroom. They went to doctor after doctor, and no one could say what was wrong. At the Children's National Medical Center in Washington, D.C., they found out that Jenesis had a rare and highly dangerous disease: pulmonary arterial hypertension. A narrowing of the arteries in her lungs was constricting her blood flow, straining her heart to pump hard enough. Her body was being starved of oxygen. **Over the next couple of years, the doctors told them, their daughter's heart muscle would weaken. Soon it would fail.**

Martine will never forget that day: "I said to the doctor, 'Surely there must be a cure.'" But there was no cure. "'Surely there must be a treatment.'" There was none, at least none that was safe and reliable. The lead physician, a specialist at the pinnacle of his profession, told them, "Every kid I've seen with this disease has died." Jenesis was ten years old and might have three years to live, five if she was lucky. Of course, she'd be added to the lung transplant list. But there were so few organs available, especially for children, that her chances were slim and none.

Martine was devastated—but far from defeated. Because that was the day she set in motion her next moonshot, to rescue her daughter. By then she knew the most critical attribute for any successful entrepreneur: total immersion and single-minded obsession. She'd absorbed how "to be able to twist that focus lens on your camera, and everything else fades to a blur and you're just targeting on what you have to do. **I had to save Jenesis. Nothing else mattered."**

Martine stepped down as Sirius CEO. She put her life's great ambition and achievement behind her for something more urgent. She sold a chunk of her Sirius shares, established a foundation, and funded ten leading doctors to find a cure for pulmonary hypertension. Six months later, none of them had made a dent. Jenesis was falling down and fainting, spending more nights in the hospital than out of it. Martine ran out of patience. There *had* to be a solution, and she would find it herself. **We're lucky to live in a time**

when anyone can become an expert in almost any subject, providing you know how to read and are willing to put in the effort. Martine decided to become an expert in pulmonary hypertension. "It was the intellectual equivalent," she says, "of the mother lifting up a Volkswagen to save her trapped child underneath a wheel."

With Jenesis in tow, Martine trekked to the libraries at Children's National Medical Center and the National Institutes of Health. She read biology, physiology, anatomy, biochemistry—one book after the next. The more she learned, the more confident she became that she'd somehow find a way to treat this untreatable disease.

"We're lucky to live in a time when anyone can become an expert in almost any subject, providing you know how to read and are willing to put in the effort."

Once again, the skeptics turned out in force. **Martine had no training in the field, the top professionals kept reminding her. If an effective medicine was out there, wouldn't the *real* scientists have already found it?** And even if she somehow stumbled onto something, pulmonary hypertension was so rare that no one would invest in it. Where would the profits come from? Who would turn a scientific solution into a commercial product?

Fortunately, **Martine has a theory that kept her afloat:** *When you do something big and bold, it takes 99 nos to get to yes.* **And you need to welcome and embrace those nos, because every one of them is one step closer to that *yes*.** As she says, "If you believe in what you do, you've just got to be persistent." After months of digging, she struck gold in an unlikely spot, an article in an obscure journal about a drug developed to treat heart failure. The drug was a total bust. **But it had an intriguing side effect. It reduced blood pressure between the heart and lungs, but nowhere else—which happened to be exactly what Martine was looking for.** She went to the developer, Glaxo Wellcome (now GlaxoSmithKline), and asked to buy their mysterious molecule. Three times they slammed the door in her face. The drug had been tried exclusively in congestive heart failure, and Glaxo didn't think it would work in pulmonary hypertension. Besides, they weren't about to license a failed medicine to a non-scientist. Finally, they had only a small amount of the drug left, past its expiration date. A possibly life-saving treatment for Jenesis was sitting abandoned in a freezer, and that's where it would stay.

A big bunch of nos, in short. That's where another one of Martine's favorite sayings came in handy: *"Identify the corridors of indifference and run down them like hell."* She needed credentials? Okay, she would get them. She recruited a team of doctors for downfield blocking and gradually wore Glaxo down. They agreed to license worldwide rights to the drug for $25,000 and 10 percent of any revenues it brought in, which they assumed would amount to zero. When the deal was done, they handed Martine a small amount of powder in a Ziploc bag, with a patent recipe that perplexed the first several dozen chemists she consulted. But as you know by now, Martine doesn't take no for an answer. She ran down a retired pharmacologist, James Crow, who thought he could make it work. In 1996, less than two years after Jenesis was diagnosed, they founded United Therapeutics. Six years after that, around the time that Martine earned her PhD in medical ethics, **they had an FDA-approved drug called Remodulin that "proved all the naysayers wrong," she says. The moonshot had landed.**

Remodulin wasn't a perfect drug. It had a short half-life, and patients had to wear a bulky infusion pump around the clock. **But it helped many of them stay alive, including Martine's daughter.** United Therapeutics later developed an inhalable version and then a pill, Orenitram ("Martine Ro" spelled backwards). **Jenesis is now 36 years old and living a full life as United Therapeutics' telepresence and digital director.**

Meanwhile, the "worthless powder" that Martine licensed for $25,000 now generates more than $1.5 billion a year in revenue. Clinical trials have proven that it reduces morbidity and mortality due to pulmonary hypertension. In short, it has radically changed the outlook for this dreaded disease. Before United Therapeutics made this breakthrough drug available, only two thousand people with pulmonary hypertension were alive in the entire U.S.—the fatality rate was that high. Today, thanks to this new treatment, more than 50,000 people are managing the condition, the vast majority enjoying normal lives. **If they can't afford the price of the drug, United Therapeutics provides it for free.** As Martine says, "That's a whole stadium of people who are living—not dying—with pulmonary hypertension. Beautiful people who have gone on to have children, to run for mayor, to become snowboard champions—you name it."

Quite a success story, right? You might call it a happy ending— except that Martine was nowhere close to finished. UT's suite of medicines slowed the progression of pulmonary hypertension, but they didn't stop it. For some, like Jenesis, the results were dramatic; for others, including some of her daughter's close friends, there was only a brief reprieve before the end. Even today, three thousand Americans die of pulmonary hypertension every year. For them—and for anyone with other end-stage lung diseases, like emphysema or COPD—there is no pharmaceutical cure.

But there *is* a solution. All it took was another moonshot.

REPLACEMENT LUNGS

"Our deepest fear is not that we are inadequate. Our deepest fear is that we are powerful beyond measure. . . . Your playing small does not serve the world. . . . As we are liberated from our own fear, our presence automatically liberates others."

—MARIANNE WILLIAMSON

One million people in the United States today have an end-stage organ disease. More than a hundred thousand are on waitlists for transplants, mainly for kidneys and hearts. Many thousands die each year before their names come up. As humanity lives longer and cars get safer, reducing the number of donor organs after traffic accidents, the shortage keeps growing more acute. Even with six of ten U.S. adults registered as organ donors, the demand far outstrips the supply. It's especially dire for people with end-stage lung disease, which steals a quarter of a million lives each year. **In 2019, there were all of 2,714 lung transplants.**[8] **The chances of a person who needed a lung getting one was barely 1 percent.**

Those odds made no sense to Martine. She threw down the gauntlet at her 2015 TED talk: **If we keep cars and planes and buildings going forever with continuous maintenance and an unlimited store of parts, "why can't we create an unlimited supply of transplantable organs to keep people living indefinitely?"** After all, you don't trash your car when you blow out a tire. You don't tear down your home when you need a new roof. If billions of people have naturally manufactured organs "since time immemorial, not to mention all the animals in the animal kingdom, then why can't we do it, too?" The concept of synthetic organs violated no known laws of physics. At its root, Martine thought, it was simply one more engineering problem.

Lungs are fragile and complex pieces of anatomy. When a registered donor dies, the vast majority of lungs are ruled out by infectious or degenerative disease. Among the few that make the first cut, 80 percent become filled with mucus and other fluids, ruined by the process of death. Like the placentas salvaged by Bob Hariri, these precious gifts of life were being thrown into the trash!

But Martine had another strategy to increase the number of healthy lungs available for transplantation. Building on the work of Dr. Shaf Keshavjee, a surgeon at Toronto General Hospital, United Therapeutics established the world's first centralized lung restoration facility in Silver Spring, Maryland. **They began taking "dead" organs that had been rejected for transplantation because of their poor condition, and pumping in special solutions to revive them under a glass dome that acted like an artificial "body," where they could last for up to twenty-two hours.** Toxic fluids and bacteria were flushed out. Tears were repaired. Once a lung was stabilized, a bronchoscope sent real-time video to surgeons around the U.S.

If the organ met their standards, it got cold-packed and flown out for transplantation. **In every single case that a surgeon remotely accepted a lung, according to Martine, the patients walked out of the hospital.**

---

8 United Network for Organ Sharing, "More Deceased-Donor Organ Transplants Than Ever."

"I've met these people," she says. "They're enormously grateful. They take me to their garage full of oxygen tanks and they say, 'We don't need these anymore.'"

This technique—"ex vivo lung perfusion," or EVLP—had been tried before, but never at the scale of United Therapeutics and its Lung Bioengineering PBC subsidiary. To date, the Maryland center, a second UT branch at the Mayo Clinic campus in Jacksonville, Florida, and similar facilities elsewhere have saved many hundreds of patients. **One of them is Heather Leverington, a former five-time national collegiate shot-put champion. By 2010, after a bout with lupus, she had begun needing oxygen to get through the day.** Two years later, on a flight to Spain with her husband, she passed out. The diagnosis: pulmonary hypertension. "She had a very, very aggressive case and blew through our medicines," Martine said. "They were not able to slow down the disease." While she was still a young woman in her 30s, Heather's outlook seemed grim.

In 2016, about to lose hope, Heather received a call from a hospital in Pittsburgh: **Would she be willing to join a United Therapeutics clinical trial and try a transplant with EVLP lungs? They didn't have to ask her twice. After the UT team revived a matched pair of lungs from a 28-year-old donor, Heather's twelve-hour surgery was a resounding success. A year later, Heather won the gold medal in the shot put at the U.S. Transplant Games. Soon after, she became pregnant and gave birth to a healthy baby,** which isn't generally possible for people with pulmonary hypertension. Her disease was effectively cured.

XENOTRANSPLANTATION: OFF-THE-SHELF ORGANS

"Never doubt that a small group of thoughtful, committed citizens can change the world. Indeed, it is the only thing that ever has."

—MARGARET MEAD

One of the big impediments for any moonshot is that human beings aren't wired for super-long-term objectives. **Martine makes her magic happen by turning moonshots into a series of "Earth shots": tangible,**

practical, bite-sized milestones that can be reached within a year or so. She chunks things down. "Then I carefully stack these one-year sub-projects," she says, "and at the end of ten years we have something that seems miraculous." For UT's moonshot to create an unlimited supply of transplantable organs, EVLP was their first Earth shot but by no means their final act. The more challenging a technology, Martine says, "the more careful you have to be about hedging your bets." **It's like diversifying a wealth portfolio among various asset classes. For maximum security, it's wiser to spread those eggs around in more than one basket.**

United Therapeutics has put tiger teams to work on at least four different platforms for organ regeneration. These groups compete with one another and cooperate toward the larger goal at the same time. One frustration with EVLP is that the organs don't always get to patients in time—after a terrible car crash, say, or when a U.S. soldier in a battle theater steps on a mine. The process relies on other people dying sudden and untimely deaths. It's unreliable, to say the least. **And Martine wondered: Why can't we build a pipeline of off-the-shelf organs, to be ready at an hour's notice?**

One solution may be found in the humble pig, in an inter-species "xenotransplant." By a fluke of nature, the organs of an adult pig are close to the size and shape of their human equivalents. (Chimpanzees might be even closer, but they're a protected species.) **In the case of heart valves, where a tight fit is all-important, porcine (pig) donors are already used for human patients. Americans eat about 130 million pigs a year. Just 1 percent of that total would more than meet the country's entire demand for replacement organs.** But there's a catch: vicious, hyper-acute rejection. Within hours—if not minutes—of a xenotransplant, pig organs "provoke a massive and destructive immune response in humans—far more so than an organ from another person."[9]

For Martine, the problem was a thrilling opportunity: Why couldn't genetic engineering delete the pig proteins that trigger rejection? Why not humanize the pig? She teamed up with Craig Venter, the master of genomic sequencing, and invested in research on editing pig genomes with **CRISPR**, a relatively new but proven technology—what *Time*

---

9 Zhang, "Genetically Engineering Pigs to Grow Organs for People."

magazine calls "by far the most precise set of molecular tools to cut, paste, copy and move genes around."[10] (You'll learn about the power of CRISPR and gene therapy in Chapter 9). The partnership discovered that a "ten-gene pig"—an animal with a mere ten problem genes knocked out or replaced by human DNA—could do the trick. As Martine told the TED assembly, this wasn't rocket science. **It was "straightforward engineering," taking on one gene at a time, not so different than her step-by-step approach in launching a communications satellite.**

The pigs are modified at a Virginia-based UT subsidiary called Revivicor, a spin-off of the British company that made Dolly the sheep, the first mammalian clone. In 2017, Martine's company agreed to fund university-based xenotransplantation programs for pig hearts, kidneys, and lungs. Before long, in preclinical trials, baboon recipients were setting survival records; by 2018, at the University of Munich, they were lasting more than six months.[11] FDA approval for human trials may not be far off. At the University of Alabama at Birmingham, researchers hope to transplant pig kidneys into human adults and pig hearts into struggling newborn children, if only to buy them more time before human organs become available.[12] "We've got a Chevy," says Devin Eckhoff, the former director of UAB's breakthrough program. "We may even have a BMW now. Do we wait for a Ferrari? There's a point where you just want to give it a test drive."[13] **Martine is aiming to kick off clinical trials for xenokidneys by 2023 ("I know folks needing kidneys I'm trying to save"), and for xenohearts by 2025. She's confident that pig organ transplants for human patients will be an FDA-approved reality before the 2020s are out: "What most people thought was impossible, they're now realizing is inevitable."[14]**

If you're wondering how fast this can happen, I'll give you a clue. As I was doing the final edits to this chapter, I received a text from

---

10 Park, "Why Pig Organs Could Be the Future of Transplants."

11 Davis, "Baboon Survives for Six Months After Receiving Pig Heart Transplant."

12 Weintraub, "Using Animal Organs in Humans: 'It's Just a Question of When.'"

13 Weintraub, "A CRISPR Startup Is Testing Pig Organs in Monkeys to See If They're Safe for Us."

14 Diamandis, "Fireside with Dr. Martine Rothblatt."

Martine. "Tony, as promised at your Palm Beach Business Mastery Event!" with a link to two reports. One from ABC News and the other from the *New York Times* reporting a breaking news story of the first time a pig kidney was transplanted into a human without triggering an immediate rejection and in fact looked like a normal kidney the following day. The procedure was done at NYU Langone Health in New York City and is the fruition of Martine's work developed by United Therapeutics. This experiment has shattered yet another obstacle in the way of organ transplant shortage, and researchers are already thinking of implications in other organ systems like skin and heart valves.[15]

Thanks to the work of eGenesis, an ambitious startup spun out of the **Harvard lab of legendary geneticist and our Life Force adviser George Church, PhD**, FDA approval no longer seems like such a long shot. The company's cofounder, Luhan Yang, figured out a way to make sixty-two simultaneous genetic edits in the pig genome—enough to strip away all of the viruses that normally reside in the genome and could possibly infect people after a transplant. **The company recently tested its virus-free pig organs in primates at Massachusetts General with impressive results.** The primates survived for nine months post-transplant, with a clear path to reaching more than a year. Other superstar scientists are attacking the problem from other angles. **At the Salk Institute in California, under Juan Carlos Izpisua Belmonte, researchers are working to cultivate human organs *inside* pigs via human stem cells.** According to James Markmann, Mass General's chief of transplant surgery, **"Everybody sees that we're at a turning point."**[16] As the *Atlantic* noted:

> Routine pig-to-human transplants could truly transform healthcare beyond simply increasing the supply. Organs would go from a product of chance—someone young and healthy dying, unexpectedly—to the product of a standardized manufacturing process. . . .
>
> Organ transplants would no longer have to be emergency surgeries, requiring planes to deliver organs and surgical teams to scramble

---

15 Rabin, "In a First, Surgeons Attached a Pig Kidney to a Human, and It Worked."

16 Weintraub, "A CRISPR Startup Is Testing Pig Organs in Monkeys."

at any hour. Organs from pigs can be harvested on a schedule, and surgeries planned for exact times during the day. A patient that comes in with kidney failure could get a kidney the next day—eliminating the need for large dialysis centers. Hospital ICU beds will no longer be taken up by patients waiting for a heart transplant.

Like Martine, Dr. Church's company, eGenesis, is also working to solve the organ shortage crisis with modified pig organs. eGenesis is focusing first on kidneys and pancreatic islet cells, though heart, lungs, and livers won't be far behind. But Church is ready to take this revolution one step further. **"We're looking to create *enhanced organs*, to produce something that is *better than we have in the body*," he says. Dr. Church imagines organs that can fend off bacterial or viral infections—or the deterioration of aging. "Some people might have issues with this kind of human 'engineering.' But if it means getting lungs as strong as Michael Phelps's, or a heart like Usain Bolt's, why not?"**

"We're doing this by making pigs more humanlike from a molecular standpoint, making them immune-tolerant, and eliminating the [internal] retroviruses in the pigs," says Church. "We call them Pig 3.0, and we've already produced two thousand of these animals for preclinical primate organ transplant trials. The primates receiving the donor organs are surviving over three hundred days thus far at Massachusetts General Hospital. It hopefully won't be very long before we switch from the primates to clinical human trials."

Though Martine shares the growing excitement over xenotransplants, she's also pursuing preclinical trials. With parallel options. Even after a pig organ is humanized, she points out, it can provoke the same long-term rejection issues as transplants from people. In other words, recipients would still need immunosuppressant drugs for the rest of their lives. Beyond some unpleasant side effects, these medications can open the door to infections or cancer. For non-emergency end-stage scenarios, where patients have a year or more to find a lifesaving replacement, **United Therapeutics is working on a third platform: building organs from scratch using the patient's own stem cells for tissue regeneration.**

Here's how it works. They start with a donor pig's lungs and strip out all the living cells. What's left is the structural framework, a scaffold of collagen, the basic protein building block for most human tissues and organs. **The beautiful thing about collagen, no matter its source, is that it's nonreactive—it causes zero immune response or rejection. Next the scaffold is *re*cellularized with either billions of human lung-type cells or the recipient's own induced pluripotent stem cells, or iPSCs, which you might recall from Chapter 2.** Derived from adult skin cells, an iPSC is reprogrammed to mimic an embryonic stem cell. It then follows instructions to become whatever type of tissue is needed.

Or as Martine explains, **"You can turn it back in time to becoming a stem cell, and then you can roll it back forward specifically to be a cardiac cell, or an alveolar cell for the lung." Since the replacement organ would match the recipient's DNA, no immunosuppressants would be needed.** The last time we checked, **UT's assembly line was churning out 500 humanized lung scaffolds per year.**

The iPSC approach is a huge step toward personalized regenerative medicine. But in Martine's big picture, it's just one more Earth shot. Her ultimate moonshot involves "on demand" organs that will be custom-designed start to finish. Easily scalable, the technology will make conventional transplants obsolete.

3D-PRINTED ORGANS

"If you're a maker, you've got to make it until you break it,
and then you've got to make it till it's better than that, until
it's flawless. And then you're making millions of them."

—MARTINE ROTHBLATT

The first 3D-printed prosthetics came out in 2010. Since then, scientists have created 3D-bioprinted skin for burn victims. They've crafted functional retinas, the part of our eyes that takes in all visual information. They've manufactured bionic ears that can pick up sounds outside the range of normal human hearing. At the Wake Forest Institute for Regenerative Medicine, pioneering tissue researcher and engineer Dr. Anthony Atala has been using stem cells

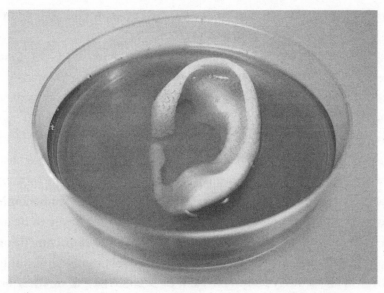

Dr. Atala has used stem cells to grow a 3D-printed human ear for a wounded warrior to replace the one that was blown off in an explosion.

to 3D-print human bladders and save lives for nearly twenty years.[17] **He is now leading research to bioprint complex tissues and organs, from cartilage to kidneys.**[18] It's all done with machines not so different than the inkjet printer in your home office, except they're the size of a refrigerator. Though Atala and others previously did similar work by hand, 3D-bioprinted tissues and organs are a huge leap forward for affordability, consistency, and precision.

The final frontier for 3D-bioprinting, the most difficult challenges of all, are solid organs like hearts, kidneys, livers—and lungs. They have dense concentrations of cells (240 billion in the liver alone), enormous structural complexity, and super-high requirements for oxygen and blood supply. **The timeframe for this achievement is usually estimated in decades. But Martine is in a hurry, as usual. In partnership with the**

---

17 Lord, "Bladder Grown from 3D Bioprinted Tissue Continues to Function After 14 Years."

18 Listek, "Dr. Anthony Atala Explains the Frontiers of Bioprinting for Regenerative Medicine at Wake Forest."

world's leading 3D-printing company, 3D Systems, United Therapeutics is gunning for FDA approval by 2028.

UT's bioprinted organs begin with a scaffold derived from tobacco leaves, genetically modified to express human collagen. No animal products are involved. **The printer lays down a "bio-ink" of induced pluripotent stem cells, layer by layer, with a carrier gel that enables the cells to spread and grow.** (Each cell somehow knows just where to go.) As Pedro Mendoza, 3D Systems' director of bioprinting, told *MIT Technology Review*, "When you see the complexity of the lung, what nature does from conception to birth, there is no way to machine that or mold it. 3-D printing is the only way we have to create that geometry."[19]

The technology is still a work in progress. **At the moment, the bioprinter can handle anatomical details down to six microns, about one-quarter of the width of a human hair, or the size of the smallest blood vessels in the lung.** That's a tremendous advance, but the lung contains other structures as small as one micrometer or even less. The organ has twenty-three descending branches; UT's printer has mastered sixteen so far. But Martine has no doubt they'll get there: "We have a disciplined engineering approach. **Every year, we've doubled the number of branches." Once the "how" problems are solved, a ready-made lung or heart can be grown more quickly than you might guess—forty-eight hours for printing the scaffold, less than a month for the finished product. And the beauty of bioprinted organs, Martine points out, is that they can be tailored for people of all ages, sizes, and shapes**: "If it's a little kid, or even a neonate, we can print a lung that's just right."

You might think that's a bold enough moonshot to crown a career. But Martine sees the world through a wider lens than most. As she told an audience of entrepreneurs at my event in Palm Beach, **"No matter how much good we do in saving people's lives, if the whole planet is sick because of overheating and over-polluting, everybody's going to go down."** Aviation contributes up to 5 percent to global warming, and that number is rising. In a single week, United Therapeutics might need eight trips by a

---

19 Regalado, "Inside the Effort to Print Lungs and Breathe Life into Them with Stem Cells."

Learjet to deliver four EVLP transplants. As the business kept growing to thousands of manufactured organs, Martine saw that it would become environmentally unsustainable. So **she amended her moonshot mission statement: "to create an unlimited supply of transplantable organs** *and have them delivered with carbon-neutral aircraft.*" Her idea is to use a delivery fleet of electric vertical aircraft, or EVAs, helicopter-plane hybrids that fly on clean electric energy. If that sounds wildly futuristic to you, join the club. Like Martine, I'm a licensed helicopter pilot myself, and I thought there was no way anything like that could happen anytime soon.

I was wrong.

Martine assembled another tiger team and entered a collaboration with Tier 1 Engineering in Southern California. **In under twelve months, with less than $2 million, they created the world's first electric helicopter! By 2017, Martine's retrofitted Robinson R44 had set a Guinness World Record for the farthest, highest, and heaviest flight of an eVTOL (Electric Vertical Takeoff and Landing) air machine.**

United Therapeutics is partnering to build a thousand of these "Wings of Life" battery-run marvels. They'll use rapid recharging pads at hospitals nationwide. On top of their tiny carbon footprint, the EVAs will be less than one-tenth as noisy as a standard helicopter. Though for now they will be piloted, the longer-term plan, subject to FAA approval, is for autonomous EVAs with a range of 250 miles. **While this might sound far-fetched, Martine points out that the technology already exists.** Indeed, her Beta Technology EVAs now fly more than one hundred nautical miles a day in test flights over New England. And, as this book was going to press, the proof-of-concept flight took place in September 2021, using a small multicopter drone to transfer donor lungs from Toronto Western Hospital to Toronto General Hospital.

In September 2018, the day of the autumnal equinox, Martine christened the 140,000-square-foot Unisphere, UT's newly rebuilt Maryland headquarters. **Powered and heated and cooled by sustainable technologies, mainly solar and geothermal, it's the largest zero-carbon-footprint building in the world.** "I did all the math," Martine says. "I knew it was practical." One of her guests was a young woman with a special interest in the company. A month earlier she'd won two gold medals and a silver at the

Transplant Games of America—just two years after her double EVLP lung transplant. "It gave me chills," said Heather Leverington. "It was really kind of surreal, seeing where everything happened, and thinking that a part of me had been there before."[20]

What's ahead for Martine? Here's yet another amazing thing about her: No matter how busy and passionate she may be in the moment, she always has a moonshot or two on tap. Lately she's been intrigued by the idea of digitally replicating the human life-form to test new medicines at warp speed. Putting her money where her mouth is, United Therapeutics established CLIMB: the Computational Lab for In Silico Molecular Biology. **Where it now takes ten years to complete a typical clinical trial, "our goal is to do ten clinical trials in one day," Martine says.** "With access to a massive genomic database, we could test a digital version of a molecule in millions of human genomes in a day—and get a much better safety profile than we could ever get in a clinical trial with a few thousand people."

Judging from Martine's track record, it's not a matter of *if* CLIMB will achieve its audacious goal. It's only a matter of *when*.

LYGENESIS—HIJACKING LYMPH NODES TO GROW ORGANS

"We're using the body's natural lymphatic system that evolved to help us fight infection, and we're leveraging all of that brilliant biology to grow these ectopic [out-of-place] organs."

—MICHAEL HUFFORD, cofounder and CEO of LyGenesis

While Martine Rothblatt and George Church and Anthony Atala have justifiably grabbed many of the headlines, we need to tell you about three more heroic ventures that hold extraordinary promise for delivering a generation of replacement organs this decade.

Let's lead off with a startup called **LyGenesis**. It comes to us from the University of Pittsburgh, where **Eric Lagasse, PhD**, the company's founder and chief scientific officer, has spent a decade learning how to repurpose a patient's

---

20 Gerber, "One Breath at a Time."

own lymph nodes. He's discovered that these cellular factories have the capacity to grow mini-organs to either support or replace a diseased organ.

The human body contains around 600 lymph nodes, aka lymph glands. What is a lymph node? It's a small organ that our immune system uses to manufacture T cells and fight off infections by trapping bacteria or viruses. That's why your lymph nodes may swell when you have a cold. They need to get larger to manufacture more immune cells.

Eric Lagasse's big idea was to turn lymph nodes into bioreactors. If liver cells are injected or engrafted into a lymph node, they will grow and multiply until they form a functional, potentially life-saving mini-liver. As LyGenesis CEO Michael Hufford explained to us, **the company is now entering a Phase 2 human clinical trial with these mini-livers in patients with end-stage liver disease**. The process begins with an ultrasound to graft a handful of donor liver cells into a few of the patient's lymph nodes. Within a few weeks or so, the nodes start filtering toxins from the blood. Over time, they Cinderella their way into full-fledged mini-livers.

LyGenesis is targeting three sets of patients. In people with partial organ failure, the mini-organs and original liver would join forces in a permanent work-share arrangement. Patients closer to total failure would rely on the mini-organs to buy time until their transplants came through. A smaller group, mainly children, would need just a small amount of donor liver mass to correct a congenital enzyme deficiency.[21]

"The beauty of this platform is that it's low-risk and low-cost," Hufford explains. "Animal trials show no serious adverse effects. **It's also super-efficient: a single donor organ can supply cells for up to seventy-five patients. It gives hope to thousands of patients now considered hopeless.**" At present, nine of ten people with liver disease are too sick even to make it onto the transplant list. But most of them can handle a thirty-minute outpatient procedure that requires only mild sedation.

What's next for LyGenesis? They're working with other organs in animals, including **a mini-pancreas and a mini-kidney**. From a healthspan

---

21 Longevity Technology, "Exclusive Profile: LyGenesis and Growing Ectopic Organs."

standpoint, the most exciting of all is a mini-thymus, which could make us biologically young again by rebooting our aging immune system.

GROWING KIDNEYS

Then there's **IVIVA Medical, which aims to develop artificial kidneys— the organ in highest demand by far—as a solution to end-stage renal disease (ESRD), a condition that afflicts over 500,000 patients in the U.S.** While many hang on with long-term dialysis, the only definitive treatment is a kidney transplant, where the supply is nowhere close to demand. To address this donor organ shortage, IVIVA is leveraging the convergence of tissue engineering, 3D manufacturing, and stem cell biology. The company was founded by Dr. Harald Ott, a thoracic surgeon at Massachusetts General who is best known for his work in whole organ regeneration.

Back in the day, Dr. Ott perfected a method for stripping a cadaver's organ of its own cells and then infusing the scaffold that remained with fresh progenitor stem cells, which can differentiate into a variety of organs. To date, his technology has been successfully applied to heart, liver, lung, kidney, and pancreas regeneration. But for people in desperate need of a transplant, the one big drawback is time—the delay in finding a well-preserved organ from a newly deceased donor, and then the wait for the stem cells to work their magic. Dr. Ott created IVIVA to remove the first of these bottlenecks by engineering a device to manufacture a scaffold. The stem cells adhere to the synthetic scaffold and create a sort of cyborg kidney. As blood flows through this biologic machine (half-biology, half-technology), it generates normal urine. IVIVA is now led by Brock Reeve, head of the Harvard Stem Cell Institute, and is pointing toward a human clinical trial in 2023. Peter and I have both become investors through BOLD Capital Partners.

DEAN KAMEN AND THE ADVANCED REGENERATIVE MANUFACTURING INSTITUTE

Our final organ regeneration hero is the legendary inventor and engineer **Dean Kamen**. Before describing his work in this area, I want to make sure you understand the breadth of Kamen's achievements. He is perhaps best known as the founder of the global high-school robotics competition, FIRST (For Inspiration and Recognition of Science and Technology), the creator of the iBOT (a futuristic wheelchair), the Segway, and the first wearable infusion pump. Kamen holds more than one thousand patents and was awarded the National Medal of Technology by President Bill Clinton.

In the last days of the Obama administration, Kamen was called to the White House and handed a challenge. As he recalls the meeting, the senior staff person told him: "There's incredible work being done in hundreds of labs throughout the U.S. **We've got the potential to grow pancreatic cells, neurons, cardiac cells, and more, but no one is integrating all of it. We want to fund an organization that puts all of this science together to create a whole new industry and manufacture replacement human organs at scale.**"

The challenge came attached with an **$80 million grant** from the U.S. Department of Defense and a **five-year mission** to demonstrate something that worked. Kamen's first step was to organize a nonprofit organization to help him move this groundbreaking technology out of the petri dish and into the factory. He named it the **Advanced Regenerative Manufacturing Institute (ARMI)**. Its mission statement? To build an industrial infrastructure "capable of manufacturing replacement human organs, from scratch, in the shortest possible time."

Today ARMI has more than 170 member organizations, ranging from top medical schools and pharmaceutical companies to industrial manufacturing control-system operations.

Just before COVID-19 struck the U.S., Kamen and his engineers had completed their first prototype machine, about twenty feet long. Here's how Dean describes its first demonstration: **"At one end of the system we dropped in a vial of frozen induced pluripotent stem cells (iPSCs), and then we didn't touch it again for twenty-two days. At the end of those three weeks, out the other end of this completely sealed system came a three-inch-long segment of freshly grown bone and ligament."** The manufactured tissue was of high enough quality to repair an actual ankle or knee. But bone and ligament segments are just a hint of what is possible.

So where does Dean want to take the ARMI system next? The next step, he says, **"is to go from iPSCs to a miniature, fully functional, beating**

pediatric heart in only forty days." They'll be sized for potential trans-plants into infants and small children. This work recently gained significant momentum **when Doris Anita Taylor, PhD**, a powerhouse researcher in regenerative medicine for replacement hearts, announced that she'll be moving her entire lab from Houston, Texas, to the ARMI facility in New Hampshire. (You'll read more about her incredible work on "ghost hearts" in Chapter 17, "How to Mend a Broken Heart".) ARMI's goal is now to have fully functioning pediatric hearts available for clinical trial by 2024.

Like Martine Rothblatt, Dean Kamen has a spectacular record of routinely making the impossible possible. So when he says, "Within this decade it will be feasible to manufacture replacement human organs from scratch," I believe him.

I can barely imagine anything more exciting than having access to a spare set of organs, ready and waiting for the time when our body parts eventually wear out. But as thrilling as that near-term future may be, in the next chapter you'll meet one of the world's leading lights in immunotherapy, a field that deploys genetic engineering to weaponize our own humble T cells and turn them into heat-seeking, tumor-destroying torpedoes. He's a man who lost nearly everything—his funding, his team, the person he loved most in the world—but somehow found the courage and resilience to stay the course. I'm inspired by his example; I think you'll feel the same way.

Let us share with you the inside story of this amazing breakthrough from the scientist hero who's led the charge to make it a reality! **Let's learn about the mighty CAR T cell. . . .**

CHAPTER 6

THE MIGHTY CAR T CELL: A BREAKTHROUGH CURE FOR LEUKEMIA

"Instead of fighting cancer from the outside, we are increasingly turning in."
—ILANA YURKIEWICZ, Stanford University oncologist

Of all the diseases one would love to avoid, with the possible exception of Alzheimer's, the C-word is probably the one feared most. *Cancer.* The war against it has been waged for decades, with only minor progress. Did you know that all of us, throughout our lives, are accumulating mutations leading to precancerous cells? As we are exposed to factors such as toxins, sun exposure, secondhand smoke, and unhealthy diets, precancerous mutations accumulate in our cells. When we're healthy and young, our immune systems destroy these cells and their damaged DNA before any harm is done. But as we age, our immune system weakens and can be overwhelmed, a term referred to as **immuno-exhaustion**, and ultimately may fail to detect cancer at its earliest emergence. That's when these precancerous cells keep growing and dividing until they become full-fledged malignancies. That's when the real problem starts.

I've already shared with you that cancer was my deepest fear when I was a kid. Then, later in life, I faced it multiple times—once with my girlfriend's mother, three other times with other people dear to me. One was a valued member of my road team; another was a business partner; a third was the wife of the longtime president of my education company. In each case, I watched them waste away, slowly but surely, and most of all painfully.

If you've ever been close to someone who's been diagnosed with a blood cancer like leukemia, then you understand how these patients are assaulted twice—first by the disease, then by the therapies. Sometimes it's hard to say which is more devastating. While chemotherapy and radiation therapy can be lifesavers, they can also have savage side effects—heart damage, liver damage, nerve damage, even subsequent cancers that show up years later.[1] So after losing three friends to the "standard of care" approach, I realized we desperately needed fresh alternatives to the medical establishment's twentieth-century solutions.

One of my dear friends, Siri Lindley, was diagnosed with a rare form of leukemia and given only a 10 percent chance of survival. She made it. Why? First, she tried an innovative treatment in combination with stem cells. Second, Siri is a unique soul, and has always had the mindset that she will not be beat. This is a woman who resolved to become the number one competitor in the sport of triathlon—at a time when she didn't even know how to swim! She unleashed her amazing will to go on to become the Triathlon World Champion. She used that same determination to fight leukemia. One year later, despite the doctors' prediction of only a 10 percent chance to live, Siri is cancer-free today and just ran her first post-cancer 10K!

So this chapter is about how the war against blood cancers is being waged with the latest technological weapons, about promising treatments that are ready for prime time! We'll talk more about how mindset impacts your biochemistry and health in the final chapter of this book. But if you've ever faced cancer, or someone you love is confronting it now, reading this chapter is a must. Let's start with the story of the hero who's created one of the most promising breakthroughs, Dr. Carl June. You're about to learn:

• How immunotherapy boosts our natural immune system with medicines made of living immune cells as opposed to chemical drugs— a welcome alternative to chemotherapy and other traditional anticancer interventions.

---

1 American Cancer Society, "Chemotherapy Side Effects."

- **How Carl June overcame personal tragedy and legions of doubters to devise what may actually be an original cure for some of the most common and deadly blood cancers.**
- **How through natural stimulation of your own immune system you can both prevent and possibly cure some of the most dreaded cancers.**

TREATING THE FIRST CAR T PATIENT

"My career has been completely unpredictable."[2]

—DR. CARL JUNE

It was the summer of 2010, and **Dr. Carl June** was desperate. Two weeks earlier, June and his colleagues at the University of Pennsylvania had **treated a cancer patient with something never tried before: infusions of the man's own white blood cells, with a twist**. June's Philadelphia lab had **genetically reprogrammed these T cells into an anti-tumor, precision-guided strike force—a set of cellular cruise missiles, if you will.**

If all went well, their subject—written off as terminal—would find a lifeline. **What's more, the experiment could open a revolutionary front in the war against cancer. June believed it could save countless people with raging blood and bone marrow malignancies, people for whom all else had failed.**

The altered immune cells were unstoppable in a petri dish. They'd racked up miracle cures in mice. But June's Patient One, a retired New Jersey corrections officer named **Bill Ludwig**, wasn't doing so well. Shortly after his third—and last—infusion for chronic lymphocytic leukemia (CLL), Ludwig ran a low-grade fever as his blood pressure plunged. Over the next five days, he got steadily worse. It seemed like the mother of all flu bugs: violent chills, sweats, nausea, diarrhea. Ludwig's core temperature skied to 105 degrees. (The nurses threw out their thermometers—they had to be broken, right?) Though the patient showed all the earmarks of acute infection, his scans and

---

2 Healio Immuno-Oncology Resource Center, "'We Have to Cure' Cancer, Says CAR T Pioneer Carl H. June, MD."

cultures came back negative—no viruses and no bacteria. Yet he kept getting sicker and weaker. His kidneys began to fail. His heart and lungs were at the brink.

Down the road, June would come to realize that Ludwig had been hit by a massive, systemic inflammatory response. **The crisis was triggered by what was initially a good thing: a massacre of the patient's leukemia cells by his immune system. As immune T cells enter mortal combat, they flood the body with inflammatory chemicals called** *cytokines.* **The collateral damage was proof that Ludwig's treatment was working— a** *feature***, not a bug.** This "on-target" side effect now has a name: *cytokine release syndrome.* In severe cases, like Ludwig's, it's called a "cytokine storm," a potentially lethal condition that became all too well known in the COVID-19 pandemic. But at the time, June admits, his team "didn't even know what that was."

Ludwig had long thought his cancer would eventually kill him; now it looked like June's trial might beat it to the punch. The crisis came to a head late one evening, after the patient's wife, Darla, had gone home. "You need to come back," a doctor solemnly told her over the phone. "Bill will not see sunrise."

"It's only a matter of time before cell-based therapy replaces high-dose chemotherapy as the front-line treatment for virtually all blood cancers."[3]

—CARL JUNE

In medical science, as in any walk of life, there are precious few truly new ideas under the sun. But **CAR T-cell therapy is completely original. It's an audacious hybrid of** *gene therapy***, where scientists edit a cell's DNA to remove a defect or insert a helpful gene, and** *immunotherapy***, which heals by boosting a patient's own natural defenses**—the intricate immune system that protects us against disease. **CAR T cells are the ultimate in personalized medicine. They're a "living drug" crafted from the patient's own tissues, and arguably the most complex cancer treatment yet invented.**

---

3 Ibid.

And here's one sure thing: **The therapy wouldn't be nearly as advanced as it is today without Carl June's intrepid commitment and maverick ingenuity.**

June is the type of scientist who gets emotionally involved with his patients. But when it came to Bill Ludwig, he had a lot more riding than the fate of a 65-year-old subject. **Today we know Carl June as a cellular medicine rock star, one of *Time* magazine's "100 Most Influential People in the World." But it wasn't so long ago when immunotherapy was the redheaded stepchild of cancer science.** Like **Dr. Michel Sadelain at Memorial Sloan Kettering and other CAR T-cell pioneers,** June was mostly dismissed by the medical establishment and ignored by the private sector. He was forced to rely on small nonprofits for funding. In the wake of the stock market bloodbath of 2008, those foundations had yet to recover from the vicious hit to their endowments. They cut back. The well was running dry.

The field was still reeling from the death of Jesse Gelsinger a decade earlier, in a trial at another Penn lab. A vigorous 18-year-old high school graduate with a rare genetic metabolic disease, Gelsinger had been declared brain dead four days after a gene transfer treatment. The FDA flagged irregularities, and the government and university paid a settlement of more than $1 million. The *Washington Post* called it "the latest in a series of setbacks for a promising approach that has so far failed to deliver its first cure."[4] **The trial had nothing to do with CAR T cells, but it impeded bedside science in genetic engineering for a long, long time.**

In 2009, June and his colleagues published preclinical data on lab mice that demonstrated the promise of CAR T-cell cancer therapy. The FDA gave its blessing to test it on human patients. But clinical trials are expensive. The National Cancer Institute, a division of the National Institutes of Health, turned down three requests for funding. They considered CAR Ts a hopeless quest, a pipe dream.

"They said, 'Cancer immunotherapy hasn't worked in one hundred years,'" June recalled. "Which was true." In 1891, a New York surgeon named William Coley injected an inoperable cancer patient with

---

4 Weiss and Nelson, "Teen Dies Undergoing Experimental Gene Therapy."

streptococcus bacteria in an attempt to rev up the man's immune system and shrink his tumor. **The method worked the first time out, but not on other patients. Over time, the immune approach to cancer gave way to chemotherapy and high-beam radiation therapy.** After the Jesse Gelsinger tragedy, the whole idea made investors skittish. **"No one from big pharma would take this on," June said. "They said it was nothing you could ever get commercialized."** From a marketing standpoint, it probably didn't help that June used a form of the HIV virus to bring the new genetic code into the patient's immune cells. It was a neutered and harmless HIV, but *still*.

June seethed with frustration. He had a radical tool and felt sure it could work, but no one seemed to be listening. There were days when he was tempted to abandon CAR Ts. He could have returned to finding better ways to grow immune cells in dishes and rodents—research that would be many years out from helping real patients, if it ever did: "It's pretty easy to just get funding for basic science."

But whenever June felt ready to give up, he remembered his wife, Cindy June, who had been diagnosed with ovarian cancer in 1996. He created a vaccine to help her, but the effects didn't last. He knew that a company called **Medarex** was developing **ipilimumab, an antibody medication that stops cancer cells from squelching immune assaults. (It was an early version of the "immune checkpoint blockade" therapy invented by Nobel laureate Jim Allison, as we'll explore in Chapter 19, "How to Win the War on Cancer"). June tried unsuccessfully to have the medicine made available for Cindy for "compassionate use," a last-ditch program for therapies not yet approved by the FDA. Cindy died in 2001 at age 46, leaving behind her husband and three children.** Ten years later, when ipilimumab finally gained approval, **June confided that his personal tragedy "gave me a real impetus to make something happen clinically,** which is a lot harder than research in mice." **And so he kept on pushing to find a way to mobilize living immune cells against cancer. For June, this was personal.**

By the time Bill Ludwig showed up at Professor June's door, **his lab was running on fumes. The year before, June had laid off most of his team, a low point in a distinguished career. He was down to his last $1 million from the Alliance for Cancer Gene Therapy, a small philanthropy.**

He'd planned his human trial for fourteen subjects, but could afford only three—just three chances to show the world that his guided-missile cells could work. Now Patient One was on the ropes. **If the worst came to pass, the trial might have to be shut down. June knew he might not ever get another shot. His life's work hung by a thread** that seemed to be fraying with each fractional spike in Ludwig's galloping fever.

But if June was desperate, he had company. Because cancer patient Bill Ludwig knew that the scientist's unproven, cell-based therapy was his last, best hope.

"It could work or it could not work. But that's the only thing I had left."

—BILL LUDWIG

CLL is the most common leukemia in adults. **It discombobulates the body's B cells, the white blood cells that make antibodies to trap foreign substances and mark them for destruction.** Once they're colonized by cancer, these cellular security guards start slacking off on the job. Worse yet, rogue B cells multiply out of control. They infiltrate the bloodstream and bone marrow, crowding out red blood cells, healthy white cells, and the platelets we need for our blood to clot. When leukemia goes unchecked, patients can die of internal bleeding or rampant infections.

Chemotherapy usually does the trick with CLL; the five-year survival rate exceeds 80 percent. **Bill Ludwig had already gone through numerous rounds of chemo, plus a clinical trial at NIH that nearly did him in. None of the treatments took.** Doctors call such patients "refractory," or nonresponsive, and with CLL their prognosis is grim. **Ludwig was down to his last FDA-sanctioned option: a bone marrow transplant, where a donor's stem cells are asked to work their wonders. Marrow transplants are high-risk procedures. When Ludwig found out it was 50-50 that the imported cells would attack his own organs, and quite possibly kill him, he passed. The odds weren't good enough.**

But when Ludwig learned of June's CAR T-cell trial, he didn't hesitate. He'd heard good things about Penn Medicine, June's hospital, a teaching institution with world-class doctors. **At that point, with his abnormal white cell count climbing sky-high, he figured he had little to lose.**

THE POWER OF YOUR T CELLS

T cells are the immune system's infantry, its essential line of defense against outsiders. From their bases in the blood or lymph nodes, "helper" T cells choreograph our immune response. "Killer" Ts find and kill infections—or, potentially, tumors. Some T cells are equipped with a memory of past invasions, an alert system that gets passed down when they divide. That's how measles or chickenpox vaccinations guard people for a lifetime. They sensitize the immune system to jump on the same microbe if it ever shows its face again.

Over eons of evolution, T cells have been trained to search out and destroy any foreign party (or *pathogen*) that might be toxic to the body. Topping the Most Wanted list are cells with foreign DNA or RNA, like viruses or bacteria. **One reason that cancer cures are so elusive is that tumor cells fly under the radar like an invasion of the body snatchers.** They look a lot like normal cells, at least from a garden-variety T cell's point of view. (After all, they share the patient's identical DNA, give or take a few mutations.) **To reliably take down cancer cells, T cells need to sniff them out—to recognize their signature proteins, or *antigens*—in a predictable way. They need a superpower gadget, a way to crack the tumor cells' camouflage—something like infrared night-vision goggles, only on a molecular scale.**

A few weeks before Bill Ludwig's first infusion, June's lab drew his blood, spun out his T cells, and mixed them with the disarmed human immunodeficiency virus, a procedure June himself had refined to guarantee its safety. The HIV would be asked to do what HIV does better than almost anything else in nature: penetrate human immune cells. **But instead of attacking Ludwig's immune system, these particular viruses were programmed to help it fight back.** Once they found a T cell's genome, they hacked their way inside and off-loaded their precious cargo. It was a snippet of customized DNA, the instruction set for making proteins that detect surface markers on specific cancer cells—in this case, Ludwig's leukemia cells.

The "CAR" in CAR T cells stands for *Chimeric Antigen Receptor*. It's an homage to the *chimera*, the fire-breathing, three-headed monster of Greek mythology: part lion, part goat, part snake. **CAR Ts are part bloodhound,**

part claw crane, and part hit man, all in one miniaturized package. The genetically doctored piece, the "receptors," are exquisitely sensitive molecular antennae. After the modified cells were infused back into Ludwig's body, they changed the game. The markers on his malignant B cells stood out like flags on a diplomat's limousine. The CAR Ts bound to them like Velcro and held fast, like turbocharged antibodies. As the T cells docked, they efficiently terminated their targets. **June proudly calls his CAR Ts**

Ludwig nearly died post-procedure when his souped-up T cells broke *down seven pounds of tumor* in a matter of weeks!

"serial assassins." *A single fortified immune cell can slaughter more than a thousand tumor cells.*

Once the battle is joined, it can be a very short war. **Ludwig nearly died post-procedure when his souped-up T cells broke *down seven pounds of tumor* in a matter of weeks! When dead cancer cells pile up faster than the kidneys can clear them, the result can be a life-threatening stew of potassium, phosphorus, and uric acid,** among other nasty ingredients.

And then Ludwig stabilized. Intravenous fluids and steroids reined in his raging immune system. His cytokine storm veered out to sea and played itself out. After four days in the hospital, June's patient went home with his wife, Darla.

One month after the treatment, his oncologist ordered a biopsy. It came back clean! Ludwig had no detectable leukemia in his bone marrow, not a single bad B cell. *Nada. Zilch!* **The readout was so improbable that the oncologist was sure the technicians must have missed something. Three days later, he asked for a second biopsy.**

That one came back clean, too.

Subsequent blood tests brought more good news. The genetically changed T cells had burrowed into Ludwig's bone marrow and were still proliferating—like jackrabbits. **From a genetic perspective, Ludwig was literally a new man!** In an exception to the usual rule, CAR T cells seemed to function even better in people than in mice.

Encouraged, June repeated the procedure with his other two sub-jects. Like Ludwig, they'd been considered lost causes. One of them matched Ludwig's total remission. The other showed significant improve-ment. Success!

Quantitatively speaking, it wasn't much of a trial. But though June's lab was just about broke, **he was sitting on a bona fide medical break-through: the first gene-based therapy to conquer cancer in a human subject.** He met for coffee with the study's co–lead investigator, David Por-

---

One month after the treatment, his oncologist ordered a biopsy. It came back clean! Ludwig had no detectable leukemia in his bone marrow, not a single bad B cell. *Nada. Zilch!*

---

ter, and decided to double down. They'd author a formal paper on their trial with Ludwig, a single patient, with brief mentions of the two others. The scientists knew they'd be flouting convention. The cancer research commu-nity tends to view such slim data with suspicion—and anyone cocky enough to report them as a showboat.

But not this time. **The June team's paper, published in 2011 in the prestigious *New England Journal of Medicine*, was a sensation.** A few brief excerpts will give you the flavor. Dry language aside, you can almost picture the authors taking a well-deserved victory lap. **Their doubters were suddenly very quiet.** Talk about vindication!

> Remission was ongoing 10 months after treatment. . . . **Genetically modified cells were present at high levels in bone marrow for at least 6 months after infusion. . . .** It was unexpected that the very low dose of Chimeric Antigen Receptor T cells that we infused would result in a clinically evident antitumor response. . . .
>
> Unlike antibody-mediated therapy, Chimeric Antigen Receptor–modified T cells have the potential to replicate in vivo [inside the body], and **long-term persistence could lead to sustained tumor control.**

The CAR T cells' "persistence," their capacity to live on indefinitely, was something not even June dared dream possible. According to the trial's consent form, the modified cells were expected to last six weeks at best. Rafts of data showed that patients will reject biological drugs that contain molecules from another species. Since a mouse antibody was one tiny piece of the CAR T cells given to Ludwig, June assumed the cells' days were numbered. "I was wrong," he said recently with a laugh. **It was like two gunmen meeting in the Wild West. The CAR T cells basically shot first and killed the cells" needed to reject them.** "That's in about three-quarters of the patients," he added. "About one-quarter do reject the CAR T cells. It's an example of acquired immune tolerance and was completely unexpected."

THE MIRACULOUS TREATMENT
OF FIVE-YEAR-OLD EMILY

"Dr. June is my hero. He saved my family!"

—EMILY WHITEHEAD

In 2010, when she was five, Emily Whitehead was diagnosed with acute lymphoblastic leukemia, or ALL. It was considered the "best" childhood cancer, the doctors told her parents, with a cure rate of up to 90 percent. But like Ludwig, Emily was a "refractory" patient, one who couldn't be helped by standard treatments. **She endured two brutal rounds of chemotherapy. Her immune system was in tatters. She developed a flesh-eating disease in her legs and nearly had to have them amputated. And then her cancer came back.**

By February 2012, with Emily's leukemia cells doubling by the day, her condition was dire. She was too far gone for a marrow transplant. **Believing the end was near, her oncologist recommended hospice and discouraged the family from enrolling her in June's clinical trial for ALL at Children's Hospital of Philadelphia (CHOP). Of course the doctor's intent was positive; he wanted to spare Emily from more pain and**

disappointment. But her parents weren't willing to give up—and nei-ther was Emily. And so they camped out at an aunt's home near the hospital and steeled themselves for the scariest ride of their lives. **Their shaggy-haired, gap-toothed daughter would be the world's first pediatric pa-tient to undergo CAR T-cell therapy.**

Like Ludwig, Emily had no problem with the infusion itself. She relaxed with an ice pop as the supercharged immune cells coursed into her blood-stream. But two nights later, her temperature spiked. Her blood pressure crashed. **She went into respiratory failure—a full-blown case of cyto-kine release syndrome. Emily's level of interleukin-6, Public Enemy Number One for CAR T-cell patients, was nearly a thousand times normal. A doctor told her father she had one chance in a thousand to make it through the night.**

The pediatric ICU put Emily on a ventilator and induced her into coma. June read the lab results and knew what they signified. **"We thought she was going to die,"** he said. "I wrote an e-mail to the provost at the uni-versity, telling him the first child with the treatment was about to die. I feared the trial was finished." Other hospitals running similar trials might be pressed to follow suit. **There was no telling how far or how long CAR T-cell therapy could be set back.**

Before June could press Send on his email, he got an idea. His own daughter had juvenile rheumatoid arthritis, an autoimmune disease. She'd recently been helped by tocilizumab, a "biologic" drug that functions as an antibody—and blocks interleukin-6. (More recently, it's helped some patients overcome the inflammation linked to COVID-19.[5]) It was just a hunch, but June played it. Luck was with them; Children's Hospital had tocilizumab on hand. **Emily received her first dose at eight o'clock that night . . . and pulled out of her death spiral. She emerged from her two-week coma on her seventh birthday, all smiles. No one there could recall a child so sick getting so much better so fast.**

Eight days later, June was gratified—but not surprised—to read the biopsy report. Emily appeared to be cancer-free. Six months later, tests

---

5 Alattar et al., "Tocilizumab for the Treatment of Severe Coronavirus Disease 2019."

confirmed that not a single leukemia cell remained in her bone marrow. By then she'd returned to school and soccer and walking her dog—to a little girl's normal life. As she told *Time* magazine: "I was a fun and energetic child. Then I spent two years in a hospital getting cancer treatment, but it wasn't working for me. . . . **Dr. June saved my life and had a huge impact on my family. Without him, I wouldn't be here today writing this—and my parents and I wouldn't be helping other kids beat cancer."**

THE NEXT STEP

"It's hard to describe someone who basically saved your life. He lost the one he loved, and turned around and saved me years later."
—BILL LUDWIG

As the media picked up her story worldwide, Emily became the poster child for CAR T-cell therapy. June's bombshell paper had already drawn the attention of Novartis, the Swiss-based pharmaceutical giant. The company was about to lose patent protection—and blow a $3 billion hole in its balance sheet—on Gleevec, its warhorse chemotherapy drug. "Their back was against the wall," June said. He'd always needed just one taker, and now he'd found them.

Novartis licensed June's CAR T-cell technology, including his production methods and dosing recipes. **In 2014, to fast-track development, the FDA designated CAR Ts as a "breakthrough therapy."** In 2015, working with June's researchers and CHOP, **Novartis launched *Eliana*, a Phase II trial with seventy-nine children and young adults with acute lymphoblastic leukemia.** The average subject arrived with a total of three failed chemotherapies or bone marrow transplants. It was a group with historically dismal outcomes. **Two years later, the results were in: 83 percent of the subjects showed complete remission—"early, deep and durable remission," said Dr. Stephan Grupp, director of CHOP's Cancer Immunotherapy Frontier Program. "We've never seen anything like this before and I believe this therapy may become the new standard of care for this patient population."**

The FDA agreed. On August 30, 2017, after a unanimous vote by an

exuberant advisory committee ("potentially paradigm shifting"), the agency gave its green light to June's modified T cells for ALL—its first approval ever for a cell-based gene transfer therapy. The Novartis brand name is **Kymriah**, a play on "chimera." In 2018, the FDA approved it to treat several types of non-Hodgkin's lymphoma. (It joined **Yescarta**, a similar product from Kite Pharma.) Based on some promising trials, it may not be long before CLL, the leukemia that launched June's pivotal pilot study, gets added to the hit list.

Altogether, approved CAR T-cell therapies can be found today in more than a hundred hospitals in the United States.

As we go to press, Bill Ludwig is 75 years old, absorbed in his travel and hobbies, doting on a young granddaughter he might never have known.[6] Emily Whitehead is 16 and recently ran her first 5K to raise more than $5,000 for the fight against childhood cancer. She has a mild case of asthma, a souvenir of her near-death experience, but refuses to let it slow her down: "I liked seeing the finish line, and I sprinted across it." Since Emily blazed the trail with CAR T cells, more than 500 children in eleven countries have been treated, the huge majority successfully.

Altogether, approved CAR T-cell therapies can be found today in more than a hundred hospitals in the United States.

Nearly a decade out from their pivotal trials, both Emily and Bill had CAR T cells patrolling their bloodstream, on the watch for treacherous B cells, ready to deploy at any time—a living vaccine. (Since CAR Ts also kill healthy B cells, patients get regular infusions of immunoglobulin, a serum of pooled antibodies, to keep their immune system up to snuff.) Malignancies are unpredictable beasts, and most doctors avoid the word "cure." They hedge their bets with terms like "disease-free survival" or "cancer-free." But of the young people who made it through the Novartis Elania trial, June believes that "most of them are probably cured."

---

6 On January 31, 2021, Bill Ludwig tragically died from an unrelated case of COVID-19.

Carl June is our cancer science hero because he persevered. No matter how bleak the circumstances, he never lost his conviction or sense of urgency. He fought back against setbacks in the lab and the clinic, some of them frankly terrifying. **He fought back against a risk-averse cancer-industrial complex.** For many years he was a lonely voice in the immunotherapy wilderness. But he kept the faith. **His daring pursuit has given hope to untold thousands of cancer patients. To people who'd had nowhere else to turn.**

In the spring of 2018, when I attended the Vatican's Unite to Cure conference, **the night got *really* emotional when rock icon Peter Gabriel dedicated his performance to the people helping his 47-year-old wife, Meabh, fight off an aggressive form of non-Hodgkin's lymphoma.** It was the first time he'd spoken publicly about Meabh's illness—the melon-sized tumors, the failed chemotherapy—and how CAR T cells had made her "remarkably well" again. **There weren't many dry eyes in the house when he thanked the assembled scientists for saving "the woman I love."**

Peter also spoke to the need to make this lifesaving treatment available to people of ordinary means. **Individualized cellular medicine is expensive, even when it's one-and-done.** The rack rate for Kymriah is $475,000, roughly the cost of a kidney transplant. The good news: **In 2019, two years after the FDA's approval, Medicare unveiled a coverage plan for CAR T-cell therapy.** Some private insurers are also on board. June predicts that **it's only a matter of time before cell-based therapy replaces high-dose chemotherapy as the front-line treatment for virtually all blood cancers.**[7] And as Caron Jacobson, director of the cell therapy program at Dana-Farber Cancer Institute, says, none of this could have happened "without the wisdom, creativity, and vision of Dr. June."[8]

I'm not here to tell you that CAR T-cell therapy is a can't-miss panacea. The risks are no joke. A handful of patients have died from cerebral edema, a swelling of the brain. More common are "off-target" neurological side effects, from headache and confusion to delirium and seizures—usually temporary, but in some cases long-term issues.

---

7 Healio Immuno-Oncology Resource Center, "'We Have the Cure.'"

8 Ibid.

Though the treatment has shown dramatic success against Emily White-head's pediatric leukemia, not every subject thrives. **For patients undergoing CAR T-cell therapy, like any other cancer therapy, the elephant in the room is the potential for relapse. According to research data, while a healthy majority of responsive patients with Emily's type of leukemia stay symptom-free for years, cancer can find its way back in one of three cases or more. Why does this happen?** One theory is that tumor cells may grow resistant to CAR Ts by shedding their surface marker molecules. (Like cockroaches, cancers excel in adapting to survive.) Without markers to target, the engineered T cells flow aimlessly through the blood, as good as blind to malignant B cells. Another possibility is that some patients lack enough "memory" T cells, the ones that prime the immune system to call out the rogue Bs. (Novartis offers a full refund for patients showing no response after one month.)

While CAR T cells are overwhelmingly effective against liquid cancers like leukemias, they've yet to prove to be of much help against solid tumors, which account for 90 percent of U.S. cancer deaths: cancers of the lung, breast, colon, and prostate, among other organs. The T cells' targets are less accessible in solid tumors because they're stashed inside the problem cells. Even when the CAR Ts get there, they're facing a hostile, low-oxygen, high-acid environment that can weaken or kill them before they can do their job. **For those solid tumor cancers, there are new breakthrough therapies we'll be sharing with you in Chapter 19, "How to Win the War on Cancer," that are up to the challenge.**

Carl June is undaunted. He and other scientists are testing CAR Ts in bone cancer, melanoma, sarcoma, and glioblastoma. At the moment, there are more than six hundred ongoing clinical trials[9] on CAR T cells—all of them spiritual descendants of June's first high-wire experiments. The work promises to advance rapidly, June believes—and CAR Ts may be only the beginning. "T cells are just one part of the immune system," he says. "We'll see engineered natural killer cells, dendritic cells, stem cells . . ."

"For immuno-oncology," June says, "we're at the end of the

---

9 Barrell, "Everything to Know about CAR T-Cell Therapy."

beginning. We finally have the tool set to talk about curing cancer." I hope this story of the power of CAR T cells is logged deep inside your brain. If someone you love ever encounters leukemia, you can return to this chapter as well as to Chapter 19 for some additional resources to consider. It could save someone's life.

Now let's turn to discover something that might sound like science fiction, but has already been used to treat more than 5,000 people suffering from Parkinson's and essential tremors—incisionless brain surgery and harnessing the power of focused ultrasound.

CHAPTER 7

INCISIONLESS BRAIN SURGERY: THE IMPACT OF FOCUSED ULTRASOUND

"I feel like a new person. I have my independence back. . . . I can do anything and everything that I want to do again."[1]

—KIMBERLY SPLETTER, Parkinson's patient

In this chapter, you're going to learn about a breakthrough tool for *incisionless* brain surgery. It sounds like science fiction, but in this chapter we'll share with you . . .

- **How more than 5,000 Parkinson's and essential tremor patients around the world have found significant relief with Insightec's focused ultrasound therapy.**
- **How this nontoxic therapy is FDA-approved for treating prostate tissue.**[2]
- **A way to destroy uterine fibroids**, a source of pain and heavy menstrual bleeding for millions of women[3]—without harming adjacent organs.
- **Proven pain relief in cases of metastatic bone cancer** where radiation is not an option. By destroying nerve tissue on the bone's outer layer, it

---

1 Focused Ultrasound Foundation, "Two Years and Countless Miles Later: Parkinson's Patient Update."

2 Cleveland Clinic, "High-Intensity Focused Ultrasound for Prostate Cancer."

3 De la Cruz et al. "Uterine Fibroids: Diagnosis and Treatment."

can ease patients' suffering and reduce the need for brain-fogging medications.

- **FDA trials are underway to use a similar approach to deliver to the brain chemotherapies and new cutting-edge medicines** that would otherwise be blocked by an evolutionary brain barrier. If the studies pan out, doctors will have a new tool to fight lethal brain cancers, depression, and even the white whale of central nervous system diseases: Alzheimer's.
- **A promising preliminary trial to calm down a structure in the brain linked to anxiety and addiction.**[4] One goal is to stop opioid overdoses, which killed nearly 70,000 people in the U.S. in 2020.[5]

A PROVEN TREATMENT FOR PARKINSON'S

When Kimberly Spletter was told in her mid-40s that she had Parkinson's disease, she was surprised—and devastated. She'd seen older Parkinson's patients who could no longer walk, "so I thought I was going to lose all my mobility."[6]

Then her fears came to pass. **Over the course of a few years, Kimberly lost the ability to run, to bike, to hike. Her toes curled spasmodically. Her left leg bounced as though it had a mind of its own.** When she'd try to cross her legs to make it stop, her left leg would hyperextend and lock. The pain was intense. **Kimberly was taking fifteen or more pills a day and just kept getting worse.** Having always been an active and athletic person, **she now struggled to dress herself.**[7] She hit a low point at a wedding, when "my dad came up and asked me to dance with him—and I couldn't get out of the chair, because my back and my foot were cramping

---

4 *WVU Today*, "WVU Addresses Addiction Crisis with Novel Ultrasound Treatment."

5 Bernstein and Achenbach, "Drug Overdose Deaths Soared to a Record 93,000 Last Year."

6 Focused Ultrasound Foundation, "Kimberly Finds Tremor Relief for Her Parkinson's Disease."

7 Michael J. Fox Foundation, "First U.S. Patients Treated in Dyskinesia Study Using Ultrasound Technology."

so bad. That's every little girls' dream, to have that dance with her dad, and I couldn't do it." Kimberly was beginning to live her worst nightmare: to be bound to a wheelchair. The situation looked grim . . . until she learned about a new, noninvasive frontier for treating disorders of the brain.

According to the Parkinson's Foundation, nearly a million people are living with Parkinson's in the U.S. alone, and 60,000 more are diagnosed each year. It's a brutal brain disease that primarily attacks the motor system. Telltale signs include rigidity, agonizingly slow movement, and—in at least one of four patients—uncontrollable shakes and tremors. Parkinson's is caused by the loss of neurons that manufacture dopamine, a natural chemical messenger that controls our muscles' movements. Dopamine also helps to regulate our sleep patterns, our recall, our appetite, and our mood and self-control. Suffice it to say that when we don't make enough of it, we're up against a really difficult and complex problem.

There has been no cure for Parkinson's, and treatment options have been limited. The frontline therapy, levodopa, won FDA approval back in 1970, which tells you all you need to know about the lack of medical progress over the last half a century. The researchers we've spoken to say that levodopa is a flawed drug at best and often causes shakes and abnormal movements of its own. And if that wasn't discouraging enough, its anti-tremor benefits tend to fade over time. For as many as half of Parkinson's patients, it doesn't really work at all.

Until very recently, the only established alternative was **deep brain stimulation**, which might not sound so bad until you find out how you get stimulated. **Surgeons drill a hole into your skull to implant an electrode, which connects to a pacemaker-like generator implanted in your chest. Complications range from infections to brain bleeds—let's just say that open brain surgery isn't for everybody.** Like a lot of people, Kimberly was waiting for something that could help her without such scary side effects.

Finally she found it: **focused ultrasound**, or high-energy sound waves precision-guided by MRIs. She enrolled in a clinical trial to evaluate the technology for treating Parkinson's motor symptoms. After twenty years of research, development, and clinical experience by an **Israeli medical device company called Insightec, focused ultrasound was approved by the**

FDA to treat essential tremor in 2016 and tremor-dominant Parkinson's in 2019. **It has alleviated these symptoms for the great majority of patients—with no incisions, no general anesthesia, next to no risk of infection, and minimal pain.**

Surgeons are laying aside their scalpels for a keyboard and a mouse. **Results are instantaneous. Patients return home, usually the same day, without ever seeing the inside of an operating room.** They regain the ability to text on their phones and to cut up their food . . . or go back to painting portraits or playing the guitar. **They're reclaiming their lives with a single two- to three-hour outpatient procedure!**

If their stunning success with Parkinson's was all the Insightec team had to show for themselves, they'd have earned their spot in this book and then some. What is the bottom line? **If Insightec can sustain its recent winning streak, millions of "hopeless" cases will be hopeless no longer.**

GETTING TO THE SOURCE WITH PRECISION ULTRASOUND

"Focused ultrasound is really a revolutionary technology that allows us to perform functional neurosurgery without any of the risk . . . of implanted electrodes or hardware."[8]

—DR. REES COSGROVE, focused-ultrasound pioneer and director of epilepsy and functional neurosurgery, Brigham and Women's Hospital, Boston

A few days before Kimberly's treatment, a CT scan was performed to measure the thickness and density of her skull and confirm that she was suitable for focused ultrasound. On procedure day, when she arrived in a wheelchair at the University of Maryland Medical Center, her head was shaved—with existing technology, hair can dilute or deflect the sound waves (Insightec is already working on a new approach that will not require shaving the head). Then she was fitted with a million-dollar halo-shaped ultrasound helmet. After sliding the patient into an MRI scanner, the surgeon applied the first

---

8 Harrison, "First Trial of Focused Ultrasound in Depression Under Way."

of a series of "sonications," or what Kimberly called "zaps"—more than a thousand sound waves that converged on a spot deep in the center of her brain. **It's the same basic technology used for imaging in pregnancies, but far more focused and powerful.** Think of a magnifying glass that concentrates energy from the sun to ignite a campfire—except with beams of acoustic energy subbing in for sunlight.

Insightec's device aimed the sound waves at a malfunctioning piece of Kimberly's thalamus, a part of the brain that governs motor control. As the surgeon gradually intensified the ultrasound, the "noisy" tissue was heated to around 130 degrees Fahrenheit. That's the minimum temperature required to disrupt the circuits that cause the involuntary movements and shaking.

Scientists isolated the source of Parkinson's-related tremor two or three decades ago. **"We've always known that was the problem,"** says Dr. Arjun Desai, MD, Insightec's chief strategic innovation officer. **"We just never had an elegant way of getting to it without cutting your head open or delivering radiation."** Insightec's revolutionary device, developed by some of the same scientists who created Israel's Iron Dome air defense system, **can pinpoint sound waves to targets the size of the tip of a pencil.** "The critical technological breakthrough," Desai says, "is our ability to target a tiny, sub-millimeter region, so we can avoid areas of the brain that control speech and other functions." It's the ultimate in precision, personalized medicine!

After each zap, followed by a round of neurological testing, Kimberly could *feel* herself "getting stronger and stronger." She experienced a sensation of heat and a little nausea, but nothing more. **Her tremor and pain were receding in real time.** After zap number fourteen, her neurologist, Dr. Paul Fishman, asked her, "If you could stay where you are now, would you call your treatment a success?"

Kimberly said, "Yes, absolutely."

The doctor said, "Then we're done!" The clinical trial director told her to get up and walk, "and I thought, **I *can* walk," Kimberly recalls. "I *knew* I could."** She rose to her feet. Lightly holding the director's hand, more for security than physical support, she slowly crossed the room without a wobble. Soon she was walking normally; her Parkinson's shuffle was gone.

Two years later, Kimberly completed a 50-mile bike ride along the

coast of Maine, a fundraiser to support the Michael J. Fox Foundation. She was babysitting three days a week with her three-year-old grandson—and, more impressive yet, keeping up with him. **Aside from some mild headaches and minor involuntary movements on her untreated right side, she remained mostly symptom-free for two years.** After that, unfortunately, some of her Parkinson's symptoms began to reappear. **But as Kimberly said, focused ultrasound "has given me a new lease on life, and I take advantage of it every day."**[9]

In a clinical trial, patients showed on average a 62 percent improvement in their "tremor score" three months after the procedure. Treatment-related side effects were mostly mild and temporary; the most common was numbness and tingling. Based on clinical findings over the last two years, **Dr. Desai estimates that up to 80 percent of Parkinson's patients show "substantial" relief from their tremor.**

Let's be clear about one thing: Parkinson's disease is progressive and degenerative, and focused ultrasound cannot cure it. It doesn't address disease-related speech issues, mood disorders, or cognitive decline. And since the therapy is so new, there's as yet no guarantee that a person's tremor or motor symptoms won't return years later. **But for the estimated 680,000 Parkinson's patients, focused ultrasound can turn back the clock and restore critical function.** Besides easing tremors, the same therapy can target another part of the brain that triggers slow and rigid movements, two other common symptoms of Parkinson's. Doctors are already using it commercially in Japan, according to Dr. Desai. The potential impact is monumental.

TREATING ESSENTIAL TREMORS

Around twenty years ago, Karl Wiedamann, a retired Florida engineer and world-class senior competitive swimmer who had held three world records in his age class, started having trouble filling out his checks. His clear handwriting turned squiggly. Then he noticed his hand shaking when he poured his morning cup of coffee. He went to a neurologist, who ran him through

---

9 Focused Ultrasound Foundation, "Two Years and Countless Miles Later."

tests to rule out conditions like Parkinson's or multiple sclerosis or some undetected brain trauma. The good news, the doctor said, was that Wiedamann had none of the above. The not-so-good news was that he had a condition called essential tremor. And it would probably get worse.

Essential tremor is the most common of all movement disorders, affecting around 10 million people in the United States. Former president Bill Clinton and retired Supreme Court Justice Sandra Day O'Connor have it. So did the late Katharine Hepburn. Yet somehow essential tremor tends to get overlooked in terms of public awareness and funding for research. Many medical professionals consider it a "syndrome"—a collection of overlapping symptoms—rather than a full-fledged disease. Some even call it "benign tremor"—but there's nothing benign about its impact on a person's daily life. Essential tremor can turn the most basic tasks into steep and jagged mountains to climb. **Though it's most common and typically most severe in older people, it strikes young people and those in middle age as well. It can derail careers and make people embarrassed, isolated, and depressed.** For a competitive swimmer like Karl Wiedamann, it threatened to steal the life he loved. "Something had to be done," he said, "so I went looking for answers."[10]

For a while Karl kept his shaking at bay with a prescription drug called primidone, an anti-seizure medication that wouldn't interfere with his intensive swim training. But then the primidone reacted with another medication and had to be discontinued. The tremor got worse. Simple activities Karl once took for granted—buttoning his shirt, tying his shoelaces—became daily frustrations. A bowl of soup was a nonstarter. When deep brain stimulation came on the scene, Karl checked it out. When he found out about the drilling, he said thanks, but no thanks—he'd hold out for something less invasive. Then came the sad day when Karl quit competitive swimming; he worried that he'd fall from the starting blocks before the race began. His future looked bleak.

After focused ultrasound gained FDA approval for treating essential tremor, in 2016, Karl connected with Dr. Travis Tierney, a neurosurgeon

---

10 Wiedamann, "Back on the Blocks: 'Focused Ultrasound Gave Me Back My Life.'"

then working at the Sperling Medical Group in Delray Beach, Florida. **(It's one of three dozen U.S. medical centers—including the Mayo Clinic, Stanford, and Penn Medicine—that collaborate with Insightec in delivering this extraordinary innovation.)** Like Kimberly, Karl underwent a series of MRI-guided sound wave zaps to burn away a small part of his thalamus. "It's a very delicate dance the surgeon is doing," he said. "He's going after a spot in your brain that's about the size of a pea—without having to physically go into your skull."[11] After each sonication, Karl was asked to trace a spiral on a pad of paper. Over the course of three hours, his drawing improved from irregular spikes to a smooth, flowing curve. **Within seconds after the treatment concluded, he was able to legibly write his name for the first time in fifteen years.**

Today Karl is back in the pool, training all out to set new world records for the breaststroke in the 80-to-84 age group. He can button his shirt without a second thought, pour a glass of wine without spilling a drop. **Friends who witnessed his old struggles are astounded. If you didn't know he had essential tremor—well, you'd have no way of knowing. Focused ultrasound, he says, "gave me back my life."**

Karl's case is dramatic but not exceptional. According to Dr. Desai, more than 5,000 Parkinson's and essential tremor patients around the world have found significant relief with Insightec's ultrasound therapy.

Clinical trial data shows that the average patient's tremor had improved by 69 percent one year after the procedure, 75 percent after two years, and 76 percent after three years. As Dr. Desai explains it, **"These people get better over time. Their brain starts firing again, the way it used to—there's neuroplasticity. People are getting better because they're back in action." The latest numbers show durable improvements for at least five years out.**

Under the protocol approved by the FDA, patients are treated on the side of the brain that controls their dominant hand—the left side for right-handers, for example. An Insightec study is underway to treat the other side as well, after allowing at least nine months for the brain to heal. Early

---

11 INSIGHTEC, "Karl Wiedamann Is Living Life to the Fullest."

returns are promising. Patients are getting the same positive impact in their second go-round on the opposite side.

Want some more good news? <u>**In the U.S., focused ultrasound is now covered by Medicare nationwide, along with Aetna and Blue Cross Blue Shield plans in more than thirty states.**</u> Given the therapy's proven efficacy and bang for the buck, other private insurers are expected to follow suit. **Which only makes sense: This technology both improves patients' quality of life and reduces the cost of their care.**

THE POWER OF FOCUSED ULTRASOUND AND ITS IMPACT ON BRAIN CANCERS

"We found we can safely open the blood-brain barrier. It's quick, reversible, and we don't see any major adverse effects."

—DR. NIR LIPSMAN, director of the Harquail Centre for Neuromodulation, Sunnybrook Health Sciences Centre in Toronto

In 2018, Paul Hudspith, an engineer and part-time cellist in Toronto, woke up in the middle of the night with the worst headache of his life. He realized pretty quickly that Tylenol wouldn't help, and he went to the hospital. Doctors found a large tumor bleeding into the right side of his brain. After surgery, they gave Paul and his wife the terrifying news. **He had glioblastoma, a hyper-aggressive and incurable brain cancer. Surgery and radiation could slow it down, but it was next to impossible to remove all the cancer cells. Typical survival time ranged from twelve to eighteen months after diagnosis.**

"I just didn't see a path forward," Paul recalls.[12] His mind was flooded with dark thoughts: Would he see his two children graduate? Would he live to be a grandfather? And what of all the plans he'd made with his wife, Francine? **Paul knew the deck was stacked against him because of the blood-brain barrier, a dense layer of cells within the tiny blood vessels that line the brain.** The barrier evolved to protect the human brain from infections in the bloodstream, which it does really well.

---

12 INSIGHTEC, "Toronto Patient Story."

The catch is that it also blocks both small- and large-molecule drugs and other medicines from doing their jobs. (Supersized molecules, like the new generation of monoclonal antibodies, have even less of a shot to get through.) **With glioblastomas, the frontline standard of care is radiation plus a chemotherapy drug called temozolomide, which can slow the growth and spread of cancer cells.** But under normal conditions, noted Dr. Graeme Woodworth, a neurosurgeon at the University of Maryland School of Medicine, "chemotherapy gets in a little but not a lot." The drug's effectiveness is severely hampered. **As a result, only 10 percent of glioblastoma patients hang on for five years.**[13]

That's where the latest Insightec technology comes in. Instead of using focused ultrasound for heat, doctors pair lower-frequency sound waves with an injection that sends microscopic bubbles into the bloodstream. As the acoustic energy pulses through the patient's helmet, it makes the bubbles vibrate and bounce around. **The molecular commotion pulls cells apart, creating a temporary opening in the blood-brain barrier.** The breach lasts six to twelve hours, long enough to infuse the desired drug. According to Dr. Desai, the hypothesis is that **focused ultrasound can boost the amount of temozolomide actually delivered to a tumor by a significant factor.**

Paul Hudspith was one of the first patients to enroll in a Phase 2 clinical study of this technique at Sunnybrook Health Sciences Centre in Toronto. As his neurosurgeon, Dr. Nir Lipsman, said, "The people who volunteer to be the first in any kind of early phase trial—there's something really unique about them. They have a kind of pioneer spirit, but they are also tremendously altruistic and selfless." Or as another member of Paul's string quartet put it: "He always thinks of other people first."

Paul came through the procedure with flying colors. He repeated the focused ultrasound process in subsequent rounds of chemotherapy. For three years after his initial operation, **he beat the odds. His brain scans were clean and he was back at his job, playing the cello and living his life.** To help raise funds for Sunnybrook's Garry Hurvitz Brain Sciences

---

13 Cohn, "University of Maryland Study Uses Tiny Bubbles in Hopes of Getting Cancer-Fighting Drugs Inside the Brain."

Centre, Paul spoke with other potential clinical trial participants and shared his journey. He never stopped thinking of others.

Sadly, in August 2021, Paul lost his battle with glioblastoma. But during those precious years after his treatment with focused ultrasound, he gained quality time with his family and friends. And Paul made scientific discovery a part of his legacy. In his memory, Paul's family has asked that donations in his memory go to support focused-ultrasound research for glioblastoma.

Though we're still in early days with this technology, it may turn out that temozolomide—and other drugs—are more effective than they've been given credit for. For example: There's a monoclonal antibody called Herceptin that has proven highly effective in treating a class of primary breast cancers. But when patients develop brain metastases from this type of breast cancer, Herceptin falls flat. Could focused ultrasound and microbubbles make the difference?

Meanwhile, Insightec has collaborated with several medical centers in opening the blood-brain barrier more than three hundred times in more than one hundred clinical trial patients—with no major safety events. **The company plans to submit this technique to the FDA to help break down the barriers to treating brain cancer, Parkinson's, and Alzheimer's disease.**

With Alzheimer's cases, the problem is more global than local. The target is different, as well. Insightec is homing in on the hippocampus, the seat of memory. **What's fascinating is that the plaque associated with dementia appears to break up and diminish wherever the blood-brain barrier is weakened—even without adding a drug to fight the disease.** (As you'll see in Chapter 22, Alzheimer's is the graveyard of failed drugs, and scientists have yet to agree on its root cause.) Dr. Desai suggests that **simply unlocking the barrier "gives more access to the immune system to go in, recognize the plaque, and destroy it."** Once Insightec gets permission to open the entire barrier, Dr. Desai can imagine a future where Alzheimer's patients get an ultrasound "haircut" every month or two "to keep your plaque burden low and stable and prevent severe progression of the disease."

But Insightec's ultimate quest isn't a stabilized patient. It's an outright cure—for cancers, Alzheimer's, Parkinson's, ALS, depression, and any other brain disorder you can name. As focused ultrasound gains acceptance as a safe and reliable technology, it will be an invaluable testing ground as a drug delivery vehicle for medicines that previously fell short, or for others now in the pipeline. The plan, Dr. Desai says, is to get them "to the right places at the right time in a really meaningful way. Think of this as the Uber for drug therapy into the brain."

Finally, the latest frontier for Insightec is opioid addiction. They've found a part of the brain that contributes to anxiety and addiction—and that lights up when exposed to drugs. A clinical trial using low-frequency ultrasound kicked off at the West Virginia University Rockefeller Neuroscience Institute.[14] **The first participant was a 39-year-old man with a long history of substance abuse with prescription opioids as well as heroin.** They placed heroin in front of him, and saw through the MRI what part of his brain lit up. They then applied focused ultrasound waves to the nucleus accumbens, a key structure in the brain involved in addiction and anxiety. He came through the procedure safely and successfully, demonstrating that the same part of the brain linked to addiction did not light up anymore. Though the evidence is still mostly anecdotal at this stage, preliminary results have been promising, which is why the WVU Rockefeller Neuroscience Institute is pursuing this study, to try and solve for one of the most challenging issues facing our society.

So now you know there's a way to have brain surgery—without a single incision. Imagine what the future will bring! Our next chapter dives into some incredible solutions that can actually not just treat but eliminate disease. I'm sure you've heard about the power of CRISPR and gene therapy. So let's take the next step in understanding about how our lives are about to radically change, and how healing can be made permanent. . . .

---

14 Rezai, "Exablate for LIFU Neuromodulation in Patients with Opioid Use Disorder."

CHAPTER 8

GENE THERAPY AND CRISPR: THE CURE FOR DISEASE

Gene Therapy and CRISPR Are Upending the Way We Treat—and Cure—Disease

"The power to control our species' genetic future is awesome and terrifying. Deciding how to handle it may be the biggest challenge we have ever faced. I hope—I believe—that we are up to the task."

—JENNIFER DOUDNA, PhD, inventor of CRISPR
and 2020 Nobel laureate in chemistry

I'm sure many of you have heard of the miracles of gene therapy. Some of you might even be confused by it. But if there's one thing I want you to understand from this chapter, it's that **gene therapy is a chance for us to literally eliminate disease, not treat it but cure it completely.** In this chapter, we'll show you that gene therapy is not twenty years in the future. We'll show you how it's being used today, and what it can be used for in the near future to make a difference in your life or the life of someone you care about.

In this chapter, you'll see some stunning examples of the many ways this ability to harness gene therapy and gene editing is being used to create more effective treatments.

For example:

- **Can you imagine that you could cure your child's congenital blindness with the mere injection of a CRISPR treatment into the back of their eye? As you'll discover, this is happening today.**

- Imagine using gene therapy to reprogram damaged heart cells (scars) and convert them into healthy beating heart cells.
- You'll learn how scientists using CRISPR restored the eyesight of a teen crooner on *America's Got Talent*, helping him to overcome his inherited genetic disorder.
- You'll read about a company that's applying CRISPR gene-editing technology to relieve Alzheimer's symptoms such as anxiety and depression—and about a researcher who's using CRISPR to block the aging process.
- You'll learn about what scientists are calling the jackpot gene, the gene that dramatically lowers your risk of Alzheimer's and can significantly enhance your longevity.

But first, let me tell you a quick story that my coauthor Peter and his writing partner Steven Kotler covered in their recent bestselling book *The Future Is Faster Than You Think*. The story is a powerful recounting of the miracle of gene therapy and its ability to cure what was previously a death sentence.

The 1970s were good for John Travolta. While the actor had broken through with a supporting role in 1972, he captured the public's attention in his starring turn in the 1975 TV show *Welcome Back, Kotter*. But it was playing the protagonist in the four-time Emmy award–winning made-for-TV movie *The Boy in the Plastic Bubble* that cemented him as a real star in 1976.

The movie was based on the life of David Vetter, a boy from Texas who suffered from "X-linked severe combined immunodeficiency," a genetic disease that destroys the immune system. Living with this condition requires living inside a bubble, a self-contained atmosphere that protects against any and all germs. Everything that passes into the bubble—water, food, clothing—has to first be sterilized. For patients with the disease, simply breathing normal air can be fatal.

About four years before Travolta took his turn in the bubble, an article in *Science* argued that a new form of treatment might hold promise for patients with severe combined immunodeficiency and other genetic diseases. Known as gene therapy, the idea was unusual yet useful. **Genetic diseases are caused by mutations in the DNA, your genome, your code for life,**

so the solution was to find a way to replace that bad DNA with good DNA. Or, in computer terms, debug the system.

But how to get that good DNA into place?

That's where viruses came into play. These microscopic parasites thrive by attaching themselves to cells. Once there, they inject their own genetic material into the nucleus, causing the host to replicate the virus's DNA—like a hijacked assembly line. Gene therapy piggybacks on this process, stripping out the disease-causing portion of a virus's code and replacing it with good DNA. **Once the virus injects the good DNA into the host cell, first the symptoms of the disease disappear, then the disease itself is cured.**

While the promise of gene therapy is tremendous, the science was not easy. It took almost two decades for the first treatments to arrive, which is when the trouble started. In 1999, an 18-year-old boy named Jesse Gelsinger, with a rare metabolic disorder, took part in a gene therapy drug trial at the University of Pennsylvania. Gelsinger's condition wasn't fatal. The combination of an extremely restrictive diet and thirty-two pills a day kept symptoms under control. But the trial had the potential to cure him completely, so he signed up. Four days after receiving the initial injection, Gelsinger wasn't cured. He was dead. The first recorded death from gene therapy.

More mishaps occurred. Not long after, in a gene therapy trial in France aimed at treating Bubble Boy disease, two out of the ten children involved developed cancer. Immediately, the FDA suspended all gene therapy trials until further notice. The dot-com crash in 2001 was the killing blow, as money from the exploding Web had been fueling gene therapy start-ups. This was the dank pit of the deceptive phase, from which many were convinced there would be no escape.

But escape did come—in the form of more science.

Even though gene therapy faded from sight, research continued. And continued. Then, on April 18, 2019, it burst back into view with a staggering announcement: **Bubble Boy disease had been cured. Ten babies born with the condition, born, technically, without immune systems, had been treated. It wasn't that their symptoms were better. <u>It wasn't that their condition was manageable. It was that they were _cured_.</u> Before treatment, they didn't have immune systems; after treatment, they did.**

The disease was gone. The missing DNA, the missing genes, had been craftily reinserted into the bone marrow of those ten babies.

Biotechnology is about using biology as technology. It's turning the fundamental components of life—our genes, proteins, cells—into tools for shaping and improving life. In a very real sense, **this story starts with the human body, which is a collection of 30 trillion cells, the function of which determines our health. Each of these cells contains 3.2 billion letters from your mother and 3.2 billion letters from your father—this is your DNA, your genome, the software that codes for "you." It's your hair color, eye color, height, a significant chunk of your personality, propensity to disease, lifespan, and so forth.**

Until recently, it's been difficult to "read" those letters, and even tougher to understand what they do. The **Human Genome Project** is a research initiative that began in 1990 with the goal of sequencing—or identifying—all of the chemical units that make up the genetic blueprint required to build a human being. It took thirteen years to complete, and is one of humankind's greatest achievements.

At the time, the goal seemed nearly impossible, and some skeptics predicted that the costs would run wild, soaring perhaps uncontrollably to hundreds of billions of dollars. But as we all know from Moore's Law, technological progress is like an unstoppable force of nature. It's an accepted truth in Silicon Valley that technology tends to grow twice as powerful every eighteen months, while the price halves.

One of the few people who foresaw with certainty that the genomic sequence could be achieved was my dear friend **Ray Kurzweil**, one of the greatest engineers and inventors of this century. Knowing how technology compounds in power and drops in cost, Ray not only recognized that the entire genome could be sequenced in under thirteen years, but even predicted the timeline and the cost, estimating it would cost $2.7 billion.

Yet after seven and a half years of intense scientific research, the international team was able to sequence only 1 percent of the human genome. Skeptics pointed to failure, and said that at that rate it was going to take seven hundred years to complete. **And yet Ray Kurzweil knew the team was exactly on track.**

How? Because 1 percent is only seven doublings from 100 percent—and it had been doubling every year. **Sure enough, less than six years later, we miraculously achieved this feat of humanity, on budget and on time!** "We don't think in these exponential terms. And that exponential growth has continued since the end of the genome project," said Kurzweil.

Since then, the price has plummeted, outpacing Moore's Law by a factor of three. **Today, what cost $2.7 billion and took thirteen years can be done in a few days and costs less than $1,000. That's such a staggering drop in price that it's a bit like being able to buy a Tesla Model X—for a nickel! In fact, a few years from now, companies like Illumina are promising to do the same in an hour and for $100.**

Why does cheaper, faster genomic sequencing matter? Because it gives us a map of how cells function, so we can design better interventions. It's a healthcare game changer. Put differently, there are a few main ways to fix a cell. **Gene therapy *replaces* defective or missing DNA inside a cell, gene-editing techniques like CRISPR allow you to *repair* the DNA inside that cell, and stem cell therapies *replace that cell entirely*. Thanks to our increasingly accurate maps, all of these interventions are now hitting the market.**

The biggest news of the last few years is CRISPR-Cas9, which has become our leading weapon in the fight against genetic diseases. **The discovery and application of this technology earned Jennifer Doudna and Emmanuelle Charpentier the 2020 Nobel Prize in Chemistry. "This year's prize is about rewriting the code of life," declared Goran Hansson, the secretary-general of the Royal Swedish Academy of Sciences, when he made the announcement of their Nobel Prize.** Considering CRISPR's wide-ranging potential, it was practically an understatement.

Technically, it's an engineering tool that allows us to target precise locations in the gene code and then edit that DNA. Want to remove the string of DNA that produces muscular dystrophy? Simple. Just target that spot in the genome, unleash CRISPR-Cas9, and snip, snip, snip—problem solved. One way to think of it is as the genetic equivalent of a trusty word processing program. **CRISPR allows its users to snip a stretch of DNA and then either disable the affected sequence or replace it with a new one.**

At this point you may be asking the same question I did: **What is the** exact difference between **CRISPR** gene editing and gene therapy? They sound very similar, don't they? Here's the key point to distinguish them. **While CRISPR gene editing fixes a typo in the existing genome, leaving the original gene with its typo corrected, by contrast gene therapy injects a completely new copy of an entire gene into the cell's nucleus. In some diseases, where the correct gene was missing altogether, gene therapy will add what wasn't there. In other cases, where there is an incorrect copy, gene therapy can add a correct copy, which helps offset the disease.**

In fact, more than 2,500 gene therapy clinical trials have been approved, are in progress, or have already been completed, as we speak.

Another key point is that CRISPR uses an editing protein discovered in bacteria called CRISPR-Cas9 (by the way, there are many different Cas proteins, Cas9 is just the most famous) to find the errant DNA and make the edit. Gene therapy, on the other hand, uses a specially modified virus as a "vector" to deliver the new, healthy gene into the target cells. The viruses act like biological delivery vans, whisking a correct copy of the gene into the nuclei of the malfunctioning cells. This may sound complex, but **gene therapy's allure can be explained very simply: <u>IT'S A ONE-TIME TREATMENT THAT CURES THE DISEASE INSTEAD OF A THERAPY THAT MUST BE REPEATED FOR THE REST OF YOUR LIFE.</u>** A quick fix instead of a lifetime of popping pills or enduring injections. **A cure instead of a patch. A patch can smooth things over, but a cure? A cure can completely reshape a person's entire life.**

I don't want these stories to merely astonish you. I want them to give you new hope. And you know what the best part is? Genetic interventions like these are not far-off, pie-in-the-sky possibilities. **In fact, more than 2500 gene therapy clinical trials have been approved, are in progress, or have already been completed, as we speak. Over the next few years, these transformative genomic technologies could change or save your life—or the lives of the people you love.**

CURING BLINDNESS WITH GENE THERAPY

"I once was lost but now I am found.
Was blind but now I see."

—"AMAZING GRACE"

Dr. Peter Marks is the director of the Center for Biologics Evaluation and Research at the FDA. It's a hugely important job, overseeing the branch of the agency responsible for approving new medications, including gene therapies and vaccines for threats like COVID-19. **By late 2020, only two gene therapies had secured FDA approval. But more than a thousand active investigational drug applications for gene therapies were pending at the agency—an indication that this technology has reached a major tipping point.** Soon, there will be gene therapies for scores of diseases.

"Even during COVID-19 times, in the first half of 2020, we were on track to receive as many or more gene therapy applications as we received in 2019," says Marks. "Gene therapy is the wave of the future."

Ultimately, Marks expects the gene therapy revolution to encompass all kinds of illnesses—for example, Alzheimer's disease, various cancers, even high cholesterol. But for now, rare diseases are the prime target. When we talk about rare diseases, you might assume that these are obscure disorders affecting a handful of people. **But would you care to guess how many people have a rare disease? Answer: 7000 rare diseases affect up to 30 million Americans. That's almost one in ten Americans impacted by a "rare" disease.**[1]

The majority of these diseases have a genetic component. What's more, fewer than 10 percent have an FDA-approved treatment. That combination—lots of sick people, not a lot of good treatment options—means that the rare disease category is ripe for groundbreaking interventions involving gene therapy and gene editing. **Zolgensma, the second gene therapy approved in the U.S., essentially cures spinal muscular atrophy. The first, Luxturna, is turning night into day, restoring sight**

---

1 National Organization for Rare Disorders, "Rare Disease Facts."

to people with hereditary blindness. To explain why I'm so excited about these medical advances, let me tell you a story.

In 2017, when **Christian Guardino was 16, he appeared on** *America's Got Talent.* He brought the house down with a soulful rendition of Ed Sheeran's song "Let It Rain." The performance left Simon Cowell speechless, which is quite a feat! Another judge, Howie Mandel, was so blown away that he awarded the "Golden Buzzer" to Guardino, automatically sending him to the next round. Guardino couldn't believe his eyes as he gazed down from the stage at the celebrity judges and the ecstatic audience. He recalls, **"Because I'd been visually impaired for so long, to be able to see those four judges sitting there, watching my performance, was amazing."**

Guardino's mom loves to tell the tale of how she discovered that her son was musically talented. One day, when he was a few months old, she sang scales to him while he splashed in the tub. He sang them back in perfect pitch, prompting her to call her mother and ask: "Is this normal?" But at around the same time, the family was hit with distressing news. **Guardino was diagnosed with Leber congenital amaurosis (LCA), a rare eye disorder caused by inherited genetic mutations.**

In the years after his diagnosis, he had a number of painful collisions. One time, he slammed into a mailbox while playing football; another time, he needed stitches after crashing into the kitchen table. He simply hadn't seen them. **Over time, his vision darkened, shadows lengthened, and he turned to music as a coping mechanism. He might not be able to see, but at least he could sing.**

Then, in 2012, Guardino learned about some cutting-edge researchers who were developing a new gene therapy. **He joined a clinical trial and received one injection of Luxturna in each eye, one week apart. "They put a gene in a safe virus, and that virus helps the gene find its missing place in me,"** says Guardino, providing a simple and accurate description of how gene therapy works. That was in June 2013.

The day after the first injection, he removed his eye patch and glanced at the floor. To his amazement, he saw diamond shapes on a carpet that he'd previously thought had no pattern. "It was pretty crazy," he recalls. Since then, he's seen countless incredible sights. The

moon. The stars. Fireworks blazing across the night sky. "It worked," says Guardino. "Boy, did it work!"

After he was awarded the Golden Buzzer on *America's Got Talent*, Guardino was heading out when Simon Cowell stopped him. Cowell had just heard Guardino's backstory from a producer. "Wow," said Cowell. "You didn't let your disability stop you. It doesn't define who you are." For Guardino, that exchange was one of the highlights of the whole unforgettable experience: "I always thought LCA *would* define me. But that night, it didn't. Simon heard my voice and he liked me without even knowing my story. It made me feel incredible about myself."

In the end, Guardino was knocked out in the semifinals. But his appearances on *America's Got Talent* led him to release several singles and perform all over the country. He still gets pre-show jitters, but nothing that approaches the pressure he felt before his most important performance to date: testifying before an FDA advisory committee about the need for Luxturna to be approved. **He recalls telling the panel of scientists: "It's either this or we go blind." In 2017, the FDA voted unanimously to approve Luxturna, making it the first gene therapy to be given the green light.**

THE HERO WHO FOUND A CURE FOR BLINDNESS

"There was no road map. We were on our own."

—DR. KATHERINE HIGH, former president of Spark Therapeutics

One person who joined Guardino on that historic day was a pioneering scientist named **Dr. Katherine High**, who was largely responsible for Guardino's ability to see the diamond-patterned carpet and the moon in the sky. **"Science will be changed forever because of what Kathy did,"** says Guardino, his voice thick with emotion. **"She changed my life."**

For Dr. High, it's a lifelong calling to help people achieve their destiny. **"People born with serious genetic defects don't have the same chance that someone else does,"** she says. **"If we can fix that and level the playing field, they have the chance to be who they were meant to be."**

High's scientific ambitions began early. When she was ten, Santa brought her a chemistry set with instructions for how to carry out more than one hundred experiments. She spent many hours mixing and tinkering alongside her father, who had big dreams for his daughter. This was in the early 1960s, when it wasn't common for a woman to enter the sciences, let alone make a name for herself. High's father wanted her to attend MIT, become an aeronautical engineer, and work for NASA. She chose a different path to scientific glory, majoring in chemistry at Harvard and then enrolling in medical school at the University of North Carolina at Chapel Hill (UNC).

After a hematology fellowship at Yale, Dr. High returned to UNC and worked on understanding the molecular basis of hemophilia. UNC had a hemophilia dog colony, and she tried using gene therapy to correct the canines' gene malfunction. Those early efforts failed. But she continued to focus on hemophilia at Children's Hospital of Philadelphia (CHOP).

In 1999, Dr. High published a landmark paper showing that her team had succeeded in curing hemophilia in a dog model using gene therapy that relied on vectors—viruses that carry the corrected gene to the spot in the genome that's malfunctioning.[2] These viruses had been manufactured by a California biotech company that folded in the 1990s, along with almost every other gene therapy startup. Back then, the science seemed promising, but the timing was all wrong. The technology sounded like science fiction—remotely plausible but a bit unlikely!

Does Dr. High sound like a person who was ready to call it quits? No way! She appealed to the CEO of CHOP, one of the nation's most prestigious children's hospitals, to set up vector production so she could continue her research. **"I figured he'd say no because no one believed that gene therapy would work,"** says High. **"But to my great and undying surprise, he said yes, with one condition." He told her: "You can't spend all this money only on hemophilia. You also have to work on** *other* **diseases that affect children."**

As luck would have it, Dr. High was friends with a scientist, named **Dr. Jean Bennett,** who also worked on dogs. **Dr. Bennett, who was**

---

2 Herzog et al., "Long-Term Correction of Canine Hemophilia B by Gene Transfer of Blood Coagulation Factor IX Mediated by Adeno-Associated Viral Vector."

researching a rare form of inherited blindness, had data indicating that a particular gene therapy corrected the dogs' vision. This raised an intriguing question. Could her research be developed so it would help humans with certain forms of inherited blindness? In 2005, High and Bennett teamed up. In 2007, they launched a clinical trial. In 2012, they moved to Phase 3 testing. In 2013, they formed Spark Therapeutics to bring this therapy—a gene that encodes an enzyme found only in the cells in the back of the eye—to market.

Dr. High became Spark's somewhat reluctant president and head of R&D, leaving "the best job in the world" in academia to turn this moonshot dream into a reality. "I was able to recruit people I couldn't have gotten had I not been willing to go in myself," she says. "I'd spent much of my academic career trying to move gene therapy forward, and this was the point when I had to say, *If this is what it takes, that's what I'm going to do.*"

It's been a long and winding road since those early days of working on dogs with hemophilia. But Dr. High's persistence has paid off spectacularly. The prize at the end of the road was Luxturna, a gene therapy product that's now used to treat patients with an inherited retinal disease caused by mutations in both copies of their RPE65 gene. When that gene doesn't work properly, the results can range from progressive vision loss to complete blindness. Some babies are diagnosed when their parents notice that they're not tracking objects with their eyes; others are diagnosed later in childhood. By age 12, most kids with this disease need to be placed in Braille classrooms.

Can you imagine being a parent in that situation and discovering that a *single injection* into each of your kid's eyes could cure your child's blindness? It's almost biblical in nature. After these injections, the cells in the retina of each eye are able to produce the RPE65 protein, which enables the visual cycle to work properly. *I ask you, what could be more miraculous?*

Dr. High, one of the great pioneers of gene therapy, expects more approvals to come with each passing year. "At Spark, our saying was *'We don't follow footsteps. We create the path.'* There was no road map. We were on our own," she says. "What's that saying . . . the early bird gets the worm, but the second mouse gets the cheese? Every product builds on the product before."

THERE HAS NEVER BEEN A GREATER TIME TO BE ALIVE

Doug Ingram, CEO of Sarepta Therapeutics, a leader in gene therapy for rare disease, says it best: "The time is now. We have an opportunity that historically has not been possible over the arc of human history—to use the tools of gene therapy and eventually gene editing to create a better life at minimum and perhaps completely transform and save lives. . . . We're trying to lead a revolution, dragging tomorrow into today, bringing gene therapy to patients who need it now."

Here's the bottom line: **If you are or someone in your family is one of the 30 million Americans living with a rare genetic disease, there has never been a better time to have hope that a treatment—or, even better, a cure—lies around the corner. Thanks to gene editing and gene therapy, diseases that have historically had no available treatments are now on the cusp of breakthroughs. Remember, more than twenty-five hundred gene therapy clinical trials have been approved, are in progress, or have already been completed. Don't resign yourself to thinking there's no solution; connect with the special interest group associated with your disease and ask if they are working on clinical trials using CRISPR or gene therapy to relieve your symptoms.** Before you know it, we will see the day when every genetic disease can be treated.

HOW GENE THERAPY CAN FIX A BROKEN HEART

"Our cells retain their youthful digital information even when we are old. To become young again, we just need to find some polish to remove the scratches."
—DAVID SINCLAIR, PhD, *Lifespan: Why We Age—and Why We Don't Have To*

I want to highlight the brilliant work of **Dr. Deepak Srivastava, a cardiologist who is president of the Gladstone Institutes,** a biomedical research organization at the forefront of the revolution in regenerative medicine. **Srivastava—a member of our Life Force Advisory Board—shared information about how he's using gene therapy to repair heart damage.**

As Srivastava explained, **"The heart is chock-full of cells that we call**

fibroblasts that normally send important signals to support the muscle, and **they also make scar tissue when the heart is injured."** These fibroblast cells produce excess collagen when activated under stress, and this has a negative impact. **But what if you could control the fate of those fibroblast cells, reprogramming them so they could perform an entirely** *different* **function within the heart? Incredibly, "that's what we've been able to do,"** says **Srivastava.** Here's how it works:

In experiments with mice, Srivastava used gene therapy to deliver a combination of genes into the fibroblast cells in the heart after the mice suffered a heart attack. **One injection of these genes was sufficient to change the fate of the fibroblast cells, turning them into beating heart cells. Peter refers to this approach as nothing less than cellular alchemy. That's right! Srivastava was able to create brand-new muscle in a failing heart by convincing fibroblast cells already in the heart to change jobs!** "We're reprogramming a cell's fate," he says.

As I'm sure you can see, the implications are mind-bending. Now that scientists have figured out how to "control the fate of cells," it's not hard to imagine using the same approach to repair tissue damage caused by everything from brain disease to liver disease.

For Srivastava, **this research took on new meaning when his father recently died after many years of living with "a damaged heart that impaired him severely. . . . We do everything with a great sense of urgency because there are people out there who are waiting and dying. I think about it every day—how we need to do everything we can to accelerate. We weren't fast enough for my father." But Srivastava hopes to be fast enough for folks like you and me, our parents, and our kids**.

The good news is that the Gladstone Institute keeps spinning out new companies to develop these regenerative technologies, so they'll be available to us in the years to come. One of these biopharmaceutical startups, **Tenaya Therapeutics, is working on curative therapies for heart disease—the world's leading cause of death. Among other things, Tenaya—which went public in the summer of 2021—is trying to reprogram fibroblasts as a way to replace lost heart cells and restore cardiac function after patients have had heart attacks.**

THE MIRACLE OF CRISPR: EDITING
THE ERRORS IN OUR DNA

"The more we know, the more we realize there is to know."

—JENNIFER DOUDNA, PhD, inventor of
CRISPR, 2020 Nobel laureate in chemistry

That goal of redefining the human race is already well under way, thanks to Jennifer Doudna, Emmanuelle Charpentier, and their discovery of CRISPR-Cas9, the gene editing mechanism that resulted in them being crowned Nobel laureates in 2020.

Remember, while gene therapy involves inserting a new, missing, or corrected gene into your cells, CRISPR gene editing involves editing an existing gene, repairing the incorrect letter that is, or letters that are, causing a genetic disease. **In other words, this tool is used to edit the genome that determines so much of who you are. In a 2015 TED talk, Doudna explained that it's "analogous to the way that we use a word-processing program to fix a typo in a document." But in this case, we're talking about changing the code of your life.**

Doudna grew up in Hawaii, where the natural beauty of the islands inspired her interest in biology. Her father, a professor of American literature, loved to read about science and gave his daughter a seminal book about the discovery of DNA's double helix structure when she was in sixth grade. Inspired to pursue a career in science at Pomona College, she had second thoughts while enrolled in general chemistry and wondered if she should switch gears and major in French. We have her French teacher to thank for encouraging Doudna to stay the course and eventually help develop CRISPR, which has revolutionized the field of genetics!

Not content with pioneering the field of gene editing, Doudna has helped to advance it further by cofounding **Mammoth Biosciences, a company dedicated to unlocking the potential of the *next* generation of the technology by discovering new proteins. You might call it CRISPR 2.0.**

You know what's really cool about these new versions of CRISPR? They are not being engineered in a lab. They're being discovered in

nature. For nonscientists like me, this whole process can seem a little intimidating. But the bottom line is simple: The fact that more of these novel CRISPR-associated proteins are being identified is wonderful, because it means that more options now exist to perform exquisitely targeted gene editing and to make multiple edits at the same time. That's great news for precision medicine.

The future is limitless, because bacteria and their proteins are everywhere. In fact, there's already another even more precise version of CRISPR-Cas9 called Prime Editing that sidesteps some of its less desirable outcomes. "In principle, the technique—called Prime Editing—could correct an estimated 89 percent genetic variants known to be associated with human diseases," declares the *Journal of the American Medical Association*.[3] That's quite a statement, isn't it? Every time you turn around, there's another huge leap forward.

In the meantime, as Mammoth continues to amass a portfolio of different versions of CRISPR, the firm is mulling where to deploy its powerful tools and how to enhance them. They've now been able to inject CRISPR straight into the bloodstream and direct it to the liver to cure amyloidosis, a disease that causes pain and fatigue, and disrupts the nervous system.

But these brilliant scientists are still striving for more. Next, they might optimize cell lines to help bring drugs to market faster. Some are beginning to target diseases, like cystic fibrosis or sickle cell anemia, that are caused by an error in a single gene. It's amazing to think that these naturally occurring tools can be deployed in so many lifesaving ways.

"We're unlocking the potential of CRISPR to tackle all sorts of diagnostics and therapeutics by unlocking new proteins," says Mammoth's CEO and cofounder Trevor Martin. "We could sit down and try to engineer this from scratch. But instead we're saying, 'Let's tap billions of years of evolution and leverage the diversity of life.'"

As it turns out, CRISPR not only *edits* the genome but can be used to *detect* DNA, too. Mammoth Biosciences is deploying CRISPR to be a DNA

---

3 Hampton, "DNA Prime Editing: A New CRISPR-Based Method to Correct Most Disease-Causing Mutations."

detective to sniff out DNA snippets that might signal viral infections, cancer, or defective genes. In 2018, it was first used to detect two strains of human papillomavirus (HPV). And now, **it has already been expanded for use in detecting bacterial infections, cancer, antibiotic resistance, and other viral infections such as COVID-19.** A separate test, using a different version of CRISPR, is being used to rapidly diagnose Zika and dengue virus. Not only that, but these tests are *rapid*, only taking *twenty minutes*.

I want you to understand the potential of this technology. **CRISPR was a scientific breakthrough for gene editing. And now, it's going to revolutionize diagnostic testing.** The world will soon see rapid, reliable diagnostic tests that are easy to use from the comforts of your own home.

THE JACKPOT GENE

Now, I need you to pay close attention here for one minute because I'm about to explain a so-called **jackpot gene that dramatically lowers your risk of Alzheimer's** is a tiny bit technical.

It's well known that the 10 to 15 percent of people who carry the **ApoE4 allele** (or version) of the **ApoE gene** are at *much greater risk* of developing Alzheimer's. **But you know what's cool? <u>The ApoE2 allele—which is the rarest version of the gene, carried by only 7 percent of the population—is associated with a *much lower risk* of Alzheimer's-related decline, not to mention enhanced longevity.</u>** Sign me up for that version! At the **Buck Institute for Aging** in Marin County, California, **Dr. Lisa Ellerby** is using CRISPR to investigate the mysterious neuroprotective role that ApoE2 plays in aging and disease. **I like to call it the jackpot gene, because, if you're lucky enough to have it, you've hit the genetic jackpot and have more protection than people without it.**

Did you know that women are at greater risk of developing Alzheimer's than men? Dr. Ellerby hopes her research will shed light on why it's more common for women to be diagnosed with the disease. She's also using gene therapy to deliver the ApoE2 gene into aged mice to see if its expression or any related treatment increases health span.[4] **If we can figure**

---

4 Buck Institute, "Exploiting a Gene That Protects against Alzheimer's."

out a way to translate this to humans, allowing us to access the magical benefits of this jackpot gene, it would be a true miracle.

As we've seen in this chapter, gene therapy and CRISPR are extraordinary tools for curing disease, but one of our advisors—**George Church, a founding father of genomics—sees gene therapy as a tool for curing the one disease that affects everyone, everywhere: aging.** "The idea with gene therapy was that you have someone with a rare genetic disease that's missing a particular protein, and you just put it back in. But the problem is, your body recognizes that protein as being foreign, and there's a chance you'll reject it." **By contrast, his strategy of using gene therapy to reverse aging involves putting in proteins that are** *already there*. **They've just diminished over time.** "We're just turning up the knob on genes that are already in your genome."

That only begins to convey the boldness of Dr. Church's ambition. What's his ultimate goal? A preventive elixir to reverse aging. I recently spoke with him over Zoom about this topic and wrapped up our conversation by saying "Thank you for your time. And thank you for your life's work." You know how he responded? He said, **"Tony, you can thank me when you're a hundred and fifty!"**

Let's turn now to hear the heroic story of the team that's paving the way for curing disease using a pathway to power. Let's learn about the wondrous WNT pathway . . .

CHAPTER 9

THE WONDROUS WNT PATHWAY: THE ULTIMATE FOUNTAIN OF YOUTH?

By Resetting the Signals to Our Stem Cells, Small Molecules Can Renew Our Body's Natural Balance—and Stop Degenerative Disease in Its Tracks

"We're reminding the body how it was when it was healthy."

—OSMAN KIBAR

On Day 2 of the Vatican's Unite to Cure conference, in a modern hall where the Pope greets bishops from around the world, we heard from one medical science superstar after the next. There were world-leading experts on the plant food revolution, next-gen genetic testing, and the stem cell "pharmacy of the future." Then a mild-mannered man with a professorial air took his seat on the dais. Wearing wire-rimmed glasses, a loosely knotted blue tie, and a shy smile, he spoke so softly that you had to lean forward to hear him. It was just before lunch, when people's attention tends to flag, and this speaker had some tough acts to follow. He didn't have a famous name or a big media profile. **But for the next twenty-two minutes, Osman Kibar—the founder and executive chair of an extraordinary startup called Biosplice—commanded that room.**

We'll soon be diving into the details of Osman's groundbreaking company and the science it believes will change the face of medicine. But first let me share with you the **"show" part of Osman's show-and-tell.** He began with **before-and-after X-rays of animal and human knees, where a single Biosplice injection grew fresh cartilage to heal bone-on-bone arthritis. You didn't have to squint to see the results; there was *visible* improvement. Then we saw before-and-after scans of an animal's colon, where angry purple masses of tumor vanished after treatment with a Biosplice pill.**

The next slides used graphs to plot the progress of eight different human tumors implanted into animals. **Over three short weeks, in an untreated control group, the tumors grew like weeds. But in each and every case, Osman said, their therapy was "able to reverse tumor growth and eliminate the tumors, both primary and metastatic."** That's a *huge* deal, because it's the *metastases*, the "secondary" malignancies that can pop up anywhere in the body, that are most elusive—and most dangerous.

There was more. **A Biosplice inhaler was healing lungs scarred by pulmonary fibrosis, which is generally considered untreatable. On deck was an Alzheimer's pill with stunning impact so far in reversing damage to brain tissue in animals. On the orthopedic front, the company was testing a lotion to repair torn tendons. Another lotion was showing strong promise with *androgenic alopecia*, which many of you know as male-pattern baldness,** the most common source of hair loss in both women and men. Osman was too modest to frame it this way, but the implications were clear: **Biosplice may have found a way to repair nearly every tissue and organ in the body—to make us functionally young again.**

The Vatican audience was no pushover, and at first you could cut their skepticism with a knife. I saw rows of crossed arms and rolled eyes—no one had heard anything like this before. But by the end of Osman's presentation, he definitely had people's attention. Many in the mostly middle-aged audience were leaning forward in eager interest, especially when he laid out a potential baldness cure!

I was sitting with friends who happened to be three of the smartest science minds around: my coauthor, Peter Diamandis; Dr. Sanjay Gupta, CNN's chief medical correspondent; and Dr. Mehmet Oz, the Emmy-winning TV host and professor of surgery at New York–Presbyterian Hospital, Columbia. They were buzzing among themselves,

midway between blown away and disbelieving: *This sounds crazy—could it be real?* Just one month earlier, the SEC had sued the top executives of Theranos, a diagnostics company once valued at $9 billion, for fraud. It was a worldwide scandal and a cautionary tale. Max Gomez, the CBS medical correspondent and Osman's moderator, voiced the general suspicion: "If something looks too good to be true, it probably is." If Biosplice had actually cracked the regeneration code, why wasn't there more data?

And so Osman explained: For the company's first eight years of existence (when it went under the name of Samumed), he and his colleagues "operated in stealth mode." To avoid tipping off the competition, they kept their data and progress to themselves—as a privately held company, they had that right. Around 2016, once Osman's executive team decided that their patents were far enough out front, they began revealing more details of their animal and human studies. And unlike the bogus blood-test machine hyped by Theranos, as Osman points out, therapeutic trials run by Biosplice fall under strict FDA reporting requirements.

By now I think you know that I'm a curious person, to say the least. I had to find out more, so I visited Osman at his company's steel-and-glass San Diego headquarters, where the parking lot is dotted with palm trees. I found out that **Biosplice has documented advances against eight all-too-common diseases: osteoarthritis, solid tumors, "liquid" tumors (like leukemias), Alzheimer's, tendinitis, degenerative disc disease, chronic lung scarring, and male-pattern baldness.**

The results looked miraculous. But Biosplice had simply found a way to **leverage our body's natural powers to renew itself—our life force. Biosplice has now presented its findings at scores of scientific meetings and in dozens of peer-reviewed journals. If their trials prove out (and there's no guarantee that they well), the winning therapy against some of the toughest cancers won't be chemotherapy or radiation or surgery. Believe it or not, it will be a once-a-day pill with minimal side effects. What's *really* exciting is that this prospective cancer remedy is just one of several radical therapies in the Biosplice pipeline.**

Since 2008, Osman and Cevdet Samikoglu (to whom Osman passed the torch as CEO in 2021) and their band of Turkish-born prodigies have been working around the clock, barely coming up for air. **Groundbreaking**

medicine is a slog. When you're out to change the world, it's usually two steps forward and one step back. Biosplice is tackling diseases that traditional medicine considers incurable or even untreatable, from arthritis to Alzheimer's. When science moves into uncharted territory, as Osman can tell you, there are bound to be wrong turns and temporary setbacks. But the fact remains that **any one of these bold therapies could become a lifeline for millions. Together they could rewrite our medical textbooks. They hold the power to change how we think about illness and—most of all—about health and healing.**

Recognizing the company's sterling safety record, federal regulators have given them a green light for eight carefully administered clinical human studies. Under the FDA's "compassionate use" policy, a program for unapproved medicines when nothing else is known to work, thousands of subjects have been treated with what Osman calls Biosplice's "secret recipe." (We'll share the ingredients with you shortly.)

While it's still early days for most of these trials, at least one set of Phase 3 results—for their landmark effort to effectively cure osteoarthritis—may be rolling out by the time you're reading this. **If the next round of data reads out as Biosplice hopes, and a single shot in the knee can offer long-term relief of chronic pain, an FDA-approved therapy could be on the market before the end of 2023. Imagine what it would feel like to regenerate your worn cartilage and walk or run without so much as a twinge. Imagine a flexible, powerful, brand-new *you*—for a cost of less than $5,000 per knee. (And then imagine how you'd feel with good-as-new shoulders or hips, the next joints on the company's hit list.)**

My coauthors and I have encountered an abundance of amazing healthspan solutions in writing this book, and here's what we need to tell you: Biosplice's proprietary molecules are demonstrating the power of regenerative medicine more dramatically than virtually anything else we've seen on the near horizon. They are showing the potential to have an extraordinary impact on humanity. You don't have to take my word for it. *Forbes* magazine put Osman on its cover and named **him one of their "30 Global Game Changers," alongside Jeff Bezos, Mark Zuckerberg, and Elon Musk.**

Some tremendously savvy people in the financial world are voting on

Biosplice with their wallets. **In April 2021, Biosplice announced $120 million in new equity financing,**[1] **on top of the more than half a billion dollars ($650 million) it raised under the banner of Samumed.**[2] **These savvy investors believe that Biosplice is more than a very smart guy's vision. So do I, which is why I also invested in the company. In fact, the venture capitalist Finian Tan, an early backer of Baidu (China's Google), believes the impact of the company's patented breakthrough could rival Alexander Fleming's discovery of antibiotics back in 1928.**[3] Does that sound a little much to you? Just slightly over the top? I might have thought so, too . . . until I heard Osman speak at the Vatican.

> *"Our small molecules can communicate with any progenitor stem cell in any tissue in the body and trigger them down any lineage . . . restoring the health of any particular tissue."*

—OSMAN KIBAR, at the Vatican's Unite to Cure conference

Sticking with the 40,000-foot version for the nonscientists among us, the gist of Osman's delivery was this: **From the day we're born until the time we die, our lives depend on the descendants of the embryonic stem cells that leave us at birth. They're called** *progenitor* **stem cells, descendants of stem cells that then further differentiate to create specialized cell types and maintain and repair every system in our body. One family of progenitor cells replenishes our blood and bone marrow. Another fixes damage to our central nervous system, a recent discovery that's given new hope to people with spinal cord injuries or Parkinson's or multiple sclerosis. A third, the epithelial family, keeps our skin supple and our hair follicles sprouting. A fourth, our** *mesenchymal* **(MEZ-IN-KIM-AL) stem cells, is in charge of muscle, bone, cartilage,**

---

1 Samumed press release, "Biosplice Therapeutics Closes $120 Million in Equity Financing to Advance Its Alternative Splicing Platform."

2 Samumed press release, "Samumed Closes on $438 Million in Equity Financing."

3 Meiling, "What's Bigger Than a Unicorn? Samumed Stuns Yet Again as Anti-Aging Pipeline Draws $438M at $12B Valuation."

ligaments, and tendons—like the rotator cuff I tore. These living cells are a core component of the life force within each and every one of us.

How does Biosplice fit into this picture? As Osman explained at the Vatican, **his company had deciphered how to utilize and impact something called the Wnt signaling pathway, a sort of relay circuit made of genes and proteins.** Our bodies have many biochemical pathways; each one is a sequence of chemical actions and reactions within our cells. But **Wnt is special. It signals our progenitor stem cells to make specific types of tissue—"when, how much, and when to stop,"** as Osman explained. **It has a huge say in how our cells** *differentiate* **and also how they** *proliferate*, **or multiply. So how important is Wnt? Let's just say it's the foundation for all animal life.** It's "the primary developmental pathway in the body," Osman says.

When we're young, up to age 20 or so, the Wnt pathway streams like a Zoom link with premium bandwidth and no hackers. Assuming normal good health, our progenitor stem cells give us what we need when and where we need it, no more and no less. **But as we age, 21st-century living takes its toll. Questionable lifestyle choices and environmental toxins and epigenetic "scratches" add up. Our Wnt signals get distorted**; they drift out of range and are drowned by static. Communication breaks down within cells and also between them. **We wind up with too much of some things and too little of others, and our healthspan takes a beating.**

But if we could retrieve the clear and timely cellular signals of our youth, or what David Sinclair calls our "lost information," we might reincarnate our optimal selves—our 20-year-old selves. The big Biosplice breakthrough is to bring the Wnt pathway back to base. Their small-molecule medicines target and penetrate particular stem cells and dial them up or down—think of the dimmer switch that controls your table lamp. When they're turned up, those tired, depleted cells in our joints or lungs or scalp will erupt in a frenzy of rejuvenation. When they're turned down, overabundant bone cells, for one example—the main cause of osteoarthritis—retreat and leave room for more cartilage. When they're turned down it also effects malignant tumor stem cells and they stop multiplying uncontrollably. Order trumps chaos.

Homeostasis is restored. Cellular creation and destruction return to their natural, healthy balance.

Venture capital isn't betting blind on Biosplice. **Osman and his team have compiled a winning track record wherever they've applied themselves, from the financial world to bench science.** In fact, Osman is a mathematical genius, something that has helped him in the analysis phase of solving some of these biochemical challenges. He even won the European Math Championship as a high school junior. In fact, shortly before launching the company, Osman entered his first poker tournament, just for kicks. He won it easily. A year later, he finished second in the World Series of Poker in Las Vegas and took home a cool $420,000. He then entered one more tournament, won again, and quit—he didn't like the mental "hangover effect," he said. What does he do for fun now instead? He reads textbooks in higher math, with meditation on the side for his own personal balance.[4]

At this point, as Biosplice continues to build on its early successes, even the professional cynics are coming around. But there's one group who never doubted Osman in the first place: the people who know him best.

"I've known him since we were eleven, and he's the smartest guy I know. If anybody's going to do something world-changing, he was my home run guy."

—CEVDET SAMIKOGLU, Osman Kibar's successor as CEO of Biosplice

Osman Kibar was born and raised on Turkey's Aegean coast. At age 11, in a high-stakes national exam involving 1.5 million students, he placed in the top one-hundredth of the top 1 percent—his ticket into Robert College, an elite American-run secondary school in Istanbul. After his triumph at the European Math Championship, "I pretty much had my pick of colleges," he told me. Smitten by California's Mediterranean climate (before the recent siege of wildfires), he chose Pomona College and the California Institute of Technology for a special dual degree program in mathematical economics and electrical engineering—your basic gut courses, right? Then it was on to the University of California, San Diego, for his PhD in biophotonics, a

---

4 Herper, "Cure Baldness? Heal Arthritis? Erase Wrinkles? An Unknown Billionaire's Quest to Reverse Aging."

futuristic field that links light technologies and medicine. Even before finishing graduate school, Osman founded the diagnostics company Genoptix.
Four years after going public, it was bought by Novartis, the pharma giant,
for $470 million.

Excited by the prospect of seeding more biotech innovations, Osman
joined Pequot Capital, a Wall Street private equity firm. One month later,
9/11 tanked the stock market and sent investors running for cover. The
high-risk, high-reward deals that Osman lived for were abandoned. "One
morning I woke up, I was an investment banker," he told me. "It had nothing to do with technology anymore." He returned to San Diego, where at
least the sun was warm.

**In a development that would change the trajectory of Osman's
career, and maybe some of 21st-century medicine along with it, the
pharmaceutical giant Pfizer proposed an audacious joint venture, a
Hail Mary incubator. They'd been working on this molecular signaling
pathway that could change** *everything*, **the Pfizer scientists said—but
there was one small problem. Since 1982, when the Wnt pathway was
first discovered, nobody could figure out how to manipulate it safely
and effectively.** Scientists knew that lots of illnesses were the result of a
dysregulated Wnt signaling—no argument there. "What they couldn't do,"
Osman says, "is come up with a way to bring it back into healthy operation."
Prior efforts failed to stay in their lane. They compromised healthy tissue.
"Modulating is easy," as Osman points out—or easy for him, at least. "But to
do it safely, that's the challenge."[5] **It goes back to a principle attributed
to the Greek physician Hippocrates: "First, do no harm."**

Biosplice was founded in 2008 as a Pfizer incubator called Samumed,
before Osman separated and struck out on his own. Osman seeded his next
success in an unlikely setting: a pickup basketball game with some of his old
Robert School brainiac classmates, the best and the brightest. Eventually
he persuaded three of them to join his startup. First on board, as CFO, was
Cevdet Samikoglu, a Harvard MBA who'd made his mark at Goldman Sachs,
Wall Street's alpha dog investment bank, and then the wildly successful Grey-
wolf Capital hedge fund. Then came chief legal officer Arman Oruc, who'd

---

5 Breakthrough: The Caltech Campaign, "Winding Back the Clock."

cofounded the Washington, DC, office of Simpson Thacher & Bartlett, one of the nation's most prestigious law firms. When Yusuf Yazici, an internationally renowned rheumatologist at NYU, got wind of what was going on, he texted Cevdet: **"You have to get me in on this. Osman has found the God pill!"** He joined as chief medical officer. All three of these old friends took steep pay cuts, with no signing bonuses. Why? Because they trusted Osman and believed he was on the verge of doing something big. The Turkish dream team was complete . . . and their dream would soon come to fruition.

Biosplice broke through where others had failed by doing two things better than anyone else. First they identified the biological targets— the signaling proteins—that could corral a Wnt pathway gone haywire. Then they chemically engineered a lineup of unique molecules to trigger their targets to jump into action. Sometimes—with hair loss or a damaged spinal cord—the goal was to stimulate stem cells that were asleep at the switch. But where there was *too* much regeneration, as in cancer or Alzheimer's, the aim was to "tell the tissue, 'Chill out, settle down, you have to do less,'" Osman said. **"That's why we call it *restorative* medicine."**

When you're tweaking an ancient evolutionary mechanism, it pays to beware of unintended consequences. The last thing you'd want to do is overstimulate someone's liver cells into a tumor or add fibrosis in a lung. **The sweet spot? Healing diseased tissue while leaving normal cells alone.** The beauty of the Wnt pathway is that it affects only undeveloped cells. Progenitor stem cells (again, these are cells that give us what we need, when we need it, and where we need it) are tuned 24/7 to the Wnt frequency. But fully differentiated adult cells don't come equipped with a receiver, and so they never get the signal. **This explains how Biosplice's proprietary molecules have rung up such an outstanding safety profile to date. It's why they can launch their D-day assault on disease without the collateral havoc of many traditional drugs. They can brighten or dim that lamp without changing the TV's volume or the heat from the radiator.**

The cherry on top is that the molecules don't stick around for very long. Many have a half-life measured in days or even hours. Once our Wnt levels snap back into equilibrium, Osman said, the molecules pass the baton to the progenitor stem cells we were born with: "They know what to do.

They've been doing it all our lives. They get jump-started, and it's a chain reaction." **Although these medicines are incredibly complex to produce, they have a fundamentally simple job: to remind our body to do what comes naturally.**

All of the in-progress Biosplice studies have one critical thing—one *astonishing* thing—in common. At the doses the company plans to commercialize, *none* **of its small-molecule therapies have caused any significant harmful side effects. They tweak their Wnt targets and call it a day. Whenever they run into healthy tissue, Osman told me, they "just float around harmlessly and then get extracted over time." Like the Lone Ranger, they take care of the bad guys and then hotfoot it out of town.**

"It doesn't matter who cures osteoarthritis. Whoever cures it
has the potential to be the largest company in the world."

—FINIAN TAN, venture capitalist

A few years back, Biosplice published a study of its treatment for osteoarthritis, a painful, debilitating condition that plagues 30 million people in the United States alone. Of 61 patients who took a solitary injection into their knee, all 61 showed visible improvement—less pain, more mobility—twenty-four weeks later. Even more remarkable, they added on average nearly two millimeters of fresh cartilage. "That's what impressed the Food and Drug Administration the most— the X-ray data," Osman told me. "We were actually able to demonstrate that causative link between the pain and function and the disease modification. Of course, we expected it, but it's such a nice thing to be able to actually show it to the FDA."[6]

By signaling a protein called beta-catenin, the Biosplice molecule—called lorecivivint—also calmed inflammation and stopped the breakdown of existing cartilage. **"We wait for six to twelve months while the mesenchymal stem cells are recruited,"** Osman said. **"They multiply, they**

---

6 Yazici et al., "A Novel Wnt Pathway Inhibitor, SM04690, for the Treatment
   of Moderate to Severe Osteoarthritis of the Knee"; McAlindon and Bannuru,
   "Latest Advances in the Management of Knee OA."

differentiate, and we are able to regenerate new cartilage. The health of the whole joint is restored back to normal." Lorecivivint is an equal-opportunity medicine; the octogenarians in the study improved as much as anyone else. "No matter how old the patient is, once the stem cells are triggered, they regenerate," Osman said. Once the Wnt pathway's signals are back in tune, there is "no difference between the regenerative capability of a forty-year-old, sixty-year-old, or an eighty-year-old."

Do you have chronic joint pain? Does someone you care about suffer with it? If so, you know just how much is riding on this startup's success. There are zero drugs on the market today—not one—that can halt osteoarthritis, let alone reverse it. Patients are traditionally left with two less than wonderful options. They can medicate their symptoms with painkillers or anti-inflammatories, which do nothing to slow the progress of the disease and come with serious downsides of their own, from liver damage to addiction. Or they can endure the pain and expense and long months of recovery from a surgical knee, or other joint, replacement.

Compared to these approaches, the Biosplice alternative—one injection—sounds awfully appealing. Since the medicine's administration is strictly "local," the company says, side effects are nil. The molecule binds to the surface of the bone, rallies the mesenchymal stem cells in the neighborhood, and spurs them to be fruitful and multiply. Over the next six months, the medicine gets excreted through the lymphatic system. It never enters the bloodstream.

What's more, the new Wnt-inspired cartilage rivals "that of a teenager," Osman says, fresh out of the stem cell factory. The progenitor cells need only a wakeup call to remember what they used to do before we were old enough to vote: "You can run, jump, whatever activity you want." After the benefits wear off and the cartilage wears down again, three years or so down the road, you can return for another shot.

If this sounds like some fantasy graphic novel, I'm with you! But I've witnessed firsthand the impact on these patients and it's blown my mind. One afternoon I was visiting with Osman and asking about new applications of their unique therapies. He took me to his computer and said, "Take a look at this." He brought up a video of adult rats whose spines had been destroyed. None of the animals could move their legs or arms.

The Biosplice researchers injected lorecivivint into the spines of half of the rats. Six months later, the untreated control group was still wasting away, while the injected rats regenerated a whole new spinal cord that was "younger and stronger" on a cellular level, Osman said, than what they had in the first place. These restored rats were racing through a maze. I literally couldn't believe my eyes. The results were so strong that Biosplice launched a clinical trial for degenerative disc disease.[7]

While animal trials must be taken with a grain of salt, in this case they certainly appear to be a justified cause for optimism. Why? Because many animal studies don't transfer to humans. However, the Wnt pathway is extremely "well-conserved," as scientists say. It's stayed intact and unchanged through hundreds of millions of years of evolution. Its signaling mechanism is basically identical in fruit flies and mice and dogs and monkeys and humans. If a Biosplice therapy works in a rodent, as Osman told us, "we believe with strong certainty that the same molecule" will work in people.

On a related point: There's another Biosplice molecule that dials up the Wnt pathway to heal damaged Achilles tendons, injured rotator cuffs, or severe tennis elbows. Delivered in a rub-on lotion, this one is also in human clinical trials. Once it sailed through a Phase 1 safety test, Osman couldn't resist becoming his own guinea pig. He'd wrecked his knee so badly playing soccer—it bent opposite the way the good lord intended—that for six months he had to sit with his leg out straight. Four days after applying the lotion, "the pain was gone," he told me. Less than a week after that, he was back on the playing field. I caution you that all of these stories are anecdotal, what really matters is what the final FDA Phase 2 and Phase 3 trials show us. But clearly Biosplice is on a pathway of discovery that could transform the quality of our lives.

---

7 Yazici, "A Study of the Safety, Tolerability, and Pharmacokinetics of SM04690 Injectable Suspension Following Single Intradiscal Injection in Subjects with Degenerative Disc Disease."

"We're not just targeting signs and symptoms. We're actually allowing the patient to not be a patient anymore."

—OSMAN KIBAR

Osman and his team estimate that an overactive Wnt signaling pathway—the result of a genetic mutation—is responsible for up to 40 percent of human cancers overall. **The percentages skew higher for more aggressive, faster-growing tumors: 93 percent of colorectal cancers, 90 percent of liver cancers, two of three pancreatic cancers, 50 percent of breast cancers.**[8] **Biosplice therapies, now in early-stage Phase 1 trials, shrink these types of tumors by blocking cancer cells from proliferating.** "Tumor cells that cannot multiply commit suicide after a matter of three or four days," Osman explains. "In three weeks, it's an exponential decline."

Unlike osteoarthritis, cancer is a systemic problem. Metastases are unpredictable and extremely challenging. In aggressive brain tumors, for example, surgeries are often out of the question. Why? Because, as scientists explain, conventional chemotherapies are pretty much useless since they're blocked by the blood-brain barrier, a border wall of specialized cells designed to contain infections.[9] **Biosplice has figured out a way to penetrate this barricade and stay biologically active in the brain. (As proof, the Wnt-modulating molecule shows up in the patients' cerebrospinal fluid.) The bottom line? The Biosplice therapy may have the potential to treat conditions now considered death sentences.**[10]

When I visited Osman more recently, he could barely contain his excitement—in his calm and low-key way, of course—over a recent discovery. It began with a small group of protein catalysts, called *kinases* (KI-nases), that govern nearly every major biological process. When the Wnt pathway is muddled, the body's stem cells are like factories with faulty switches. They generate useless kinases or even harmful ones.

---

8 Beaupre, "A Study Evaluating the Safety and Pharmacokinetics of Orally Administered SM08502 in Subjects with Advanced Solid Tumors."

9 Canadian Cancer Society, "Chemotherapy for Brain and Spinal Cord Tumors."

10 Melão, "Samumed's SM07883 Can Prevent Tau-Mediated Neuroinflammation, Neurodegeneration in Mice, Study Shows."

After years of research on a few critical kinase families, **Biosplice has gained an even deeper understanding of regenerative science—***why* **and** *how* **their medicines can manipulate the Wnt pathway.** The upstream factor is something called the *alternative splicing mechanism*. It's how stem cells transcribe their DNA into messenger RNA (or mRNA), which in turn determines which proteins get manufactured and what the cells become. (It also explains the company's new name.) Most DNA-to-mRNA transcriptions are hardwired, but a significant minority are subject to mutations, the source of rogue proteins and a glitchy Wnt signaling pathway. As CEO Cevdet Samikoglu explained to us, "You get aberrant mRNA or too much of an mRNA you don't need or too little of an mRNA you do need." The Biosplice molecules can't stop mutations from happening, but they can silence the rogue proteins before they do their damage.

While other biopharmaceutical companies have also targeted the alternative splicing mechanism, the Biosplice approach has "much broader applicability," Cevdet added. The company's compounds are "highly selective" in homing in on a particular branch of a kinase family tree, **"but once you zoom into that branch, they are hitting everything." The rifle becomes a shotgun.** On the one hand, the Biosplice platform has extraordinary promise to combat complex diseases caused by multiple mutations, like cancer, where more than one switch may need fixing. On the other hand, the molecules' selectivity figures to limit adverse side effects, like the gastrointestinal issues that come with standard cancer treatments.

The goal of the next generation of Biosplice therapies is to attack different tumors with laser precision. The lower-hanging fruit are six of the more common malignancies: cancers of the prostate, breast, lung, ovaries, uterus, and colon. (Pancreatic cancer, an even more intricate problem, will be tackled down the road.) The company's custom molecules will give the relevant stem cells "a nudge in the right direction," Osman says. "Once the correct composition of proteins is generated, the cell is healthy again."

As you can see, Biosplice is a long way from being satisfied. They have in their sights almost every leading cause of death and disability. They aim to restore damaged cardiac muscle, post–heart attack, by delivering a Wnt-stimulating molecule through a special stent. Cardiac progenitor cells will bathe in the elixir and regenerate the injured tissue. **What's more, they believe that a pill-delivered molecule can revive brain neurons ravaged by Alzheimer's.**

Looking farther to the future, Osman and Cevdet are confident that a way will be found to awaken dormant stem cells to impact or cure Parkinson's and ALS, and perhaps even macular degeneration. Other targets would be traumatic brain injuries, and hearing loss, and dozens of "orphan diseases" that afflict hundreds of thousands of people but have yet to find a therapeutic market.[17] **They have an internal "library" of more than 50,000 small molecules that can modulate the Wnt pathway.** Used in different combinations, these medicines could potentially treat an unlimited number of conditions.

In other words, the company's trials to date have barely scratched the surface. Frayed joints, dimmed retinas, raging tumors, immune systems gone bonkers—all are fair game for this revolutionary approach. **"We have not encountered any tissue that is not renewable," Osman says.** How exciting is that? When I hear about these latest breakthroughs, the transformations that lie in the not too distant future, I can only wonder: How can the Biosplice team get to sleep at night?

And before I forget, let me bring you up to date on the company's work on androgenic alopecia. Ongoing studies in Turkey have established that **a Biosplice lotion-based molecule increases hair follicle counts—and with none of the side effects, including sexual dysfunction, that some men experience with the widely prescribed finasteride (Propecia). In the pictures they shared with me, patients had noticeably fewer bald spots.** Though the therapy may take a while to cross the regulatory divide between Europe and the U.S., it's just a matter of time.

And how about this for a bonus? The same progenitor "dermal" stem cells that grow hair also go to the rescue of aging skin.

"We call our platform a fountain of youth, but piece by piece."

—OSMAN KIBAR

Biosplice has a large vision, but it comes in two parts. For now the company is going after one disease at a time, Osman says, using their Wnt toolbox to "restore the health of patients piecemeal and thereby increase their quality of life and healthspan." **The next step is even more ambitious: to turn back our biological clock. To make our aging bodies limber, supple, and free of pain. Osman isn't content with the concept of "anti-aging." Biosplice is all about *"de-aging,"* he says: "We define health not just as lack of disease, but what our optimal health was when we were younger." He sees the Wnt pathway as a basic tool (though not the only one) to not just stop or slow the aging process, "but actually to reverse it. We believe we are going to make us younger."**

This is where the enormity of Biosplice's potential grows almost beyond imagining. **Once lorecivivint receives the FDA's blessing as a prescription osteoarthritis drug (as I said, they're in Phase 3 trials now and are hoping for an approval if all goes well), physicians will be able to legally and ethically prescribe it "off label" for any use they see fit. "The population that can benefit from more cartilage is tenfold the population that has osteoarthritis," Osman noted.** "At the age of forty we start losing cartilage, whether we have osteoarthritis or not. Same thing with tendons. I cannot jump like I used to when I was twenty." **He envisions a day when Biosplice will be marketing "cartilage regenerators" and "tendon repairers" for healthy middle-aged people. "Just put a few drops on each joint," he says, and we'll be like new.**[11]

Remember, there's no guarantee that their next approach will succeed. But the most advanced approach is the Phase 3 trials, and that should be completed around the time that this book becomes available. If they do succeed, you'll have the opportunity to have a single injection that will regrow your cartilage in as little as twelve months, literally like new! If for some reason this formulation doesn't pass, here's one thing you can be certain of—Osman and the Biosplice team will not rest until they find the exact formulation that creates the impact on the Wnt pathway to create regeneration, revitalization, and repair.

Like Peter Diamandis, Osman believes that our species has the capacity to live well beyond the historical limit of 120 years. As he told me that

---

11 Biosplice Therapeutics, "Biosplice Licenses Rights to Lorecivivint, a Novel Phase 3 Osteoarthritis Drug Candidate, to Samil for the Republic of Korea."

day in San Diego, "If you wear out your car's tires, you replace them. In theory, you could replace every part of the car indefinitely. After a while, there is nothing of the original, but it's still your car." **By rebalancing the Wnt pathway, Biosplice plans to do the same for our bodies—and not 100 years from now in some far-off future, but sooner than you may think. Over time, there might be relatively little left of your original tissues. But it would still be you. You, rejuvenated to your 20-year-old self—you, restored.**

Again, there's no guarantee of success in their endeavors, but as you can see from all of the heroes mentioned in this section, their level of absolute resolve and commitment to find answers are already changing our understanding of the human body's healing capacity and providing alternative solutions to some of our largest health challenges.

So let's recap!

You've learned about the miracle of organ regeneration and creation, the power of gene therapy and CRISPR to actually cure disease at the source, and how incisionless brain surgery using ultrasound is transforming Parkinson's and tremor patients, crossing the blood-brain barrier to help treat cancer, and even showing promise in combatting addiction. You've also learned about the mighty CAR T cell, and now the power of the wondrous Wnt pathway.

So where do we go now? Let's talk about the very specific things you can do right now to immediately transform the quality of your life even if you don't have any significant challenges. As we turn to Section 3 we'll introduce you to . . .

- **Chapter 10: Your Ultimate Vitality Pharmacy:** the power of hormones, peptides, and some of the most impactful pharmaceutical-grade nutraceuticals that scientists are using to create massive changes in health and performance.
- **Chapter 11: How to live pain-free**, and the most powerful tools available without drugs to free you from the ravages of physical pain.
- **Chapter 12: The power of simple lifestyle changes in a longevity diet**, tools that cost you nothing and can help you prevent disease and restore your body to its highest levels.

- **Chapter 13: The power of sleep,** which sounds so basic, and was something I didn't truly understand until recently. Learn how optimizing this third pillar of health can dramatically change your life.
- **Chapter 14: A quick guide to transform your strength and performance and increase muscle mass,** one of the most important factors when it comes to aging and warding off many diseases, including cancer.
- **Chapter 15: We'll also show you how to enhance your visible vitality,** and reveal the greatest breakthroughs in beauty that science is offering.
- **Chapter 16: And then finally, we have a special chapter on women's health,** so that we can dispel myths and provide empowering solutions for women to live full, healthy, and vibrant lives.

So let's move forward to Section 3, and discover the latest breakthroughs and technologies that are available NOW, and how they can improve your life. . . .

WHAT YOU CAN DO NOW

Discover the best breakthrough tools today in maximizing energy, optimizing our hormones, and transforming your vitality and strength, including . . .

- **The power of peptides, hormones, and key nutraceuticals**

- **The most powerful tools available to eliminate pain** once and for all, without surgery or medication by addressing the source of pain instead of just treating the symptoms.

- Uncover how **a handful of "low-risk" lifestyle choices can literally add 12 or more years to your life.**

- Discover the third pillar of health, sleep, and how to increase your daily focus, boost your mood, and experience greater vitality without caffeine or other stimulants.

- Simple tools and techniques to **increase your strength and muscle mass, boost your metabolism, and increase your bone density up to 14 percent.**

- The latest **anti-aging breakthroughs in beauty** to help you look and feel your best.

- Discover the latest breakthroughs and empowering **solutions for women** to live full, healthy, and vibrant lives.

CHAPTER 10

YOUR ULTIMATE VITALITY PHARMACY

The Power of Peptides, Metformin, Hormones, NAD+, and Key Nutraceuticals

"Every man desires to live long, but no man would be old."
—JONATHAN SWIFT

It's been quite a journey so far, wouldn't you agree? We've heard firsthand from our scientific heroes on some of the boldest regenerative breakthroughs that are currently in clinics and others that are following close behind, moving through clinical trial pipelines. From stem cells to CAR T-cells to the wondrous Wnt pathway, some of these amazing therapies are approved and available today. Others are charging through clinical trials and should be widely accessible within two or three years. Before the decade is out, the doctors and researchers we've interviewed are convinced that they'll transform the face of everyday medicine—of how we age and how we heal.

Now, are you up for a brief but important detour? **Let's pivot to some vitality-enhancing and healthspan-extending remedies on the market *right now*, accessible for anyone ready and willing to take action.** To be clear, this chapter is not giving you medical advice. Before you begin using any of these therapies, it's always important and appropriate to seek the guidance and supervision of an expert physician.

Your ultimate vitality pharmacy contains a wealth of options to turn back your biological clock and make you feel more vibrant and *alive*.

We're talking about concrete steps you can take _today_ to retrieve the energy and pain-free functionality—even the appearance—of youth.

Peter and I were committed to finding an expert in nutraceuticals— someone we could trust to be at the unique intersection of clinical, regulatory, and ingredient expertise. And we were fortunate to know **Dr. Hector Lopez, MD,** who we trust with our own supplement lists.

Not only does Hector have a diverse medical background, in sports medicine, nutritional biochemistry, and integrative and regenerative medicine, he is now primarily focused as a research scientist on dietary supplements and foods. His deep expertise spans a decade as a physician-scientist, and then transitioning away from medicine for the last fifteen years as a leader in ingredient innovation, clinical research, regulatory/safety, and more recently AI machine learning–driven natural product technologies.

Worried that a supplement may not be safe or pure? So were we, which is why we turned to Dr. Lopez. Hector is a key opinion leader in **safety and regulation. He has cofounded companies to further clinical research in the supplement space, as well as a major regulatory compliance company. Even more so, he holds the expertise to discover, develop, and bring new bioactive compounds to market for licensing.** Think dietary supplements, food ingredients, beverages, and natural products. He oversees signing off on the safety of these ingredients. **Personally, he's given me an unfair advantage in a very complex and sometimes confusing ocean of supplements and health claims.**

For a taste of what's in store in this chapter, here are of the most promising therapeutics and medications **you'll learn about that have the potential to change your life for the better:**

1. Have you heard of peptides, those bioactive molecules that build lean muscle mass and revitalize sexual desire and function in both men and women? Surprisingly, they're modeled after mini-proteins found in common foods—and their safety profile is outstanding.

2. You'll learn about a widely prescribed, pennies-per-dose medication that safely treats and prevents diabetes—and, experts say, just might protect you from cancer, heart disease, and Alzheimer's.

3. **We'll explore how restoring your hormones to an optimal level can revitalize you and strip years away from your biological age.**

4. Are you aware that widely available **dietary supplements are demonstrating tangible benefits for cellular longevity, healthspan, and a peak performance lifestyle**—both inside and outside the gym? Many of them are used by high-level athletes—and now promising science is emerging on their crossover benefits for healthy and vital aging for the rest of us.

As you'll see, **some of these tools are sold as over-the-counter supplements, where the FDA regulations don't require pre-market approval. Others, classed as medicines, are already FDA-approved, and they simply require a physician's prescription. If you want more information, you can always visit LifeForce.com, where we have telemedicine physicians who can work with you to understand your needs and provide you with guidance.**

Because Peter and I are always looking for the cutting edge, every time that we see a breakthrough study, our first call is to our colleague, Dr. Lopez, in order to draw on his deep experience in ingredient innovation, supplement safety, quality assurance, and clinical research. That's how he's become a leader in developing breakthrough, next-generation nutraceuticals. Peter and I use the nutraceuticals he created for our own personal regimen, and we don't utilize anything without his analysis. For that reason we've asked him to join us in advising on this chapter to make sure that we can bring you the best scientifically sound insights in the areas of energy, strength, and longevity.

Here is the roadmap for the chapter ahead. **We'll be diving into what we consider the five key therapeutic areas that you can focus on, today, to increase your energy and vitality:**

1. Peptides
2. Metformin
3. Hormone optimization therapy (HOT)
4. NAD+ precursors
5. Key nutraceuticals

Most of these interventions, according to the scientists, appear to have few if any serious side effects. We'll clarify what the science shows, so that you can inform your own decisions. While we'll never tell you that any treatment is risk-free, you may find some to have a compelling *asymmetrical risk/reward*. In other words, some of these interventions involve very little risk for a potentially big upside. It's the secret all great investors use to make money— and the same principle can also help guide you to greater strength, vitality, and health than you might have thought possible, once you have the facts.

We'll drill down into the upsides and downsides to help you make up your own mind after exploring these options with your medical practitioners. Sound fair enough to you? Then let's get started in seeing what some of the freshest breakthroughs offer us today!

THERAPEUTIC #1: PEPTIDES—LITTLE PROTEINS, BIG IMPACTS

Back in the 1960s, at the peak of the Cold War arms race, the Soviet Union had a problem. To keep pace with America, they were pulling out all the stops to expand their nuclear program. But they couldn't stop their reactors from leaking—a big problem in military submarines. Sailors were dropping like flies with terminal cancers. In 1973, the generals tapped a young doctor and gerontologist named Vladimir Khavinson to find a solution.[1]

Khavinson's research team focused on the mini-proteins called peptides, the short chains of amino acids that help regulate cell division and gene expression. They're also a big part of our repair kit for every tissue and organ in our body. As signaling molecules, peptides bind like keys in a lock to protein receptors on a cell's surface. The Soviet scientists devised ways to isolate and extract and purify these protein fragments. **Then they injected them into the at-risk sailors, who stopped dying. They suddenly seemed to have vastly improved immune systems—and it wasn't a fluke. Years later, after the Chernobyl nuclear power plant**

---

1 Bulmash, "The Unknown Russian Revolution—Has the Fountain of Youth Already Been Discovered?"

disaster, local residents who received peptide treatments had far lower cancer rates.[2]

We absorb peptides—to a point—from meats, fish, and plant-based proteins (beans, wheat, oats) in our diet. **But as our bodies' peptide stockpile diminishes with age, it can lead to a loss of function and a weakened, vulnerable immune system.**

More than 80 peptides have been approved by the FDA to treat one or more diseases.[3] Dozens more are in the regulatory pipeline. **Unlike chemical drugs, peptides preserve the body's natural feedback loops and restore our homeostasis, our natural balanced state. If you're healthy, they can help you reach and sustain your physical peak. If you're ailing, there's a good chance they can help make you better; they're accepted as low-risk therapeutics for diabetes, cancer, and cardiovascular disease.** Applications are in the works for neurodegenerative illnesses like Alzheimer's. Maybe most exciting, peptides are emerging as a valuable tool in battling autoimmune conditions and out-of-control inflammation, the root of all degenerative disease.

Over the last five years, **Dr. Mitchell Fleisher, a Virginia-based family physician who specializes in regenerative medicine, has successfully prescribed peptides to dozens of patients**. A few months before we spoke, one of them, a 48-year-old truck driver, had a serious traffic accident. The injury threw the man's inflammatory response out of whack and sent his multiple sclerosis—an autoimmune disease that attacks the nervous system—into relapse.

"When he came to me, he was using a cane and dragging his right foot," Mitchell said. The man was lethargic, weak, achy, and barely living: "He couldn't drive—he couldn't even work in his garden. He spent most of his time on his living room couch." Though his patient had an acute fear of needles, Mitchell persuaded him to try a cocktail of three commonly used peptides: **thymosin alpha 1, thymosin beta 4, and BPC-157. Six weeks later, the man walked up to the reception desk with a big**

---

2 Peptides Store, "An Interview with Professor Khavinson."

3 Muttenthaler et al., "Trends in Peptide Drug Discovery."

grin—and his cane held high above his head. "If this keeps up, Doc," he said, "I might dance an Irish jig!"

I know this sounds like hype, but the body has an amazing ability to heal when you provide it with the key ingredients it needs. This is why the FDA has approved more than 100 peptides. Their impact can be dramatic.

To stave off feeling and looking older, millions of people have turned to the peptide supplement market for bodybuilding, performance enhancement (both athletic and sexual), and skin rejuvenation. As weapons in the war against aging, peptides have tremendous potential. As of 2019, their global market had grown to $70 billion.[4]

Properly administered, peptides are about as safe as you'd expect natural substances to be. Since their molecules are mostly smaller than biological proteins or antibody medicines, they're less likely to set off immune system alarms and provoke inflammation. **And since they hit their targets more selectively than chemical drugs, serious adverse side effects are rare, says Dr. Hector.** Once their signaling is done, says Horst Kessler of the Institute for Advanced Study at TU Munich, peptides **"can be recycled by the body—no accumulation, no complicated detoxification."**[5]

Since most peptides would get broken down by our gastrointestinal enzymes, they need to be injected in fatty tissue just under the skin, typically in the lower abdomen or upper arm, with tiny ultra-fine insulin needles (similar to those used by diabetics who self-administer insulin). Recent advances, like fail-safe, auto-dosing, prefilled syringes, have made these shots simple and easy to apply. A new generation of synthesized peptide variants can be taken less frequently—once a week, say, instead of daily. And more of them are now available orally, as a nasal spray, or as topical creams.

At the same time, we need to share two caveats. For starters, you'll need to seek out a reputable source. The black market is bad news, an online minefield. By one estimate, four of five peptides sold on the web

---

4 Lee et al., "A Comprehensive Review of Current Advances in Peptide Drug Development and Design."

5 Technical University of Munich, "Breakthrough for Peptide Medication."

"are adulterated or outright fakes."[6] The better way to go? A *compounding pharmacy* that fills customized prescriptions by licensed physicians or healthcare providers in a highly regulated, sanitary environment. Staffed by licensed professionals, these facilities meet strict federal standards for pharmaceutical-grade ingredients and quality-controlled processing.

Then you'll need to find the right doctor. Peptides are *pleiotropic*, which means they have multiple effects, and you'll want someone experienced in supervising their use. Doses vary from one patient to the next. Freelancing is a really bad idea. **Overdoses can wipe out a peptide's benefits—in terms of impact, *more* can actually be *less*.** And sometimes it can even be dangerous if overdone. **The International Peptide Society can refer you to a certified medical practitioner if you need one. A good compounding pharmacy should be able to do the same.** And of course, if you'd like we can connect you to a medical expert at Lifeforce.com.

One last piece of advice: **Though the FDA affirms that peptides "play a significant role in providing necessary medications for the public,"**[7] the agency's rules for these vital therapies are in constant flux. Many peptides are still in the agency's new drug approval process, so you'll need to consult your doctor or pharmacy on their regulatory status and accessibility. But for anyone who's curious about these intriguing healthspan boosters, we'd like to offer a starter information kit. Speaking personally, I've found great value in peptides myself, including several on the list below.

Since peptides' names are technical mouthfuls, we'll break them down into categories and give you quick summaries as a basis for further research by you and your regenerative physician.

1. TO REDUCE APPETITE, PROMOTE FAT LOSS, AND RE-BALANCE OUR METABOLISM:

- **The peptide <u>semaglutide (and other glucagon-like peptide-1 agonists)</u>** have aced four-year-plus clinical trials, with **subjects routinely losing 15 percent of their body weight—or 30 pounds**

---

6 Powell, "At the Heart of a Vast Doping Network, an Alias."

7 FDA, "Impact Story: Developing the Tools to Evaluate Complex Drug Products: Peptides."

for someone weighing in at 200. Generally well-tolerated, with a terrific safety profile, GLP-1s can be game-changers when added to a healthy diet, exercise, and other lifestyle changes. Occasional side effects: nausea, diarrhea, and flatulence. May not be suitable for individuals with a history of thyroid gland tumors.

- <u>MOTS-c and Humanin</u> are derived from the mitochondria, our cells' power packs. Among other things, they may revitalize our carbohydrate and fat metabolism. This category of mitochondrial peptides is a potential wellspring of future innovation for longevity, healthspan, and peak performance!

2. TO STRENGTHEN OUR IMMUNE SYSTEM AND COMBAT ITS AGE-RELATED DECLINE:

- **The peptide thymosin alpha-1 (Zadaxin)**: As we age, our thymus gland gradually turns into fat tissue and stops producing the robust battalions of T cells that fight off infections or eliminate rogue cancer cells. **If we had to choose a single peptide to help address immunological aging, according to Dr. Lopez, thymosin alpha-1 might be the one.**
- <u>TA-1</u> has proven its ability to stimulate the immune system in both animal and human studies. It's also racked up promising data in fighting liver and kidney disease and rheumatoid arthritis and is **FDA-approved for malignant melanoma, hepatitis B, and hepatitis C. Its safety record is outstanding.** And as a potent anti-inflammatory and antioxidant,[8] it may help keep you from getting sick in the first place.

3. TO BOOST SEXUAL AROUSAL AND SATISFACTION FOR BOTH WOMEN AND MEN:

- **The peptide <u>PT-141 (bremelanotide)</u>** binds to receptors in the brain that are believed to be a central nervous system "hub" for sexual arousal and libido. This peptide has also been tested in clinical trials

---

8 Qin et al., "Proliferative and Anti-Proliferative Effects of Thymosin Alpha1 on Cells Are Associated with Manipulation of Cellular ROS Levels."

as an **intranasal spray and is FDA-approved for low sexual desire disorder in premenopausal women.** <u>Not</u> recommended for those with uncontrolled hypertension or heart disease.

4. **TO HEAL THE GUT, LIGAMENTS, TENDONS, AND SKIN:**
   - **The peptide <u>BPC-157</u>** may promote speedier recovery from ligament tear reconstruction and rotator cuff tendon injuries. **As we've already mentioned, <u>this peptide has shown outstanding results in treating debilitating gut problems.</u> I found that out firsthand after my bout with mercury poisoning, which does brutal things to the body. BPC-157 was one of the tools I used to help rebuild my gut, and it was extraordinarily effective.**

5. <u>**TO INCREASE MUSCLE MASS, STRENGTHEN BONES, REVITALIZE SKIN, AND RESTORE YOUTHFUL METABOLISM:**</u>
   - **The two peptides <u>sermorelin</u> and <u>tesamorelin</u> mimic the action of growth hormone–releasing hormone (GHRH),** a hotbed for new drug development. GHRHs stimulate the pituitary gland to secrete natural growth hormone. They're **a lot cheaper than synthetic human growth hormone (HGH)**—and, unlike HGH, can be legally prescribed off-label. What's the downside? If you take growth hormone or these peptides, you should be aware that growth hormone elevates levels of insulin-like growth factor-1, which has been shown in some studies to have "a modest association" with cancer risk.[9] So it's critical that you work closely with your physician to determine what options are best based on your symptoms, blood work, and careful monitoring.

6. **TO REVIVE OUR SKIN AND RESTORE OUR HAIR:**
   - **The peptide <u>GHK-Cu</u> is a topical foam that can be used daily to erase fine lines and wrinkles.** It counteracts cosmetic aging by **boosting collagen synthesis up to 70 percent.**[10] According to Dr.

---

9 Weroha and Haluska, "IGF System in Cancer."

10 Interview with Ryan Smith, February 2, 2020.

William Seeds, chairman of the International Peptide Society, **GHK-Cu also stimulates wound healing and "amazing" hair growth.**[11]

- **Melanotan I (Scenesse)** darkens our skin by stimulating the production of melanin pigment production. **Melanotan I is FDA-approved for treating skin damage in people with light intolerance, and may also help those struggling with mold toxicity. For the rest of us, it offers aesthetic benefits while protecting against damaging ultraviolet radiation.** It also has some intriguing potential **side benefits: reduced appetite, higher fat metabolism, and increased sex drive.**

We could go on and on, as there are countless peptides either in use or in the pipeline, for just about every organ system and tissue in the body, from head to toe. **I believe without a doubt that peptides deserve your consideration, whether you're looking to regenerate your body, prevent or recover from injuries, optimize your metabolism, improve your performance, or rejuvenate your immune system.** Once again, we can help you locate professional medical experts at Lifeforce.com, or you can turn for assistance to the International Peptide Society, as mentioned above. The table below is a quick summary to help you evaluate (with your regenerative physician) which peptides might be right for you. We've included the six mentioned above as well as four additional ones. You'll see the name, the benefit, the category of use, and the way it's applied.

Peptide / Molecule	Category/Benefit	Form of Delivery	Target Mechanism
Semaglutide	Weight Loss peptide; insulin/ glucose management peptide	Injection (SubQ)	Targets the pancreas, liver, muscle, and fat
PT-141 (bremela-notide)	Sexual health peptide	Intranasal spray or Injection (SubQ)	Triggers parts of the brain that are believed to be a "hub" for sexual arousal and libido Melanocortin receptors

---

11 Ben Greenfield, "Peptides Unveiled."

Peptide / Molecule	Category	Form of Delivery	Benefit/Target Mechanism
BPC-157	Regenerative peptide; tissue remodeling	Oral or Injection (SubQ)	Activates growth factors Activates FAK-paxillin and growth hormone receptors Acts on fibroblasts and tenocytes
Thymosin alpha-1	Immuno-modulation	Injection (SubQ)	Thymus Designed for T-cell, B-Cell, and dendritic place maturation
Sermorelin; tesamorelin	Mobilizes stored body fat for fuel; Improves muscle mass: fat ratio and body composition; Recovery from exercise; Revitalizes skin	Injection (SubQ)	Optimizes IGF-1 Stimulates synthesis and release of GH from pituitary
GHK-Cu	Skin, hair, and regenerative peptide; remodeling	Topical cream or Injection (SubQ)	Anti-inflammatory Promotes extracellular matrix Collagen synthesis
Ipamorelin	Mobilizes stored body fat for fuel; Improves muscle mass: fat ratio and body composition; Faster recovery from exercise; Revitalizes skin	Injection (SubQ)	Optimizes IGF-1 Promotes secretion of your own GH; activates ghrelin receptor; stimulates synthesis and release of GH from pituitary
MK-677 (investigational new drug)	Mobilizes stored body fat for fuel; Improves muscle mass: fat ratio and body composition; Faster recovery from exercise; Revitalizes skin	Oral	Optimizes IGF-1 Promotes secretion of your own GH; activates ghrelin receptor; stimulates synthesis and release of GH from pituitary
MOTS-c / humanin	Energy metabolism; physical working capacity	Injection (SubQ)	Mitochondrial peptides Activates liver, skeletal muscle, and brain
Melanotan I	Skin and hair aesthetic / cosmetics Off-target effects to decrease appetite and improve metabolism	Oral	Activates alpha-MSH receptors

THERAPEUTIC #2: METFORMIN—
THE LOW-RISK WONDER DRUG

"Metformin may have already saved more people from
cancer deaths than any drug in history."[12]

—LEWIS CANTLEY, director of the Meyer Cancer
Center at Weill Cornell Medical College

Now let's take a look at another amazing medicine, one that our friend Dr. David Sinclair and millions of other people utilize every day . . . *metformin.* The FDA-approved, first-line treatment for type 2 diabetes, **metformin, is wildly popular in the longevity field.** My coauthors Bob Hariri and Peter Diamandis have been taking it for years. So have futurist-par-excellence Ray Kurzweil and biotech entrepreneur Ned David. And so does Nobel Prize winner James Watson of double-helix fame, who once went so far as to say that metformin might be "our only real clue into the business" of beating cancer. **When a recent anti-aging forum of 300 people was asked who was using this medicine to extend their healthspan, half the audience raised their hands. As David Sinclair says, metformin "might work on aging itself."**[13]

A **generic medicine modeled after a plant called French lilac, metformin has an unparalleled safety record over more than sixty years.** It's used off-label to treat prediabetes and other endocrine, cardiovascular, and metabolic problems.

How does metformin work? Like intermittent fasting and intensive exercise, it stresses the mitochondria. It throws the body into hunker-down-and-repair mode. With a three-pronged mechanism involving our liver, gut, and muscle cells, it lowers blood sugar, a critical factor for anti-aging. The beauty of metformin, as opposed to insulin or other diabetes meds, is that it won't drive the body into *hypoglycemia* **(low blood sugar), a dangerous condition. If your level is healthy to begin with, metformin will keep it that way.**

---

12 Apple, "Forget the Blood of Teens. This Pill Promises to Extend Life for a
    Nickel a Pop."

13 Sinclair, "This Cheap Pill Might Help You Live a Longer, Healthier Life."

Because metformin has been used so widely for many decades, it's been widely studied. **Time and again, the studies suggest that metformin may reduce cancer risk and mortality by up to 40 percent, particularly for tumors of the lung, colon, pancreas, and breast.**[14] According to Lewis Cantley, the cell biologist who directs the Meyer Cancer Center at Weill Cornell Medical College, "Metformin may have already saved more people from cancer deaths than any drug in history."[15]

The bombshell study that spotlighted metformin came out of Cardiff University in Britain, in 2014.[16] **They discovered the diabetics on metformin were outliving the non-diabetics—by a lot! The presumably healthier group was dying 15 percent sooner. Here was evidence "that metformin may confer benefits in non-diabetic people."**

Who should consider metformin? If you're a non-diabetic looking for help with disease prevention, it boils down to a negotiation between you and your doctor. If you decide to move forward, metformin won't break the bank. It's covered by most insurance and costs pennies per pill.

Even better, Metformin has **minimal side effects**. When there are side effects, the most common are diarrhea, nausea, and bloating. But these tend to lessen over time. Metformin has been correlated with vitamin B12 and B6 deficiencies, which can lead to anemia, so be sure to monitor your vitamin levels and supplement as needed. Lactic acidosis, which is no joke, has been weakly associated with metformin. But this is mostly in people with acute kidney or liver failure.[17]

A controlled study out of the University of Kentucky found that metformin limited the growth of muscle mass in healthy people over 65 after fourteen weeks of resistance (weight) training.[18] (Though their muscles did get bigger.) Since muscle mass is a well-known factor for healthspan and

---

14 Ibid.

15 Apple, "Forget the Blood of Teens."

16 Bannister et al., "Can People with Type 2 Diabetes Live Longer Than Those Without?"

17 Salber et al., "Metformin Use in Practice: Compliance with Guidelines for Patients with Diabetes and Preserved Renal Function."

18 Walton et al., "Metformin Blunts Muscle Hypertrophy in Response to Progressive Resistance Exercise Training in Older Adults."

longevity, we asked **Dr. Nir Barzilai**—director of the Institute for Aging Research at Albert Einstein College of Medicine—about it. He responded that the exercisers taking metformin showed equivalent improvement in muscle *function* to the placebo group, and that the **many anti-aging benefits of metformin—in clearing out zombie "senescent" cells, for example, or reducing inflammation—more than outweighed the muscle mass factor**.

But what highlighted metformin more in recent years was its anti-inflammatory impact on the hallmarks of aging, from epigenetic changes to stem cell exhaustion. An article from *Science* said **metformin "turns down the cell's metabolic thermostat." It's slowing down our biological clock.**

In 2015, Barzilai won the FDA's blessing to run a radical, unprecedented study called TAME, or "Targeting Aging with Metformin"—a paradigm shift away from conventional whack-a-mole medicine. With partial funding from the American Federation for Aging Research, a private nonprofit, TAME will be the first randomized, controlled clinical trial to take aim at the riddle of aging itself. We'll have those results by 2025, to see if metformin can give us an edge against aging.

Based on metformin's sterling track record, Barzilai feels confident it will pass with flying colors. But TAME is only the beginning, a proof of concept. The long game is to compel the FDA to recognize aging as a disease, or "indication," and open the door to developing even better, next-gen drugs. The advance of anti-aging therapies "will be dramatically accelerated," Barzilai predicted. "Biotech is almost ready, and the pharmaceutical companies will be jumping in. **Most importantly, it will make life much better for the elderly. And it will have a huge economic longevity dividend." If metformin can delay aging, extend healthspan, and increase life expectancy by as little as 2.2 years, it would save the U.S. an estimated $7 trillion over the next half century.**[19]

---

19 Goldman et al., "Substantial Health and Economic Returns From Delayed Aging May Warrant a New Focus for Medical Research."

THERAPEUTIC #3: HORMONE OPTIMIZATION THERAPY—GETTING BACK TO OUR BEST SELVES

The importance of hormones can't be overstated. These natural chemical messengers regulate our growth and development early in life, our blood pressure and blood sugar, our sex drive and capacity to procreate, our sleep cycle, and just about all of our body's core functions.[20] **As people get older, a common occurrence is that hormone levels get off-kilter. This can lead to fatigue, insomnia, and depression. We're more vulnerable to stress and less interested in sex. Our skin loses its youthful appearance; we lose muscle mass and accumulate body fat.**

We touched briefly on **hormone optimization therapy (HOT)** in Chapter 3, "Diagnostic Power," but to restate: By addressing an individual's complete clinical picture and lifestyle with truly personalized, precision medicine, HOT can help you avoid many downstream age-related conditions long before they set off biomarker alarms on a blood test. Unlike doctors using conventional hormone replacement therapy (HRT), physicians and allied health teams trained in HOT can paint a clinical picture of the best "biological" version of each patient. They diagnose the individual's current physical, biochemical, and occasionally genomic data and psychological state, consider their lifestyle, nutritional status, exercise capacity, medical history, and then craft a unique and customized program to restore the individual to their best self. HOT doesn't wait until something's broke to fix it; it's the epitome of preventive, proactive healthcare.

Dr. Hector Lopez sorts HOT therapies into four buckets:

1. <u>Male sex hormones:</u> When optimized, according to Dr. Lopez, **testosterone** has broad and enormous benefits for <u>both men and women</u>. Here are just a few: **restored and enhanced energy levels, mood, sexual drive, exercise capacity and recovery, stress resilience, and bone health. It can even reduce your risk of heart disease!** <u>DHEA</u>, a precursor to both testosterone and estrogen, may also be

---

20 Johns Hopkins Medicine Health, "Hormones and the Endocrine System."

supplemented—**your body's production of it peaks in the mid 20s and declines from there.**[21]

2. **Female sex hormones** are essential to female health and quality of life, but they're also critical for men's libido, cardiovascular and brain protection, bone and joint function, and multi-organ system health. As Dr. Lopez notes, clinical findings have confirmed that **progesterone can promote general calm and restful sleep, a healthy sex drive, and balanced blood sugar and fat metabolism.**

3. **Thyroid and adrenal hormones** match energy supply with demand. **They regulate our body temperature and sleep cycle, protect us against stress, and fortify our immune response.** Thyroid optimization therapy, administered orally, centers around the two main thyroid hormones—T4 and T3—that govern overall cellular and tissue metabolism, from our brain to our cardiovascular system to our skin and GI tract. **Pregnenolone and DHEA, adrenal gland hormones, while having health benefits themselves, are building blocks for many other hormones, including estrogen, testosterone, progesterone, and cortisol.**

4. **The human growth hormone (HGH)/insulin-like growth factor-1 (IGF-1) axis** acts via the hypothalamus and pituitary gland to regulate **whole-body organ and tissue repair, remodeling, and regeneration.** Carefully monitored HOT in this area **can rejuvenate a patient's muscle-to-fat ratio, skin appearance, brain health, sleep quality, and daytime energy.** IGF-1 is the active molecule and biomarker that offers most of the benefits of both HGH-stimulating peptides and HGH injections—**more lean muscle mass, more efficient fat-burning, quicker recovery from intense exercise, even improved brain function.** The HGH-stimulating secretagogues or peptides have often provided most of the reliable benefits of HGH and IGF-1 itself—with **fewer side effects** or risk.[22, 23]

---

21 Ratini, "DHEA Supplements."

22 Langridge, "The Truth About Using Peptides and How They Impact Your Health."

23 McLarnon, "Tesamorelin Can Improve Cognitive Function."

Well-trained physicians and allied health teams who have embraced HOT over conventional HRT recognize that no intervention is "risk-free." However, according to Dr. Hector Lopez, "Many of these risks have been overstated, and fears that hormone treatments cause cancer or heart disease are largely unsubstantiated from flawed interpretations of the clinical research."

As Dr. Lopez described, the Women's Health Initiative (WHI) study caused a chilling effect on hormone therapies for women around the world, but "an objective analysis of the WHI and Million Women Study data revealed that when utilizing the appropriate dose and administration form, HOT may actually be **cardio-protective**, **neuro-protective** and help stem the tide of physiological aging." In fact, women's health and their hormonal profiles are so important that we have an entire chapter on women's health written by the Buck Institute's Jennifer Garrison and Dr. Carolyn DeLucia, a practicing OB-GYN for more than thirty years, to guide the women reading this book.

In fact, declining estrogen, progesterone, and other hormones are associated with increased risk of cardiovascular disease, osteoporosis, type 2 diabetes, and even dementia. Physicians practicing HOT utilize protocols that combine the best practices of evidence-based guidelines from around the world with each patient's unique clinical picture, the presence of any "red flags," detailed lab analysis of many biochemical and nutritional biomarkers, careful monitoring, well-balanced dosing, routes of administration, age, and other risk factors. According to Dr. Lopez, "Our hormone optimization protocols draw upon an extensive database of successfully managing thousands of patients, navigating the potential risks while providing enormous upside health and peak performance benefits."

Likewise, in men a careful assessment of clinical symptoms, physical examination, lifestyle factors, and biochemical lab data are all necessary not only to determine if you are a candidate for HOT with true testosterone deficiency, but also to rule out any important red flags that would require a deeper investigation and may lead to alternative therapeutic options. A HOT approach that incorporates updated guidelines from the Endocrine Society and other leading organizations, alongside integrative, comprehensive, and customized solutions with careful monitoring, serves to guide our patients to maximizing health outcomes, while managing any potential risks.

Ultimately, HOT practitioners carefully weigh potential benefits with potential risks, and the opportunity costs of various Rx, lifestyle, and nutraceutical interventions, to inform and empower patients as partners in optimizing their health and performance journey. Most importantly, the focus with HOT as opposed to conventional HRT has now shifted from a reactive, sickness-based, fragmented model to the proactive, preventive, and integrative care model, in an effort to promote longevity and enhance healthspan and peak-performance living!

If it seems like there's a lot of overlap among these four categories of hormones, that's a good thing—it means you've been paying attention!

THERAPEUTIC #3: NAD+ SUPPLEMENTATION— RECHARGING OUR CELLULAR BATTERIES

"NAD replacement is one of the most exciting things happening in the biology of aging."

—DR. NIR BARZILAI, director of the Institute for Aging Research, Albert Einstein College of Medicine

Here's a refresher from Chapter 4, "Turning Back Time": **NAD+ is a helper molecule—a "coenzyme"—found in every cell in our body.** It partners with our **sirtuin vitality genes**—those signaling proteins that regulate cell metabolism and longevity genes—to keep those cells in good working order. Specifically, **it helps process nutrients into ATP, the power "currency" of our cells. NAD+ is an essential component of all living things; we'd be gone without it.**

As molecules go, NAD+ is so big and bulky that it can't get past a cell's outer membrane. To keep us up and running, a variety of smaller "precursors molecules" that can enter a cell are naturally converted to NAD+ once they pass through our cell's outer membrane into our cells. (They're actually versions of **vitamin B**3, also known as **niacin**.) For the most part, this process works just fine when we're younger. **But by middle age, for reasons scientists are still figuring out, we lose half or more of our NAD+ reserve.** Poor sleep, unhealthy eating, too much alcohol, and prolonged low-grade inflammation deplete us even more. Here's a short list of the consequences: obesity, chronic fatigue, diminished brain function . . . and accelerated aging.[24]

Our cells absorb small amounts of NAD+ precursors from certain foods. But it would be a tall order to drink enough milk or eat enough salmon or mushrooms to make up for our age-driven shortfall. **So what's the solution? It's twofold.**

The first solution, according to Dr. David Sinclair and other top scientists in the age reversal space, lies in NAD+ supplements. Sinclair's supplement of choice is nicotinamide mononucleotide (NMN).

What we're seeing in animal trials has been nothing short of spectacular. **Older mice on NAD+ precursor supplements became slimmer, with improved insulin sensitivity and more youthful stem cell function. They return to more youthful circadian rhythms and sleep cycles.[25] Other rodent studies have shown dramatic impact on dementia, kidney and liver disease, osteoporosis, noise-related hearing loss, and cancer.** A few have shown increased mouse lifespan.[26] An Australian study published in *Cell* found that small doses of NMN, dissolved in drinking water, dramatically improved egg quality and increased the ratio of live births among older female mice: **"Our findings suggest there is an opportunity to restore . . . female reproductive function using oral administration of NAD-boosting agents—which would be far less invasive than IVF [in vitro fertilization]."[27]**

Scientific interest in NAD+ (and its precursors) has exploded, and dozens of other preliminary human studies—from sleep and cognition to premature skin aging—are now in progress.

While NAD+ precursors have satisfied the FDA's criteria for supplement safety, a few studies point to possible long-term risks. It is critically important to know where you are getting your supplements from—the source has to be safe, stable, and vetted. As mentioned in

---

24 Imai and Guarente, "NAD+ and Sirtuins in Aging and Disease."

25 Hill, "NAD+ and the Circadian Rhythm."

26 Zhang et al., "NAD+ Repletion Improves Mitochondrial and Stem Cell Function and Enhances Life Span in Mice."

27 University of Queensland, "Scientists Reverse Reproductive Clock in Mice."

Chapter 4 (and it's worth saying again), a quick visit to Google or Amazon will reveal at least a dozen different brands selling what they claim to be NMN with prices ranging from $24 to $95 for 60 tablets. The challenge is that a lot of these supplements do not in fact contain actual NMN when tested in the lab. And in many cases, it isn't a stable form of the molecule and can degrade in under sixty days.

In 2019, the Wistar Institute found that higher NAD+ levels increased inflammation from senescent cells in mice, which in turn provoked the growth of pancreatic and ovarian tumors. NAD+ supplements for anti-aging, the researchers concluded, "should be administered with precision."[28] **While Sinclair agrees that the Wistar findings merit further exploration, he's not overly concerned. "My lab has been studying cancer in mice for the last three years," he told us, "and we haven't seen any evidence that NAD boosting makes any cancer worse—if anything, it slows the cancer down. . . . I want to be the first person to know if there is any risk, because my whole family takes this stuff. If there is ever a day I find toxicity, I'm going to tweet it out to all my followers and stop taking it."**

There is a second solution for restoring NAD+ levels in our aging bodies that involves preventing its loss in the first place. Dr. Hector Lopez believes the available data strongly supports the notion that there is a "leaky sink" whereby NAD+ levels decrease as a result of chronic inflammation and aberrant immune activation. He and his partners at JUVN3, a company that leverages molecular data-driven technology to discover and develop novel ingredient solutions that address longevity, healthy aging, immune health and neuro-cognitive and metabolic wellness, have introduced a promising new player to restore healthier levels of NAD+ called **NAD3.**

What exactly is NAD3 and how does it work?

NAD3 is a patent-pending nutraceutical containing a unique *Wasabi japonica* extract, theacrine and copper(I)-niacin complex. Preliminary preclinical and human studies suggest that it **turbocharges enzymes that**

---

28 Nacarelli et al., "NAD+ Metabolism Governs the Proinflammatory Senescence-Associated Secretome."

boost the conversion of NAD+ precursors, such as NMN, to NAD+, while *also suppressing* the activity proteins that deplete NAD+. Dr. Lopez explains, "NAD3 co-supplementation with any NAD+ precursor (such as NMN) is like playing both on offense and defense at the same time."

As we're writing this, a pivotal **human clinical trial** of over sixty subjects taking a daily 312mg dose of **NAD3** is being completed. Dr. Lopez is measuring all the health-related biomarkers, including cardiovascular risk factors; lipids such as VLDL, LDL; triglycerides; telomere length; and gene expression, plus other molecular hallmarks of aging. Once it's completed, and in publication, we'll be sharing all the exciting data with you on Lifeforce.com.

What we can see already is **that NAD3's effects seem to reach beyond the mere increase in NAD+ levels. There are also other non-NAD+-dependent molecular hallmarks of aging, vitality, and human performance that are being impacted. As Dr. Lopez shares, "NAD3 has preliminarily been shown to slow down inflammatory signaling and telomere loss and improve antioxidant responses, lipid metabolism, and genomic instability (remember that we accumulate DNA damage over our lifespan)." NAD3 also plays "offense" again and hits the accelerator to amplify the molecular signature or gene expression profile of genes associated with healthy cellular aging, longevity, and resilience.**

The technology behind NAD3 set out to mimic the biochemical profile or signature associated with longevity-geared activities like exercise, fasting/refeeding, Mediterranean diets, sauna thermal stress, healthy sleep and circadian alignment, stress management, and social connection. While it's "early days" for NAD3, and much about how NAD+ influences human health and the biology of aging remains to be studied, Peter and I each take NAD3 every day, and remain enthusiastic and excited given the potential upside and relatively safe profile. The developers of NAD3 have invested heavily into the pipeline of mechanistic, pre-clinical science and human clinical research, as they are committed to providing a solid body of evidence. This approach will push the forefront, advance the field of longevity, and make an undeniable impact on human healthspan for society.

THERAPEUTICS #4: NUTRACEUTICALS—SAFE AND NATURAL HEALTHSPAN ENHANCERS

Let's next go beyond NAD+ supplementation, peptides, metformin, and hormones, and ask the question, what else should you consider taking that is safe, and has a compelling risk/reward ratio? To answer this, Dr. Lopez shared with us a list of over-the-counter nutraceuticals that can significantly boost healthspan and performance. But before we review that list, Dr. Lopez wanted to pass along two caveats:

1. **Although all of these nutraceuticals are freely and widely available, and have strong safety profiles, it's a good idea to discuss them with your health professional before adding them to your daily regimen.** Every individual has a unique healthspan history and game plan. And each nutraceutical has its relative risk, accessibility, potential efficacy, and body of scientific data.

2. **No matter which nutraceuticals you ultimately decide to explore, their impact will be universally enhanced by healthspan-promoting activities: regular aerobic exercise and strength training, a healthful diet (and time-restricted eating when appropriate), optimal sleep, social connection, and stress management and mindfulness techniques.** Here's one thing to keep in mind as you read this book: **A healthy lifestyle is the bedrock foundation for all regenerative medicine and healthspan-enhancing interventions.**

Here's Dr. Lopez's list of 8 key nutraceuticals, most of which you've probably heard about and may already be taking.

1. **Vitamin D3** boasts a strong safety profile, along with broad and deep evidence that links it to brain, metabolic, cardiovascular, muscle, bone, lung, and immune health. New and emerging research suggests that vitamin D supplements may also slow down our epigenetic/biological aging.[29, 30]

---

29 Chen et al., "Effects of Vitamin D3 Supplementation on Epigenetic Aging in Overweight and Obese African Americans With Suboptimal Vitamin D Status."

30 Zhu et al., "Increased Telomerase Activity and Vitamin D Supplementation in Overweight African Americans."

2. <u>Omega-3 fish oil</u>: Over the last thirty years or so, the typical Western diet has added more and more pro-inflammatory omega-6 polyunsaturated fatty acids versus anti-inflammatory omega-3 PUFAs. **Over the same period, we've seen an associated rise in chronic inflammatory diseases, including obesity, cardiovascular disease, rheumatoid arthritis, and Alzheimer's disease.**[31] Rich in omega-3s, fish oil is another incredibly versatile nutraceutical tool with multi-pronged benefits from head to toe. By restoring a healthier PUFA ratio, it especially helps your brain and heart. Regular consumption of fatty fish like salmon has been linked to a lower risk of congestive heart failure, coronary heart disease, sudden cardiac death, and stroke.[32] In an observational study, omega-3 fish oil supplementation was also associated with a slower biological clock.[33]

3. <u>Magnesium</u> deficiency affects more than 45 percent of the U.S. population. Supplements can help us maintain brain and cardiovascular health, normal blood pressure, and healthy blood sugar metabolism. They may also reduce inflammation and help activate our vitamin D.

4. <u>Vitamin K1/K2</u> supports blood clotting, heart/ blood vessel health, and bone health.[34]

5. <u>Choline</u> supplements **with brain bioavailability**, such as CDP-Choline, citicoline, or alpha-GPC, can boost your body's storehouse of the neurotransmitter acetylcholine and possibly **support liver and brain function**, while protecting it from age-related insults.[35]

6. <u>Creatine</u>: This one may surprise you, since it's often associated with serious athletes and fitness buffs. But according to Dr. Lopez, it's "a bona fide arrow in my longevity nutraceutical quiver for most individuals, and

31 Patterson et al., "Health Implications of High Dietary Omega-6 Polyunsaturated Fatty Acids."

32 Rimm et al., "Seafood Long-Chain n-3 Polyunsaturated Fatty Acids and Cardiovascular Disease."

33 Lu et al., "DNA Methylation GrimAge Strongly Predicts Lifespan and Healthspan."

34 Pearson, "Vitamin K1 vs K2: What's the Difference?"

35 Raman, "Acetylcholine Supplements."

especially older adults." **As a coauthor of a 2017 paper by the International Society for Sports Nutrition, Dr. Lopez, along with contributors, stated that <u>creatine not only enhances recovery, muscle mass, and strength in connection with exercise, but also protects against age-related muscle loss and various forms of brain injury.</u>**[36] There's even some evidence that creatine may boost our immune function and fat and carbohydrate metabolism. Generally well tolerated, **creatine has a strong safety profile at a daily dose of three to five grams.**[37]

7. <u>**Omega-3 optimizer: SmartPrime-Om**</u>**:** With his partners, **Dr. Lopez has leveraged artificial intelligence to identify a cocktail of methylation pathway nutrients and plant-based bioactive ingredients** found in sesame seed oil extract that can expand the benefits of fish oil and increase activity of genes and enzymes responsible for increasing the body's "pool" of omega-3s like DHA, DPA, and EPA. SmartPrime-Om also promotes delivery of omega-3s in the ideal biochemical phospholipid package to increase benefits for most cells, tissues, and major organs.

8. <u>**23Vitals**</u> **for nutraceutical immune optimization** was formulated to shore up our bodies on a molecular level and rejuvenate our immune system. **It contains 23 bioactive ingredients, covering more than fifty human clinical trials showing immune system bolstering, and other ingredients to support our digestive tract, respiratory, and cardiovascular health, and muscle and joint recovery from exercise stress.** It's designed to promote a healthy immune response when we need to fight off a challenge, and then **tone down inflammation** once the threat has been neutralized and the "wave" has receded. Available in a ready-to-mix powder. I use this personally, and am also an investor in the company.

This is not intended to be an exhaustive list, but it should give you a taste of some powerful steps you can take to enhance your body's extraordinary

---

36 Kreider et al., "International Society of Sports Nutrition Position Stand: Safety and Efficacy of Creatine Supplementation in Exercise, Sport, and Medicine."

37 Antonio et al., "Common Questions and Misconceptions about Creatine Supplementation: What Does the Scientific Evidence Really Show?"

capacity—things that you can do now. To learn more about advanced nutraceuticals, hormones, and peptides and to explore a custom regimen for
improving vitality and performance, simply visit our website.

We're living in exciting times, and technology is speeding up the evaluation of every medicine and form of nutrient known to man. New formulations are being created at a breakneck pace. The opportunity for us to
support our bodies in being their best for decades beyond what we have in
the past is now with us.

**Decide if any of these are right for you. Are there some peptides
that might make sense? Should you be tested for your hormones so
that you can make sure that you're at your optimum? Is the power
of NAD+ important to you?** Dr. Lopez has created three formulations
containing these key nutraceuticals to take throughout the day: **Peak Rise,
Peak Healthspan, and Peak Rest.** I use all three of these, as does Peter.
Our mission is to make it easy and convenient for you to live the best life
that you possibly can. You have a great checklist to consider evaluating with
your health professional. And again, you can have a telemedicine consultation with one of our medical experts at Lifeforce.com. We'll also continue to
publish new breakthroughs here after the publication of this book.

In the end, let me be crystal clear. In the race to find a safe and effective
silver bullet against aging, you'd be hard-pressed to predict a winner. Will
it be metformin? NAD+ boosters helping out your sirtuin proteins? The
Wnt signaling pathway? Genetic reprogramming? Or perhaps some synergy
between two or more of these tools? After all, as Francis Collins, director of
the National Institutes of Health, reminds us, aging is "a complex process
controlled by more than one protein encoded by one gene."[38] It stands to
reason that the longevity fix will be equally complex.

Still, Dr. David Sinclair is confident that "somebody is going to do it."
There are just too many ongoing clinical trials, he says, for *everybody* to
strike out. Sooner than later, according to Sinclair, aging will become just
one more treatable disease.

**I know this is like taking a drink of water out of a fire hose, so
thanks for sticking with me! Let's continue our journey!** In the next

---

38 Collins, "Less TOR Protein Extends Mouse Lifespan."

chapter I'm going to dive into a topic that almost everyone has to deal with in their life—physical pain. Because of my ten-inch growth spurt and a lot of other challenges I've faced in my life, I've found some incredibly effective tools that I use that have gotten me out of pain. Let's discover how to live a truly healthy and pain-free life. . . .

POWERFUL SENOLYTIC MEDICINES: THE JURY IS STILL OUT

Read this only if you're an anti-aging geek or a passionate biohacker! We'd like to give you just a few notes on two therapies that could have huge healthspan and longevity benefits . . . **but based on the current research, they may have too much risk without enough certain corresponding reward.** We're only bringing these to you because if you start studying things in the anti-aging space, you're sure to hear about these. However, many experts believe, as do we, that more research is needed to establish a favorable benefit-to-risk ratio. In any case, we'll definitely be keeping an eye on these two therapies and as new science comes forward will bring you more updates on our website.

<u>First, Senolytic Medicines.</u> Senescent cells are the **"zombie" cells** that refuse to die and that inflame surrounding cells, tissues, and organs. They're on the Most Wanted list for contributing to type 2 diabetes, Alzheimer's, and certain cancers.[39] **Senolytics are therapies that eliminate these cells, help stave off degenerative disease—and possibly disrupt the mechanism of aging at its source, before it moves downstream.**

In the anti-aging arena, **Dr. James Kirkland at the Mayo Clinic** is leading research on **dasatinib,** an anti-leukemia drug, in combination with the plant-based supplement **quercetin.** In a small human pilot study, this cocktail improved mobility and stamina in patients with idiopathic pulmonary fibrosis, a progressive and lethal scarring of lung

---

39 Childs et al., "Cellular Senescence in Aging and Age-Related Disease: From Mechanisms to Therapy."

tissue.[40] **But no peer-reviewed study has yet to show that senolytics actually reduce the number of senescent cells in people. And while many scientists believe the overarching strategy is sound, dasatinib can have serious off-target effects: vomiting, bleeding gums, anemia, heart arrhythmias.**

One promising alternative: fisetin, a plant-based substance that is far more powerful than quercetin. In a pre-clinical study by Dr. Kirkland's team at the Mayo Clinic, fisetin extended the lifespan of aging mice by close to 10 percent.[41]

The second treatment is rapamycin and has been used since 1999 to prevent transplant patients from rejecting their new organs. In 2007, it won additional FDA approval to treat metastatic renal cell carcinoma, the most common kidney cancer. Off-label, it's widely called upon to protect against graft-versus-host disease and to coat coronary stents.

But what has the healthspan and longevity world buzzing is rapamycin's unmatched anti-aging track record in animal trials. The National Institute on Aging's Intervention Testing Program has tested middle-aged mice with dozens of drugs, supplements, foods, plant extracts, hormones, and peptides. **Only six substances have shown significant lifespan benefits.** Resveratrol, fish oil, and green tea all failed the test. Aspirin did a little better. **But rapamycin beat all comers, extending median survival by as much as 18 percent for females and 10 percent for males.[42] When combined with metformin (which had little impact on its own), rapamycin racked up a 23 percent average survival dividend for both sexes, plus a sizable increase in** *maximum* **lifespan.**

In a study by Dr. Matt Kaeberlein at the University of Washington, a three-month course of rapamycin increased remaining

---

40 University of Texas Health Science Center at San Antonio, "First-in-Human Trial of Senolytic Drugs Encouraging."

41 Yousefzadeh, "Fisetin Is a Senotherapeutic That Extends Health and Lifespan."

42 Miller et al., "Rapamycin, But Not Resveratrol or Simvastin, Extends Life Span of Genetically Heterogeneous Mice."

life *expectancy* in middle-aged lab mice by *up to 60 percent*.[43] In the healthspan arena, Dr. Kaeberlein and coauthor Veronica Galvan concluded, **rapamycin "delays, or even reverses, nearly every age-related disease or decline in function in which it has been tested** . . . including cancers, cardiac dysfunction, kidney disease, obesity, cognitive decline, periodontal disease, macular degeneration, muscle loss, stem cell function, and immune senescence."[44]

<u>So what's the catch?</u> At typical clinical doses, rapamycin is part of a powerful immunosuppressant regimen for transplant patients that makes people significantly more vulnerable to bacterial infections. It can impair wound healing. And as yet, <u>there's no clinical trial data</u> <u>to show that its remarkable lifespan-enhancing results in animals</u> <u>can be replicated in people.</u> A highly publicized human trial by the biopharma startup resTORbio, focused on respiratory illnesses, and immune response to a vaccine challenge was promising, yet inconclusive. **Even so, scientists like resTORbio cofounder Joan Mannick believe that rapamycin—or synthetic facsimiles known as rapalogs— will ultimately break through as a safe and effective anti-aging therapy. The key, Dr. Mannick says, is to use lower and more intermittent dosing than the standard for transplant patients.**[45]

---

43 Bitto et al., "Transient Rapamycin Treatment can Increase Lifespan and Healthspan in Middle-Aged Mice."

44 Kaeberlein and Galvan, "Rapamycin and Alzheimer's Disease: Time for a Clinical Trial?"

45 Zhavoronkov, "Women in Longevity—Dr. Joan Mannick on Clinical Development for Aging."

CHAPTER 11

LIVING PAIN-FREE

You Can Take Control of Your Pain Without Surgery or Medication by Addressing the Source of the Pain Instead of Just Treating Its Symptoms

"The pain passes but the beauty remains."
—AUGUSTE RENOIR

Pain is a fact of life. We all experience pain at some point in our lives. For me, it started in childhood, when I went through an otherworldly growth spurt, every inch of my body stretching out painfully as I sprouted up nearly a foot in the course of a year due to a pituitary tumor. For others, pain occurs as a result of an accident—sharp and fast and traumatic—or creeps in slowly as the years pass by, growing from a minor annoyance into chronic discomfort that cries out to be managed over the long term.

Pain is also big business, which makes a lot of sense when you consider that chronic pain is estimated to affect 20 percent of people at some point in their lives. There's an entire medical specialty called pain medicine. And there's an entire arsenal of medications to counteract pain, both over-the-counter and prescription drugs prescribed by doctors who are trying to help their patients manage pain that keeps them from living the lives they're meant to live. Of course, you know all about the opioid crisis that has resulted in more than 450,000 Americans dying in the past couple decades. **Last year, according to the CDC, more than 150 million opioid prescriptions were filled in the United States. <u>That's 46 prescriptions for every 100 people.</u>** But opioid use isn't new. Would you believe it stretches back thousands of years to ancient times? The Sumerians cultivated opium in Mesopotamia as early as 3400 BC. The colonial English were so enamored of opium that they went to war with China to maintain their access to it.

What exactly are opioids? You may be wondering. **Opioids, including oxycodone (commonly sold as OxyContin) and fentanyl, are powerful painkillers that are highly effective at relieving pain after surgery or trauma.** The downside is that they are also highly addictive—so addictive that Purdue Pharma, maker of OxyContin, is named in countless lawsuits that claim they aggressively marketed these painkillers as safe and effective while knowing just how addictive these substances are. Even over-the-counter painkillers can be suspect. Take Tylenol, for example. A tremendous marketing campaign has made Tylenol one of the most trusted brands for pain relief. But according to **Dr. Erika Schwartz**, author of the book *Don't Let Your Doctor Kill You*, **each year, acetaminophen overdose is responsible for 56,000 ER visits, 2,600 hospitalizations, and 458 deaths due to liver failure. In fact, just taking one or two pills above the recommended dosage for two weeks can be deadlier than if you tried to overdose. Shockingly, the <u>leading cause</u> for calls to poison control centers isn't kids accidentally ingesting cleaning supplies; it's accidental acetaminophen overdose!** Close to 50 percent of cases of acute liver failure in the U.S., as well as 20 percent of liver transplant cases, can be traced to acetaminophen poisoning.[1]

At the same time, some researchers wonder whether acetaminophen is <u>impacting</u> something as critical and fundamental as our emotions. One Ohio State researcher who examined this found that study participants who received acetaminophen versus a placebo had a harder time feeling "positive empathy" for strangers, which matters because the ability to experience empathy is associated with more stable romantic relationships and more successful careers. **"Just like we should be aware that you shouldn't get in front of the wheel if you're under the influence of alcohol, you don't take [acetaminophen] and then put yourself into a**

---

1 Yoon et al., "Acetaminophen-Induced Hepatotoxicity: A Comprehensive Update"; Larson et al., "Acetaminophen-Induced Acute Liver Failure: Results of a United States Multicenter Prospective Study."

situation that requires you to be emotionally responsive—like having a serious conversation with a partner or coworker," Dominik Mischkowski, an assistant professor at Ohio University who studies the relationship between pain and social behavior, told the BBC.

Americans have been programmed to believe that there's always a magic pill to cure whatever ails us. Just take a peek at any drugstore aisle with a dizzying array of over-the-counter (OTC) drugs and supplements competing for your hard-earned dollars, and you'll see the proof. It's buyer beware: A few years ago, a doctor told me to take Zantac, a common heartburn medication, following a bout of food poisoning, but guess what happened in April 2020? The FDA ordered manufacturers to take Zantac off the market due to concerns that it could contain dangerous levels of a chemical that may cause cancer in humans. Another example is the commonplace practice of aspirin therapy to lower cardiovascular risk. In October 2021, new research issued by the U.S. Preventative Services Task Force overturned this recommendation, as recent evidence suggests that the risks for those over 60 outweigh the benefits, and could actually cause harm, including bleeding in the stomach, intestines, and brain –which can be life-threatening.

A study published in the *Journal of the American Medical Association* (*JAMA*) analyzing how advertising changed when four prescription drugs became available over the counter found that the drugs' benefits were emphasized more while mention of their side effects plummeted—from 70 percent to 11 percent!

In medical school, doctors-in-training don't learn much, if anything, about over-the-counter meds. After all, if you don't need a doctor's prescription to buy them, why should medical school instructors spend time educating future physicians about their effects? **But this gap in knowledge has led to the false belief that OTC drugs are harmless cure-alls; often, patients don't even think to mention to their doctors that they're taking them!** But some OTC drugs can be downright dangerous.

By now, it should be pretty clear that with so many people experiencing pain and with current treatments so woefully inadequate, we need some new approaches. Fortunately, there are groundbreaking new tools to control pain that I'm going to share with you. You won't be surprised that these breakthroughs are coming from people outside the industry who thought outside the box. **There's a reason that so many breakthroughs come from out-siders: because it's these folks who are able to look at a situation with fresh eyes and fresh perspectives to find fresh solutions.**

Remember, as we told you earlier, German philosopher Arthur Schopenhauer said: "All *truth* passes through three stages.

First, it is ridiculed.

Second, it is *violently opposed.*

Third, it is accepted as being self-evident."

All this is to say that if you're in pain, don't despair! There are tools to help, and we're going to share with you how to access them and how to self-advocate. Over the years, I've learned that no one is going to care as much about your health as you do. No one is truly going to be able to put themselves in your shoes and understand the depth of the pain you're feeling. It's up to you to take matters into your own hands and advocate for what you need to feel your best. **Although I spent decades with severe pain in my back and spine, I never stopped looking for ways to live a more pain-free life and to help others do the same.** Today, my life is completely transformed in this area, and I want yours to be as well. I've been on this crusade for more than forty years. Let me tell you how it all started. . . .

GROWING PAINS: MY PERSONAL HISTORY OF HURT

"It is easier to find men who will volunteer to die than to find those who are willing to endure pain with patience."

—JULIUS CAESAR

Everyone has heard about growing pains, right? I'm here to tell you that they're not some abstract theory; they're the real deal and they're excruciat-ing. **After I grew ten inches in one year because of that pituitary tumor, I experienced the impact of that growing spurt for decades.** My natural growing process was entirely out of whack. My bones grew too fast for the rest of my body to adjust, leaving my muscles stretched, my joints stressed, and my whole body imbalanced. Even walking could be unbearable. Like a lot of people, I learned to suck it up and just deal with the pain. I'd ice everything, doing my best to cope with the discomfort with only the help of some frozen water! Because I wasn't willing to numb the pain—I wouldn't even take aspirin for a while there—I was forced to continue seeking solutions. I went from one doctor to another, hoping that eventually one of them would find a solution to my problem.

I was in my 20s when things became less manageable. I got injured playing football. Then I was rear-ended twice in four months. The first time, I was on my way to racing school, just ten minutes from the track, when a car hit me at 35 miles an hour. I suffered minor whiplash. I was still very much in the healing phase when the second crash occurred. It was a few months later, and I was waiting at a stoplight when I looked in the rearview mirror and saw headlights coming at me full speed. I remember thinking, *That guy better slow down.* He didn't. He fell asleep at the wheel, and I got rear-ended again, only this time at 70 miles per hour. Everything happened in slow motion. The cassette player exploded past my face and out the back window. The first thing I remember was being pulled from the car by firefighters who wanted to take me to the hospital. I didn't think there was any need for that. "No, no, I'll see my chiropractor tomorrow," I said. "Look, I can walk."

But the next morning, I couldn't. In fact, I couldn't even stand. My hips snapped underneath me and the level of pain was off the charts. I started doing therapy after therapy after therapy, and I began to get a little better. But I never knew what would set me back. **At 23 years old, I was doing my trademark strategy seminars, where I was used to running and jumping for ten, twelve hours a day. But now as soon as I'd take a step up the stairs to the stage, searing pain would course through my body.** I'm a guy who normally roams around the stadium, absorbing and radiating energy, but now I felt like an 80-year old man, confined to a chair because standing was too excruciating. I'd start to get better, then I'd get worse. It was an endless cycle of massive pain.

I found small solutions along the way, but as the years went by and I put even greater demands on my body, I had to find more powerful solutions. Thankfully I did, and I'll be sharing these with you in this chapter. But to help you imagine what it's like and the demands on my body, let me give you a simple example. **I happened to attend a concert by Adele** at a venue I would be speaking at a few weeks later. I was so touched by what an extraordinary performer she is, and to see her captivate 15,000 fans, but then **I realized her entire show was just two hours; I, on the other hand, would be in the same building in a couple of months with the same-size audience, but on my feet for fifty hours over four days in a row—the equivalent of twenty-five straight concerts in one weekend**. Then I'd do it all over again two weeks later. So obviously it wasn't an option not to find a solution to deal with my pain.

Even back in the early days of my career, I realized that I was working my body to the bone, and that was the initial wake-up call. It forced me to take responsibility for my own pain and take control of my own health. I went on a quest to find innovative treatments and solutions. In this chapter, I'm going to share the best of what I've learned, starting with **the unavoidable truth that to get out of pain, you have to get to the source of it**. On this journey, you'll meet the visionaries who are liberating people from pain—pain specialists, doctors and therapists who have spent decades developing and refining leading-edge treatments—including therapies that the greatest athletes in the world swear by. **You'll gain a new perspective on how you can manage your pain, or better yet become pain-free for life, so that it no longer saps your vitality or keeps you from living a full life.**

In this chapter, you'll learn about six tools that I've found to be extraordinary ways to attack pain and reclaim function. For example:

1. You'll see how pain disappears when electromagnetic energy—so-called lighting in a box, or PEMF, pulsed electromagnetic field, therapy—is harnessed as a restorative therapy. Its incredible impact has been demonstrated in thousands of studies.

2. We'll share with you the incredible story and dedication of a Vietnam veteran who returned home with a Purple Heart and combat wounds that left him in unbearable chronic nerve pain that doctors were unable to alleviate. He was told that his injuries were irreversible and he'd have to live with his pain for the rest of his life. Because he

wouldn't settle, he found a solution based at the source of his pain, and not only went on to heal himself, but over the last 40 years has become one of the most sought-after experts to eliminate pain in the world. He's worked with everyone from sports teams like the San Francisco 49ers to the best golfer of all time, Jack Nicklaus.

3. You'll learn that a simple but powerful repositioning of the body called "postural therapy" can actually have an immediate impact on chronic pain.

4. You'll discover a microscopic drainage system that flows through the body, one that can be tapped to help release toxins and inflammation even though scientists didn't even know it existed until recently.

5. You'll read about a doctor who has combined ultrasound, a tiny injection, and a cocktail of bioactive molecules to unleash a powerful new treatment for pain.

6. You'll marvel at how virtual reality can actually be used to block pain signals from making their way to your brain and retrain your brain to no longer react to that pattern of pain.

These tools and technologies are all grounded in the same core belief: that treating pain without first getting to the root of the problem is the wrong way to go. **For the best results, you must drill down and find the source of the pain instead of merely treating symptoms.** Sometimes, the source can be traced back decades. You may have forgotten the knee you sprained in college or the muscle you pulled in your back from a pickup basketball game a decade ago, but your body hasn't. And not only has your body not forgotten, but it may still be trying to adapt to those injuries, forever compensating for the dysfunctions they created.

You see, the body is hardwired to protect and make concessions for injured, overused, weaker parts of itself. It's why your right hip might come to the rescue of a weakened left knee without your ever being aware, or why a seemingly minor car accident is inhibiting your breathing years later. **At**

first, this seems like a good thing, that stronger body parts can take over the heavy lifting from weakened ones. But over time, compensations develop into imbalances and dysfunctions that cause tightness and tension and pain. The breakthroughs you'll learn about in this chapter are intended to turn back time and restore your body to pain-free living.

LIGHTNING IN A BOX

"The great art of life is sensation, to feel that we exist, even in pain."

—LORD BYRON

Have you heard of pulsed electromagnetic field therapy? It relies on the idea that Earth is basically one big magnet—an idea supported by gravity, the oceanic tides, and the perpetual rotation of the planet. This massive magnet that is Planet Earth is charged with electromagnetic energy and electrified by the roughly 8 million lightning strikes that occur each and every day. (It's true: Lightning strikes the Earth more than a hundred times per second!)

Not to get too metaphysical with you, but energy is what sustains human life. Our bodies rely on a charge of energy to fuel every cell; likewise, an optimal level of magnetic energy is required for optimal health. That energy is maintained when we consume the nutrients and minerals we need, get quality sleep, and stay active and energetic by moving our bodies. Of course, no matter how healthy our lifestyle, we lose some of that charge as we age. **That's where PEMF comes in: It restores our body to a peak level of energy.**

PEMF therapy was first introduced as a way of encouraging broken bones to heal; in fact, veterinarians were early adopters of the technology, using it to try to knit together racehorses' broken legs. These days, PEMF is used for a broad spectrum of applications in humans—everything from cervical fusion surgery, to depression, to musculoskeletal pain. **I'm living proof that PEMF machines, which administer a controlled pulse of electromagnetic energy, really work. Not a day goes by when I don't use my PEMF machines.** That should tell you something.

Let me tell you how I first learned about PEMF. Remember when I described the agonizing snowboarding accident that left me with a torn rotator cuff and pain that felt like a 9.99 out of 10? It was so excruciating that I could barely breathe. I flew to see a doctor experienced in platelet-rich plasma (PRP) therapy, a special injection of my own platelets to accelerate healing. As luck would have it, he was a huge personal fan of mine. He told me his life had turned around thanks to me. But then he dropped a bomb. After looking at my spine, he diagnosed severe spinal stenosis. That plus my torn rotator cuff compelled him to say, **"One good hit, you know, from another snowboarding accident or jumping or being aggressive with squash and hitting a wall and you could be a quadriplegic."**

I was dumbfounded, truly in shock, but I accepted his offer to inject PRP to see if it would ease the pain temporarily. Sure enough, it numbed the agony completely, but it also rendered my right arm useless. Hours later, with my arm dangling uselessly by my side, I had to explain to my audience of 8,000 people that I'd had a procedure. I asked for their grace and understanding, but less than three hours into my presentation, the pain roared back worse than before. Still, I had to keep my promise to take pictures with one hundred VIPs in the audience. **I'm 6'7", so people see me and think I'm indestructible, but in my head, I was screaming out in pain as they'd give me a hug or a friendly smack on the back.** But there was one woman who didn't do that. She was staring at me and analyzing every time someone hugged me. She knew what was going on. She had my number.

"You're in pain," she said. "What happened?" I briefly told her the story. **As fortune would have it, this woman was a spinal surgeon. She told me, "Surgery isn't the answer; it usually isn't in these situations." What was the answer? "In the short term, you need to get the pain to a level where you can deal with it," she advised me. "In the long term, you need to get a PEMF machine."** This surgeon explained how electricity would enter my body and literally calm my frayed nerves, circulating the lymph fluid, stimulating my body to heal itself.

I flew out that night but could barely sleep; I was bleary-eyed with pain. But the next day, I found a PEMF practitioner, who came to my hotel with his own PEMF machine. It looked like something out of a science fair project, with electric pads that wrapped around me. **I got on the table and within 20 minutes, my pain went from a 9 to a 4.5.** Over the next month or two, I continued using the machine daily and making great improvements before I eventually flew to Panama, where as I shared with you earlier, I had the stem cell therapy that completely healed my shoulder.

These days, I remain a staunch believer in the healing power of PEMF and its therapeutic magnetic field. I've since bought at least a dozen PEMF machines, including an upgraded one from a company called Pulse Centers in Georgia. **These machines are a godsend in terms of pain relief and healing. But I also use them for entirely different reasons: The machines boost my energy and concentration levels and improve my sleep.** It has had a big impact on my overall daily function. And it's not just me: **Studies have shown that PEMF decreases pain, swelling, and inflammation, and improves cellular metabolism and energy.**[2]

Recently, my 83-year-old aunt Carol fell down and was rushed to the hospital. As she was unable to move, in massive pain, and very fearful to be going home in that condition, I got her a PEMF machine that got her out of pain and helped her heal at an incredibly rapid pace, shocking even her doctor. I've used it with professional athletes I coach as well. Of course, PEMF isn't the only method of healing I employ; I've got an entire toolbox! I have my own **hyperbaric oxygen** machine, and I'm also a huge fan of **cryotherapy,** which can be a phenomenal tool for reducing inflammation and which we'll discuss more in depth in Chapter 15, on visible health and vitality. But PEMF is my go-to.

I don't want you to think that PEMF is something that only professional athletes, CEOs, and those in unbearable pain have access to. The therapy is increasingly being offered by holistic practitioners, physiotherapists, chiropractors, and doctors. In fact, the eGym locations we will talk about in Chapter 14, on strength, have PEMF machines. I personally recommend that you get yourself an experience with one, and you'll be sold on its power and impact. Most people will do three sessions of twenty to sixty minutes and see significant positive changes. But I felt the impact, and many

2 Kubat et al., "Effect of Pulsed Electromagnetic Field Treatment on Programmed Resolution of Inflammation Pathway Markers in Human Cells in Culture"; Martino et al., "The Effects of Pulsed Electromagnetic Fields on the Cellular Activity of SaOS-2 Cells."

do, after just the first session, and I'm willing to bet you'll notice a positive change. **PEMF devotees affectionately call it "lightning in a box," and it just may be the right way for you to decrease both acute and chronic pain, increase circulation, and boost your overall energy while recharging your health.**

THE MIND-BODY CONNECTION

Pain doesn't happen in a vacuum. Maybe you got injured. Maybe your body is stressed. Perhaps you're dealing with trauma. **Pain occurs when your body gets out of alignment. Think about it: Our body's number one job is to keep us upright, balanced, and in sync.** When something gets in the way of that, we hurt.

It can be helpful to think of the body as a spiderweb, a vast and delicate map where all roads, big and small, intersect. We've got muscles and joints and nerves and blood vessels and capillaries that form the scaffolding, blood that nourishes, and lymph that detoxifies. They're all working in tandem until this smooth functioning is disrupted: You might overwork your biceps at the gym and suddenly your lower back hurts.

I'm no stranger to overworking my body. In addition to my fourteen-hour-a-day, four- to ten-day marathon speaking events, I'm an adventure enthusiast, a thrill-seeker. I love pushing myself beyond my limits. But after being in those two car accidents I told you about, within the span of four months, I could barely function. I was lucky to be alive, especially after the second car crashed into me at full speed.

At the time, I wasn't even 25, but I felt three times my age. So I kept looking for answers. And that's how I found **Pete Egoscue.** Now a bestselling author, pain expert, and radio host, Egoscue had dealt with similar challenges in his time as a Marine in Vietnam. **He has actually figured out how to crack the pain code.** Let me tell you how he did it: **When Egoscue came back from serving in Vietnam, he returned with a Purple Heart—and, from his combat wounds, unbearable chronic nerve pain** that none of the doctors back home could alleviate. **They couldn't figure out how to help him, so they told him he'd just need**

to live with the pain. You know that Marines aren't the type to give up, so what did Egoscue do? He set out to heal himself.

As he dug into researching his own tools for self-healing, he began to discover different types of exercises to restore the body's equilibrium. **He started with a fairly straightforward but completely profound insight: In order to heal, he would first need to find the source of his pain—his posture and balance. You see, Egoscue believes that the human body is perfectly designed; pain creeps in only due to overuse, injury, or underuse that puts the body out of balance and sets us up for injury.**

Egoscue's approach to body mechanics, which I was lucky enough to discover after I was immobilized with pain from those two accidents, is all about being in balance. He believes our biomechanical well-being starts with alignment, and that most of us are out of alignment in one way or another. So **he developed the Egoscue Method, a kind of "postural therapy" designed to banish chronic pain** caused by everything from sports injuries and car accidents, like those I experienced, to commuting, typing, and aging in general. Brian Bradley, who worked alongside Egoscue for decades, puts this in context, explaining that even minor injuries wreak havoc over time. "If you sprain your right ankle playing basketball in high school, you're now dealing with a nervous system that remembers the ankle injury and compensates by putting a heavier load on the left side. So now that left knee suffers, in some cases for years. You've got to start going after the cause versus the symptom."

I highly recommend that you read Pete Egoscue's bestselling book, *Pain Free: A Revolutionary Method for Stopping Chronic Pain*. In it, he lays out the exercises—he calls them "E-cises"—that can realign posture and return the body to a balanced, more functional state. He believes no one knows more about our bodies than the people who inhabit them. Here's what he tells clients: **"We'll never know as much about your health as you do. So my job is to get out of the way and give you the tools to maximize your well-being."**

I first went to Pete to cope with my pain from those accidents. I had already spent a year in physical therapy, and nothing had worked, but by the third session I had with Pete, I literally had no pain in my body. I couldn't believe it! But it made so much sense, because we dealt with the source of the problem, instead of reacting to the pain. I was doing great, until later, being the crazy man I am, I was being overly aggressive in a polo game and was jettisoned from my horse. The injury was devastating. **But within three days, Pete got me back to my old self.**

Now, more than three and a half decades later, I'm still doing his exercises to keep my body in peak form and alignment. They're a part of my daily routine and help me handle the incredible demands that I place on my body so that I can continue performing at the highest level. **These exercises aren't time-consuming.** They take just a few minutes, but the results are incredible, allowing me to do the things I want to do and feel great doing them.

Egoscue has worked with some of the greatest athletes in the world, including golfer **Jack Nicklaus**, the late great **NFL linebacker Junior Seau**, and the **San Francisco 49ers**, coaching them to be **pain-free** and reach **peak performance** by addressing chronic pain and dysfunction at its source rather than attempting to treat it with surgery or painkillers. My athletic skills aren't in that league, but the Egoscue Method is helpful for anyone. **After working with Egoscue for so many years, I've learned that injury compounds from a series of stressors in our daily life.** Craning our necks to see our phones and hunching our shoulders to type lead to a stacking of small insults, which leads to chronic accumulated pain. So even if you don't get rear-ended twice like I did, modern life doesn't treat our bodies kindly. If you want to show your body some compassion and get yourself out of the chronic pain rut, I can't recommend the Egoscue Method enough. **Pete is a dear friend of mine, having made such a difference in my life for forty years, and he's offered to do a free postural assessment for readers of this book. You can do it on Zoom or on your phone; simply go to www.Egoscue.com and put in the code PAINFREE. Information is also available on our Lifeforce.com website.**

After three decades following the Egoscue regimen, I know that pain isn't a foregone conclusion. I know how to eliminate it. Of course, this isn't my only tool. . . .

EASING PAIN WITH COUNTERSTRAIN

"Pain is weakness leaving the body."

—CHESTY PULLER

I've had every kind of bodywork you can imagine, and it all has some value. At the right time, a skilled chiropractor or masseuse is priceless. **Most kinds of bodywork are based on the theory that pushing on tissue—massaging or kneading it—is fundamental to getting it to relax. So what if I were to tell you that the secret to easing pain lies in something as simple as some gentle repositioning?** You might think: "Tony, that's ridiculous." But I'm here to tell you that it's true—and to tell you all about this magical modality known as **Counterstrain**. I was first introduced to it by a 75-year-old competitive tennis player. He competed at a national level in amateur tennis at that stage, and as you may guess, at his age, there were times when he would get injured from the demands of that sport. I shared with him some of the tools that had helped me and he told me about counterstrain. **He said, "Tony, it's painless, it's quick, and it's life-changing." I tried it out and found it to be truly extraordinary.** Let me share with you the story of how it was created and a little bit about how it works so you can decide for yourself whether this might be something you'd like to try as well.

Let's go back more than half a century to 1955, when **Dr. Larry Jones, an Oregon osteopath and the go-to guy for pain** in his area, experienced success with a patient who was in so much discomfort that he wasn't able to stand upright despite having been treated by a couple of local doctors. This unfortunate fellow couldn't even get comfortable enough to sleep at night, so Dr. Jones spent half an hour experimenting with various positions that might make this guy more comfortable. **When he moved the patient's legs up toward his head and shoulders and off to one side, the patient was amazed: no pain!** Dr. Jones excused himself to treat another patient then returned to find his first patient had drifted off to sleep, right there in the exam room. Upon awaking, this young man could stand soldier-straight. He was glowing with relief.

The next person to experience sleepless nights was Dr. Jones himself, as he turned this amazing and unexpected turn of events over in his head. What exactly had happened? After a few weeks of pondering this, he decided that **the repositioning had triggered the relaxation of a protective reflex that had gone into overdrive. Experimenting with different positioning had stopped the spasming, helping the body unload tension so it could relax. It had actually reset the nervous system!** Building on that insight, Dr. Jones continued to experiment with creating new techniques that hinged on the simple premise of finding a comfortable, pain-free position. And Counterstrain as a modality was born.

Importantly, Dr. Jones discovered more than 180 "tender points" that intersected with each unique treatment position; with proper positioning, these tender points of pain would simply vanish! This discovery was too consequential to keep quiet about. As Dr. Jones spread the word through speaking engagements, a book, and trainings, he began applying his approach to patients in more than five countries, including the U.S., Canada, Germany, Japan, and Australia. As the father of counterstrain, Dr. Jones inspired a **young physical therapist in Maryland, Brian Tuckey**, who saw that counterstrain resulted in a huge improvement in range of motion. Tuckey worked with Dr. Jones for more than a decade, learning how to administer counterstrain with precision. Eventually, as Dr. Jones aged, he passed the counterstrain torch to Tuckey.

Forty years after Dr. Jones's eureka moment with the sleeping patient, Tuckey made another startling discovery that would extend the fundamentals of counterstrain. He discovered that Counterstrain can be applied to all inflamed painful tissues, not just muscle. **This includes organ, vessel, and nerve tissue, which enabled Tuckey to expand counterstrain from 180 to over 900 treatments. Counterstrain works by releasing trapped inflammation in the interstitial pathways, the deep fluid-filled channels that surround our cells.** These pathways are part of the interstitium, which accounts for 20 percent of all the fluid in the entire body.

(Science didn't even know the interstitium existed until twenty years ago! Now some experts consider the interstitium to be the body's largest organ, larger than the skin.)

Remarkably, even bone can be treated with Counterstrain, as it can be utilized to alleviate vasospasm (reduced blood flow) in the "nutrient" blood vessels that transport blood to and from our bones. The two pictures below demonstrate resolution of chronic osteomyelitis (bone swelling) in a patient who suffered for three years with swelling and pain during everyday activities following fracture and toenail removal. The swelling (bone marrow edema) was verified via multiple MRI studies from 2016 to 2019, and it had persisted despite multiple medical interventions. One medical practitioner even went so far as to suggest that the patient have the end of her great toe amputated to alleviate the pain. A singular Counterstrain treatment performed in October of 2019 resulted in marked improvement and allowed the patient to return to trail running within seventy-two hours. A post-treatment MRI (November of 2019) was utilized to objectively verify the results, which can be noted by the reduction of swelling (bright white area).

Persistent inflammation can cause chronic muscle knots called "trigger" or "tender" points; in fact, Tuckey says that **unresolved inflammation can underlie everything from tendonitis, sciatica, and bursitis to irritable bowel syndrome, chronic headache, and vertigo.** This is a new medical concept recently described in detail in the peer-reviewed medical journal *Frontiers in Musculoskeletal Pain.* The manuscript titled **"Impaired Lymphatic Drainage and Interstitial Inflammatory Stasis in Chronic Musculoskeletal and Idiopathic Pain Syndromes: Exploring a Novel Mechanism,**

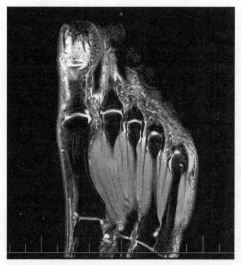
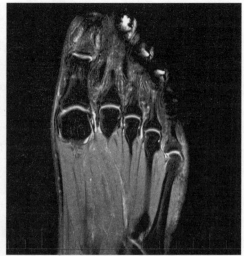

Tuckey B., Srbely J., Rigney G., Vythilingam M. and Shah J., was published in August 2021, is a must-read for any medical practitioner who wishes to understand the latest theoretical rationale behind peripherally generated chronic pain and multiple other poorly understood medical conditions.

With that in mind, here's what a Counterstrain treatment looks like: Practitioners palpate the body for "tender points" then decompress the involved tissues using only their hands, releasing trapped inflammation back into the bloodstream, disrupting the chronic pain cycle. **The key to Counterstrain is targeting the source of the problem rather than the surface muscle response.** Unfortunately, most bodywork does the opposite, targeting the surface muscle spasm, not the underlying inflammatory source, which yields only temporary results. **Amazingly, Counterstrain releases take only about forty seconds and often produce lasting relief. "It's kind of like rebooting your computer," Tuckey says. "Shut off the pain reflex, wait a few seconds for the swelling to resolve and voilà."**

You can understand why the work of practitioners like Tuckey could be key in treating, even eliminating, certain diseases related to chronic inflammation. Best of all, **Counterstrain is completely painless;** no more mashing on trigger points or enduring the pain of dry needling and foam rolling. It's clear the Counterstrain revolution is **changing how people deal with pain, digestive problems, and chronic inflammation at the same time that it's reshaping the power and scope of hands-on therapies.**

Like the Egoscue Method, Counterstrain has attracted high-profile athletes, including star Portland Timbers midfielder Diego Valeri. Injuries had taken such a toll on Diego's body that in 2015, he came in last on his soccer team's pre-season functional movement test. Suffering the strain of years of high-level athletic competition, he was no longer able to jump, as his ankles had essentially fused from repeated sprains. **But eighteen months later, following Counterstrain therapy, Diego had improved markedly and was named Major League Soccer's 2017 MVP, shattering the Timbers' all-time scoring record with twenty-one goals and ten assists.** Ten of those goals were jumping headers, an impossible task for Diego prior to receiving Counterstrain treatment.

But Counterstrain isn't just for elite athletes. It's a critical tool in the pain-free toolbox for you and me. I can't recommend counterstrain

enough. To make an appointment with a Counterstrain practitioner trained by Tuckey, **you can go to https://counterstrain.com/clinics/ or simply go to our website where all of the resource links in this book are listed.** As Tuckey puts it, alleviating pain and restoring function is about restoring hope. **"When you restore hope after it's been gone so long,"** he says, **"you can open doors for people to do anything."**

RESTORING CONNECTIVE TISSUE, FROM HEAD TO TOE

"The world breaks everyone, and afterward,
some are strong at the broken places."

—ERNEST HEMINGWAY

When **Major-League baseball legend Miguel Cabrera** could no longer take the pain in his right ankle, he didn't turn to a sports medicine doc or an ankle specialist. He'd already tried them, with limited results. Instead, he paid a visit to **Dr. Abhinav Gautam, an anesthesiologist trained** at the University of Miami/Jackson Memorial Hospital. A former tennis player, Dr. Gautam developed RELIEF, a natural treatment for pain, limited mobility, and stiffness designed to restore damaged connective tissue in our hips, ankles, knees, back, shoulders—really anywhere—so that we can quickly vanquish pain. RELIEF **uses ultrasound and artificial intelligence to zero in on scarred, damaged tissue and locate entrapped nerves within the interstitium—there's that new organ again!—and across the body's connective tissue, liberating those nerves and repairing tissue without ever coming near a scalpel.**

Cabrera, a two-time American League MVP and 2012 winner of the MLB Triple Crown, is a staunch believer. **His pain decreased as soon as he began treatment, and his ankle mobility improved from 20 percent to 90 percent.** If he chose surgery, he was told, the most he could hope for was 50 percent rehabilitation. He'd simply have to deal with the pain. But, just like Pete Egoscue, he refused to accept that. And Dr. Gautam—his patients call him Dr. Abhi—assured him he didn't have to. "I was like, go to sleep—pain. Wake up—pain. Go to the field—pain. Go to the gym—pain,"

Cabrera said in a video endorsing Dr. Abhi's work. **After treatment, the pain vanished. "When I wake up, I don't feel pain. I feel free."** Cabrera's ankle was not his only issue; in 2019, **four specialists diagnosed him with a chronic right knee injury. Told he would have pain and limited mobility for the rest of his career, Cabrera again turned to Dr. Abhi. Within weeks, he regained the ability to jump on his right knee, run pain-free, and hit with the same force as earlier in his career.**

For years, the sports medicine world has known about the importance of fascia, that pliant web of connective tissue that surrounds the body's muscles and tendons like an elastic hairnet. The fascia is what your trainer is trying to loosen when he gives you a foam roller before your workout. The fascia can bunch up and dehydrate over time. Nerves can get stuck, causing pain. And accumulated scar tissue can inhibit mobility. **All of this can clog up the interstitium like a traffic jam on the way to the beach on a Friday afternoon in August.**

In fact, Dr. Abhi had experienced this blockage himself. After years of competitive tennis, he had built up scar tissue in his left shoulder. Years later, the tightness still hadn't resolved. One day, he used his ultrasound machine to zoom in on his shoulder and recoiled at what he calls "stiff-looking, disorganized tissue." Then, Dr. Abhi got to work . . . on *himself*. "I was like, 'Let me see if I can stick a needle in and, you know, rejigger things.'"

He rejiggered to the point that he was able to break up the scar tissue and restore the fascial planes enough that his shoulder loosened up and returned to a range and ease of motion he hadn't felt in years. And despite the fact that the needle hurt like hell—leave it to a professional anesthesiologist to forget to anesthetize himself before sticking himself with needles!—it immediately felt like a breakthrough. (He now provides a local anesthetic for all his patients so the experience is as close to pain-free as possible.) **"It was a real Aha! Moment," he says, "this feeling of space being created inside your body."**

Dr. Abhi's goal is to create "volume" in the body, restoring the tissue planes and establishing some much-needed separation for previously entrapped nerves. He uses needles—I'm here to tell you that you can't feel them thanks to lidocaine—to break up the scar tissue and create more space. **Then to further promote growth and regeneration and open up the**

space where the connective tissue has hardened, he injects a specially formulated cocktail of proteins, collagens, and growth factors derived from healthy donated human placental tissue. "We're trying to trick the body to act like it's still back in the womb, when it was busy creating new healthy tissue," Dr. Abhi explains.

After Dr. Abhi applied RELIEF's techniques to Bob, a patient in his mid-60s with a long history of hip and lower back pain and immobility due to a horrific car crash, **Bob got up and walked fluidly around Dr. Abhi's office,** his gait returned to normal now that the scar tissue in his back and hips had been released. He was incredulous and overjoyed. "I just can't believe it," he said.

Dr. Thomas Michael Best, past president of the American College of Sports Medicine, couldn't believe it either at first. Dr. Best is a sports medicine doctor, a biomedical engineer who earned his PhD at Duke University and serves as the Miami Marlins' team physician, but he engaged with RELIEF on a personal level after suffering with hip pain for a decade. At first he was dubious, but Dr. Best observed immediate improvement after a thirty-minute treatment. Three months later, his hip range of motion remained intact and he was running pain-free. "My functional improvement was correlated to structural changes around the hip joint that were easily visible on ultrasound," he marveled.

When I first went to see Dr. Abhi, I shared Dr. Best's initial skepticism. As Dr. Abhi moved the ultrasound wand across my left ankle, which I'd injured jumping twenty years ago, he showed me how the nerves were trapped by this connective tissue that covers the interior of our bodies. **I became a believer as I watched on ultrasound while Dr. Abhi gently inserted a needle and coaxed a nerve to pop free.** Up until that day, I'd always cautioned my masseuse to steer clear of this ankle. Touching it made electric shocks course through my body. But after Dr. Abhi's manipulation and protein potion, I haven't had any problems at all with the ankle. **RELIEF literally opened tissue that had been locked up for twenty years.**

Dr. Abhi has now trained others in this breakthrough treatment, and there are many experts around the world who are also using a similar technique to eliminate pain. One of these pioneers is Dr. Dallas Kinsbury, an internationally known musculoskeletal ultrasound practitioner who independently developed a similar modality while he was teaching residents at NYU Langone Medical Center, and is now part of the Fountain Life medical team. Dr. Dallas is a board-certified physical medicine and rehabilitation doctor who is also board-certified in sports medicine. He is pioneering further work with the placental biologic material being developed by Dr. Bob Hariri and his team at Celularity and has now instituted all of the pain relief protocols that he's been using for a decade at all Fountain Life centers. This is what my father-in-law had done to his hip if you recall from our Chapter 3.

Thanks to Dr. Abhi, I've learned that we don't have to blindly accept that aches and pains are just part of getting older. "You start to think, 'Well, my neck is supposed to feel a little stiff or I'm supposed to feel this tightness' because we think that's just what aging is," says Dr. Abhi. "We accept it. But I can tell you now that's completely not true."

MIND OVER MATTER

"Pain is temporary. It may last a minute, or an hour, or a day, or a year, but eventually it will subside and something else will take its place."

—LANCE ARMSTRONG

The sad truth is that there's some chronic pain that just won't go away, despite all the best tools. When that happens, all is not lost. In these cases, the key is learning how to use your mind effectively. That's exactly what's being done at **Cedars-Sinai Medical Center in Los Angeles**, where research in 2019 showed that virtual reality (VR) can lessen pain experienced by hospitalized patients. **When patients suffering from any number of problems, from orthopedics to cancer, donned VR goggles with a choice of relaxing scenarios, they rated their pain significantly lower than patients who watched the health and wellness channel on their hospital room TVs. Imagine that: An artificial world can offer a drug-free way to reduce pain!**

We've talked about these incredible results elsewhere in this book. But it bears repeating because **it's truly mind-blowing that virtual reality both distracts the mind from thinking about pain and also blocks pain**

signals from communicating with the brain. Other experts are exploring how VR games actually rewire the brain so that it responds differently to pain. "I believe that one day soon VR will be part of every doctor's tool kit for pain management," says **Dr. Brennan Spiegel, director of Cedars-Sinai's Health Service Research**, who introduced VR to the hospital.[3] You may note that I'm including websites for all of these pain solutions, and there's a reason. **If you're in pain right now, I want you to get the answers you need immediately.** So if you want to learn more about how VR is relieving pain, you can visit https://www.cedars-sinai.org/newsroom/virtual reality-as-medicine-an-interview-with-brennan-spiegel-md/ or through the resources section on our website.

AN ADDITIONAL TOOL FOR SPEEDING UP THE HEALING PROCESS AND BECOMING PAIN-FREE

Another innovative option for pain management? I'm sure you've heard about the powerful healing impact of **therapeutic lasers**. They were used initially in animals and horses and are now used by peak performance athletes and sports teams.[4] Because of the nature of my work, I've had the opportunity to use some of the best. My favorite is the **Genesis One laser,** which we'll share more about in Chapter 15, on beauty. It's one of my trusted go-to tools for pain relief. My wife and I have several of these lasers, developed by my friend **Dr. Antonio Casalini**, one of the foremost experts in the field. He created and licensed the well-known THOR laser for tissue healing, reducing inflammation, pain relief, and healing wounds. But Dr. Casalini didn't stop there; he is now producing wider-spectrum, more powerful lasers in his Genesis One line. I take his lasers on the road with me

---

3 Dascal et al., "Virtual Reality and Medical Inpatients: A Systematic Review of Randomized, Controlled Trials"; Birckhead et al., "Recommendations for Methodology of Virtual Reality Clinical Trials in Health Care by an International Working Group: Iterative Study"; and Aubrey, "Got Pain? A Virtual Swim with Dolphins May Help Melt It Away."

4 Genesis Performance Chiropractic, "Deep Tissue Laser Therapy."

as a must-have, because they help me counteract the tension and pain that comes from running, jumping, and standing on my feet for more than 12 to 13 hours per day, for four days in a row. They've helped me so much, I've become an investor in the company.

Studies have backed up lasers' effectiveness when it comes to decreasing pain, inflammation, and swelling. They work by delivering energy to the body through light photons, which encourages self-repair. **In fact, laser therapy has the unique ability to ignite and regenerate the body, just as plants absorb the UV rays of the sun and convert photon energy into chemical energy.**

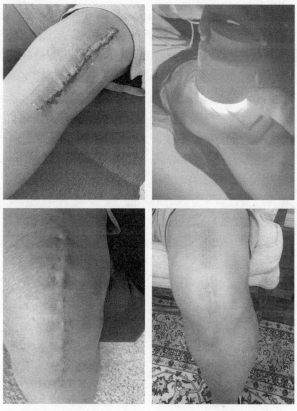

Example of the impact of Genesis One laser used for healing post surgery, shown at the top left on first day of treatment, top right at 10 days, bottom left at 30 days, and bottom right at 90 days. Pretty extraordinary!

Laser energy penetrates deep within the body. It's so incredibly effective that we're offering laser treatments for pain and rapid tissue healing, sports recovery and injuries, concussions and PTSD at Fountain Life. In fact, Fountain Life's COO, Dr. Matthew Burnett, is teaming up with Dr. Casalini to work on new evolutions in the field and develop even more powerful tools. I can't wait to see what revolutionary next-gen treatments emerge from their partnership.

All these exciting innovations that we've talked about in this chapter can change your life from a world of hurt to living without pain. Whether you are seeking out **the healing power of electromagnetic frequencies found in PEMF machines, the postural therapy of the Egoscue Method, the gentle and precise repositioning of counterstrain, the dismantling of scar tissue to restore mobility, or the technological wonderland of virtual reality, these are some of the best anti-pain tools I know.**

Of course, stem cells are one of the best plans of attack, one of the greatest solutions for true healing for so many ills. And you remember Chapter 9, on the Wnt pathway? Perhaps by the time you're reading this, if their final Phase 3 trials go well, you'll soon have the opportunity to wipe out osteoarthritis with a single injection. If all goes well, FDA approval is expected by the fall of 2022 or early 2023. Depending on when you're reading this, the treatment might already be on the market!

Here are three quick tools to be aware about, and then we'll wrap up this chapter together!

TOOL #1: AVOIDING ADDICTIVE OPIOIDS IN THE EVENT OF AN EMERGENCY

by Dr. Roberta Shapiro, assistant clinical professor,
Columbia University Medical Center, Department
of Rehabilitation and Regenerative Medicine

Before you ever find yourself in the hospital, read below on alternatives to addictive opioids, and new technology that is helping break the opioid addiction.

As we've discussed, the management of acute pain has been a frustrating challenge. One that has led to gross mismanagement and ultimately addiction. Most of us are "painfully" aware of the opioid epidemic facing the United States, but few realize that there is an alternative to opioids for acute pain, in most cases.

Some years ago, I had firsthand experience of this when I fractured three ribs and was in severe pain. The emergency room administered morphine, which in fact had no pain-relieving effect for me. **I asked them for intravenous Toradol (ketorolac), a nonsteroidal anti-inflammatory, which by the way they were happy to administer. My pain literally was gone for more than three hours!**

So why is it that when someone goes to the emergency room with pain, they are often given Vicodin (hydrocodone), Percocet (oxycodone), morphine, or Demerol, to name a few? They are then sent out with a prescription for opioids. Same goes for postoperative pain, for which patients often awaken on a morphine pump, are transitioned to an oral pain medication, and then sent home on the same.

Toradol is an extraordinarily safe, nonaddictive, anti-inflammatory alternative with excellent analgesic effects that can be administered intravenously (IV) or intramuscularly (IM) in addition to orally (oral for up to five days). By having the IV or IM options, we can avoid the potential for gastrointestinal side effects. **Because Toradol is an anti-inflammatory, we must always be aware of**

the potential blood thinning effects and monitor renal function, but overall the risks are exponentially less than the risks of opioids.

Opioids have so many negative potential side effects, from constipation, to altered consciousness, mood changes, and obviously addiction, and the list goes on. Toradol has none of these.

I suggest there IS an alternative, if not otherwise contraindicated. I educate every one of my patients regarding this and have done so for more than twenty years. The patients get relief, I do not create a potential for addiction, and the hospital-based doctors are more than satisfied with this request.

Now, I am not in any way discounting that there is a role for opioids, but rather, why not choose a safe alternative first?

TOOL #2: A PROMISING FDA-AUTHORIZED SOLUTION FOR TREATING ADDICTION

But let's say you are one of those struggling with addiction. First, you are not alone! Second, a breakthrough company called Pear Therapeutics has created ombi, the first prescraiption digital therapeutic to receive FDA authorization for substance use disorder. The app is used as a supplement to provide cognitive behavioral therapy (CBT) in an innovative way.

The app contains a dashboard of information for both the clinician and patient. This includes lessons, patient-reported substance use, cravings, triggers, medication use, rewards, and lab results. Even if it feels overwhelming to have so many eyes on your care, it's a community approach to healing.

How does it work exactly? People struggling with addiction often have an overactive dopamine circuit in their brains. Pear Therapeutics uses that dopamine to retrain a reward system to enforce lasting behavioral change. The app causes a release in dopamine through a simple reward system **just by interacting with the app**. It'll give the user a smiley face, a $2–3 gift card, even the rare $50-plus gift card in response to different actions. This keeps people engaged and incentivized. And in weeks, it lays the foundation for a rebuilt dopaminergic circuit.

Only four hours per week of talk therapy and use of the app more than doubled the rate of abstinence across all patients. <u>Thirty to forty percent of people achieve abstinence after twelve weeks!</u> And even better, people started to **feel better after only a month**. I know that can still seem like a long time, and no one said it would be an easy road to recovery, but this breeds hope that there are promising solutions out there. I'm so passionate about finding real solutions to addiction that I invested in the company as well.

TOOL #3: THE POWER OF THE ANCIENT ART OF ACUPUNCTURE

By Dr. Jie Chen, experienced practitioner, lecturer, and researcher of Chinese medicine, founder of Gaya's Clinic based in Modi'in, Israel

Why does at least a mention of the ancient healing art of **acupuncture** belong here alongside the cutting-edge medical breakthroughs at the vanguard of the future frontier? Because traditional acupuncture isn't just a relic of antiquity, it's still one of the most masterful therapies in existence. My patient, Tony Robbins, has found great value in its healing powers. . . .

Acupuncture is an essential part of Chinese medicine therapeutics whose history dates back almost 3,000 years. Traditionally, acupuncture is performed as a therapy to mediate with *Qi*, which is **Life Force in Chinese language.** Life force circulates along energetic highways known in acupuncture as meridians. These meridians are the body's intelligent network whose priority is to integrate the body's interior organs and exterior parts into a unified form. The communication between organs via the meridian network allows the body systems to cooperate in synchrony as a holistic masterpiece. Using needles, acupuncture taps into life force locations and stimulates its stronger gathering and flow. Using various techniques, needles can direct life force to flow into targeted regions and promote more active interactions among systems, the practice of which always aims at helping the body maintain a state of equilibrium.

For centuries, acupuncture has been practiced popularly worldwide, especially for chronic disease management. However, it also proves to be highly efficient and effective in emergency care, to relieve pain, ease convulsions, aid menstruation and conception, stabilize vital signs, resuscitate cardiac system, and revive the patient to consciousness after an event like fainting, shock, or coma. This is another interesting observation reflecting how quickly acupuncture can preserve and redirect the circulation of life force back to the essential organs and connect a person's body and mind with the environment again.

Besides the traditional practice, acupuncture's analgesic effect has been developed into a new feature of therapy—acupuncture anesthesia, which is a notable breakthrough of modern practice. By needling before and during surgery, the pain can be safely and effectively suppressed at the operation site. Such techniques have been used alone or with traditional anesthesia for operations on the head, neck, chest, abdomen, limbs, and in various invasive examinations. Patients remain conscious during the operation, as a result they cooperate better with surgical process, and enjoy the benefits of less anesthesia side effects, in-time protection for the essential organs, and immunoregulation, and faster post-operative recovery.

Another exciting finding of modern research is acupuncture's positive influence on stem cells. Many animal studies done in the brain, spine, and bone marrow have brought forth encouraging results showing that acupuncture may increase expression of stem cell genes, promote the proliferation and differentiation of the injected stem cells, and improve stem cell migration into the host system. These results indicate that the combined intervention of injecting stem cells with acupuncture provided a better outcome than stem cell transplantation alone.[5] Acupuncture has been used for millennia and is still as dependable today. Its integration with breakthroughs in this book may lead this ancient healing art to a future role in regenerative medicine.[5,6,7,8,9,10,11,12,13,14,15,16]

5 Pawitan et al., "Various stem cells in acupuncture meridians and points and their putative roles."

6 Ho et al., "The possible role of stem cells in acupuncture treatment for neurodegenerative diseases."

7 Ding et al., "Electroacupuncture promotes the differentiation of transplanted bone marrow mesenchymal stem cells overexpressing TrkC into neuron-like cells in transected spinal cord of rats."

8 Ding et al., "Electro-acupuncture promotes survival, differentiation of the bone marrow mesenchymal stem cells as well as functional recovery in the spinal cord-transected rats."

9 Yu et al., "Electro-acupuncture at Conception and Governor vessels and transplantation of umbilical cord blood-derived mesenchymal stem cells for treating cerebral ischemia/reperfusion injury."

10 Kim et al., "Potential benefits of mesenchymal stem cells and electroacupuncture on the trophic factors associated with neurogenesis in mice with ischemic stroke."

11 Dubrovsky et al., "Electroacupuncture to Increase Neuronal Stem Cell Growth."

12 Chen et al., "Electro-acupuncture improves survival and migration of transplanted neural stem cells in injured spinal cord in rats."

13 Yan et al., "Electro-acupuncture promotes differentiation of mesenchymal stem cells, regeneration of nerve fibers and partial functional recovery after spinal cord injury."

14 Zhu et al., "Electro-acupuncture promotes the proliferation of neural stem cells and the survival of neurons by downregulating miR-449a in rat with spinal cord injury."

15 Chen et al., "Electro-acupuncture exerts beneficial effects against cerebral ischemia and promotes the proliferation of neural progenitor cells in the cortical peri-infarct area through the Wnt/□-catenin signaling pathway."

16 Ogay et al., "Identification and characterization of small stem-like cells in the primo vascular system of adult animals."

What I really hope you realize now is that there is no shortage of tools to implement and explore to control and eliminate pain. So don't doubt that we're living in the right time to deal with your pain. **Whatever you do, don't just sit and suffer.** Sure, surgery might be necessary. **But before you head to the operating room, you might want to try something less extreme that you've discovered in this chapter—something that can free you from pain—that doesn't require such extreme intervention.**

Hopefully you're as optimistic as I am about the prospect of living pain-free. But it requires more than optimism; it requires a commitment to test new approaches because breakthroughs are coming out every day. One of the most important things I've learned is that **we have to be willing to look beyond the traditional approach to find solutions that work and practitioners who are willing to find the root of the problem and not merely treat its symptoms.**

Luckily for us, we're living in an age of medical revolution, where **a generation of independent-minded mavericks are finding better ways to combat pain without surgery or pharmaceuticals.** Like so many other ideas and treatments in this book, it's all about finding ways to increase your well-being so you can continue to do all the things you love—and feel strong, healthy, and pain-free doing them for many years into the future.

Now let's move on to discover simple lifestyle changes that you can make, at no cost, that can have a profound impact on your energy, focus, and quality of life. Let's discover, the longevity lifestyle and diet. . . .

CHAPTER 12

THE LONGEVITY LIFESTYLE & DIET

A Few Simple Lifestyle Changes Can Dramatically Improve Your Energy, Health, and Longevity

"While the science is complex, our application of it is both straightforward and practical: eat well, stress less, move more, and love more."

—DR. DEAN ORNISH

This chapter doesn't require you to spend any extra money. It doesn't require a major commitment of time. You won't need a doctor's prescription to implement any of the solutions that you're going to learn about here. **And yet the simple lifestyle changes that we're about to share with you can have an immediate and enduring impact on your vitality, your energy, your strength, and your quality of life.**

The good news is that these actionable insights are available to you right now. **All you need is a solid grasp of what works and a commitment to harness that understanding in ways that will dramatically increase your chances of living a long, vigorous, and healthy life.**

The trouble is, there's so much misinformation and conflicting advice out there that it's easy to get confused and knocked off course. Our goal is to cut through all of that noise and nonsense, so you can move forward with a new sense of clarity and awareness. After all, awareness—combined with effective action—is the foundation, the *bedrock* of a healthy and vibrant lifestyle.

To guide us on this journey, we've assembled a dream team of experts with an unsurpassed depth of insight based on decades of rigorous scientific research. Who better to lead this team than my great friend and Life Force adviser **Dean Ornish, MD? He's often hailed as the father of lifestyle medicine,** a field that uses lifestyle changes to prevent, treat, and reverse disease.

As Dr. Ornish explains, it's "very empowering" to realize how quickly and decisively you can improve your health by simply modifying your own behavior. The truth is, most of us wildly underestimate the power of our basic lifestyle choices. But the latest science is so compelling that it's impossible to ignore. For example, we'll explain:

- **How a handful of "low-risk" lifestyle choices can add twelve or more years to your life.**
- **How moderate exercise can literally *halve* your risk of dying from heart disease.**
- **How smart dietary decisions can *reduce your risk of death from any cause by 36 percent*, while poor dietary choices can *increase your risk of death by 67 percent*.**
- **How you can take advantage of the regenerative benefits of fasting without putting yourself through needless misery!**
- **We'll also show how understanding your microbiome can help you customize your diet for increased health and vitality.**
- Finally, I'll share with you **two of my favorite biohacks that can truly transform the quality of your life** in ways that you might not even believe is possible. **The power of heat and the power of cold. Two natural stressors that can lower your blood pressure, cut your chance of heart disease in half, improve your mood, and even give you a moderate exercise effect without having to do much movement!**

This subject of lifestyle is so central to your health and well-being that we're going to continue exploring it over the next two chapters as well. In those chapters, you'll learn how to optimize your life force by improving everything from how you sleep to how you build muscle mass.

The fundamental truth underlying the chapters in this section is so simple that it's easy to underestimate their critical importance. **In short, your basic, day-to-day lifestyle choices will have a profound impact on your quality of life, your healthspan, and your lifespan—and those choices are entirely in *your* hands.**

PHYSICIAN, HEAL THYSELF

"You are the cause of your own joy or your own misery. You hold
that power. You are your own friend and your own enemy."

—SWAMI SATCHIDANANDA

When Dr. Ornish was a 19-year-old premedical student in college, his life began to unravel. "I was suicidally depressed," he recalls. "I came about as close to committing suicide as you can without actually doing it." The stress from striving to excel overwhelmed him. Surrounded by gifted students who seemed so much smarter than him, he felt like an imposter, a dumb fraud whose inadequacy would be exposed for everyone to see. He feared that he'd fail to get into medical school, that he'd disappoint his parents, that nobody would "love and respect" him.

Worst of all, he was filled with a sense of total futility. Even if he achieved a measure of success, he was convinced that *nothing* would ever bring him lasting contentment. Unable to sleep, sit still, or focus on his studies, he tried to calm himself by taking tranquilizers and drinking alcohol. The future seemed so bleak that he even contemplated crashing his car into the side of a bridge, so his death would look like an accident. In the end, he was saved by sickness. Slammed by mononucleosis, he barely had the energy to crawl out of bed. "My parents saw what a wreck I was and took me home to Dallas," he says. "My plan was to get strong enough to kill myself."

His sister had experienced some striking health benefits from practicing yoga with an Indian spiritual teacher named Swami Satchidananda. So Ornish's parents decided to host a party for the swami in the living room of their home. Dressed in saffron robes and with a billowing white beard, Satchidananda delivered a life-changing lecture. **He explained that nothing external can bring lasting happiness and that a wiser path is to focus on quieting down the mind and body enough to experience a deep sense of inner joy and peace.** "This was back in 1972," says Dr. Ornish. "*Today* it would be weird in Dallas. But it was *especially* weird then." Still, he could see that Satchidananda "was glowing and I was miserable. It was, like, what am I missing here?"

Desperate to ease his suffering, Ornish was willing to try anything. So he learned to meditate, studied yoga, and started to use breathing and visualization techniques that helped to calm his mind. Inspired by Satchidananda, he also changed the way he ate. Renouncing the juicy steaks and cheeseburgers of his youth, he gave up his high-fat American diet and became a vegetarian.

Feeling healthier, happier, and more focused, Ornish returned to college and became first in his class. After that, he aced medical school and landed a fellowship at Harvard. **He eventually became a professor of medicine at UC San Francisco,** the author of bestsellers like *Dr. Dean Ornish's Program for Reversing Heart Disease*, and a pioneering researcher whose studies have been published in the most prestigious medical journals. **He also built a nine-week "lifestyle medicine program" that's been scientifically proven to reverse heart disease and other chronic illnesses by optimizing four factors: how you eat, how active you are, how you respond to stress, and how much emotional support you receive.** Not so "dumb," after all.

Like so many of the scientists in this book, Dr. Ornish took his own pain and used it as the inspiration for a career in which he's lifted so many other people out of *their* pain.

When Dr. Ornish looks back now on what he's learned over four decades about the causes—and prevention—of disease, he's struck by what he calls "a blinding flash of the obvious." He explains: "I was trained like all doctors to view heart disease, diabetes, prostate cancer, breast cancer, and even Alzheimer's disease as being fundamentally different diseases, different diagnoses, different treatments."

In reality, says Dr. Ornish, "they really are the *same* disease just manifesting and masquerading in different forms. They all share the same underlying biological mechanisms: things like chronic inflammation, oxidative stress, telomeres, angiogenesis, and so on. And each of those mechanisms is directly influenced by what we eat, how we respond to stress, how much exercise we get, and the psychosocial support we get."

That realization has profound implications. "It radically simplifies what we advise people to do," says Dr. Ornish. **"For the vast majority of chronic diseases, it's the same lifestyle recommendations because, again, they really are the same disease."**

One of his favorite examples involves telomeres, which are the protective caps at the ends of your chromosomes, much like the plastic tips on your shoelaces. As you age, your telomeres tend to shorten, causing your cells to malfunction and die. Shorter telomeres are associated with an elevated risk of premature death from many illnesses, including heart disease, Alzheimer's, type 2 diabetes, and a rogues' gallery of cancers. To put it bluntly, as your telomeres get shorter, your life gets shorter, too.

Are you powerless in the face of this decline? Not at all!

It turns out that your lifestyle—including how you eat, exercise, and handle stress—has a huge impact on your telomeres. **Ornish's Preventive Medicine Research Institute teamed up with Dr. Elizabeth Blackburn, a Nobel Prize–winning scientist who's famous for her research on telomeres, to conduct the first controlled study showing that lifestyle changes can *lengthen* your telomeres. A group of patients who went through Dr. Ornish's lifestyle program for just three months displayed a 30 percent increase in telomerase—the enzyme that repairs telomeres.**[1] **After five years, telomere length had increased by 10 percent, instead of *decreasing* with age. The editors at *Lancet Oncology* described this as "reversing aging at a cellular level."**[2]

Another research team has shown that adults who exercise consistently have significantly longer telomeres than those who lead sedentary lifestyles. They found that "highly active" adults who jogged for thirty to forty minutes a day five days a week had a "biologic aging advantage" of nine years over sedentary adults.[3] Yes, you read that right! **Biologically, it was if they were *nine years* younger, just because they made the commitment to exercise on a regular basis!**

We're seeing this pattern again and again in scientific studies. **Simply put, the impact of the most obvious, commonsense lifestyle choices**

---

1 Ornish et al., "Increased Telomerase Activity and Comprehensive Lifestyle Changes."

2 Ornish et al., "Effect of Comprehensive Lifestyle Changes on Telomerase Activity and Telomere Length in Men with Biopsy-Proven Low-Risk Prostate Cancer."

3 Tucker, "Physical Activity and Telomere Length in U.S. Men and Women: An NHANES Investigation."

is staggering. In 2018, a research team from the Harvard School of Public Health published a landmark study titled "Impact of Healthy Lifestyle Factors on Life Expectancies in the U.S. population."[4] **They showed the effect on more than 120,000 people of five "modifiable" lifestyle factors:** *never smoking*; *moderate alcohol intake*; *regular physical activity* (at least thirty minutes a day of "moderate to vigorous exercise"); *"a normal weight"*; and *"a healthy diet."*

The study also found that people who adopted a healthy lifestyle had an 82 percent lower risk of dying from cardiovascular disease during a follow-up period and a 65 percent lower risk of dying from cancer.

What did they discover? **In midlife, say at 50 years old, men who followed all five of these "low-risk" guidelines could expect to live *12.2 years longer* than men who followed none of them, while women could expect to live *an extra 14 years*. The study also found that people who adopted a healthy lifestyle had an 82 percent lower risk of dying from cardiovascular disease during a follow-up period and a 65 percent lower risk of dying from cancer.** The authors emphasized that cardiovascular disease, cancer, and other chronic illnesses "are the most common and costly of all health problems, but are largely preventable."

Just think about that for a moment. **The biggest threats to your health are largely preventable. Once you've truly internalized that essential idea, you can begin to zero in on some more specific questions. For example, what constitutes a healthy diet?**

---

4 Li et al., "Impact of Healthy Lifestyle Factors on Life Expectancies in the US Population."

EAT WELL, FEEL GREAT, LIVE LONG

"If it's a plant, eat it. If it was made in a plant, don't."
—MICHAEL POLLAN

There's fierce disagreement about the negatives and positives of countless diets—from Keto to Paleo, Nordic to Mediterranean, GOLO to Jlo. It's almost as bad as listening to politicians bickering about everything under the sun! Dr. Ornish has been a valiant warrior in these nutritional debates, duking it out in public with controversial figures like the late Robert Atkins, MD, who created a high-fat, low-carbohydrate diet that many experts (Ornish included) consider harmful.

But Dr. Ornish has had enough. "I'm not doing these diet wars anymore," he says. "It was just confusing people and providing a platform for people who really don't have the science to back up what they're saying." He's choosing instead to lay out clearly what he's learned about nutrition over four decades, based on published research (by himself and others) and his successful results with thousands of patients. **"The studies are there for anyone who really wants to look through them,"** he says, and there's **"an emerging consensus"** about how to eat healthily. "If you want to do it, here's how you do it. If you don't want to do it, that's fine, too. But it works really quickly and you'll experience the benefits in your own life if you try this approach."

First of all, the evidence shows emphatically that the typical Western diet *isn't* working. Many of us consume too much sugar, too much meat, too much fat, too much salt, too many calories, *too much everything*—and these choices are making us sick.

"Most Americans eat way too many refined carbs," adds Ornish. That includes white bread, white rice, pizza, pasta, pastries, fruit juice, and sodas brimming with high-fructose corn syrup. "It's like mainlining sugar. It goes straight into your bloodstream, so your blood sugar spikes, your pancreas makes insulin to bring your blood sugar back down, which is good. But the insulin accelerates the conversion of those calories into fat. **It causes chronic inflammation and many of these mechanisms that underlie some of these chronic diseases."**

The question is, what should you eat instead, if you're ready to cut back on those "bad" carbs? "I'd love to be able to tell your readers that pork rinds and bacon and sausage are good for you, but they're not," says Ornish. That may sound sacrilegious to most Americans, and we're not suggesting you give up meat if you're a dedicated carnivore! As we'll explain shortly, **one of the advantages of the newest DNA testing is that it helps us understand why different people thrive on different types of diets.** Now, you have to be careful, as DNA is not absolute, it's the epigenome that impacts us most, but it can be impacted by diet as well.

For example, whether your body tends to primarily burn carbohydrates, fats, or proteins can help you understand why certain diets work better for some people. But there are still fundamentals. We all need the same core ingredients and still need some universals like vegetables and greens. **It is important to note though that many studies have found that diets high in animal protein—especially red and processed meats when not accompanied by fruits and vegetables——are associated with increased risks of illnesses like breast cancer, prostate cancer, diabetes, and heart disease.**

Dr. Ornish's solution is to replace those "bad" carbs with "good" carbs—mostly fruits, vegetables, whole grains, legumes (like beans,

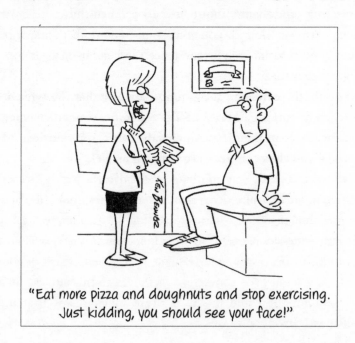

"Eat more pizza and doughnuts and stop exercising.
Just kidding, you should see your face!"

chickpeas, and lentils), and soy products (like tofu and soy milk). Most good carbs are low in fat, high in fiber, and do a better job of filling you up than bad carbs.

What's more, says Ornish, good carbs "don't provoke these repeated insulin surges," which can "lead to metabolic syndrome and, ultimately, type 2 diabetes." **Good carbs also contain "thousands of protective substances that have anti-cancer, anti–heart disease, and anti-aging properties," including bioflavonoids, polyphenols, retinols, lycopene, carotenoids, isoflavones, and other goodies with equally obscure names!**

The protective qualities of vegetables are particularly mind-blowing. For example, studies have shown a stunning range of health benefits from cruciferous vegetables like broccoli, cauliflower, kale, and brussels sprouts.[5] They've been linked to lower rates of everything from cardiovascular disease to breast and prostate cancer. <u>What's the secret? One factor is that these veggies contain sulforaphane, a compound that reduces inflammation and can even slow the growth of tumors.</u> Given what we're learning about sulforaphane's mighty powers, Popeye should load up on raw or steamed broccoli sprouts, along with his spinach.

The point is, when you eat fewer *harmful* foods and replace them with *protective* foods, you gain what Ornish views as a "double benefit." In dietary terms, it's the ultimate win-win.

None of this is particularly complicated. **"It's essentially a whole foods plant-based diet that's naturally low in fat and sugar and refined carbs," says Ornish.** His preference for "whole" foods (like fruits, vegetables, and beans) is worth emphasizing. As you'd expect, it's usually healthier to eat high-quality foods in their natural, organic state than packaged products processed by ingenious people in white lab coats.

But these are really just general guidelines to help you decide for yourself how to eat, based on reliable research about the expected effects on your health. In one of his books, *The Spectrum: A Scientifically Proven Program to Feel Better, Live Longer, Lose Weight, and Gain Health*, Ornish categorizes food into five groups, listing the healthiest in

---

5 Zhang et al., "Cruciferous Vegetable Consumption Is Associated with a Reduced Risk of Total and Cardiovascular Disease Mortality."

Group 1 and the unhealthiest in Group 5, which is where you'll find "the usual suspects: the processed meats and donuts and so on." But **he's not saying, "Eat this" or "Don't eat this." He's simply demystifying the science so you can make educated choices, given your own health, tastes, and willingness to change.**

"If you're just trying to stay healthy, lose a few pounds, get your cholesterol or blood pressure or blood sugar down a bit, it's not all or nothing," says Dr. Ornish. **"What matters most is your *overall* way of eating. So, if you indulge yourself one day, it doesn't mean that you're 'good' or 'bad.' It just means, eat healthier the *next* day."**

On the other hand, says Dr. Ornish, "if you're trying to reverse a life-threatening disease, that's a lot harder," and you'll need "to make even bigger changes."

Let's say you're at risk from heart disease—a largely preventable illness that's the world's leading cause of death. Maybe you or someone you love is overweight or sedentary or has other common risk factors like high blood pressure, high blood sugar, and elevated LDL cholesterol and triglyceride levels. If you reduce your intake of refined carbs and saturated fats (say, by cutting back on red meat, whole milk, cheese, and baked goods), you're likely to see significant improvements on all of these fronts.

If you boost your intake of whole grains, vegetables, and fruits, you're further reducing the threat of heart disease, it's that simple. Add in some moderate exercise and the picture brightens even more. One study found that **simply walking for thirty minutes a day five days a week can lower the risk of premature death by *20 percent*, compared to people who remain sedentary.**[6] **Another study found that women who walked briskly for sixty to ninety minutes per week *halved* their risk of dying from heart attack and stroke.**[7]

You can expect a similar pattern if your goal is to prevent or reverse the

---

6 Arem et al., "Leisure Time Physical Activity and Mortality: A Detailed Pooled Analysis of the Dose-Response Relationship."

7 Lee et al., "Physical Activity and Coronary Heart Disease in Women: Is 'No Pain, No Gain' Passé?"

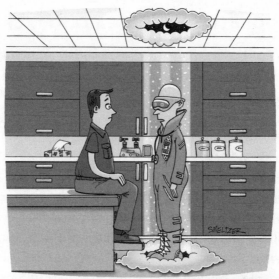

"I'm a doctor from the future, with revolutionary
health advice. Exercise, drink plenty of water
and eat your veggies."

progression of many other chronic diseases. **In one study, 926 men with prostate cancer were followed for about fourteen years after their diagnosis to assess the impact of diet on their mortality.**[8] **It turned out that men who ate a Western diet filled with red and processed meats, high-fat dairy, refined grains, and sugary desserts had a** *250 percent higher risk* **of dying from prostate cancer and a 67 percent higher risk of death from any cause.** I'd like you to pause for a moment to let those appalling numbers lodge permanently in your beautiful brain. As you probably know already, sugar is a silent killer.

By contrast, men who ate a "prudent" **diet filled with vegetables, fruits, legumes, whole grains, soy products, oil-and-vinegar dressing, and fish had a** *36 percent lower risk of death from any cause.* In a classic display of scientific understatement, **the study concluded that "modifications to diet" may "influence survival."** I don't know about you, but I'd bet my life on it.

---

8 Yang et al.,"Dietary Patterns After Prostate Cancer Diagnosis in Relation to
   Disease-Specific and Total Mortality."

SAY GOODBYE TO THE "HEART ATTACK DIET"

*"Dietary interventions can not only delay diseases but
actually eliminate a major portion of chronic diseases in mice,
monkeys, and even humans to extend longevity."*

—DR. VALTER LONGO, director of the Longevity
Institute, University of Southern California

Valter Longo, PhD, was born and raised in Italy. Longo had no intention of becoming a longevity guru. He started out wanting to be a rock star. At 16, he moved to Chicago with his guitar in hand, planning to study music while living with an aunt. He soon discovered that many inhabitants of his new hometown had adopted some pretty unhealthy habits! **It was perfectly normal to start the day with a breakfast of bacon, sausages, and eggs—and it wasn't unusual to eat meat at *every* meal. Longo was also introduced to Chicago-style pizza, which was smothered with enough cheese to sink a battleship, and he saw people washing it all down with vast sugary drinks, then topping it off with mountainous desserts.** Some of his relatives in Chicago were dying of cardiovascular disease, and he'd later describe this way of eating as the "**heart attack diet.**"

Longo moved to Texas for college, where he eventually made the leap from learning to play jazz guitar to studying biochemistry. In those student years, he fell into the habit of fueling himself with a steady supply of hamburgers, French fries, and the cheesy delights of Tex-Mex. **By his late twenties, his cholesterol and blood pressure were so bad that his doctors recommended that he take statins and hypertension drugs. Instead, he fixed his health by altering the way he ate.**

How? He essentially returned to the style of eating he'd grown up with in Liguria and Calabria, two regions of Italy where the cuisine was famously healthy. **It was a diet that revolved around complex carbs like vegetables, beans, nuts, and fruit, along with *moderate* portions of pasta, plenty of olive oil, and some fish. As a kid, says Longo, meat was a "once-a-week treat." It was no coincidence that these areas of Italy were home to an unusual number of centenarians.**

Longo became fascinated by the connection between nutrition and "healthy longevity"—a subject that he's now explored for more than thirty years. Today **Longo** is the director of the **Longevity Institute at the University of Southern California** in Los Angeles, and a leading expert on the biological mechanisms of aging. **He describes nutrition as "the most important factor you can take control of to affect how long you live, whether you will be diagnosed with certain major diseases, and whether you will be active and strong or sedentary and frail in old age."**

Longo has met with hundreds of centenarians, interviewing people like Emma Morano, an Italian who lived to 117. He's studied "longevity hotspots" everywhere from Sardinia to Ecuador, looking to uncover what they have in common. In the laboratory, he's also investigated the relationship between nutrition and the key genes and pathways that accelerate aging. **His mission? To reveal how dietary interventions can minimize disease, repair our bodies, and keep us young for decades longer. "I'm in the business of making people live to 110 and helping them to get there in good health," says Longo.**

In one of his studies, Longo and his collaborators examined the effects of protein consumption on the mortality of 6,381 people over the age of 50.[9] During an eighteen-year follow-up period, he found that **people aged 50 to 65 who ate high levels of protein were more than _four times_ as likely to die of cancer than people who ate low levels of protein. The group that ate high levels of protein also had a _74 percent increase_ in their risk of dying from any cause.**

But what really mattered was whether the protein they ate came from _plants_ (for example, beans, peas, nuts, seeds, and whole grains) or _animals_ (for example, meat, eggs, milk, and cheese). The study found that, for people aged 50 to 65, plant-based proteins were healthy, whereas "high levels of animal proteins promote mortality."

Dr. Longo's research has led him to develop what he describes as a **"Longevity Lifestyle and Diet."** It consists _almost entirely of plant-based foods_, making it broadly similar to Ornish's style of eating. **But Longo also**

---

9 Levine et al., "Low Protein Intake Is Associated with a Major Reduction in IGF-1, Cancer, and Overall Mortality in the 65 and Younger but Not Older Population."

recommends eating fish a maximum of two or three times a week, being careful to avoid types that contain notoriously high levels of mercury, including tuna and swordfish.

Dr. Longo favors those fish that are rich in omega-3 fatty acids, such as salmon and Atlantic mackerel. **What about meats like beef, lamb, and chicken? He avoids them.** Should you follow his lead? You don't have to. Remember these are *your* choices. But don't buy into the myth that you *have* to eat meat because it would be hard to get enough protein from a plant-based diet. The reality is, many of the healthiest and most energetic people on earth stick largely (or even exclusively) to a diet that's dominated by plants.

Take my friend Tom Brady, the best quarterback who ever lived. He primarily fuels himself with fruits and vegetables. For snacks, he likes nuts and seeds. And he eats *modest* servings of lean protein from fish or chicken. Tom sums up his dietary principle in two words: "Mostly plants."

Dr. Longo adds that there are striking similarities in the diets of the many centenarians he's met: They don't eat high quantities of saturated fats from meat or cheese. They don't eat heaps of sugar, either. Instead, they tend to consume lots of complex carbs like beans and vegetables, along with plenty of healthy fats from nutritious sources like olive oil and nuts. Another trait they have in common is that they're not that self-indulgent. **"Maybe once or twice a week they had some meat,"** says Dr. Longo. "They couldn't overeat usually because they didn't have the money to overeat."

I hope by now that you're seeing some clear patterns that will provide you with a few of the most fundamental guidelines. Remember, it doesn't need to be complicated. When the celebrated food writer Michael Pollan set out to answer the question of how humans should eat to be "maximally healthy," he managed to sum it up in seven words: **"Eat food. Not too much. Mostly plants."**

THE REJUVENATING POWER OF FASTING

"Fasting is the greatest remedy—the physician within."

—PARACELSUS, sixteenth-century physician

As Dr. Longo sees it, eating a nutritious, plant-rich diet is only half the story. **The other half of his strategy for preventing disease and staying young for longer may sound more radical, but it's extraordinarily effective. It involves harnessing the healing and protective powers of letting the body rest from the constant consumption, breakdown, and digestion of food. In other words, practicing what's known as "intermittent fasting."**

When Dr. Longo recommends that people adopt the habit of fasting, they often respond about as enthusiastically as if he'd suggested sleeping on a bed of nails. "They see it as a crazy idea," he says. "Lots of people are still in the camp of eat-all-the-time, and if they go one or two meals without eating, they think they're going to die!"

Time Restricted Eating: eat an early dinner (ideally, you finish your meal three hours before you sleep), and then eat nothing at all for at least the next twelve hours.

In most parts of the world, it's now standard to eat throughout the day, typically consuming at least three big meals, plus snacks. **In the U.S., says Longo, "people tend to eat over a period of about fifteen hours, without ever taking a sustained break. But when you think about human evolution, you realize that we were never built to live like this—for example, having instant access to meat in this superabundant, continuous way."**

Dr. Longo, who started his career by studying organisms like yeast and bacteria, remarks, "Most organisms on Earth are starving all the time. Then, when they're lucky once in a while, they get some food—and then they go back to starving. So obviously, we're the first species that got away completely from that."

Back in the 1980s, Longo observed in laboratory experiments that

when you starve yeast and bacteria, "they live longer." That revelation launched him on the path of researching whether fasting might also enhance the lifespan of humans. **Since then, he and many other scientists have conducted a number of studies in animals and humans suggesting that fasting can be a powerful weapon against illnesses like obesity, diabetes, hypertension, cancer, asthma, arthritis, multiple sclerosis, cardiovascular disease, Parkinson's disease, and Alzheimer's.**

Part of the challenge, says Dr. Longo, is to find practical ways of fasting that not only promote health and longevity but are manageable, "so people can actually *do* it." One popular approach that he recommends is a strategy called "time-restricted feeding."

It simply works like this: **He suggests that you eat an early dinner (ideally, you finish your meal three hours before you sleep), and then eat *nothing at all* for at least the next twelve hours. It's easy because most people are asleep for six to eight hours of the fast!**

There are many other variations of intermittent fasting. For example, fans of the 5:2 diet cut out around 75 percent of their calories on two nonconsecutive days each week and eat normally the other five days. **Another common approach, which many people find reasonably easy and sustainable after a week or two of adjustment, is to skip breakfast and fast for sixteen hours every day. Peter Diamandis practices a more intense version of time-restricted eating: He fasts for nineteen hours a day, typically eating in a five-hour window between 1 p.m. and 6 p.m. "Fasting gives me control," he says, "and I have a tremendous amount of mental clarity and physical energy during my mornings because my blood is not rushing to my gut to digest a big breakfast or lunch."**

Dr. Ornish agrees that fasting for twelve hours or more each day is "a great idea." Similarly, Dr. David Sinclair, the Harvard longevity expert we spotlighted in Chapter 4, routinely skips breakfast and lunch and waits until dinner for his only meal of the day.

As you'd imagine, many people are attracted to intermittent fasting as a way to lose weight. But longevity experts are also fascinated by the ways in which fasting can be used to slow aging and treat or prevent diseases. For example, Dr. Longo's research suggests that a

combination of prolonged fasting and chemotherapy can be highly effective in fighting various cancers, since cancer cells (which rely on glucose as a source of energy) become more vulnerable when weakened by starvation.

It's not easy to convince people who are battling cancer to take part in studies that require them to consume nothing but water for days on end. So, with funding from the National Cancer Institute, **Dr. Longo developed a five-day "fasting-mimicking diet" that's less grueling than a water-only fast.** On the first day, it consists of 1,100 calories. For the next four days, that drops to 800 calories a day, largely in the form of vegetable soups. As purists will tell you, this isn't *truly* a fast. But it's designed to have the same benefits without as much hardship. **So far, says Longo, more than 200,000 people have tried his fasting-mimicking diet, which is marketed by a company called L-Nutra as a rapid way to lose fat and "enhance cellular renewal."**

Why put yourself through all this misery? **Having fasted on a regular basis throughout my life, I can tell you that it's really not that difficult—especially after the first day or two—and you quickly begin to realize that so much of your desire to eat is tied to your habits and driven by your mental and emotional patterns.** Freeing yourself from those patterns can be incredibly liberating. And when your body isn't constantly engaged in processing foods, it has a chance to revitalize itself, so you can rediscover the natural energy that's already available inside you.

Dr. Longo explains that prolonged fasts like his five-day fasting-mimicking diet can have a profoundly restorative effect on your health. How come? To put it simply, your energy reserves are depleted after two or three days of fasting, and your body undergoes a metabolic shift from a sugar-burning mode to a ketogenic state in which you use fatty acids and ketones for fuel. Faced with the stress of fasting, "cells shrink," adds Longo, and enter a "protected" state. When you eat normally again, "they have an opportunity to rebuild." **Dr. Longo explains that this cycle of "starvation and refeeding" triggers a "regenerative and self-healing process" that can reduce the "biological age" of your cells and organs. How cool is *that*?**

In a clinical trial involving 100 people, Longo's team tested the effects of doing his fasting-mimicking diet for five days a month over

three months.[10] **Participants with risk factors for diabetes, cancer, and cardiovascular disease displayed an array of impressive results. For example, their Body Mass Index improved, their glucose levels were lowered, their blood pressure decreased, their cholesterol and triglyceride levels fell, and their levels of insulin-like growth factor 1 (which is associated with aging, cancer, and diabetes) dropped. "In most cases,"** says Dr. Longo, participants who started out being prediabetic **"came back to normal." It's worth noting that Dr. Longo does the fasting-mimicking diet twice a year in the belief that prolonged fasts are beneficial even for people in good health.**

These three simple moves—eating healthily, exercising regularly, and fasting intermittently—work wonders!

If you take full advantage of the insights we've discussed so far, the impact can be truly transformative. **These three simple _moves—eating healthily, exercising regularly,_ and _fasting intermittently_—work wonders!** Best of all, they work beautifully together. **But there isn't one "right" way to do it. So you want to find a balance that feels practical and sustainable for you, based on your lifestyle and preferences. Remember: These are time-tested guidelines, not rules.**

THE POWER OF WATER AND OXYGEN

"Everyone knows that water is 'good' for the body. They seem not to know how essential it is to one's well-being. They do not know what happens to the body if it does not receive its daily need of water."

—F. BATMANGHELIDJ, MD, author of *Your Body's Many Cries for Water*

There are two other key ingredients that I want to mention briefly because they're so fundamental to your health. The first is the most essential

---

10 Wei et al., "Fasting-mimicking Diet and Markers/Risk Factors for Aging, Diabetes, Cancer, and Cardiovascular Disease."

nutrient of all: *water*. **You can't think of your diet solely in terms of food because none of us can live without water.** It plays a crucial role in many functions of the body, whether it's transporting proteins and carbohydrates through your bloodstream, lubricating your joints, flushing out waste through your urine, regulating your body temperature when you sweat, or serving as a shock absorber for your brain.

For adult women, about 50 percent of the body is made of water. For adult men, it's about 60 percent. So it's not surprising if your body starts to malfunction and your energy levels crash when you're dehydrated. Scientists have shown that even mild dehydration can cause a significant impairment of concentration, memory, alertness, and physical endurance.[11] In fact, when your mind is foggy or you're exhausted, it's often because you're dehydrated. That's why I constantly remind people at my events to keep sipping water, so they function at their best.

Ironically, many people suppress their need for water by drinking sodas and coffee, which actually dehydrate them! In truth, water is the only liquid nutrient you need. How much should you drink? A simple guideline is to divide your weight (in pounds) by two and drink that amount of water (in ounces) each day. If you weigh 180 pounds, you'd drink 90 ounces of water per day—a little less than three liters. A review article on the importance of "hydration for health" recommends that **"healthy adults in a temperate climate, performing, at most, mild to moderate physical activity" should drink 2.5 to 3.5 liters of water a day.**[12]

Here's what I do. I weigh 282 pounds, half of my bodyweight in ounces is 141. So every morning, I fill 8 glass bottles that are 18 ounces each for my full quota of water for the day, and I number them so that I can make sure I'm on track. I often add some fresh lemon, as an easy and tasty way to improve digestion and manage appetite, and protect the body from cell damage caused by oxidation. I also add a pinch of Celtic sea salt to one of those bottles, which helps the body to absorb and

---

11 Jéquier et al., "Water as an Essential Nutrient: The Physiological Basis of Hydration."

12 Perrier et al., "Hydration for Health Hypothesis: A Narrative Review of Supporting Evidence."

retain water, optimizing hydration. Simple, right? Yet this one seemingly small decision to drink enough water can have a huge impact on your health.

There's one other basic lifestyle choice that I want to share with you here because it's produced such profoundly positive changes in my own life: <u>the power of breath</u>. You can't live without oxygen, just as you can't live without water. What's more, your breathing affects the *quality* of your life. So you can't think about health without thinking about breath.

As yogis have taught for thousands of years, the way that we breathe produces different emotional and physical states. I'm sure you've experienced times when your breathing was constricted. For example, do you ever notice when you're feeling stressed you breath really shallow or not at all? In more extreme cases, when people are having a panic attack, they can't catch their breath, and they go into a specific breathing pattern that makes them hyperventilate. **We can even become addicted to our anxiety because the body releases dopamine to cope with these challenges.**[13] **The way we breathe can also create painful problems inside the gut.**

Fortunately, you and I can improve our breathing by becoming more conscious of it. Many years ago, I began experimenting with different breathing patterns, including a number that I learned from a book that I'd highly recommend: *Breathwalk* by Gurucharan Singh Khalsa, PhD, and Yogi Bhajan, PhD. **They explain how to rhythmically synchronize your breath and your steps while walking, so you can change your mood and energy.** For example, one breathing pattern entails inhaling for four seconds, holding your breath for four seconds, exhaling for four seconds, and holding your breath for four seconds—**a "segmented" 4/4 pattern that you can continue for several minutes while you walk in order to boost your energy and mental clarity**. In fact, a very similar pattern of breath is also taught to **Navy SEALs** to calm their minds and emotions and increase their focus.[14] **Often they're taught to inhale for four breaths through the nose, and exhale a count of four breaths through the mouth in order to calm their nervous system in stressful situations.** Another pattern entails inhaling for eight seconds and exhaling for eight

---

13 Hadhazy, "Fear Factor: Dopamine May Fuel Dread, Too."

14 Nazish, "How to De-Stress in 5 Minutes or Less, According to a Navy SEAL."

seconds as you walk, repeating this for several minutes—an 8/8 pattern that can reduce stress and foster calmness.

Decades ago, a doctor who was a lymph specialist taught me another basic breathing pattern that uses a ratio of 1:4:2. I utilize this strategy to train the body to fully oxygenate by holding the breath longer and exhaling twice as long as you inhale, in order to eliminate toxins and stimulate the lymph system. I've found it an invaluable tool to enhance my energy, my state of mind, and my sense of well-being. **In my case, I inhale for eight seconds, hold my breath for thirty-two seconds, and exhale for sixteen seconds. You could do 7:28:14 or whatever is a natural capacity for you at this stage.** I use this breathing technique at least once—and often three times—a day. I start by doing it once in the morning, shortly after waking up; I repeat it once again if I'm feeling stressed in the afternoon; and I often do it one final time to relax before bedtime. In my experience, it's a wonderful way to oxygenate the body, get the carbon dioxide and toxins out of your system, reduce stress, and break your mental pattern when you need a reset. I also use a more explosive breath when I'm tired and need to snap myself into a peak state right before getting on stage. I drink my water, do my breathing, and I'm ready to rock 'n' roll!

As you'll quickly discover for yourself, these breathing patterns offer a powerful and instantly accessible way to upgrade your mood, your vitality, and your health. These ancient techniques are a reminder of a simple truth that any of us can choose to harness right now: Oxygen is life.

THE POWER OF YOUR MICROBIOME AND DIET

"There is no such thing as an average person, we are all genetically and biologically unique."

—DR. JEFFREY BLAND, father of "functional medicine" and author of *Biochemical Individuality*

So far, we've discussed a number of basic lifestyle choices that, broadly speaking, will benefit anyone. Intellectually, most of us already know that these rules of the road make sense. If you lounge around on the sofa every day and rarely move, you know that your body will eventually stop functioning like a well-oiled machine. If you regularly opt for deep-fried chicken and hot fudge sundaes over vegetables and fruit, you know that you're raising your odds of an unhappy life—and, perhaps, an unhappy ending. If you constantly swig sugary sodas and sweetened juices instead of water, you know that you're more vulnerable to threats like obesity and diabetes. General guidelines like these are pretty obvious, even if we don't always abide by them.

Besides the blood chemistries and body imaging we discussed in Chapter 3, "Diagnostic Power," there is another critical check of your biology that is important to make, and that is a measurement of your microbiome and genes (DNA). As the old saying goes, "What gets measured, gets managed." It's important to note though, that this technology is still evolving, and is not absolutely accurate yet.

One company at the vanguard of this revolution is **Viome**, which studies the effects of different foods on the gut. Did you know that there are roughly 40 trillion organisms living in your digestive tract?

This hidden ecosystem of bacteria, viruses, and other microbes plays a vital role in maintaining your health. Scientists have shown that these squatters inside your gut have a complex influence on your metabolism, digestive efficiency, brain function, immune system, susceptibility to disease, and even your mood. When your microbiome (the technical term for this community of microbes) is out of balance, your body can't absorb nutrients properly, which may cause inflammation—an underlying cause of many chronic diseases.

After collecting a stool sample from its customers, Viome (which Peter and I invested in through his venture firm, BOLD Capital Partners) uses its genetic sequencing technology to identify trillions of microbes in the gut and analyze their activities, including their biochemical interactions with the foods you eat. (Another great company that does biome analysis is called GI Map.) "There wasn't even a supercomputer that was built ten years ago that could have analyzed this massive set of data," says Viome's CEO, **Naveen Jain. Using advanced artificial intelligence, Viome crunches that data to offer individualized advice on which foods and supplements may positively or negatively affect your microbiome.**

Viome's website lists "common foods" that would be best for all of us to avoid, including sugar, processed meat, processed cheese, white flour, French Fries, and corn syrup. But the personalized recommendations the company provides are much more nuanced. For example, a friend of mine was recently told to avoid tomatoes and cucumbers because of two specific viruses that Viome detected in his microbiome.

What excites me most are the cases where people with debilitating or deadly diseases can see life-changing improvements simply by modifying what they eat. This is one way to treat imbalances in the gut microbiome, such as obesity, diabetes, irritable bowel syndrome, and Crohn's disease.

A good example of how changing diet can radically change your health involves Viome's founder and chief science officer, Momchilo "Momo" Vuyisich. He developed the company's foundational technology while leading the applied genomics team at the Los Alamos National Laboratory, which famously developed atomic weapons during World War II. Vuyisich was on a personal mission to "understand the root cause of chronic diseases" because he suffered from one himself: rheumatoid arthritis. In his thirties, he got so sick that his doctors recommended a drug that would cost $30,000 a year, but warned that he'd *still* wind up in a wheelchair. His response: "I found that unacceptable."

Thankfully, Vuyisich stumbled on a "simple nutritional intervention" that would transform his life. **After studying research by Ajit Varki, a distinguished professor at UC San Diego, Vuyisich realized that his immune system was triggering a disastrous inflammatory response to one particular sugar that he consumed regularly in meat and dairy. So, in 2015, he quit eating "any products from mammals." The result? "My symptoms went away. My joints were cured. And I literally have no residual disease left." Vuyisich is the perfect example of how we can benefit from understanding the precise workings of our own unique physiology.**

THE POWER OF ALIGNING YOUR DIET WITH YOUR DNA

Another useful tool to determine how your body utilizes carbohydrates and fats is a genetic test like the one my wife and I used from

DNAFit. In a two-year study comparing the effects of a genetically matched diet versus a ketogenic diet, they found weight loss after the first twelve weeks was nearly identical. **But after two years, the participants in the ketogenic group began to gain their weight back as they struggled to stay consistent.** Those who ate according to their genotype not only lost significantly more weight but also reduced total cholesterol, increased the beneficial HDL cholesterol, and improved fasting blood glucose levels.[15] It appears that humans from different ancestral backgrounds utilize carbohydrates and fats differently.

Why is this? International travel is a new occurrence. It's been only over the last century that humans began to travel in masses. **Prior to this, cultures married within the same population, so the gene pool was similar.** Consider the Inuit who reside in the harsh Artic climate. For centuries they consumed a diet mainly of fat and protein from fatty coldwater fish, seals, and caribou, with very little in the way of plants, no agricultural or dairy products, and was unusually low in carbohydrates. Compare this to the traditional Caribbean Islander diet, which is the polar opposite of the Inuit—high in plant-based carbohydrates derived from fruits and roots and very low-fat seafood. **Now, what happens when these two groups have children? What about when their children have children?** There's only one way to find out for sure—genetically test to see what traits they inherited. This type of testing offers important data that can help eliminate the trial and error of what your body's genetically preferred fuel source is— carbohydrates, fats, or a combination of the two.

My wife, for example, burns carbs incredibly rapidly. As a result, she can eat without gaining a lot of weight, but she also can get hypoglycemic if she doesn't eat throughout the day. Carbs burn very quickly, like lighter fluid. Whereas I burn fat as a primary source of energy, which burns more slowly, like burning coals on a barbeque, so I can go sometimes eleven to fourteen hours without seeing much of a drop in my energy.

Although microbiome and genetic testing are early in their infancy, they

---

15 Vranceanu et al., "A Comparison of a Ketogenic Diet with a Low GI/Nutrigenic Diet Over 6 Months for Weight Loss and 18 Month Follow-up."

may be able to provide some helpful information to make better choices and offer clues to the best approach for you.

Companies like Viome, WHOOP, and Oura are leading us into a data-driven future that makes these *individualized* interventions possible. Increasingly, you and I will be able to optimize the way we eat, fast, exercise, rest, and sleep because we'll know with more clarity than ever before what impact to expect when we fine-tune our behavior. We'll still need to understand the *general* rules of the game. But this is the dawn of a new golden age of precision and personalization.

THE HEALING POWER OF HEAT & COLD

Last, **I'd like to share my top 2 biohacks that have had a profound impact on my well-being, and science is now showing that they can stimulate your immune system, lower your blood pressure, sooth inflammation, increase cardiovascular strength, and reduce your chance of having a stroke or heart attack—all in 20 minutes!**

Saunas are nothing new. Bathing oneself in heat for the purposes of purification, cleansing, and healing is an ancient practice, dating back thousands of years and observed across many cultures. But now, for the first time in history, **scientists can actually** *prove* what many cultures around the world have long suspected: regular sauna use can have a profound and powerful impact on your health, your well-being, and your healthspan.

Dr. Rhonda Patrick, PhD, one of our Life Force Advisory Board members, a published scientist and health educator, and founder of the website Found My Fitness, has been studying the benefits of exposing the body to hormetic stressors, such as through sauna use or heat stress, as well as various forms of cold exposure for years. She shares that, appropriately, much of this groundbreaking research has been conducted in Finland, where a population of 5.5 million uses an estimated three million–plus saunas!

How dramatic are the benefits? **Well, one study involving 2,315 middle-aged Finnish men found that <u>those who used a sauna four</u>**

to seven times a week were 50 percent less likely to die from cardiovascular disease than men who used a sauna only once a week.[16]
That's right! **By regularly sitting in a sauna for around 20 minutes
at a time, these men *halved* their risk of cardiovascular disease—a
scourge that causes nearly one of three deaths globally.**

In case that's not enough to grab your attention, consider this: **these
frequent sauna users were also 40 percent less likely to die from
all causes of premature death.** But there's more—*much* more! Researchers have also found that **frequent sauna use radically reduces
the risk of cognitive disorders such as dementia and Alzheimer's
disease.** Regular sauna bathing, as it's often called, has also been
shown to alleviate everything from arthritis to skin diseases to
depression. **In another Finnish study, men and women who used
a sauna four to seven times per week also lowered their risk of
stroke by an astounding 61 percent** compared to those who visited
a sauna just once a week.[17]

What's the theory behind this magic? Dr. Patrick explains that saunas
generate heat stress responses within the body, including the activation
of **heat shock proteins.** This protein family is produced by our cells in
response to stressful conditions, such as excessive heat, and are important
to many cellular processes, including regulation of the cell cycle, cellular
signaling, and functioning of the immune system. Multiple studies have
shown that heat shock proteins increase in response to heat exposure in
people as they do in animals. **Studies show that to get the results described above, all you need to do is 4 to 7 days per week, all you need
to do is take 20 minutes at 73°C (163°F). A 2012 study showed that**

16 Laukkanen et al., "Association Between Sauna Bathing and Fatal Cardiovascular
    and All-Cause Mortality Events."

17 Kunutsor et al., "Sauna Bathing Reduces the Risk of Stroke in Finnish Men and
    Women."

people who stayed 30 minutes in a heat chamber at 73°C (163°F) saw a <u>49 percent increase in heat shock protein</u> levels as well.[18]

Dr. Patrick explains that short-term exposure to extreme heat can deliver a wide range of benefits to your body's natural healing mechanisms. She pointed out in a recent study in *Experimental Gerontology*,[19] <u>saunas have been shown to stimulate the immune</u> <u>system, lower blood pressure, reduce inflammation, and improve</u> <u>cardiovascular function.</u> Sitting in a sauna can also boost your heart rate in much the same way as medium-intensity exercise—but with far less effort! Plus, there's the emotional bonus of taking time to relax, rejuvenating in peace on your own or in the company of friends and family.

The good news is that you don't have to be extreme to experience the life-enhancing power of intense heat. In fact, Finnish researchers found that **men who used a sauna just two to three times a week reduced** **their risk of dying from cardiovascular disease by 27 percent.**

Statistics like these are so compelling that more and more people around the globe are visiting the gym exclusively for saunas four times a week, or are fitting their homes with a sauna. Some opt for traditional steam saunas while others favor infrared saunas, which use light to create heat that warms the body from within. The best infrared saunas heat the organs as well as the skin. I already owned a traditional steam sauna, which I enjoyed but rarely used. But after getting up to speed on these benefits, **I decided I wouldn't let a week go without going in** **at least four times for 20 minutes at 163°.** To make it even easier, I decided to get an infrared sauna. I have no investment in the company, but my favorite is **Health Mate Sauna** (www.healthmatesauna.com). That said, one advantage of traditional Finnish saunas versus infrared saunas is that they tend to be hotter, which may explain their healing power. One brand worth checking out is **Almost Heaven Saunas**

18 Iguchi et al., "Heat Stress and Cardiovascular, Hormonal, and Heat Shock Proteins in Humans."

19 Patrick, "Sauna Use As a Lifestyle Practice to Extend Healthspan."

(www.almostheaven.com), which specializes in making steam saunas in the Finnish tradition.

Before you go any further, you should definitely consult a physician, since saunas aren't recommended for everyone. But if you're given the green light, one excellent option is to sit in a sauna about four times a week, aiming for at least 20 minutes per session at 163 degrees. Your heart and brain will soon come to relish this regular infusion of healing heat.

I'll tell you, in the beginning it feels difficult. You can start with 10 to 12 minutes and build to 20, but once you do it's extraordinary. My habit is to do it 4 to 7 times a week just before I go to sleep late at night. The heat cleanses and relaxes my whole body, and I find that my sleep is much deeper. Plus, I get all the benefits you've already read about above—and even more so when I add my second biohack, daily cold plunge or cryotherapy session.

The Power of Cold: Daily Cold Plunge & Cryotherapy

If you've ever played competitive sports, you've probably used ice to relieve the pain in your inflamed and achy joints. Back in my youthful days of playing baseball, I was constantly strapping ice packs onto my pitcher's arm. And after a bruising game of football, I'd frequently immerse my entire body in an ice bath on and off for twenty minutes or more of Arctic-style misery! Shivering like crazy, you couldn't help but ask yourself: isn't there a better way?

Well, nowadays there is! It's called whole-body cryotherapy. In my experience, it's been a total godsend. When I've just spent thirteen hours tearing up the stage, running up and down the stairs of a stadium to keep tens of thousands of people involved, it takes quite a toll on my body. The inflammation can be extreme. For me, nothing provides quicker, more efficient, and more dramatic relief than stepping into a cryotherapy chamber. After just two and a half minutes in there, I find that almost all of my pain and inflammation is gone!

Dr. Patrick is also a fan of the cold, and reveals the benefits include improved metabolic health, improved mood and cognition, increased mitochondrial biogenesis in skeletal tissue, altered gut and microbiome activity, activation of antioxidant enzymes, and decreased inflammation.

How does it work? Basically, you stand inside a cryotherapy chamber that's filled with mind-blowingly cold gas, exposing yourself to temperatures as low as minus 240 degrees Fahrenheit while wearing little more than your underwear and some protective coverings for your feet, hands, and ears. It may sound brutal, but this short, sharp shock to the system can stimulate an amazingly rapid recovery.

Initially, I would go to centers all over the world in almost any major city where you can pop in for five or ten minutes and be done, feeling incredibly rejuvenated. Because I used it so much I actually purchased one for my own recovery at events and in my home. As you might expect, many of the most ardent fans of this technology are professional athletes, who routinely use cryotherapy to treat strains, sprains, and fractures, accelerating their recovery from injuries and overuse. But interest in cryotherapy has also spread far beyond the athletic community. There are high-end spas, gyms, and wellness centers that now offer whole-body cryotherapy. There's increasing interest. And if you don't have access to whole-body cryotherapy, you can submerge in an ice bath as well to activate the power of cold stress. In addition to my cryotherapy unit, I've built cold plunges in my home that I keep at 50 degrees. If you do this for 2 minutes you can feel a transformation as well. There are many companies that make self-contained units that stay cold. Dr. Rhonda personally uses The Plunge (www.TheColdPlunge.com).

Are you convinced? **Try testing out the power of heat or cold for 30 days and see what you think. The science shows that you'll be glad that you did!** For more information on the power of heat and cold, visit FoundMyFitness.com.

So now, let me ask you a question. . . . What lifestyle choices are you going to make right now to maximize your health, energy, and vitality? Based on what you've learned in this chapter, why not commit to two or three simple changes that will propel your life to the next level?

- Are you going to cut your meat consumption down a bit—perhaps to one, two, or three times a week—or possibly even eliminate it entirely from your diet? Or at least ensure that it's from a clean source?
- Are you going to commit to exercising for 150 minutes per week—just 20 to 30 minutes a day, five or six days a week—so you can experience the energy you'll have for your family, your friends, your work, your mission, and your own enjoyment of life?

YOUR LONGEVITY HEALTH, FITNESS & LONGEVITY WEEKLY CHECKLIST

1. **Hydrate.** Drink half your body weight in ounces of water per day. Add some fresh lemon and a pinch of Celtic sea salt to optimize your hydration and electrolyte balance.
2. **Eat foods closest to their natural source.** Avoid processed carbs, and low quality processed meats.
3. **Decrease Disease Risk.** Consume at least one serving of cruciferous vegetables per day including broccoli sprouts, cauliflower, broccoli, brussels sprouts, or kale.
4. **Commit to a structured eating window.** Consume meals in an 8 to 12 hours and fast for 12-16 hour window each day.
5. **Stay consistent with sleep.** Go to sleep and wake up at about the same times each day.
6. **Get strong.** Perform three resistance training sessions per week.
7. **Strengthen your heart, lungs, and build endurance** with 3 cardiovascular exercise sessions of 20 to 30 minutes each session.
8. **Consider the power of using heat and cold** to use positive stressors to lower your blood pressure, reduce inflammation, reduce your risk of Alzheimer's, and cut your risk of cardiovascular disease by up to 50%.
9. **Train your brain with daily breathwork and meditation** 5–20 minutes per day.

- Are you going to explore the restorative power of intermittent fasting by restricting your eating to eight hours a day and fasting for the other sixteen? Eating 3 hours before you go to sleep, adding to your 6 to 8 hours of sleep so that your digestive system gets a rest? Or perhaps try Dr. Longo's full-immersion five-day "fasting mimicking diet"?

    By the way, if you'd like to experience a 5-day program of transformation, you can always attend our Life Mastery event in person or in digital form. It includes the transformation of your mind, emotions, and your body and you can make these physical changes together with others. Visit TonyRobbins.com for more information.

- Are you going to commit to drinking half your body weight in ounces each day so that you're still fully hydrated and experience the energy and mental clarity that comes with it?

- Are you going to breathe in a specific pattern three times a day? A ratio of 1:4:2 or 4:4:4 to revitalize your mind, body, and soul? If so it would be great to set an alarm on your phone so you follow through and it becomes a habit.

- Will you consider using the power of heat and cold, using a sauna four times per week or more, to cut your chance of heart disease in half? Or cryotherapy or cold plunge to reduce inflammation?

Whatever you choose, write it down now. Make a commitment to stick with these simple yet powerful lifestyle changes for the long term. And then feel the momentum. These little shifts in behavior may not seem like much. But as the science shows, the impact on your energy, your health, and your longevity is extraordinary.

And now let's turn to another core component of a healthy lifestyle—one that most of us neglect in ways that are incredibly damaging. To be honest, it's a subject that I've never focused on until recently: sleep. As you're about to learn from the world's most renowned expert, **sleep affects your health, your vitality, your immune system, and even your sexuality. What you're about to read will shock you. But it will also show you one of the simplest ways to transform your energy, your vitality, and the quality of your life. Let's wake up to the power of sleep. . . .**

CHAPTER 13

THE POWER OF SLEEP: THE THIRD PILLAR OF HEALTH

This One Factor Is Fundamental for Your Energy, Your Happiness, Your Sexuality, and Your Resistance to Life-Threatening Illnesses Like Diabetes and Heart Disease

"Proper sleep has helped me to get where I am today as an athlete, and it is something that I continue to rely on every day."

—TOM BRADY, the only NFL quarterback to win
a Super Bowl in three different decades

I don't know about you, but my wife loves to sleep. For her, eight hours a night would be an ideal minimum, if we weren't so busy so much of the time. Most days, she wakes up looking perfectly refreshed and revitalized, bright-eyed and glowing with good health. For me? In the past, I usually grab five or five and a half hours of sleep. And I'll admit, there are times when my schedule is so intense that I might go two to five days without sleeping more than four and a half hours a night.

I don't recommend this, and I know that it's not good for the body. In preparing for this book, I've since changed my habits significantly. But for a long time, I prided myself on the hard-charging mindset "I'll sleep when I'm dead." Why waste a third of your precious life when time is short and there's so much to do? If you're an overachiever like me, you may well feel the same way. But let me tell you: Boy, was I wrong!

One of the many miracles of modern science is that it's become possible to measure more accurately than ever the many benefits of

sleep—and the devastating effects of sleep deprivation—on our biological mechanisms. The health implications are so remarkable that sleeping better has become an urgent priority for me, Peter Diamandis, Bob Hariri, and many of the most high-performing people we know.

For us and millions of others around the world, this change of attitude is largely due to one scientist, **Matthew Walker, PhD,** who is the hero of this chapter. **Dr. Walker, a friend of Peter's, is the most persuasive sleep evangelist on the planet. More than anyone, he's played a starring role in waking the world up to the critical importance of this all-natural healthcare intervention, which costs you nothing and—unlike many drugs—has no unpleasant side effects.**

When it comes to sleep, there's no greater authority than Dr. Walker. He's best known as the author of a blockbuster book, *Why We Sleep: Unlocking the Power of Sleep and Dreams*, **which has been translated into more than forty languages.** He's also a professor of neuroscience and psychology at UC Berkeley and the founder-director of the **Center for Human Sleep Science**. He's spent more than two decades as a sleep researcher, published more than one hundred scientific studies, and served as a sleep consultant for athletes from the NBA, the NFL, and England's premier soccer league. **One of his more unusual titles is "sleep scientist at Google," which goes to show that some of the world's most dynamic businesses now recognize that sleeping well is vital not only for health, but productivity and creativity.** And finally, we're proud to have him as an adviser for this book.

In a sense, humans have always known that sleep is essential for our health, happiness, and well-being. Almost four hundred years ago, William Shakespeare wrote in *Macbeth* that sleep is the "chief nourisher in life's feast." Scientists now believe that he was probably right. **In fact, if you're looking to live a long and healthy life, sleep might just be the single most important ingredient of all.**

Think of it this way: If evolution could have done away with sleep, it would have done so. While you're asleep, you're vulnerable to attack, you're unable to procreate, and you can't hunt for food. Yet sleep has survived, despite all of the evolutionary pressure to devise a safer and more productive use for our time! As Dr. Walker explains in his book, "sleep would appear to be the most foolish of biological phenomena," which means that it can have persisted only because it provides "tremendous benefits that far outweigh all of the obvious hazards and detriments."

Dr. Walker says he used to regard sleep as "a third pillar of good health," along with eating well and exercising regularly. **"But I think I've changed my mind: I'd now suggest that sleep is probably the** *foundation* **on which those other two pillars of diet and exercise sit.** It's the Archimedes lever. It's the superordinate node that if you inflect change there, all of the other health systems fall into line. . . . **Sleep is the tide that seems to raise all of the health boats."**

Later in this chapter, Dr. Walker will share with you a series of extremely practical tips about how to radically improve the quantity— and quality—of your sleep. But first, it's important to understand why sleeping well *must* **be a top priority for you, me, and everyone we love. To put it simply, why is sleep such a big deal?**

Well, let's consider a few startling pieces of sleep data that I'm guessing will shock you as much as they shocked me.

Twice a year, many of us take part in what Dr. Walker calls "a global experiment on 1.6 billion people in about seventy countries." That's his description of daylight savings time, when clocks move forward an hour each spring and back an hour each fall. Many of us complain when we lose an hour of sleep on the night in March when this switch occurs. But we all know that it's trivial, right? As Dr. Walker says, "How much damage could just one hour of lost sleep really do?"

Actually, a lot! By studying daily hospital records, **researchers discovered "a 24 percent increase in heart attacks"** the following day, says Walker, **and a similar surge in traffic accidents. "In the autumn, when** we *gain* **an hour of sleep, there's a 21 percent** *reduction* **in heart attacks the following day.** To me, that's so striking because that's just one hour of lost sleep opportunity."

Unbelievable, isn't it? Just *one hour of lost sleep for one night* causes that much harm. Doesn't it make you wonder what might happen if an entire country were chronically sleep deprived?

Well . . . **in 1942, the average American adult slept for 7.9 hours a**

night, and that figure has since plunged to about 6.9 hours. That's almost a 13 percent reduction in how much we sleep. To put this in context, the World Health Organization and the National Sleep Foundation suggest that adults need an average of eight hours sleep per night. You don't have to be a math genius to recognize that this is a drastic shortfall! And if the *average* American loses out on about sixty minutes of sleep a night, you know for sure that millions of us scrape by on much less, turning ourselves into zombies in a healthcare horror story.

Like me, I'm sure you've experienced this yourself—the stark contrast between those nights when you slept terribly and woke up feeling sluggish and blurry-eyed, versus those nights when you slept deeply and woke up naturally without an alarm, feeling fully rested and alive. The difference in your energy level and your readiness to face the day couldn't be more obvious.

Walker, who is English, emphasizes that our modern "epidemic of sleep deprivation" isn't just an American phenomenon, but a global issue that's especially bad in rich countries. In the UK, he says, 70 percent of the population sleeps less than eight hours. In the U.S., 79 percent of people sleep less than eight hours. In Japan, 90 percent of the population sleeps less than eight hours.

One reason is that many economically advanced societies tend to regard sleep as shameful—and doing without it becomes a "pernicious" way to communicate that we're "busy and important." Dr. Walker explains, **"Sleep has an image problem. We associate people who are getting sufficient sleep with being slothful or lazy.** It's surprising to me in some ways because nobody looks at an infant sleeping during the day and says, 'What a lazy baby!' And that's because we know that sleep at that time of life is fundamentally, non-negotiably essential." As adults, we seem to forget that truth. To make matters worse, many of us face extreme pressure to juggle long hours at work, a time-consuming commute, and our responsibilities at home. No wonder sleep gets squeezed.

As you know, we don't all need the same amount of sleep. You might wake up after seven hours of blissful slumber and feel ready to take on the world, while your partner or friend (let alone your teenaged kid!) might need nine hours of sleep before they can speak coherently. "There's definitely a range," says Dr. Walker. "**But when adults routinely start to get less than eight hours of sleep, their risk for serious medical conditions increases significantly. . . . Once you get below** *seven* **hours of sleep, the brain stops being able to perform in a cognitively optimal way.**" I'm sorry to tell you, but this is about to get worse. . . .

As Dr. Walker explains, **when people regularly sleep for less than six hours a night, they become more vulnerable to a whole host of serious health problems. For example:**

- Their **"ability to regulate their blood sugar is markedly impaired,"** intensifying the risk of type 2 diabetes.
- **"Measures of cardiovascular function" are also negatively affected, says Dr. Walker, including worrisome increases in hypertension and blood pressure.**
- **In his book, he adds this stark warning: "Routinely sleeping less than six or seven hours a night demolishes your immune system." And as we've seen during the COVID-19 pandemic, there's no better defense against viruses, the flu, and many other threats to our health than to maintain a robust immune system.**

Not convinced yet?

A lack of sleep is also associated with a heightened risk of developing Alzheimer's disease and dementia. It even contributes to psychiatric conditions like depression and anxiety and significantly reduces the "ability to experience pleasure and positive emotions."

Speaking of which, sleeplessness also affects our sexual energy. After one week of sleeping four or five hours a night, men have been found to have the testosterone levels of someone *ten years older*. Okay, gentlemen: If that doesn't get your attention, maybe this will. . . . **When alpha males brag about how little sleep they get, Dr. Walker enjoys informing them that "the less and less sleep an individual has, typically the smaller and smaller their testicles."**

As you'd expect, sleep is also vitally important in terms of women's health and sexuality. For one thing, women need to restore the body in different ways as it transforms throughout the menstrual cycle. But here's an interesting fact that's *not* well known. **According to Dr. Walker, scientists have found that "for every hour of sleep that a woman will lose, she has about a 14 percent decrease in her desire to be physically intimate with her partner."** The lesson? Ensuring that you and your partner get enough sleep can greatly enhance your sensual intimacy.

Summing this all up, Walker explains the importance of sleep as bluntly and simply as possible, declaring, "The shorter your sleep, the shorter your lifespan." In fact, there are so many ways in which our health is affected by sleep that he describes it as "the greatest health-care insurance policy that's freely available to society."

DR. WALKER'S PRESCRIPTION FOR A GREAT NIGHT'S SLEEP

"There does not seem to be one major organ within the body, or process within the brain, that isn't optimally enhanced by sleep (and detrimentally impaired when we don't get enough)."

—DR. MATTHEW WALKER, *Why We Sleep*

Now that we have your attention, what practical steps can you take to improve your sleep?

1. FIRST OF ALL, YOU NEED TO ASSESS WHETHER OR NOT YOU'RE GETTING ENOUGH SLEEP. How can you get a general sense of how sleep-deprived you might be? **"One simple way of doing this,"** says Dr. Walker, **"is by asking yourself:** *If your alarm didn't go off in the morning, would you sleep past it?* **If you would, then clearly your brain isn't done with sleep and you need more."**

Another simple question that's worth asking is: *Are you trying to sleep longer at the weekend than you do during the weekdays?* And if that's true, it probably means that, during the week, you're not meeting your sleep need. It's also revealing to **ask yourself:** *Can I function properly without caffeine before noon?*

2. IF YOUR SLEEP DEPRIVATION SEEMS EXTREME, CONSULT A DOCTOR. In certain situations, says Dr. Walker, it's important to ask your doctor for a referral to a sleep clinic. **For example, a sleep clinic can help you if you're concerned that you might have a serious sleep disorder like severe insomnia or sleep apnea—a condition in which your breathing is repeatedly interrupted.** The most common form of this last disorder is obstructive sleep apnea, which occurs when the muscles in the back of the throat relax. This narrows or closes the airway, making it hard to inhale enough air. One of the biggest risk factors for sleep apnea is obesity, though it's also more common among men, smokers, and people with conditions like high blood pressure, congestive heart failure, and Parkinson's disease.

For years, I woke up so many times each night that I ended up visiting a sleep clinic to get myself checked out. Sure enough, a doctor there told me that I had extreme sleep apnea. He warned that this condition could shorten my life unless I took action. His solution? He recommended that I use a continuous positive airway pressure (or CPAP) machine every night. For many people, these devices are lifesavers. But I can't say that I was enthusiastic about using one. It consisted of a noisy bedside machine that pumped air into a tube connected to a mask that I'd have to wear every night. It felt like I was strapping a vacuum cleaner onto my face as I climbed into bed. Not the best aphrodisiac!

So I consulted several doctors to see if there was any alternative. In my case, at least, I was told that having surgery to fix my deviated nasal septum could help. Thankfully, the surgery worked beautifully, and I was able to breathe easily once more without wearing that sexy vacuum cleaner! When I went on stage again, my energy levels were so improved that I felt like Hercules. It was great for me, but a little scary for my audience!

There's another option that also works well for many people: a mandibular advancement device (or MAD). Basically, this is a mouth guard that pushes your lower jaw forward, shifting the placement of your tongue while you sleep. MADs are small, easy to carry when you travel, and can be customized to provide a perfect fit for your teeth. They stop you snoring and also serve as a night guard if you've been told that you grind your teeth.

Peter, who used to use a CPAP machine but found it difficult to lug along on his travels, now swears by his mandibular advancement device.

In any case, if you think that you might have sleep apnea, it's not something you want to ignore, because it can increase the risk of heart disease, metabolic syndrome, type 2 diabetes, fatty liver disease, depression, and reduced sexual desire. What are the symptoms of sleep apnea? They include heavy snoring, episodes in which your breathing stops, and occasionally gasping for air as you sleep.

3. SET YOURSELF A REGULAR BEDTIME AND WAKEUP TIME.

"We're designed for regularity," explains Dr. Walker. "If you feed your brain regularity, which is what it wishes for and expects, the quantity and quality of sleep will improve. So it's really trying to get in lockstep with your biology's expectation, because when you fight biology, you typically lose—and the way that you *know* you've lost is usually through disease and sickness."

How can you set up the right sleep schedule, given that we each have our own "genetically imprinted circadian rhythm"? Walker suggests imagining that you're alone on a desert island, then asking, *What time, typically, do I think I'd probably end up going to bed, and what time would I probably wake up?*

A recent sleep study involving 2,115 physicians in their first year of training found that those with irregular sleep times also reported more feelings of depression than those with regular sleep patterns— another indication that our bodies and minds thrive on regularity.[1] The study concluded that "variability in sleep parameters substantially impacted mood and depression" and that "sleep consistency" could "improve mental health."

4. FOCUS ON GIVING YOURSELF A LONG ENOUGH "SLEEP OPPORTUNITY" EACH NIGHT. For most of us, it takes time to

nod off, and we're often wakeful at certain points during the night. You should factor in that lost sleep time when you're figuring out your bedtime. **Dr. Walker, who recommends setting a "get-in-bed" alarm each night,**

---

1 Fang et al., "Day-to-Day Variability in Sleep Parameters and Depression Risk."

insists on giving himself an eight-and-a-quarter-hour sleep opportunity, so that he can sleep a minimum of seven hours. What's his typical sleep schedule? "I'm a 10 p.m. to 6.30 a.m. kinda guy. If you knew of all the health dangers I know of, you'd do nothing other than give yourself that chance to sleep. I don't want to invite disease into my life any earlier than it has to be there. . . . I don't want to live a shorter life."

5. IMPROVE THE *QUALITY* OF YOUR SLEEP, NOT JUST THE *QUANTITY*. How? "You need to get cool to get good sleep," says Dr. Walker. "Aiming for a bedroom temperature of sixty-five to sixty-seven degrees Fahrenheit is going to be optimal for an average adult." One helpful piece of technology that Peter uses religiously is a cooling mattress pad called a ChiliPAD. He sets it for sixty-five degrees—the same temperature as his bedroom air-conditioning.

Dr. Walker adds that you should also try to avoid going to bed "too hungry" or "too full," and be aware that alcohol often causes "fragmented" sleep. What about coffee? Drink as much as possible. Just kidding! It's smart to limit coffee, especially in the afternoon and evening. Dr. Walker, who drinks one cup of decaf coffee in the morning, says, "Caffeine has a quarter life of twelve hours, which means that if you have a cup of coffee at noon, a quarter of that caffeine is still swirling around in your brain at midnight. . . . Even if you fall asleep and stay asleep, caffeine can also decrease the amount of deep sleep you get by up to 15 to 20 percent. For me to take that amount of deep sleep away from you, I'd have to age you by about twelve to fifteen years. So, that's one of the problems with caffeine."

6. PUT DOWN YOUR PHONE. One common cause of sleeplessness is "the invasion of technology into our bedrooms," says Dr. Walker. This frequently leads to "sleep procrastination. You're sleepy and have the opportunity to sleep, but you do things that get in the way, like watching a few more YouTube videos or the next episode on Netflix." All right, I confess! I'm not immune to sleep procrastination!

Another problem is that your computer, tablet, and mobile phone bathe you in blue LED light, which "fools your brain into thinking it's still daytime" and delays the release of melatonin, a sleep-signaling hormone. "It's not just electrical devices," he adds. "Indoor lighting is a problem, too. We need darkness."

What's the solution? Dr. Walker suggests not only avoiding electronics at night, but turning down the lights in your home when your alarm alerts you that it's time for bed. **This signals to your brain that it's night and helps to trigger the release of melatonin. He also recommends installing blackout curtains in your bedroom. Another simple way to block out the streetlights or the morning sunrise is to wear a blackout mask. The one that Peter loves and often gives as a gift is called the Manta sleep mask. Personally, I love the Mindfold sleeping mask.**

These simple recommendations might lead you to believe that technology is the enemy. But Dr. Walker thinks it could also be "the salvation of us." **In the future, he expects to see innovations like smartbeds with sensors that will listen to your breathing, diagnose sleep apnea, and keep your body at the optimal temperature. "Your car right now is full of intelligent sensors, but your mattress is about as dumb as it was fifty years ago," he says. "There's a vast amount we could be doing with that."**

In the meantime, if you're looking for technology that can help you now, "sleep trackers are a good place to start," says Dr. Walker, because "what gets measured gets managed."

Among tech-savvy friends like Peter, one of the most popular wearable devices is a high-end sleep tracker called the **Ōura Ring**. A technological marvel designed in Finland, it's a lightweight titanium finger ring that contains about ten embedded sensors, including two infrared LEDs, an infrared detector, a gyroscope, three temperature sensors, and an accelerometer to measure your movements.

Every morning, the Ōura Ring delivers to you an overall sleep score that gamifies your sleep, along with delivering a detailed analysis of the previous night. It tells you not only how long you slept, but how much deep sleep and REM sleep you had, how restless you were, and how ready you are for the day ahead (based on measurements such as your heart rate variability). It's a dream come true for biohackers, athletes, and health-conscious data junkies.

As Peter explains, sleep is so important that the Ōura Ring is one of the first devices that members of Fountain Life use regularly once they join. It's also why we've invested in the company via BOLD Capital. Why? When it comes to this pillar of vitality, it's invaluable to know precisely where you stand. Then you can measure the effects of different habits and choices on your sleep and can see what helps or harms you.

The data definitely isn't flawless, but it's precise enough to provide precious insights into the many ways in which our own behavior affects our sleep. **Harpreet Rai**, the CEO of Ōura Health, says the company has sold more than half a million of its second-generation rings and gathered over 1 million nights of sleep data from its users. **"The most important thing,"** he says, is that tracking devices like this help you to **"understand what choices you made and how that resulted in good or bad sleep—and that ultimately means making better decisions daily."**

Many people who wear the Ōura Ring have reported sleeping better after making some of the basic changes recommended by Dr. Walker, whether it's sticking to the same bedtime every night, not eating or drinking late in the evening, or banishing electronics from the bedroom. **Similarly, says Rai, "we've seen so many people actually cut out that three o'clock or four o'clock cup of coffee and see really large improvements to the quality of their sleep."**

Rai knows firsthand how sleep loss can contribute to ill health. **Early in his career, when he was an investment banker, he routinely pulled one or two all-nighters every week. "I started to get gray hair at the age of twenty-two or twenty-three," he says. "I gained about fifty pounds in my first year . . . and my blood labs indicated that I had a ton of cortisol and a ton of cholesterol."**

Years later, while working at a hedge fund, Rai bought an early version of the Ōura Ring. Once he started tracking his sleep, its impact on his health and well-being became too glaringly obvious to ignore. **He soon realized that, when he slept for seven to eight hours, "my performance was**

better, I was more productive, and I was in a better mood." As luck would have it, he met one of Ōura's Helsinki-based cofounders while shopping in a Whole Foods store in New York City—a chance encounter that ultimately led to him running the company.

Having experimented with many strategies, Rai discovered that a handful of changes consistently improve his sleep:

- **"I don't have coffee after 11 a.m.,"** he says, and he's cut back to **"one or two cups, instead of three or four."**
- **He sleeps better when he exercises earlier in the day, not in the evening.**
- **It helps when he finishes dinner by 6 p.m.**
- **He rarely drinks alcohol.**

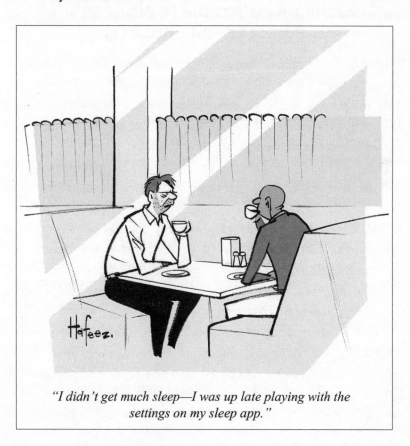

"I didn't get much sleep—I was up late playing with the settings on my sleep app."

- He keeps his bedroom cool.
- And if he can't resist using his iPad before sleeping, he wears a pair of glasses that are specially designed to block the blue LED light emitted by electronic devices. They don't work for everyone, but Rai found that he was "tossing and turning way less" after he began wearing them.

But here's the thing. You and I shouldn't expect to respond the same way to LED light, caffeine, alcohol, the timing of meals and exercise, or countless other factors that can influence our ability to sleep. **So what matters, says Rai, is that you learn to "listen to your body."**

ONE OF MY FAVORITE BIOHACKS FOR SLEEPING: NUCALM

We all know what it feels like to get a good night's sleep. However, as we age, a good night's sleep becomes more elusive which accelerates the aging process. As I've shared, getting enough sleep was not always something I focused on. **One of my favorite biohacks that I use regularly is a simple device called NuCalm.**

Developed by Solace Lifesciences, this device is changing the world through patented, clinically proven neuroscience solutions that allow you to change your mental state on demand without drugs, and without side effects. **For the past 12 years NuCalm has helped the U.S. military, the FBI, more than 50 professional sports teams, and thousands of doctors and their patients, pilots, business executives, moms, dads, sons, and daughters lower their stress and improve their sleep quality without drugs.**

Using biochemistry and physics, NuCalm safely and predictably slows down your brain waves into alpha and theta, where the body and mind can restore, recover, get back into balance and build resilience. **In fact, research at Harvard Medical School** shows a 45-minute treatment of NuCalm may give you the benefits equivalent to 2–5 hours of deep, restorative sleep by balancing your autonomic nervous system and restoring you to optimal health.[2]

They also have programs that induce Ignite Warrior Brain brain waves into gamma regions of high frequencies resulting in high intensity, mistake-free focus. And of course Deep Sleep predictably slows down brain waves to the lowest frequencies and into the deepest depths of dreamless deep sleep.

NuCalm, Ignite Warrior Brain, and Deep Sleep are easy to use and have cumulative benefits that can put you back into control of your life and empower you with certainty to live your best life! To find out more about NuCalm's new software tracked solutions, simply reach out to them at their website, www.NuCalm.com.

Widespread access to tiny, inexpensive sensors in devices like the Ōura Ring and the **WHOOP Strap** (a superb sleep and exercise tracker that is my favorite health monitoring device) provides new ways to listen, so you can modify your behavior, track the effects, and see for yourself what benefits you the most. Excitement about the power of these wearable devices has grown to such an extent that Ōura was recently valued at $800 million and **WHOOP was valued at $3.6 billion.**[3]

Finally, your cell phone might also help you to sleep better—if you use it the right way. If you don't believe me, check out a groundbreaking product called **Somryst** that's delivered through an app on your smartphone or tablet. **Somryst has been authorized by the FDA as a prescription-only "digital therapeutic" for adults over the age of 22 who are wrestling with chronic insomnia.**

How does it work? **Over six to nine weeks, the Somryst app guides you through a six-part program based on the principles of cognitive**

---

2 Dental Excellence Integrative Center, "Harvard Research Update."

3 Kruppa, "Wearables Company Whoop Valued at $3.6 Billion after SoftBank Investment."

behavioral therapy—a form of therapy that's clinically proven to be effective in treating insomnia. Among other things, the Somryst program trains you to identify and change thought patterns that lead to sleep disruption; teaches you to create a more efficient "sleep window" that increases the amount of time you actually sleep while you're in bed; and guides you to fix environmental factors (like excessive noise and light) that contribute to sleep problems. Like the Ōura Ring and the WHOOP Strap, the Somryst app also tracks your progress along the way, so you can see for yourself what's working.

In a clinical trial of more than 1,400 adults with chronic insomnia, patients who used Somryst experienced a 45 percent reduction in the time that it took them to fall asleep, a 52 percent reduction in the time they spent awake at night, and a 45 percent reduction in the severity of their insomnia symptoms.[4] Pretty impressive, right? You bet! To learn more, visit Somryst.com. Once you've filled out a sleep questionnaire, you can set up an online consultation with a board-certified healthcare provider to see if you're a suitable candidate for a prescription to use Somryst.

Now that you've read this chapter and understand the importance of sleep, what are you going to do to improve the sleep you get each night? Let's come up with a sleep challenge—a firm commitment that will deliver transformative benefits. What are you willing to try for a minimum of ten days—or, even better, for twenty-one days, which is usually enough to get you hooked on a positive new habit? **Pick two or three simple things that you're prepared to commit to, then see the difference that these small changes make to your energy, your dynamism, and your mood.**

Believe me, I'll be right there with you because there's no question in my mind that enhancing my sleep is one of the greatest gifts I can give to myself. In fact, the quality and quantity of my sleep has already improved significantly, thanks to the WHOOP Strap, which we'll talk about more in

---

4 Ritterband et al., "Effect of a Web-Based Cognitive Behavioral Therapy for Insomnia Intervention."

the next chapter. Just remember, focus creates change. What you measure tends to improve.

And now let's turn to another core component of a vibrant and joyous life: We're going to guide you to some of the best tools available to you right now for increasing your strength, enhancing your mobility, and maximizing your strength, fitness, and performance. . . .

CHAPTER 14

STRENGTH, FITNESS & PERFORMANCE: YOUR QUICK GUIDE TO MAXIMUM RESULTS

How to Optimize Your Energy and Performance by Building Muscle Mass, Bolstering Bone Density, Enhancing Mobility, and Increasing Endurance

"My attitude is that if you push me towards something that you think is a weakness, then I will turn that perceived weakness into a strength."

—MICHAEL JORDAN

What if I told you there was something you could do for just a few minutes a day that could . . .

- Reduce your risk of cancer by 40 percent
- Cut your risk of a stroke by 45 percent
- Slash your risk of diabetes by 50 percent
- Halve the risk of premature death from heart disease
- And if you're a woman, protect you from osteoporosis. Known as the "Silent Killer" since you often don't know you have it until a bone is broken, it effects one in three women over the age of 50.

What is this nectar of the gods? The answer is, exercise. Yes, exercise. When I say you literally can't live without it, it's the truth: <u>Exercising just fifteen minutes a day can slash the risk of death by 14 percent and</u>

boost life expectancy by three years on average, according to a study in the *Lancet*.[1]

Most people think about working out as a chore, something they really ought to do, but they don't truly understand how transformative it is. We all know we should work out, but most people don't want to: We're pressed for time. We're tired. We're frustrated or confused about how to achieve results. So we just give up because we don't realize how essential it is to not only do aerobic exercise, keeping our hearts strong, but actually build the muscles that make everything work.

With that in mind, I'm going to show you how to grow stronger, fitter, and shapelier than ever—in as little as ten minutes a week, using new insights from science and new tools created by entrepreneurs around the world. **This chapter is all about learning how to promote and harness your body's vitality, so I'm going to introduce you to four of the most simple, effective, and transformative training strategies and breakthrough technologies** that can give you the power and energy you deserve in far less time than you ever dreamed possible. For example:

- You'll discover how to **get the greatest results in the shortest amount of time by utilizing a machine that top athletes use to fortify their muscles and bones in just ten relatively sweat-free minutes per week**. The machine measures your output and maximizes the ideal amount of muscle stimulation so that your muscles grow as you rest over the next week. **(You don't build muscle when you're working out; you build muscle when you're recovering!)** This isn't some silly infomercial; it's backed up by science and will give you the muscle strength you want while enabling you to build muscle nearly effortlessly and keep making gains.
- Most people over train, and as a result they get injured or burn out. **Learn how to determine the perfect dosage of exercise, intensity, and recovery to maximize your energy** and boost your outcomes.

---

1 Wen et al., "Minimum Amount of Physical Activity for Reduced Mortality and Extended Life Expectancy: A Prospective Cohort Study."

- You'll marvel at the way **artificial intelligence fine-tunes a workout to yield peak efficiency and maximize progress** in a minimum amount of time. The key is the right dose of exercise for the right result.

- You'll see how the very simplest of tools makes sure your back stays strong—an unbelievably low-tech series of **foam arches can realign the spine, banishing back pain and boosting mobility to the extent that your actual breathing pattern changes**.

- You'll be energized by the way that **virtual reality makes working out a blast, even for people like me who aren't gamers. Use it to connect and work out with other users anywhere, at any time. I was skeptical, but Black Box VR** is so much fun that you don't even realize you're working out. When you're having that much fun, you stick with it. It makes working out addictive.

- For people who can't exercise due to an injury or disability, we'll share a promising new oral medication that's currently being tested. Taken once a day **mimics the biological effects of a strenuous work out, giving you chemically the jump-start you need to start exercising and get all the rewards.**

Too much pain is *not* gain. Achieving the right dose of exercise and effort is the key to success. What's more, these tools and technologies are not complicated or hard to implement. Nor do they require a huge time commitment or superhuman Herculean effort. **Did you know that simply walking twenty to thirty minutes a day could cut the chance of dying prematurely from heart disease in half?**[2] (*Really, Tony, you're going to tell me to go for a walk?* Yes, I am—and I'm going to encourage you to take it to the next level, too.) **Dial it up just a little bit by turning that walk into a jog and you reap even more benefits: One study found that adults who jogged five days a week for thirty to forty minutes a day had a "biologic aging advantage" of *nine years* over sedentary adults.**

If you stop and think about it for a moment, those are pretty startling statistics. **Just imagine if a Nobel Prize–winning scientist developed a pill that could make your body nine years younger, while also halving your**

---

2 *The Guardian*, "Brisk Daily Walks Can Increase Lifespan, Research Says."

risk of dying prematurely from heart disease. Wouldn't you take this miracle pill? Of course you would. Now, what if it wasn't a pill but a lifestyle choice? Consider that researchers have shown that regular physical activity significantly reduces the risk of a wide range of potentially devastating illnesses, including coronary heart disease and stroke, hypertension, diabetes, breast and colon cancer, kidney disease, and dementia.

The point is, **sometimes the simplest interventions work just because our bodies need to be challenged in order to get stronger, healthier, or revived. If you don't use it, you lose it.** I'm not saying that you need to look like some bulging Adonis, flexing your well-oiled biceps on the beach. **But muscle strength matters for many reasons beyond your appearance.** It drives your physical performance to a whole new level; **improves your metabolism, helping you burn fat and look and feel athletic, powerful, and sexy; and if you're in a later stage of life, it also gives you the balance and stability to protect against falling, which is a growing risk as we age. So no matter what your stage of life, there are benefits that you want to take advantage of.**

In 2018, a prestigious medical journal reported that muscle mass is just as important to health as blood pressure and how much you weigh!

Now, what if you could have this kind of vitality throughout your entire life, not just in your twenties and thirties? Let me introduce you to a friend of mine, **Bob Weir, the legendary co–lead singer and rhythm guitarist for the Grateful Dead. At age 74, he maintains a fitness regimen that incorporates interval training, TRX Suspension Training, and tossing around a twenty-pound medicine ball.** The guy is a bundle of rippling muscles who knows that regardless of whether you're in your twenties or your seventies, strength matters. Staying active and toned as you age is vital to your well-being, physically and emotionally.

In fact, <u>in 2018, a prestigious medical journal reported that muscle mass is just as important to health as blood pressure and how much you weigh! The study in the *Annals of Medicine* found that people with</u>

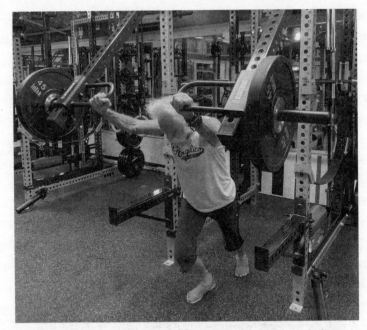

Bob's workout at age 74 consists of interval training, including a
set of 10, 20-second sprints, followed by a 20-second walk on a
45 degree incline, overhead rotations using a 20 pound medicine
ball, and strength training using TRX bands.

**low muscle mass had outcomes that were associated with more surgi-
cal complications, longer hospital stays, and poorer quality of life.** The
difference in outcomes between people with low versus higher muscle mass
were so stark that the study's author, **Carla Prado, PhD, a professor at the
University of Alberta,** remarked, "**Muscle mass should be looked at as
a new vital sign.**"

**Muscle mass should be considered a new vital sign because it gives
you youth and energy and strength. It makes you look better. It makes
you feel better. Whether you're a man or woman, increasing muscle
mass is within your reach, no matter how old you are.** Just imagine what
it's like to feel strong and vital and energized and powerful at any age and
not experience age-related decline at 40 or 50 or 60 or even 70 years old.
It's possible today with the right type of stimulation and training. "This is
something guys my age can do," Weir told *Men's Health*, "and it will make an

immense difference in what they call your golden years if grace and happiness are goals of yours."[3]

Grace and happiness are certainly goals of mine, so my mission is simple. **I am going to show you how to get more by doing less.** How are you going to achieve better results, greater strength, energy, and vitality, with less time training than you ever thought possible? Let me tell you about OsteoStrong.

THE SIMPLE THINGS

"We don't even know how strong we are until we are
forced to bring that hidden strength forward."

—ISABEL ALLENDE

There's a good chance that you and those you love are not moving enough. The World Health Organization defines sufficient physical activity as one hundred and fifty minutes of moderate activity—that's two and a half hours—in a whole week! Or seventy-five minutes of vigorous activity per week, which again is only one hour and fifteen minutes in an entire week (or any equivalent combination to make up the two and a half). How many of us meet that relatively modest target? **A 2018 study found that more than a third of people in high-income Western countries don't get enough physical activity, a shockingly high percentage given that physical inactivity is the fourth leading risk factor for global mortality.**[4]

It doesn't help that so many of us lead increasingly sedentary lives, commuting to work by car or subway or immobilized by COVID work-from-home policies, sitting at a desk all day and staring at screens even in our leisure time. In Chapter 12, I introduced you to my friend Dr. Dean Ornish, a pioneer of "lifestyle medicine" and a member of the Life Force Advisory

---

3 McCammon, "The Grateful Dead's Bob Weir is 72 and Still Working Out Like a Beast."

4 Carlson et al., "Percentage of Deaths Associated with Inadequate Physical Activity in the United States."

Board. Ornish and his wife, Anne, wrote a terrific book, *UnDo It!: How Simple Lifestyle Changes Can Reverse Most Chronic Diseases*, in which they warn that **"the combination of both sitting more than six hours a day and being less physically active was associated with a 94 percent increase in all causes of premature death rates in women and a 48 percent increase in men compared with those who reported sitting less than three hours a day and being most active."** In other words, <u>sitting is the new smoking</u>.

One obvious solution is to use a walking desk with a treadmill, so you can keep moving while you work. I was an early adopter of these desks and found mine so transformative that I recommended it to everyone, including my friend Salesforce CEO Marc Benioff, who popularized this way of working to all his entrepreneur friends. I also encouraged my dear friend Paul Tudor Jones, the hedge fund tycoon, who saw his traders' output increase after getting them these standing desks. **There have been many days that I've spent up to four hours a day walking and working, logging fifteen miles a day while having meetings.** It's the ultimate in multitasking!

"The combination of both sitting more than six hours a day and being less physically active was associated with a 94 percent increase in all causes of premature death rates in women and a 48 percent increase in men compared with those who reported sitting less than three hours a day and being most active."

But even if you don't have access to one of these desks, **you can boost strength without investing a lot of time through a scientific breakthrough called OsteoStrong that produces the greatest results in your body with a minimum amount of time.**

When I was a kid, I remember doing tons of push-ups and not seeing much in the way of results. I evolved into a gym rat. I'd visit the gym five days a week, pushing myself like crazy to lift heavier and heavier weights. Then, inevitably, I'd hit a plateau and stop improving. I couldn't understand why this huge investment of time and effort didn't pay dividends. It was exasperating. I felt like Sisyphus pushing his immense boulder up a hill, only to watch it roll back down again and again!

I decided what I really wanted was energy and strength in as little time as possible. After years of overtraining, I found hope in a **muscle-building strategy called static contraction**, a way to boost muscle growth faster than anything science had previously identified.

I heard about a study involving thousands of bodybuilders who mirrored my gym rat behavior. They'd pump iron five, six, seven days a week. But they wound up plateauing. Then, after suffering injury or illness and taking ten days or more off, they almost inevitably set new personal bests upon their return. **This led the researchers to conclude that people like me had been overtraining, essentially draining the body's energy systems in ways that actually weakened us. That's because muscle does not grow just because you stimulate it; it grows because you stimulate it intensely enough. And then—here's the most important key—you rest enough for the body to recover and rebuild enough to respond to the next stimulation.**

I learned all about this counterintuitive approach—that **less is more** when it comes to getting stronger—from the source himself: Peter Sisco, the bodybuilding pioneer behind static contraction. I'm going to explain what I did initially, and then share the groundbreaking strategies that Peter taught me. Then I'll show you how technology has come up with a solution to do this faster and easier.

You see, the fastest and most efficient way to increase strength is to hold the maximum weight you can handle in a static position—in other words, with no range of motion. You can't hold the weight for more than a few seconds because the stimulus is so extreme. As a result, the entire workout is over in a matter of minutes!

At first, I couldn't believe it. How could building power and strength require so little time? But I saw the proof at Gold's Gym, where I went with my camera crew. I watched as a gray-haired woman in her late sixties, slid onto a leg press machine after a chiseled twentysomething guy, dripping sweat, agreed to let her knock out a quick set. I was still watching as this guy's eyes grew huge with disbelief when **the woman added 50 pounds to his already hefty load and banged out a set, holding for just a few**

seconds each time. "I don't want to build big muscles, but I like feeling strong," this powerhouse of a grandmother told me. "It feels like all my screws are tightened. This changes my life; I can carry bags, open and slam the trunk with just a few fingers!" she said with a smile.

I became convinced of the value of this in short order and began to practice it. I couldn't believe how much my strength that was increased. **These short bursts of outrageous intensity done once every week to ten days proved so powerful that I built 16 pounds of additional muscle in a matter of months.** At the time I was 32 years old. I remember having fun walking into Gold's Gym with my camera crew and leg-pressing 1,225 pounds, all the weight they had plus two men sitting on the leg machine. The manager at Gold's Gym said, "That's unbelievable! You did that with your mind, man!" I laughed and said that anyone could do this through gradual building and effort.

But as the weight got heavier and heavier, I ran into a challenge. When I was bench-pressing for example, one arm was slightly stronger than the other. Things got out of balance and I'd injure myself, and it impacted my ability to do my live events, so I reluctantly dialed back, because I couldn't afford to be hurt; after all, I make my living bounding around a stage. I realized I was pushing the envelope, and the challenge was to balance the weight.

So while I love static contraction and the super-efficient strategy of going all out for a few minutes and producing extraordinary results, working out once or twice a week and taking several days off to recover, what I really wished for was a safer and more balanced way to get stronger. Eventually, I hoped someone would find a way to do this where you wouldn't get injured. I finally found it in a company that took these principles and implemented them with technology. The company is called **OsteoStrong**, and they have developed some of the most innovative strength-building equipment on the planet.

OsteoStrong takes its cue from static contraction, offering state-of-the-art machines that safely strengthen your entire musculoskeletal system in a workout that lasts *less than ten minutes just once a week*! You don't need to change out of your regular clothes or even wear sneakers if you don't want to. Most of the time you won't even break a sweat. How's *that* for maximum efficiency and minimum hassle? And it doesn't put

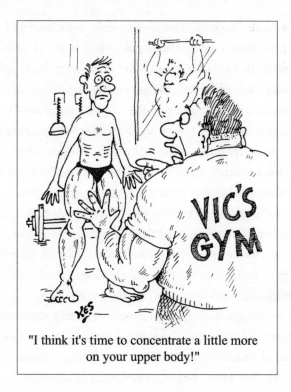

"I think it's time to concentrate a little more
on your upper body!"

you at risk of being out of balance, as the machines measure the effort and there's no weight on you; it's a computer-pressurized system.

One of the main reasons that OsteoStrong appeals to elite athletes is that they are constantly seeking an edge by maximizing the strength of their bones and muscles. **What most people don't realize is that the strength of your bones determines how big your muscles can become.** The bones are usually the limiting factor. In fact, **athletes who supplement their regular training regimens with weekly OsteoStrong sessions consistently report big performance gains, moving faster and jumping higher**. Case in point: Two loyal fans are world triathlete champion Siri Lindley and her partner, Rebekah Keat. These elite Ironman competitors are also widely regarded as among the world's top triathlon coaches.

OsteoStrong attracts people from virtually every generation—not just athletes looking to push farther and faster but young adults who want to be stronger, businessmen and -women who need a strength and energy boost to face the challenges of their lives and careers, and middle-aged people pulled in a dozen different directions who want to take care of their bodies but need to do so in a way that is as time-efficient as possible. Otherwise their workout gets set aside for other demands.

OsteoStrong not only strengthens your muscles but simultaneously strengthens your bones, making it the perfect antidote for staving off osteoporosis, which causes bones to become brittle and weak. Remember, this is an extremely important concern for women over 50. In fact, **a woman's risk of breaking a hip is equal to her combined risk of breast, uterine, and ovarian cancer.**[5] When you push, the machine measures the pressure and calibrates it in accordance with what your body can handle.

As a result, **I've seen continued development in my muscle strength at age 62 to the extent that I can lift and push with an intensity that outweighs what I did when I was 30.** But what's truly mind-blowing is seeing how it changes people's lives, starting with my own wife! Sage has been blessed with incredible metabolism. She could eat almost twice as much as me and remain totally lean. She doesn't have to exercise to stay slim, but she got addicted to our OsteoStrong machines because she was concerned about her bone density. For example, she started out at 125 pounds in a chest press and got up to 250 pounds within a year. And she didn't get lumpy, as female bodies respond differently to the stimulation. Her muscles were supple, sleek, and strong, and she feels strong and powerful as a result. She witnessed herself improving, and she was sold.

What's most addicting with OsteoStrong is that you only work out once every week or ten days, and you get to see the improvements continuously, if you don't improve, you actually take *more* rest. Remember, the body needs time to regenerate. My wife became addicted because she had exercised before and never saw improvements, but here she saw continuous progress.

As for me, I use it every 7 to 10 days and it's been life-changing. And if you do love to lift weights or work out like I do, you can still do that, and this can supplement it. **But for the 95 percent of the population that does not enjoy spending hours at the gym, OsteoStrong can transform your body in a matter of minutes.**

---

5 Bone Health and Osteoporosis Foundation, "What Women Need to Know."

All of this is possible because of an ingenious biomedical engineer and concerned son named John Jaquish.

Jaquish developed the OsteoStrong technology after his mother, Marie-Jeanne Jaquish, was diagnosed with osteoporosis. Osteoporosis is especially common among post-menopausal women, but it affects millions of people, female *and* male. **The International Osteoporosis Foundation estimates that one in three women over 50 and one in five men over 50 will experience fractures related to osteoporosis.** Hip fractures alone are extremely debilitating; a full 40 percent of survivors can't manage to walk independently one year later.

Before her diagnosis, Marie-Jeanne was an active woman in her 70s who loved to hike, bike, and play tennis. John saw how devastated she was by the prospect of a future constrained by broken bones, hospital stays, and declining strength. Even though he had no medical training, he started to investigate bone density, hoping to devise a solution that would help his mom and millions of others confronting the same dire future.

For most of us, bone density peaks by age 30. **Once we hit 40, we begin to lose up to 5 percent of our bone density each decade. It turns out that one of the secrets of developing muscle strength is that we must also maintain—or even increase—our bone density.** But how?

John Jaquish started answering this question by asking: *Who has incredibly strong, abnormally dense bones?* Answer: gymnasts. **Think about Simone Biles sticking a landing: The intensity of the impact helps strengthen her bones.** Did Jaquish ask his mom to start launching herself off the parallel bars or cartwheeling off the balance beam? Of course not.

His idea was to create a machine that could deliver a similar impact in a more controlled manner. He designed a prototype that resembled four standard weight-lifting machines, including a leg press and a shoulder press. But he converted them to static contraction, so the user would apply extreme force without actually moving the weights. **Imagine pushing your hands or feet as hard as you can against a brick wall (but one that moves slightly) for fifteen seconds and you'll have a rough sense of how it feels.** Again, these devices respond to your ability in real time with a computer.

John tested his device on his parents, instructing them to exert maximum effort, performing each exercise for ten to fifteen seconds, while he measured the force they generated. The whole circuit took less than ten minutes. They recovered for a week then repeated the routine. After a month or two of these weekly sessions, Marie-Jeanne had gotten her life back. Her strength output had improved dramatically. She resumed hiking and tennis. **As her son put it, "She went from having the bones of an eighty-year-old to those of a thirty-year-old."**

Her osteopath, a physician named Dr. Eleanor Hynote, was astonished by the results of Marie-Jeanne's bone scans. **It seemed unthinkable, but she had completely reversed her osteoporosis!** Dr. Hynote was so impressed that she sent more than 200 patients to Jaquish and ended up writing a book with him, *Osteogenic Loading*—the term Jaquish uses to describe the process of strengthening bones by imposing a heavy demand on them.

What this means for you is that if you're at risk of osteoporosis or have already developed this debilitating disease, OsteoStrong's patented machines could be a godsend. In 2015, Jaquish coauthored a study of fifty-five postmenopausal women with osteoporosis. **Over six months, they did five seconds of static contraction on each of his four machines just once a week. At the end of this twenty-four-week trial, the women in the study saw bone density increases of 14.9 percent in the hip and 16.6 percent in the spine.**[6] What's more, their musculoskeletal functional ability also improved dramatically, making it possible to perform routine tasks like walking, climbing stairs, picking up groceries, and driving golf balls with a much-improved range of motion and mobility.

I've found this technology so transformative that I use it every week and also invested in the company, helping to finance its expansion. I am such a fan that I encouraged them to open centers around the world, which they've done with remarkable success. OsteoStrong is already available in more than 120 locations in the U.S. and abroad, and it's spreading rapidly, even gaining fans in the UFC.

It's easy to get people to try it, because it takes just ten minutes, and it's great whether you're in your twenties or your eighties since

---

6 Hunt et al., "Axial Bone Osteogenic Loading-Type Resistance Therapy Showing BMD and Functional Bone Performance Musculoskeletal Adaptation Over 24 Weeks with Postmenopausal Female Subjects."

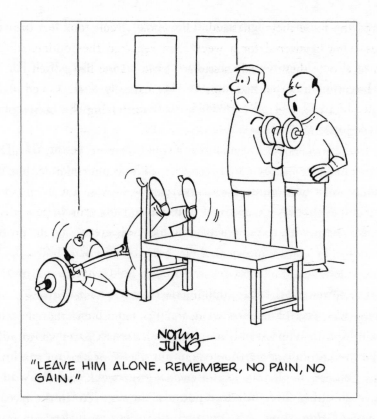

"LEAVE HIM ALONE. REMEMBER, NO PAIN, NO GAIN."

it measures where you're at with precision and adjusts to your level of demand. It's safe and amazingly effective. Readers can check it out free for a month by going to www.OsteoStrong.me/Lifeforce. Just look in the resources section and you'll be directed to a studio near you for your complementary thirty-day trial. **Whether you're a competitive athlete, a fitness enthusiast, or simply looking to optimize your bone density, this technology can safely harness the magic of static contraction to boost your strength, balance, mobility, and metabolism in just ten minutes a week.** Now, that's powerful!

QUICK AND EFFECTIVE WORKOUTS YOU CAN DO ANYWHERE

Say you don't have access to OsteoStrong. You can still get stronger, but the key, the essence, is getting yourself to train effectively. Because most of us start to lose muscle strength around the age of 35, it's vital to take matters into our own hands.

Just ask my longtime personal friend and trainer Billy Beck III, a fitness legend who's twice won the "World's Best Personal Trainer" and has coached hundreds of high-performing athletes and helped train people like Dwayne Johnson, The Rock.

If you're looking for a straightforward, inexpensive, yet highly effective program for building strength, here's what Billy recommends. **He suggests focusing on a minimum of four exercises—squats, lunges, push-ups, and planks—that are guaranteed to increase your muscle power if you perform them with the correct form and consistently try to do more each time.** "Start with one squat, if you have to," he says. "Hold a plank for ten seconds, if that's the most you can do. Just hold it a little longer tomorrow. The power and the strength build over time, so be patient."

Billy, who received his first set of weights and a punching bag as a gift from his dad when he was only four years old, has access to the most sophisticated strength-building technology on the planet. But everything he does is based on the simple principle of *gradual progression*. **"You don't all of a sudden go lifting three hundred pounds," he says. "You start by adding one pound, then three. It's the relentlessness that makes you strong. Challenge creates change. You must do enough to stimulate the body but not annihilate it. It's the little things done consistently and relentlessly that lead to massive results over time."**

Don't overdo it, as I used to do: As Billy says, "stimulate, don't annihilate the muscles." Less is often more. Spending less time working out, but doing it on a regular schedule that allows for plenty of time for your muscles to recover, will achieve even greater results. The secret to success is in creating the habit and sticking to it.

Billy's most basic strategy is developing the habit of working out for just ten minutes per day—a **micro-workout**. Some people work out for an hour, then can't walk for three days and stop their routine. If you do a minimum of ten minutes per day *consistently*, you'll become addicted to the good feeling that pushing yourself and increasing your strength creates. No one has an excuse not to spend ten minutes!

MY GIFT TO YOU

I understand not everyone reading this is a beginner, and strength training is an entire study in itself. So as a personal favor to me, Billy Beck III has created free beginner, intermediate, and advanced training programs so that you can get started wherever you are, and safely and effectively improve your strength, muscle, and body composition. **Simply visit BillyBeck.com/Tony.**

"It's difficult to change overnight, but if you are persistent and take one step at a time you will see results!"

—JACK LALANNE

Still skeptical about the value of having strong muscles? Try performing the sitting-rising test to evaluate your muscle power, joint flexibility, balance, stability: **Sit on the floor, then try to get up using the least support necessary. Begin with a maximum score of ten and subtract one point for each support you need as you sit and rise—for each hand, forearm, knee, or side of the leg you require along the way. You lose another half point if you execute the test unsteadily, partially losing your balance.** Ready? Go!

To put it bluntly, **you can't ace this test if you lack muscle.** No amount of cardiorespiratory fitness will earn you a high score if you lack the muscular strength and mobility to maneuver yourself down to the ground and up again in an efficient manner. It may sound laughably easy—like child's play. But for many of us, this simple act of sitting and rising exposes all sorts of unexpected weaknesses. Billy says the test is an excellent measure of three critical elements of human function: **"It measures balance, mobility, and muscular strength—and in putting all of that together, it tests your likelihood of falling, which is the number one cause of injury-related death for people over sixty-five."**

This basic test is even more revealing than it seems. **Researchers tested** the performance of more than 2,000 people aged 51 to 80, followed up a few years later, and discovered that their scores in the sitting-rising test helped predict their "all-cause mortality." Those with the lowest scores had a three-year-shorter life expectancy than those with the highest scores. That's right. If you performed well in this test, you can expect to live significantly longer than those who performed poorly. Why? **Because musculoskeletal fitness really matters!** And you know what else makes a difference? Measuring your results. You've got to know your baselines in order to know how much you're improving.

TECHNOLOGY THAT TRACKS AND ACCELERATES YOUR PROGRESS

"If you can't fly then run, if you can't run then walk, if you can't walk then crawl, but whatever you do you have to keep moving forward."

—MARTIN LUTHER KING JR.

As you just read, OsteoStrong's power derives from applying just the right amount of stimulus—not too much, not too little. **You don't want to over-stimulate; that's what tears you down. But if you understimulate, you'll never achieve results. The key is being able to measure your ability to recover** and understand the amount of stress you're creating, so you can stay on track. I'm going to be honest—it can be challenging for me to not overextend myself, to not push myself too hard. It's just my nature. If you're a type A personality like me, I'm sure you understand exactly what I'm talking about. **But you will burn out eventually if you constantly exert yourself and don't build in enough recovery time.**

One of the best ways to accelerate your progress is to harness the power of wearable devices, regardless of whether you're a hardcore athlete, a new convert to exercise, or you've simply gotten off track and want to start fresh. **There are lots of great tools for this, but one of my favorites is the WHOOP Strap.**

Over the last decade, we've seen an explosion in wearables containing tiny sensors that monitor every move you make, every calorie you burn, every beat of your heart, and the quality of your sleep, among many other measures of your health and performance. You may already be an ardent data analyst, obsessed with your Apple Watch or your Fitbit! If so, great! All of the most popular wearables have their virtues (and limitations), and they're improving all the time. But I have to confess, I love my WHOOP Strap, a comfortable band that you wear on your wrist or bicep, and now even inside your sock or shoe. **WHOOP connects to an app on your phone that collects and analyzes an impressive array of physiological data, including body temperature, heart rate variability, resting heart rate, respiratory rate, deep sleep, and REM sleep.**

But here's what's really special about it: **It gives you all the details you want, but more importantly, it distills those metrics to provide you with two key scores: one for *strain*, one for *recovery*.** As you already know from OsteoStrong, you need to push yourself beyond your comfort zone or you won't see any growth or improvement, but you also need to have enough time to rest and recover so that the body can make progress. That's why WHOOP emphasizes strain—a term for the intensity of your workout or the effort you put out in just your daily routine. But it also measures the recovery from those intense stress loads. WHOOP has actually changed my patterns, helping me make sense of the data it collects. Because it's not enough to just have the data; the data has to mean something. **WHOOP's data helps me determine the right dosage of exercise and demand or stress, or strain as they call it, versus the amount of recovery time needed, sleep and rest. This is priceless information that will change your quality of life because what you can measure, you can focus on. And what you can focus on, you can improve.**

WHOOP gathers data continuously twenty-four hours a day, seven days a week, measuring precisely how hard your body is working and how well you're recovering through sleep and rest. When I've slept badly or racked up a long string of tough workouts, WHOOP tells me to take it easy. And you know what? I've learned to listen because I've seen for myself the difference between my performance on days when I was running on fumes and days when I'd recovered properly. **When I wake up and WHOOP says I'm in the Green Zone, it means my body is primed for peak performance, so I can get more out of my workouts. If it's yellow, I know I've got to be a little more careful. And if it's red, that's a signal that I have**

to pause, which is tough for a guy like me who's always striving to do more. But I know that ultimately, taking a break will pay off in terms of better performance.

The beauty of wearables like WHOOP is that they measure your progress over weeks, months, and years, so you can *accurately track the impact of the lifestyle choices you've made.* Let's say you currently exercise twice a week and decide to ramp it up to five times a week, including a couple of strength-building sessions. Now imagine what you'll see reflected in your metrics six or twelve months from now. **There's nothing more inspiring than watching your biomarkers get better and** *knowing* **that your own behavior improved everything from your resting heart rate to your sleep quality.**

You can also share this data with your doctor or trainer, so they can help you interpret the information and provide you with personalized guidance. It's a bit like flying a plane through the night sky with the assistance of gyroscopic instruments, an experienced copilot, and air traffic control. Given a choice, why would you opt to fly blind, relying primarily on your own instincts?

Along the way, **there are also times when your body sends you urgent messages that you might have missed if your tracking device hadn't picked them up on your behalf.** In 2020, a professional golfer named Nick Watney got tested for COVID-19 before playing a tournament with hundreds of the world's top players. The test came back negative. Then, three days later, his WHOOP Strap data showed a sudden surge in his respiratory rate after remaining steady for nearly a year at a much lower level. That spike was an early warning signal that Watney, a five-time PGA Tour winner, was fighting something—even though he had no symptoms like fever, cough, or shortness of breath. **That prompted him to take another COVID test, which led to him becoming the first player to test positive on the Tour.**

Watney immediately withdrew from the tournament and avoided infecting any of his fellow players. **How did the PGA respond? By procuring 1,000 WHOOP Straps, for all of the players, caddies, and other essential personnel on the Tour.**

Will Ahmed, who captained the Harvard University squash team and founded WHOOP in 2012 in his college dorm room, says that "there are secrets that your body is trying to tell you. The reality is there are biomarkers that may indicate something that's very different than how you feel."

Of course, Watney is an extreme example. But his story is a reminder that **technology can now unlock the secrets of your physiology in ways that were previously unimaginable. When I wear the WHOOP Strap, I make better decisions. No matter what exercise I do, it helps me determine the right amount of effort and the right amount of time so that every single day I can balance the perfect dose of demand with recovery.** On top of that, WHOOP also helps elevate what we talked about in Chapter 13—the quality of sleep you're getting. When your sleep is enhanced, your mind, your body, your emotions, and your energy are at their peak, allowing you to maximize your quality of life, whether you're a stay-at-home mom, a businessperson, a student, an entrepreneur, or a retiree who wants to crush it and continue to live life to its fullest. It's better living through data. I have to tell you, I've added greater depth in my sleep, but also nearly an hour more since I started using this. Again, what you measure you tend to improve.

HARNESSING AI FOR POWER AND PROGRESS

"I do not fear computers. I fear the lack of them."

—ISAAC ASIMOV

Now let me introduce you to a third innovation that also relies on data to help you emerge stronger and get more out of your workouts. **Technogym Biocircuit is an artificial intelligence-driven workout that determines the right dosage of exercise delivered in the most efficient way so you can achieve maximum results in a minimum of time. It's yet another tool to help you reach your strength and performance goals.**

Technology has improved almost every aspect of our lives, apart from our attention spans. Yet the experience of going to the gym has barely changed in decades. Your mobile phone is now a supercomputer. So why is the gym still just the *gym*? Well, that's actually not the case in the more than twenty markets around the world where Biocircuit is available.

Picture this: You enter a gym featuring eleven **Biocircuit** Smart Strength machines. You scan in by waving your wristband in front of a sleek interactive screen. **The AI-powered Smart Strength system remembers the personal profile you set up when you first registered to use the machines, and like OsteoStrong, it instantly pulls your profile from the cloud, along with your personalized workout plan. This computerized system has also stored every detail of your past workouts—the level of resistance you chose, the effort you exerted—and can predict what you'll be able to achieve.**

You start at the first level "stations" and follow the circuit in a preordained sequence, instead of wrestling to decide whether to work your chest before your arms or shoulders. **The entire circuit gives you a full and balanced body workout in just thirty minutes.** You don't have to wonder if you're neglecting your glutes in favor of your quads or favoring exercises you like over ones you dread, since Smart Strength AI doesn't give you a choice. **When you arrive at each machine, it automatically adjusts to your ideal settings, so you don't have to fuss and fiddle with the height of the seat or the position of the hand grips. The machines are engineered to help ensure that you maintain the proper form. And as you grow stronger, they automatically add resistance, calibrating the challenge so it's achievable while also pushing you to keep improving.**

Amazing, right? All the guesswork and wasted time has been eliminated, leaving you free to concentrate exclusively on training in the most efficient way imaginable. **Once again, the right amount of demand or strain is paired with the right dosage for your current level of recovery capacity.** No searching for an unused set of dumbbells or a spare bench press. No struggling to remember how many reps you were meant to do or whether it's your second or third set of bicep curls!

Everything is streamlined and simplified—and fun because the whole experience is gamified. The Smart Strength AI machines have a built-in video game screen, which allows you to guide a ball through an undulating obstacle course by controlling the resistance of the machine. Imagine yourself on the leg press, where you push to extend your legs, raising the ball in the process. You then lower the ball gradually by slowly bending your knees. The better you control the weight, the higher your score and the more progress you'll make.

The gaming aspect isn't just a gimmick. **Numerous studies have established a reliable correlation between gamification and exercise. It's simple: Humans hit the gym with more sustained effort and consistency if they know they're making progress—and even more so if they know that others are *watching* them make progress.** A 2017 study by the *Journal of the American Medical Association* tracked more than two hundred families, some of whom were using a game-based fitness app that encouraged them to compete with other families. The groups using the app exceeded their daily walking goals by nearly a mile more than the control groups. *One extra mile each day!*

Over the next few years, you'll be able to find more and more Biocircuits as this playful AI concept catches on. In fact, Peter, Bob, Bill and I are so excited about it that we've already begun putting these machines at our Fountain Life centers. You can also find these machines and other AI-driven workouts in special gyms in most major cities around the world. And keep your eyes open, because technology is going to improve all this drastically over the next 3 to 5 years.

STRETCH YOUR SPINE

"Notice that the stiffest tree is most easily cracked, while the bamboo or willow survives by bending with the wind."

—BRUCE LEE

The fourth innovation that I want to share with you is something incredibly simple. It's called the Backbridge—and it's so simple and low-tech that it's hard to believe how effective and powerful it can be. **It takes less than five minutes a day so it's easy to incorporate into your life. Yet most find its effects so profound that they do it every single day, I'm one of them.**

As you already know, it's great to be *aerobically fit*, but it's not enough. Similarly, it's not enough merely to have *muscular strength*. You need both.

But there's a third component of fitness and performance that's equally important: *flexibility and mobility*. **Whatever you do, you have to do your best to keep increasing your flexibility and mobility at the same time that you're increasing your strength.**

Having grown ten inches in one year, my body was out of balance, and as a result I suffered from searing back pain for more than a decade. So I know firsthand how hard it is to embrace life fully when your back is killing you and it's hard to move. **At my seminars, I often ask the audience if they have back pain. Three-quarters say they do, including many people under the age of thirty!**

Much of the problem is that most of us spend our days seated and staring down at our phones and computers, so the Backbridge tackles one of the challenges of modern living: sitting. Remember earlier in this chapter when we said **sitting is the new smoking**? Because we spend so much of our day sitting while hunched over a phone or an iPad or a computer, we tend to roll our shoulders forward, cutting off oxygen flow and sapping our energy.

Our bodies become habitually overstrained when they're constantly in flexion, hunched over with head, neck, and shoulders tilted forward, gut compressed, oxygenation plummeting because we're shutting down our diaphragms. Our bodies were built for flexion *and* extension—a fancy way of saying that we need to bend *and* straighten. We were designed to be in balance, but our modern tech-centric lifestyle is gradually contorting us into twisted human pretzels.

How can we straighten this problem out? One solution is to effectively and efficiently stretch for a few minutes every day to maintain a healthy equilibrium in our body, especially as we age and our muscles shorten and become less elastic. **We need to pay special attention to our back health— most notably, the spine. Enter the Backbridge, an inexpensive invention that's the brainchild of Dr. Todd Sinett, a New York–based chiropractor, applied kinesiologist, and author of** *3 Weeks to a Better Back.*

Sinett designed the Backbridge as a way to decompress and realign the spine, restore proper posture, and eliminate back pain. Like Osteo-Strong's machines and the Biocircuit Smart Strength system, the Backbridge delivers outsized benefits in a minimal amount of time. **You're supposed to**

use it for just two minutes every morning and two minutes every evening. *A four-minute commitment!*

How does it work? It could hardly be simpler. The device consists of five soft foam arches. You choose how many of them to stack on top of each other, adjusting the height from a base level of two inches to a maximum level of seven inches, depending on how flexible you are. **You place the Backbridge on the floor and lie with the highest point between your shoulder blades, while your arms rest on your chest or above your head.** And then? *Relax. Breathe. Savor the sensation of this gentle stretch, which extends your spine to counteract the slumping flexion, corrects the imbalances in your core, and repairs the damage you've done to the biomechanics of your back.*

You'll see the benefits over weeks and months and will probably need to raise the height of the Backbridge as your flexibility improves. In the morning, those two minutes of stretching your spine feel like a fresh start. In the evening, they feel like the perfect ending.

After using the Backbridge daily, I'm able to stand tall without effort. I experience my entire breathing pattern change. This deceptively simple tool is incredibly valuable, but it's not the only tool out there. Similar benefits are also available using a BOSU ball or a fitness ball. Always make sure to control how slowly you lean back as you adjust your body. You don't want to push yourself. This is a time to let the body settle in and open up gently. Remember, always talk to your health practitioner before doing anything strenuous in this area. What you can expect is a burst of renewed energy as your chest and shoulders drop back, your breathing becomes more full and natural, and your entire body becomes more oxygenated.

There is no doubt that there will be more of these tools that make exercise more efficient, more measurable, easier, and more fun. Keep your eyes open because while I've told you about a few, including some that I'm involved with directly, there will be so many more hitting the market in the next few years, including an exercise format whose secret ingredient is fun.

FUN AND GAMES

"Do anything, but let it produce joy."

—WALT WHITMAN

When it comes to building strength over time, one of the most motivating aspects is really pretty simple: It's all about having fun. If you're having fun, you're much more likely to keep working out and stick with your training. Now, I'm the first to acknowledge that I'm not much of a gamer, so it would have been easy for me to overlook Black Box, which is based on virtual reality. I'm not going to lie: the virtual reality component of **Black Box, an exercise platform whose results match or beat those of traditional fitness formats,** seemed complex at first. But when I got into it, it was extraordinary. **I felt like I was singularly focused and incredibly energized; I felt purposeful and powerful at the same time. It was an incredibly intense workout, too.** When it was over, I was soaked and had worked every last muscle. But here's the key: It didn't feel like work! It felt like pure fun, and the time just disappeared. I couldn't wait to do it again.

The secret sauce is not that the core element of Black Box workouts is radically different from standard hit-the-gym sessions; it's that even the most dedicated gym rats can have trouble staying motivated. Black Box is inspired by the fact that gyms are packed every January but empty by March. **The Black Box product incorporates the addictive qualities of a video game into a virtual reality eSports–style fitness module that entices enthusiasts to show up day after day, consistently building muscle, increasing their endurance, and boosting their overall wellness.** Black Box is so engaging that it makes people stick to their workout schedule, which means they achieve their fitness goals.

Black Box users spend just thirty minutes getting fit as their workout stats are automatically tracked. **You can even engage in friendly competitions with other Black Box users anywhere, which is great for people like me who thrive on competition.** The technology is available only at official Black Box VR gyms or at commercial gyms that participate, but within a few years, a home version should be ready. I have to be honest, I couldn't wait to get my hands on one, so I invested in the company and have the commercial version in my home and it's a blast!

In terms of VR and fun exercise there's one more game worth checking out that Peter Diamandis swears by and uses as a cardio complement to his goal of 10,000 steps per day. It's called **Supernatural VR Fitness** and its available as a subscription on the Oculus. Supernatural is so fun and engaging that you'll probably consider canceling your gym membership.

At the start of your workout you'll be teleported to one of a number of gorgeous "photo-real" locations on Earth. Imagine opening your eyes and finding yourself standing before the Great Wall of China, Machu Picchu, the Galapagos Islands, Iceland, or Ethiopia's Erta Ale Volcano. Before you is your exercise coach (a real person) speaking into your ear, encouraging you to swing your bats (that you're holding, one in each hand) toward the pairs of black and white targets flying your way. A rousing soundtrack consisting of musical hits that you know and love is blasting at an increasing rhythm. Soon, you're breathing hard and breaking out into a sweat as you squat, spin, and swing in time with the music. There are large number of workouts you can choose from, ranging from a quick eight-minute burst to an elongated thirty-minute workout.

P39: A FUTURE SHORTCUT TO BUILDING MUSCLE MASS WITHOUT EXERCISE?

We all know how important exercise is. But what if there's a reason you can't—rip-roaring arthritis, an injury, etc.? That can't be the end of the story. **You shouldn't accept that your body can't reap the rewards of a good workout.** If you google for exercise mimetics (things that simulate exercise), you will find that the most promising is a small molecule, AICAR. *But we have something better for you.*

But first, let's understand the chemistry of exercise. It turns out that a molecule called adenosine monophosphate (AMP) is the most important molecule you make when you start to exercise. It informs the entire body you are exercising. The AMP causes muscle cells, brain cells, and liver cells to break down stored glycogen and fat to use as energy. This leads to the key question, **"If you could deliver low levels of AMP to targeted organs, could you mimic the effects of exercise?"**

The answer is yes. One current analog of AMP, called ZMP, has been shown in animal and human studies to **increase endurance, slow muscle loss, decrease inflammation, and decrease fat-to-lean body mass index.** So why isn't this used? In order to achieve these effects, it must be IV-infused with the small molecule AICAR, in large amounts.

Skylark Bioscience has discovered a first-generation product, code-named P39, that is much more efficient at delivering ZMP than AICAR. "It is **one hundred times as potent and can be taken orally. Instead of getting large infusions, you can just take a small 25mg pill every day, and** *get most of the biological effects of strenuous exercise.*" **This will be the jump-start you need to start exercising chemically and get all the rewards from exercise. Skylark's Oliver Saunders notes, "**<u>The molecule is not available yet</u>**, and is just now beginning trials but we are hopeful that it will become available in the next few years!"**

Well, we've covered a lot of territory in this chapter. I hope what you pull from everything you've learned is that **muscle is a "must" for quality of life and that you don't have to be a gym rat to build and sustain it.** You can take advantage of short workouts and still get *tremendous* results instead of making excuses or feeling guilty that you aren't pushing yourself to work out.

· **Remember that you want the right dosage of exercise for the greatest result.** Otherwise, you don't get results and you'll just burn out from waste of time. Your challenge is to create a sense of demand on your body and its muscles, **as simple as just ten or fifteen minutes of demand at least a few times a week.** What are you going to choose? **Are you going to design your own strength-based workouts for 15 minutes per day, or perhaps use OsteoStrong so that you can get stronger and expand the demands over time? Will you optimize your performance and daily life with the help of a WHOOP Strap? Will you find an AI-fueled** circuit to maximize your results or a VR playground like Black Box or Supernatural VR fitness? Or are you going to slash your risk of death by 14 percent and add 3 years to your life by exercising just 15 minutes per day?

Whatever you decide, <u>there is truly an opportunity here for you to change your quality of life today in every way—mentally, emotionally, physically, even sexually—everything from your sense of attractiveness and your sense of power to your sense of health and vitality.</u>

Why not commit right now? Decide on one, two, or three things you learned in this chapter that you want to make a habit. Come up with a ritual, a simple habit that you can do 10 to 15 minutes per day, 2 or 3 times per week. Rituals make it real. Once you develop a habit, you'll start feeling, and it will become easy and you'll want to keep going. Maybe it's something that you do with a friend, or get a trainer. But do something right now and commit yourself—send a text to someone who can hold you accountable. If you do, you'll emerge stronger and more determined not only for your health and well-being, but you'll find that this simple discipline around your body will provide greater power and discipline in every area of your life. **The way we feel determines the way we perform, the way we interact, and how much we enjoy. As I've said many times, it's not enough to make a decision; at the moment you make it, you need to take action to convince yourself to follow through.** Lay out a quick plan, schedule it. I always tell people: When you talk about something, it's a dream; when you envision it, it's possible; when you schedule it, it's real.

This chapter has highlighted some invaluable tools, but these aren't the only ones out there. **Find the right tools that work for you, your body, and your goals and prepare to be amazed at how you'll revitalize your energy, rejuvenate your body, and maximize your life force.** I'm someone who relies on these tools to enrich the quality of my day-to-day experience, so take it from me that **building your strength translates to building an extraordinary life.**

Now let's move on to discover the latest breakthroughs for rejuvenation of our visible health and vitality. . . .

CHAPTER 15

BEAUTY: ENHANCING YOUR VISIBLE HEALTH & VITALITY

Want to Look and Feel Younger? Cutting-Edge Technology Can Rejuvenate Your Body, Skin, and Hair in Ways That Once Seemed Unimaginable

"If I'd known I was going to live this long,
I'd have taken better care of myself."

—EUBIE BLAKE

Can you remember a time when you returned from a vacation feeling well rested and happy, with a visible glow? You noticed it, and everyone else did, too, didn't they? Or the last time you came in from an invigorating run, a revitalizing yoga class, or an exhilarating day of skiing. Your cheeks were flushed with good health. Your eyes were bright and clear and alert. It felt like you could tackle the world—and you probably could!

The point is, your external appearance isn't superficial, after all. It's a reflection of your inner health and vitality. For example, skin, which accounts for about 15 percent of your weight, is the biggest organ in the body—and the quality of your skin reveals the quality of your internal systems. Redness, puffiness, and other visible problems serve as red flags warning you that something is wrong with your diet, medications, or autoimmune system. In other words, your overall well-being is reflected right there on the surface of your skin. Think of it as the canary in the coal mine of your body.

If you're dehydrated, it also shows in your skin. When you've slept badly or have consumed too much alcohol or unhealthy food, you wear that, too. And you know it, even as you try to cover it up with sunglasses or a baseball hat. **We might be able to hide our habits, but they reveal themselves in the way we look. That includes psychological wellness, especially stress.**

Can I ask you a personal question? When you stand in front of the mirror, how do you feel? Do you like the way you look? Do you love yourself unconditionally in all of your glorious imperfection? Or do you sometimes look at yourself with concern, upset or even dismayed about the subtle (and not so subtle) side effects of time on your body? Some people feel their muscle tone has softened or their waistline has expanded. Others notice that their hair has thinned, exposing areas of their scalp that had never previously been viewed by humankind. Or maybe their face has become more wrinkled—a living testament to decades of sunshine and laughter!

Sooner or later, we all experience these moments when time seems to be catching up on us. It's a natural part of growing older and wiser, right? Anyway, we all know that our appearance isn't the real measure of our worth. It's your heart and soul that truly make you beautiful.

But whether we admit it or not, most of us care a good deal about our appearance as well. It's not just a matter of vanity or social conditioning, although that's obviously part of it. It's also a question of survival. From an evolutionary standpoint, humans are hardwired to assess the appeal of potential mates, appraising their looks for physical clues about their health and status.

Appearances matter in the workplace, too. Researchers who study the effects of the so-called "beauty bias" or "beauty premium" have documented a correlation between attractiveness and career success. **A 2019 article in the _Harvard Business Review_ sums it up like this: "Physically attractive individuals are more likely to be interviewed for jobs and hired, they are more likely to advance rapidly in their careers through frequent promotions, and they earn higher wages than unattractive individuals."**[1]

It isn't fair, and it isn't always true. But this research suggests that it literally pays to look your best. Imagine that two people are interviewing for the same job. One has radiant hair, glowing skin, gleaming teeth, and

---

1 Chamorro-Premuzic, "Attractive People Get Unfair Advantages at Work. AI Can Help."

body weight proportionate to their height. The other has limp hair, gaunt cheeks, and darkly circled eyes. Basically, the second applicant looks halfway recovered from a bender. All other things being equal, who do you think will land the job? You and I both know that what really matters is qualities like intelligence, communication skills, leadership abilities, work ethic, and passion. But the thing that's *not* equal—your appearance—can sometimes tip the scales.

A better reason to care about how you look is that it can strongly affect how you feel about yourself. You radiate confidence when you look and feel your best. That sense of physical well-being is the serotonin of self-esteem.

I'm not arguing that you should obsess about your appearance, since there are so many things that matter more. But why *wouldn't* you want to look your best as much as possible, so you can relish that vibrant sense of well-being on every level, both inside and out? The good news is that looking great doesn't require you to spend your life savings on the type of dramatically invasive interventions that we tend to associate with movie stars of a certain age. Instead, what we're talking about here are breakthrough technologies that turn back time in surprisingly *gentle*, *kind*, and *natural* ways—yet also turn out to be incredibly effective.

As you'll discover in this chapter, beauty-related technology is advancing so rapidly that it's now possible to:

- **Grow new hair at any age without drugs (and their side effects) through plant regimens and cellular regeneration.**
- **Dramatically rejuvenate your skin with products customized specifically for you, taking into account your DNA, the bacteria on your face, your lifestyle, and environmental factors like the weather conditions and pollution levels in your neighborhood.**
- **Melt away unwanted body fat in minutes using radio frequency— and then use ultrasound waves to fix the excess skin that's left behind.**
- **Control your weight with the help of a nonchemical, FDA-cleared appetite suppressant that's entirely natural, so it's not even classified as a drug. This comes at a time when over 70 percent of adults in**

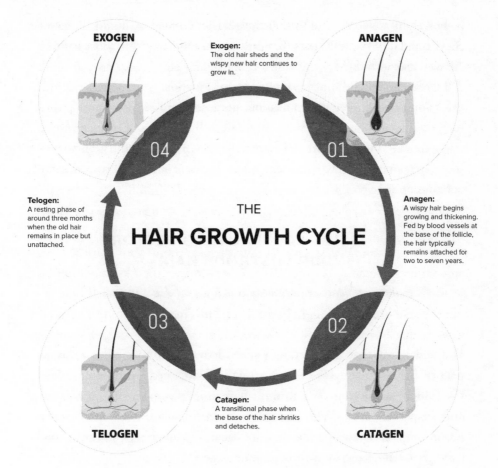

EXOGEN

Exogen:
The old hair sheds and the wispy new hair continues to grow in.

ANAGEN

04

01

Telogen:
A resting phase of around three months when the old hair remains in place but unattached.

THE

HAIR GROWTH CYCLE

Anagen:
A wispy hair begins growing and thickening. Fed by blood vessels at the base of the follicle, the hair typically remains attached for two to seven years.

03

02

Catagen:
A transitional phase when the base of the hair shrinks and detaches.

TELOGEN

CATAGEN

the U.S. are overweight and 39 percent are obese—a reminder that our appearance and our health are inextricably linked.

Of course, the rich and famous have always had access to the most sophisticated beauty treatments and technologies. Believe me, it's not *just* a genetic miracle when celebrities look decades younger than their biological age! I've seen friends of mine emerge from the most exclusive spas and cosmetic surgeries looking like they'd just bathed in the Fountain of Youth!

But what's exciting about the innovations we're going to discuss is that they're increasingly accessible and affordable for the average person. You don't have to be a movie star in Beverly Hills to experience cellular-level skin rejuvenation or fat-burning therapies. You don't have to be a millionaire to buy restorative hair and skincare products designed exclusively for you. They're readily available, part of a new movement toward what's known as "mass personalization."

Here's the catch. You need reliable information to benefit from this explosion of technological innovation, because there are so many options to choose from—and the results often fail to live up to the hype. So we're going to take you on a short and extremely selective tour of the beauty landscape, introducing you to a few remarkable breakthroughs that truly deserve your attention.

ALL IS NOT LOST! HOW TO RESTORE YOUR LUSTROUS HAIR

"To lose confidence in one's body is to lose confidence in oneself."

—SIMONE DE BEAUVOIR

Did you know that the average person loses 50 to 100 hairs a day as part of the normal cycle of hair growth? That's not a problem, unless the follicle starts to grow a thinner hair in its place, becoming smaller and wispier in each cycle. In case you're in the mood for a brief science lesson (nope!), here's how the healthy cycle of hair growth works in four easy steps. Each hair passes through four stages:

Every hair on your head is at a different stage of the growth cycle. Over time, the length of the anagen stage decreases and the hair comes in weaker and thinner until it's gone, at least to the naked eye.

What causes hair loss? The biggest culprits are aging and genetics. But there are other contributing factors, including stress, diet, various illnesses and autoimmune disorders, medications, and treatments that damage the scalp. By age 50, about 85 percent of men and 50 percent of women have experienced significant hair loss. In 2020, Ricki Lake—the actress who found fame as the star of the original non-musical movie *Hairspray*—revealed her own struggle with hair loss, as did Massachusetts representative Ayanna Pressley. **In the U.S. alone, about 30 million women suffer from noticeable hereditary hair loss, compared with 50 million men.**

Fortunately, there's never been a better time to find safe, effective, and affordable ways to reverse hair loss. That's a tremendous relief for folks like Beth Ann Corso. A few years ago, when she was 62, this Connecticut mother of three grown children noticed that her hair was thinning. Not a little, but a lot. She tried pulling it up in ways that might hide the wispy places, but it was no use. Her scalp was becoming visible at her temples and on the crown of her head.

Beth Ann suspected that her hair loss had its origin in stress, and with good reason. Her then husband had been convicted of white-collar crime, caught stealing $5 million from his accounting clients. And in the process of the highly publicized legal case, she learned that he had a second life—and a second relationship—in Las Vegas, where he'd racked up significant debt.[2]

Beth Ann knew that she had to find a way to turn stress into healing. Through Facebook, she found a small group of women whose spouses had been convicted of similar crimes, and she set off on a cross-country driving adventure to visit fifteen of them. She calls the experience "life-changing," infusing her with a new sense of courage and self-worth. It didn't stop her hair falling out. But when she got back home, it gave her the psychological boost to do something about it.

Like many of us, Beth Ann didn't want to flood her body with chemicals. **So she ruled out treatments using minoxidil (the active ingredient in Rogaine) and finasteride (which was originally sold under the brand name Propecia and is now used in products like Keeps and Hims). Finasteride is FDA-approved for men with thinning hair. It's also used by many women, but is recommended only for those past childbearing age because it's been linked to birth defects.** Truth be told, there can be some pretty unpleasant side effects for men, too, including impotence and loss of libido.[3] **One man told me, "You have hair, but you don't care!"**

Then Beth Ann read about **Harklinikken**, whose hair loss clinics have gained a devoted following among European royalty and Hollywood celebrities. **The company's Danish founder, Lars Skjoth, has spent decades working with plant extracts and products made from cow's milk,**

2 Eaglesham, "Mob-Busting Informant Resurfaces in SEC Probe."

3 Mysore, "Finasteride and Sexual Side Effects."

combining these natural ingredients to create his own line of shampoos, conditioners, and night serums—**all of which are customized for each client**.

The result? **As Beth Ann learned, Harklinikken clients routinely saw a 30 to 60 percent increase in the volume of their hair, based on the company's precise measurements of hair mass and the quantity and diameter of hair in the treated areas. She saw similar results.** Her reddish-blond hair now falls full and fluffy to her shoulders—a striking contrast to photos from her cross-country trip, when her hair lay limp against her head. I remember being shocked seeing her after she'd experienced approximately a 50 percent increase in the volume of her hair. She was beautiful and had such a youthful, vibrant, and joyful glow about her that I would have sworn that she was at least a decade younger than the 62 years old she claimed to be!

SunHee Grinnell, a former beauty director at *Vanity Fair*, had a **similarly striking** experience. After surgery for a medical condition, she was alarmed to find herself losing her hair, which had been long and thick her entire life. SunHee was so ecstatic that Harklinikken restored her hair (and, as she puts it, gave her back her "mojo") that she agreed to appear in a video featuring her before-and-after photos. **Other Harklinikken clients in the video included a young blond woman in her 20s, with portions of her head nearly completely bald. Seeing her hair restored to its former thickness and vibrancy without surgery was truly moving, not to mention the impact it had on all these individuals' lives.** We sometimes forget that hair loss and even balding can happen to people when they're really young like this, possibly due to stress or chemicals in the environment. Whatever the reasons, I can't tell you how touching it is to meet these clients and see how happy they are to walk into a room with renewed confidence, instead of worrying that everyone will notice their thinning hair.

The Harklinikken founder knows a thing or two about this anxiety himself. In his early twenties, Skjoth had a scalp condition that required many visits to a dermatologist, and he **began to lose hair because of it**. He was able to reverse the condition, but that experience left him with an enduring desire to help others who are unhappy about their hair loss. **"It's a massive attack on your self-image when you lose your hair,"** he says.

"It's like losing an organ you took for granted. And then suddenly it's under brutal attack, and you find yourself in this hopeless situation and desperate for help."

Lars gave up his dream of becoming a pilot to pursue his new passion, which led him to earn a master's degree in nutrition and biochemistry. He launched his first hair loss clinic in Copenhagen in 1992 and now has locations in Germany, Iceland, and Dubai, as well as Los Angeles and Tampa. More recently, he launched his U.S. flagship clinic in New York City. **Harklinikken also offers online consultations for a nominal fee over FaceTime and Skype.**

Located in a loft overlooking Fifth Avenue, the New York clinic feels more like an apartment or cooking school than a treatment center for hair loss. An elevator opens directly into the clinic's "kitchen," where a marble center island with barstools is surrounded by two walls of shelves and cabinets lined with bottles of products. On the countertop next to the sink, a row of beakers filled with different colored liquids might as well contain salad dressings. Consultations with clients take place at a long wooden table with ten chairs beneath a modern chandelier shooting off bulbs like a molecule. An adjacent seating area is decorated with a sofa and chairs, soft lighting, black-and-white photography. It's the embodiment of *hygge*, that Danish concept of cozy living.

It's no accident that the atmosphere is so warm and inviting. **"I think getting your hair back has much less to do with vanity than with life quality," says Lars. "There are a lot of people for whom hair means more than just tissue on your head, and they're surprised how much of an emotional reaction they have to it. For many women who come in, can you say they're vain just because they want hair? Or that they're afraid to be looked at as if they're ill?"**

Lars estimates that women account for 80 percent of his practice. When it comes to hair loss, women are typically more willing to seek help than men, who tend to believe that balding is just part of life. Still, I know loads of men who are horrified by their headlong descent into baldness! Take **Andre Agassi**, a friend and former client of mine, who's one of the best tennis players of all time. **Andre felt so self-conscious when he started going bald at 19 that he opted briefly to wear a big shaggy wig on** the court. In his memoir, he confided that he probably lost the 1990 French Open because he was so worried that his wig would fall off, exposing his hair loss to the world.

A few years ago, I noticed that my own hair was thinning, too. Nothing dramatic. Just a small spot on the left and right temples and a little on the crown of my head. Luckily, people had to be *really* tall to see what was going on up there! But I'm not someone who waits passively for things to get worse, and I enjoy finding high-quality solutions that I can share with others to improve their lives. When I discovered Harklinikken, I was amazed at how easy the process of restoring hair can be.

Lars's treatment regimen starts with a consultation to determine the extent of hair loss. He measures the density of hair in different parts of the scalp and tries to identify the reason why it's thinning. **He believes that the problems of hereditary hair loss can be transformed by rejuvenations through changes to your environment and habits, including a reduction of stress, and with the right mix of root-plant extracts and proteins, fatty acids, and cow's milk.** A few of his favorite ingredients

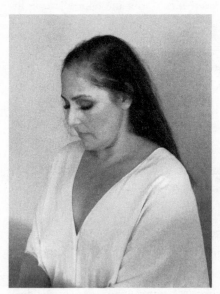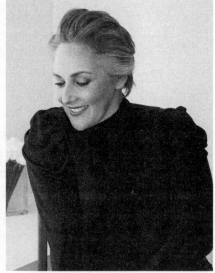

Ricki Lake struggled with hair loss for three decades and had tried everything from Rogaine, prescription medications, to PRP therapy. Nothing worked. Through her journey with Harklinikken, she rediscovered her confident self.

include extract of whey, marigold, and burdock root. **Each of his clients is given a mix that's formulated specifically to suit their own needs. But the goal is always the same: to revitalize the follicle, which is literally the root of hair health.**

For me, the results were amazing. Instead of *losing* hair as I age, I'm *regaining* it! In fact, Harklinikken's measurements show that **I have 40 percent more volume of hair, and it's thicker than it was**! And all it takes is rubbing a few natural ingredients onto my scalp before bed each night and using Lars's customized shampoo whenever I shower. What could be easier?

For Beth Ann Corso, Harklinikken's magic potions have been a godsend. All she has to do to keep revitalizing her hair is continue using the company's shampoo, conditioner, and serum indefinitely as an ongoing part of her hair rituals. If she stops, she risks losing her hair again. Her maintenance cost is about $100 a month. I know plenty of people who'd prefer to keep the money and lose their hair! Still, $100 a month is a far cry from, say, $15,000 or more for hair replacement surgery.

Beth Ann says it's been worth every cent. **"I don't live the lavish life, no massages or spa treatments, and I even cut my own hair. But I'd pay for these products over food on the table,"** she laughs. "I don't mean it to sound superficial, because your looks aren't who you are. But when you look better, you feel confident, and you feel better about yourself facing the world and trying new things. I have a confidence I didn't have before."

HOW STEM CELLS CAN REJUVENATE YOUR HAIR

> *"The dogma was that you were born with the total number of hair follicles that you were ever going to have. Their loss was considered permanent. Now, we know it's not."*

—DR. GEORGE COTSARELIS, cofounder of Follica

What I love about Harklinikken's plant-based approach to hair restoration is that it's so simple, low-key, and noninvasive. In a sense, it's the opposite of surgical hair transplants, which are not only expensive but can be painful and (if you're unlucky) can cause infections and scarring. In many cases, people also fail to warn you that the benefits of surgery may well be impermanent.

But we're also starting to see unbelievable breakthroughs from scientists who are tackling the problem of hair loss from an entirely different direction. Their mission? To harness the power of stem cells to repair and stimulate the scalp, so your hair can grow back again.

As we've discussed in previous chapters, stem cells derived from amniotic fluid and placentas that might otherwise be thrown away are revolutionizing the way we treat and heal our bodies, making it possible to replace and rejuvenate all sorts of damaged tissue—a biological magic trick! This concept of cellular regeneration can also be applied to restore your youthful beauty.

This is where things get especially interesting—and competitive. Right now, at least ten companies are locked in a global race to prove that they've found the best scientific solution for growing hair. Labs in Japan, Sweden, France, the UK, and the U.S. are all jockeying to finish first in clinical trials, so they can hit the market as soon as possible. Several are getting close.

One of the front-runners is **TissUse**, which has developed a proprietary Smart Hair Transplant technology. The process involves extracting thirty hair follicles from the back of the scalp and multiplying them to create 10,000 "neopapillae," which are then injected back into the scalp. Neopapillae are hair-promoting cells that can grow new hair follicles and rejuvenate weakened ones. TissUse has been licensed to **J. Hewitt**, a regenerative medicine company in Japan. That's an advantage because Japanese regulations offer fast-track approval for stem cell technologies.

Another trailblazer in this race is a Boston-based biotechnology company, **Follica**. It's developed a process that uses a proprietary "skin disruption device" to create micro-wounds on the scalp during a series of short office-based treatments. Sounds brutal, right? In fact, the healing process creates a precious "embryonic window" of opportunity for new follicles to grow out of the epithelial (surface lining) stem cells. The idea of using abrasions to stimulate the skin isn't new. What *is* new is Follica's approach of introducing a topical compound during that window of opportunity so the cells are persuaded to form hair, instead of forming epidermis. That's right! **The tech wizards at Follica have figured out a way to influence a stem cell on your scalp so that it makes the decision to become a cell that grows new hair!**

This regenerative effect, which is called *hair follicle neogenesis*, originated in the research lab of Follica's cofounder, Dr. George Cotsarelis, who is chair of the dermatology department at the University of Pennsylvania. **As he declares on the company's website, "The dogma was that you were born with the total number of hair follicles that you were ever going to have. Their loss was considered permanent. Now, we know it's not."**

In 2019, Follica reported the results of a pivotal trial, which showed an astounding 44 percent improvement of visible hair count after three months of treatment.[4] The company points out that there are currently two approved drugs in this field, which offer a modest 12 percent improvement of visible hair count. In other words, Follica's technology promises a *huge* leap forward, not a minor incremental advance. The next step? To demonstrate in the critical Phase 3 stage of clinical trials that its groundbreaking treatment for hair loss works effectively on a larger scale.

A slew of other companies are in hot pursuit of the same prize, and it's still anyone's guess who'll win. For example, **RepliCel** is working with beauty giant **Shiseido** on a treatment that cultures a person's own follicle cells, creating millions that can be implanted around the head. **Biosplice Therapeutics**, whose extraordinary work on cancer and other diseases we discussed earlier, in Chapter 9, is developing a topical solution to activate the **Wnt pathway** to pass signals through surface receptors, signaling the growth phase of the hair cell. **L'Oréal** is a key player, too. It's collaborating with a bioprinting company, **Poietis**, on 3D-printing hair follicle organoids in a dish. What does that mean? In essence, it means that L'Oréal is moving us one step closer to the Holy Grail of hair cloning.

If you're a little lost, I get it. All of this sounds a lot like an adult episode of Bill Nye the Science Guy. But here's the bottom line: **If your hair is thinning, you're already living in the greatest moment *ever* to do something about it. And the next few years will be infinitely better!**

---

4 Burns et al., "A Pilot Evaluation of Scalp Skin Wounding to Promote Hair Growth in Female Pattern Hair Loss."

WHAT ABOUT YOUR SKIN?

"Nature gives you the face you have at twenty; it is
up to you to merit the face you have at fifty."

—COCO CHANEL

The beauty-related applications of cellular regeneration won't stop there. After all, if stem cells can be used to grow new hair, why can't they also be used to rejuvenate your skin? Sure enough, this is already happening at anti-aging medical spas like the **Beverly Hills Rejuvenation Center**, which boasts about 50 locations across the U.S. Its co-owner, Dan Holtz, is often hailed in the media as a "Wellness Expert to the Stars" because he's helped folks like Superman (Dean Cain) with his knees and Miss USA (Ali Landry) with her back pain.

These days, Holtz is fascinated by the regenerative power of stem cells derived from umbilical cords. Cord blood has a high concentration of mesenchymal stem cells (MSCs), which are used for regrowth in all kinds of tissue repair. The connective tissue of umbilical cords, rich with MSCs, is called *Wharton's jelly*. That may sound like something you'd spread on a slice of toast. But it's now prized as a potent substance that can be injected throughout the body to heal injuries.

"When you have cells from a newborn—those very, very young growth factors—that's as youthful and good as it gets," says Holtz. "It can be used in regenerative joint and tissue repair. But there are also opportunities to use those growth factors in facial rejuvenation, hair restoration, overall skin rejuvenation." Holtz was so intrigued that he tried a Wharton's jelly *facial* on himself, and he liked the results so much that he was determined to offer this innovative therapy to the public.

As you can imagine, there's white-hot interest within the beauty industry in developing anti-aging rejuvenation therapies like this. It helps that the FDA is eager to encourage innovation that pushes the boundaries of what we know, so it's made the approval process relatively easy. In 2016, as part of the 21st Century Cures Act, the FDA offered a shortcut for drugs and devices that are classified as **regenerative medicine advanced therapy (RMAT)**. Human cell and tissue-based products are considered RMATs, so they don't require premarket authorization. Bottom line? Folks like Holtz, who are working on regeneration, gained an E-Zpass to approval.

Landry, who became a successful actor after winning the Miss USA title in 1996, shares Holtz's openness to new treatments. **She'd already received injections of Wharton's jelly in her back and was thrilled to find herself free of the pain that had plagued her ever since an accident two decades earlier.** So Holtz invited her to try a **Wharton's jelly facial**, which would entail having these growth factors injected in her face. Landry was game. **"These mesenchymal cells, they're like little missiles that go where you need them to go to tackle inflammation,"** she says. "I don't mind being a guinea pig. I like experimenting. Let's go for it, and share the information!"

The procedure was filmed for a TV show, *The Doctors*, and Landry came on afterward to discuss the experience, armed with before-and-after pictures. **Her verdict: "When I first saw the pictures side by side, I was shocked. I didn't know everything was drooping—the jowls and eyelids, and the pores enlarging . . ."** I don't know about you, but I suspect that she didn't look too shabby even *before* those stem cell injections! But Landry has no doubt that the treatment had a positive impact. **She raves, "I couldn't believe the results we got—the years we knocked off."**

But what if you don't fancy the idea of having stem cells injected into your face? Well, there are plenty of other cutting-edge therapies to revitalize your skin. As we discussed in our Diet & Lifestyle chapter, cryotherapy is a powerful tool for tackling inflammation that left unchecked can turn into a devil's playground for pain and swelling.

Imagine applying the same principle to rejuvenate the skin on your face. Cryofacials work like this: You recline with protective glasses, and a practitioner stands over you with a handheld wand. It blows a beam of vaporized liquid nitrogen slowly around your face and neck. The blast causes blood vessels to constrict, tightening enlarged pores, reducing puffiness, and exfoliating the outer layer of dead skin cells. When it's over, the rush of returning blood flow delivers a surge of nutrients and flushes out all sorts of unwelcome stuff, including environmental toxins and bacteria. The regenerative effects come from the "emergency" message that kicks the natural functions of cells into high gear, boosting the production of collagen—a protein layer of the skin that breaks down over time due to aging and sun damage.

Friends of mine have tried it tell me that a cryofacial is a much more pleasant experience than it sounds. The cold is apparently no worse than a bracing ride on a chairlift in a ski resort, and you emerge with a smoother complexion, reduced pigmentation, and a red-cheeked glow. People who like these results tend to get cryofacials regularly, the way some folks go for manicures or pedicures. And the cost is about the same.

Another popular option is to use lights to combat the effects of aging on the skin. **Lasers, which deliver a small focus of high-intensity light, are brilliant for minimizing all kinds of skin damage—from wrinkles and pigmentation to scars, veins, and precancerous growths.** And the variety and specialization of lasers keep getting better.

Dr. Ellen Marmur has no fewer than forty different lasers, and she wields them like an artist. For example, she uses **Fraxel** for fine lines around her patients' eyes and **PiQO4** for brown spots on their hands and faces. Before opening **Marmur Medical** in New York, **she was the first female chief of dermatologic surgery at Mount Sinai Hospital**. Since then, she's become a media darling on programs like *Good Morning America* and the *Today* show because she has a gift for explaining complex science while also delivering commonsense advice about sunscreen. **As a skin cancer survivor herself, she knows her subject from every angle.**

When she became one of Marmur's patients, Lauren Quinn was wrestling with the aftermath of skin cancer, which had been diagnosed when she was only 38 years old. The surgery had left Quinn with a significant hole on the bridge of her nose, 170 stitches, and a substantial graft using skin removed from her forehead. "I looked like a monster," she says. "I looked horrific."

After eight more surgeries, Quinn was remarkably mended. But she still had to keep a close watch for new growths. When a small precancerous spot appeared, Marmur treated it with photodynamic therapy, which combines light energy with a drug. She also gave Quinn a take-home LED device—a technology that delivers varying wavelengths of light to penetrate the skin at different levels. **LEDs (light-emitting diodes) have been shown to help significantly in healing wounds, reducing pain and inflammation,**

improving acne and rosacea, softening scars, increasing blood flow and oxygenation, and relieving pain.[5]

Quinn's LED therapy, which involved twenty minutes of blue light each morning for her abnormal cells and twenty minutes of red light at night for her inflammation, worked beautifully. Months after she was done with treatment for the spot, she still uses her LED device religiously because it so improves the overall quality of her skin. **"You notice the difference immediately," she says. "It shrinks the pores and tightens up the skin. . . . I saw my old dermatologist in California, and she was like, 'Look at you. What are you doing? You look great!'"**

Therapies using LED lights have surged in popularity recently, partly because the full-body machines found in medical spas have been reproduced in smaller sizes for home use. But what makes LED light therapies especially alluring is the accessible concept—different colored lights serve different purposes—combined with a soothing sense that you're sitting in a sunny window.

"There are all the skin benefits: building collagen and improving acne and sun damage, reducing redness and hyperpigmentation. But there are so many different utilizations," says Marmur. **"We know they have great impact on insomnia and circadian rhythms, seasonal affective disorder, and calming heart rates. It gives you this radiance, all kinds of healing."**

Marmur is just one of many experts breaking new ground in the realm of medical lasers. Another leader in this field whom we introduced in the Pain Free chapter is **Dr. Antonio Casalini, an electrical engineer and inventor whose lasers have helped me and many of my professional athlete friends and clients. The impact has been priceless to me and them.** He used to design medical lasers for corporations, for medical doctors, and for veterinarians. In fact, one of the most renowned lasers in these types of practices is the **Thor** laser, and after designing lasers for corporations, Dr. Casalini built increasingly complex and effective models of the Thor for

---

5 Ablon, "Phototherapy with Light Emitting Diodes: Treating a Broad Range of Medical and Aesthetic Conditions in Dermatology."

904 Laser, his group practice in Orange County, California, which specializes in **anti-aging treatments and pain management.**

Most lasers have one to four waves; Dr. Casalini's have nine to seventeen synchronized waves, with varying levels of power. They have built-in ionizers to pump your blood with fresh, pure oxygen. They even have timers, in case you get so relaxed that you fall asleep. Some of his clients, including professional athletes, buy their own bespoke lasers to use at home. **"Our lasers give you multi waves, meaning they're multipurpose,"** says Dr. Casalini. **"So you can work on pain treatment, scar tissue, anti-aging, all in one unit, because each wave gives you a different power."**

Having bought several of Dr. Casalini's lasers for me and my wife, Sage, and having invested in his company, here's what I can tell you. It's crazy how many different things they can accomplish. **They can accelerate the healing of wounds, relieve pain, combat inflammation and swelling, and reduce tension. On lower cosmetic settings, they can also repair scars and hyperpigmentation, smooth the surface of the skin, and reverse some effects of sun damage. There are all kinds of studies that show this.**[6] Imagine looking in the mirror, seeing a new wrinkle or discolored patch, and being able to do something about it on the spot. They also work wonders after a grueling day on stage. I only wish this technology had existed back when I played football!

FREEZE YOUR FAT?

"The shoe that fits one person pinches another; there is no recipe for living that suits all cases."

—CARL JUNG

One of the best examples of this trend toward low-key interventions involves the freezing of stubborn pockets of body fat, which tend to accumulate in hard-to-exercise areas once we reach middle age. We're talking here about your thighs, your back, your love handles, or possibly under your

---

6 Karmisholt et al., "Laser Treatments in Early Wound Healing Improve Scar Appearance."

chin! Some people used to go under the knife to get rid of this excess fat. **But today's treatments require no incisions or anesthesia, no collateral damage of bruising or scarring.**

Instead, you've probably heard of a noninvasive technology called **CoolSculpting**, which will weaken your fat storage cells by exposing them to extreme cold. The fat cells die, and your body then naturally eliminates the waste through the urine. How cool is that? **And would you care to guess how CoolSculpting was discovered? By two Boston doctors who noticed that kids lost dimples of fat inside their cheeks from** *eating popsicles*! **Incredible but true.**

Other devices (with macho names like **Thermage** and **Vanquish**) take the opposite approach, using radio frequency waves to *heat and kill fat by melting it*! One high-end device, **Exilis Ultra, works its cosmetic wonders by combining radio frequency waves with ultrasound waves to melt unwanted fat while also tightening the stretched-out skin that's left behind.** The device uses a layering effect, delivering energy to varying depths, from the superficial layer to deep tissue. **Again, these treatments are much less intrusive than surgery. If treated by a skilled professional, patients typically come away with nothing more unpleasant than temporary swelling or redness.**

Crazy, isn't it? If you were writing a sci-fi novel, this is the type of technology that you'd dream up in your fertile imagination—and your readers might think it was too far-fetched! *No pain, no surgery, no recovery time.* **Just something you can do effortlessly during your lunch break.**

PERSONALIZED PRODUCTS DESIGNED SPECIFICALLY FOR YOU

"Always remember that you are absolutely unique. Just like everyone else."
—MARGARET MEAD

There's one last trend that I want to mention here because it will transform the products you use over the next few years. We're now hurtling full speed into an era of "mass personalization." What does that mean? **It means that companies will increasingly create customized products that are** tailored to suit the idiosyncrasies of your body, your lifestyle, and your environment. Instead of taking a one-size-fits-all approach, they're already fine-tuning products to take into account everything from the bacteria on your face (your microbiome) to the humidity in your hometown.

Consider a leading-edge brand like **SkinCeuticals**. **It now offers a personalized product called Custom D.O.S.E., which** *Time* **magazine named a top 100 innovation of 2019.** (In case you're wondering, D.O.S.E. stands for Diagnostic Optimization Serum Experience.) The experience begins with a consultation in which a skin specialist assesses your needs with the help of a patented diagnostic tool. Then, in less than ten minutes, you watch in wonder while an elegantly designed compounding machine mixes and dispenses a "corrective serum" *exclusively for you*, blending the ingredients after considering more than 250 possible combinations of skin traits. The process is said to involve more than 2,000 algorithms.

L'Oréal, which owns SkinCeuticals, is a driving force in beauty research, and its Technology Incubator is responsible for some of the industry's most intriguing advances. At the 2019 Consumer Electronics show, L'Oréal launched **Perso**, a smart device that cooks up customized skincare products *in your own home*. The process starts with you taking a photograph of your face. **The Perso app then uses artificial intelligence to analyze the condition of your skin. The app also considers environmental factors like local weather conditions, UV radiation levels, and pollution.** Once you've inputted some additional details about your skincare goals, **the device dispenses a single-dose formula on the spot, based on your needs on that specific day!**

For the cosmetics industry, one attraction of AI is that it can be used to analyze mind-bending quantities of data in order to provide customized product recommendations. Take a company like **PROVEN Skincare, which won the MIT Artificial Intelligence award in 2018**. The business was founded by **Ming Zhao** (a high-flying private equity executive who was worried that the effects of exhaustion were starting to show on her skin) and **Amy Yuan** (a data scientist with a PhD in computational physics).

With the help of machine learning and AI algorithms, Zhao and Yuan analyzed more than 20,000 skincare ingredients, 100,000

products, **4,000 scientific journal articles, and millions of consumer reviews to figure out how various ingredients affect different people.** That mountain of information is stored within their **Skin Genome Project**, which is nothing less than the world's most comprehensive skincare database.

How do they mine that vast treasure trove of data? The company's customers take a **Skin Genome Quiz**, which enables PROVEN to construct a detailed profile of their skin, incorporating about forty-five factors ranging from age and ethnicity to environment and diet. **AI then makes it possible for the company to trawl through its enormous database at warp speed and recommend skincare products that are personalized to suit that customer's specific profile.**

There are many other players in the personalization game, and each one is going at it a little differently. Some track your zip code to gauge the hardness of your water. Some use sensors and biometric data to track your hydration and sunscreen needs. **One company, LifeNome, can even help consumers choose the right beauty products based on their DNA.** Ali Mostashari, one of LifeNome's founders, remarks, "There's a lot you can tell from the blueprint of a person's DNA about how their aging will be impacted by their environment and their habits."

LifeNome's technology is seriously sophisticated. But the underlying principle is simple: *You and I are different. So why should we expect the exact same product to work equally well for both of us? Wouldn't it be smarter to buy products designed specifically for you, based on your genetic makeup, where you live, and how you live?* Nonetheless, says Mostashari, **"Most people try to follow the same recipes that work for other people. And that's actually disastrous."**

Finally, there's one other groundbreaking company in this field that I want you to know about because it's driving the science of skin rejuvenation in a new and hugely promising direction. Its name is **OneSkin Technologies,** and it was cofounded in 2016 by a pioneering team of four female PhDs. They include CEO **Carolina Reis Oliveira** (an expert in stem cell biology) and chief science officer **Alessandra Zonari** (an expert in skin regeneration), who dazzled the audience at a recent event hosted by Peter Diamandis on the science of longevity.

The trailblazing scientists at OneSkin are obsessed with the biology of aging. Based on this fundamental knowledge, they believe that they can reduce the molecular age of your skin cells. **To put it another way, their mission is to revitalize your skin from the inside and extend your "skinspan"—the period in which your skin remains healthy and youthful.**

How? **"We're targeting what we believe is the root cause of skin aging,"** says Dr. Reis Oliveira. **As she explains, the chief culprits are senescent cells, which are damaged cells that build up in the body, contributing to aging and age-related disease. As senescent cells accumulate in our skin, they create wrinkles and sagging, produce inflammation, and also make us more susceptible to skin cancer. So OneSkin set out to kill them.**

The company developed a powerful screening mechanism that made it possible to evaluate about 1,000 small peptides to see if any of them would eliminate senescent cells. **They hit the jackpot, discovering one highly effective small peptide that they christened OS-01. OneSkin's experiments have shown that this proprietary peptide can significantly decrease the level of senescent cells, reducing the age of the skin by several years at a molecular level.**

This discovery led the company to release its first product toward the end of 2020. It's a topical supplement containing OS-01. You apply it to your face, neck, and hands twice a day like a moisturizer after cleansing your skin. **Unlike most skin treatments, OneSkin's product is not a superficial short-term fix, though it certainly makes your skin look great! Rather, it's designed to reduce the accumulation of aged cells, repair damage, and improve the overall cell function of your skin. In short, it's all about long-term restoration and rejuvenation.**

As I hope you can see by now, the beauty of beauty today is that your options are endless. If you want to enhance or revitalize some aspect of your appearance, almost anything is possible. But believe me, **I'm not suggesting that you** *need* **to do anything at all. For many people, smile lines, crow's feet, and other visible signs of aging are badges of honor, representing a lifetime of experience. Wear them with pride!** Andre Agassi, for one, ultimately decided to embrace his baldness, shaving his head completely at

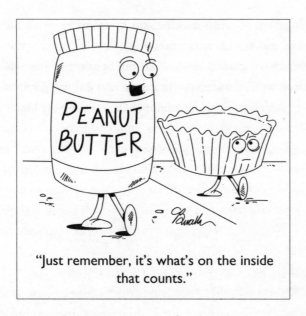

"Just remember, it's what's on the inside that counts."

the grand old age of 25. Looking back many years later, he declared, "When I did that, I never felt freer in my life."

But if you *don't* want to go quietly into that good night, the decision is yours. The technology is now available for you to choose how you want to look and how you want to age, regardless of your birthdate. Isn't it empowering to know that so many effective and painless solutions are available to you right now? So check out some of the companies we've discussed, research a few of their most innovative treatments and therapies, and then **decide for yourself whether it's time to *reverse time* by revitalizing the very cells of your magnificent body.**

Now, before we finish this third section of the book, we have one final chapter specifically written on women's longevity and reproductive health. As I'm not the expert in this field, I asked **Dr. Jennifer Garrison, PhD, founder of the Global Consortium for Reproductive Longevity and Equality and assistant professor of cellular molecular pharmacology at the University of California, San Francisco, School of Medicine along with Dr. Carolyn DeLucia, MD, who has been a practicing OB-GYN for nearly thirty years and is a specialist in the field.**

While this chapter is designed for women, if you're a man and you want a deeper understanding and appreciation for the feminine cycle of life, and the unique challenges and opportunities in women's reproductive health, you might find the chapter interesting.

Then we'll move onto Section Four, "Tackling the Top 6 Killers," and reveal the latest breakthroughs in prevention and combatting the "big six": heart disease, cancer, strokes, autoimmune disease, obesity and diabetes, and Alzheimer's.

With that, let's continue our journey. . . .

CHAPTER 16

WOMEN'S HEALTH: THE CYCLE OF LIFE

This chapter is specific to women's well-being, female longevity, vitality, lifespan, healthspan, and reproductive aging. It's such an important subject. While twenty or so pages isn't nearly enough to encompass all of the wondrous complexities and miraculous capabilities unique to women, note that there is no such male-specific chapter in this book.

I have so much respect for women, and I live in awe of the gifts they possess which made it possible for each and every one of us to be here now. There is not a human being alive who did not come into this world without the courage, endurance, and commitment of a woman's spirit and soul, or the wondrous faculties of a woman's physical body ushering them into life.

Women's biochemical oscillations and cycles are indeed intricate indications and biomarkers of total body health—which is part of the reason why **reproductive aging in women is perhaps the most important *and simultaneously* the most understudied field of medicine.** It's also the reason why I won't attempt to interpret secondhand the breakthroughs that have been made in this field.

I'm passing the torch to **Dr. Jennifer Garrison, PhD, faculty director of the Global Consortium for Reproductive Longevity & Equality and assistant professor at the Buck Institute for Research on Aging.** She is writing with advice from **Dr. Carolyn DeLucia, MD, and Dr. Lizellen La Follette, MD, who have been practicing OB-GYNs for 25 and 30 years, respectively.** The three of them are far better suited **than I am to address** this critical area of health that affects more than half the population and all of us who love and adore them.

WHY WOMEN'S LONGEVITY MATTERS TO US ALL BY DR. JENNIFER GARRISON, PHD, DR. CAROLYN DELUCIA, MD, AND DR. LIZELLEN LA FOLLETTE, MD

Most people don't realize that the age at which a woman goes through menopause is correlated with her overall lifespan. Put simply, a woman who goes through *menopause later* will tend to *live longer.* The science of reproductive longevity is just now starting to take off. Not only does it have the potential to dramatically improve women's health, fulfillment, well-being, and enable them to enjoy a high quality of life well into old age, it also has the potential to yield groundbreaking insights on why we age in general.

In this chapter, we'll share with you . . .

- The common myths about women's health, and the truths, and the work in progress that can set you free!
- Why the science of female reproductive longevity may be the single most under-explored key to unlocking the secrets of aging
- Why your period is an invaluable vital sign of your underlying health
- Things you can do right now that will have a profound impact on your life, vitality, hormonal health, total body wellness, and fertility, whether children are part of your future plans or not

THE LINK BETWEEN LONGEVITY AND OVULATION

"Ovulation has been recognized as an event linked with reproduction; however, recent evidence supports the role of ovulation as a sign of health."

—DR. PILAR VIGIL, MD, PhD

For the first time in our history there will soon be more people over the age of 65 than there are under the age of five. According to the World Health Statistics report of 2021, **women around the world can** expect to live an average of five years longer than men. In fact, females of most species live longer lives than their male counterparts. The confirmed world record holder for human longevity was a French woman who lived to the ripe age of 122 before she passed away in 1997, and the oldest living person in the world at the time this book is going to press in 2022 is a 118-year-old Japanese woman. (For comparison's sake, the oldest living man is *only* a spry 112.) **Studies suggest that women possess a genetic advantage over men that partly accounts for a longer lifespan,** but differences in sex hormones and social factors also play a role. **But even though women live statistically longer than men, they spend more of their lives in poor health (thirty-four years on average) compared to men (twenty-six years).**

While there's still a lot we don't understand, it seems there's one thing researchers are certain of: For women, aging is closely tied to reproductive aging. Why? Because studies show evidence that menopause accelerates the aging process in a woman's body.

By now, you're familiar with Horvath's clock, a way to determine someone's biological age. Horvath's team discovered that menopause speeds up cellular aging by an average of 6 percent. **The research and resulting arguments "very, very strongly suggest that the loss of hormones that accompanies menopause accelerates or increases biologic age," said Horvath to** *Time* **in 2016.**

The thing is, women born today have a predicted lifespan of nearly 100 years.[1] **Think about that; that means that soon women will live more of their lives** *after* **menopause than before.** While many women come to dread "the change of life" because the end of the reproductive era can unleash a cascade of effects in even a healthy woman's body—like increasing risk of heart disease, stroke, cognitive decline, insomnia, depression, weight gain, osteoporosis, and arthritis, combined with other symptoms that affect at least 75 percent of women *during* menopause, including hot flashes, brain fog, insomnia, and sexual dysfunction. Any one of these could decrease

---

1 Tergesen, "Is 100 the New Life Expectancy for People Born in the 21st Century?"

a woman's quality of life (as many women reading this chapter may be all too familiar with!), but there is a bright side.

While many will agree that menopause can feel bleak, most women find that post-menopausal life (after one year has elapsed since the last period) is one of nature's best kept secrets! Many women say that after menopause, as hormone levels stabilize either naturally or through hormone replacement therapy (more on that later in this chapter), symptoms disappear, and they feel the best they have felt in years. It's different for every woman.

The good news is, great problems provide great opportunities. Women's lifespans are already extensive, and while there are unique challenges later in life, scientific research is finally stepping up to provide real solutions for a sustained healthspan that will make life worth living long into the golden years.

Many women say that after menopause, as hormone levels stabilize either naturally or through hormone replacement therapy (more on that later in this chapter), symptoms disappear, and they feel the best they have felt in years.

Before we get to the latest developments that are providing revolutionary solutions, it's important to understand ovulation as a marker of health, the story a woman's cycle is telling, and what is happening in a woman's body well before menopause.

DEMYSTIFYING MENOPAUSE

"My mother always used to say 'The older you get, the better you get. Unless you're a banana.'"

—BETTY WHITE

In the United States most people learn about the hormonal changes that happen during puberty from that awkward sex ed class in grade school, but there's not really a time in our lives as mature adults when we get any kind of formal guidance around healthy menstruation, ovulation, fertility, or menopause. Women's fertility has long been relegated to the shadows as a taboo subject that women hardly discuss even with close friends.

Silence and a lack of reliable information has led to menacing myths and misunderstandings about women's health. Most people don't realize that while men produce sperm throughout their lives, **female humans are born with their lifetime supply of eggs**. That's right, while still in the mother's womb in fact, a female fetus has already developed a reproductive system, which contains around 6 million eggs (oocytes) in the ovaries. So, although Dr. Garrison was born in the 1970s, the egg that she came from was already in the fetus that became her mother, *in her grandmother's womb in 1956*. Like real life science fiction! The number of eggs a woman has declines precipitously, and long before she ever wants to use them, dropping to approximately 1 million at the time of birth, then to about 350,000 by puberty. **At that point, eggs start dying off at a rate of approximately 1,000 a month with each menstrual cycle.**[2] **All in, only about 400 mature eggs go through ovulation in a lifetime** (released from the ovaries, through the fallopian tubes, and into the uterus).

Menopause happens when the ovaries cease functioning because they have run out of eggs. Suppressing ovulation with hormonal contraceptive medications (like the pill, patch, injections, IUDs, rings, etc.) does nothing to slow the loss of eggs. <u>As a result, 10 percent of women are infertile by the time they turn 35, and just five years later, at the age of 40, women have only a 5 percent chance of becoming pregnant in any given month.</u>[3] In fact, women who become pregnant after age 35 are classified by the medical community as being of "advanced maternal age." How could that be when they are predicted to have some sixty years of life left?! Obviously, that's an outdated classification,. Especially with the help of the powerful science of development of assisted reproductive technologies (ART) means that rates of women getting pregnant in their 40s are

---

2 Wallace and Kelsey, "Human Ovarian Reserve from Conception to the Menopause."

3 Broekmans et al., "Ovarian Aging: Mechanisms and Clinical Consequences."

increasing. **Nearly 20 percent of births are to women over the age of 35.**[4] **Research suggests that it may be possible to delay menopause in women using cryopreserved tissue grafts to replace hormones in physiological concentrations.**[5] This has already been successfully accomplished in mice, but we have a long way to go to make this a reality for humans. Beyond that dream scenario, researchers are working on many different ideas to extend women's reproductive span. Imagine if we could delay the timing of ovarian failure? This would be game-changing for women's overall health, not to mention fertility.

NOW LET'S BUST A FEW MEGA MYTHS

The chart depicting the dramatic decline in egg quantity and quality with age—which is characterized by a single point of inflection then a descending cliff—is burned into women's brains as an inevitable truth. While there may be some truth to that depiction *on average*, at the level of the individual

---

Nearly 20 percent of births are to women over the age of 35. Research suggests that someday stem stem cells could be used to grow new egg cells and thus delay menopause in women.

---

this is not true at all. **Every woman has her own unique reproductive span trajectory. Fertility is not like a bank that only goes in one direction; rather it is stochastic and cyclical. Young, healthy women often go through periods of infertility, while some women have random spikes of fertile periods well in to their 50s.**

As for that twenty-eight-day cycle that you were taught was "normal," that's another myth! Only 12 percent of menstrual cycles are twenty-eight days long. Like everything related to female reproductive

---

4 Mathews et al., "First Births to Older Women Continue to Rise."

5 C Yding Andersen et al., "Fertility Preservation Freezing of Ovarian Tissue and Clinical Opportunities."

longevity, **"normal" cycle length is variable at the level of the individual and changes with age; your natural cycle varies responding to stress, nutrition, exercise, illness, light exposure, and many other lifestyle factors.**

And how about the main event—**ovulation**—which is widely taught (and believed) to fall on Day 14 of the cycle. Consider that a study measuring 1,060 menstrual cycles in 141 women found that **only one-quarter of participants experienced their fertile window (ovulation) between Days 10 and 17 of their cycle.**[6] **That means 75 percent fell outside of that "normal" range, meaning what's** *actually* **"normal" when it comes to the menstrual cycle is considerable variability!**

And while we believe every woman should have access to birth control anytime she wants, there's one myth that's both so deceptive and popular that we want to point it out here; many women think that contraceptives keep them from losing eggs. But the single egg that's ovulated each month isn't the only one you lose. With each cycle somewhere around 1,000 eggs die no matter what, even if you're on birth control or pregnant. So **taking birth control pills does nothing to slow the rate of ovarian aging.** In addition, there is emerging data on the side effects of long-term hormonal birth control use, so it's important to speak with your doctor and educate yourself about all of your options and what's best for you.

The great news is, there are many non-hormonal contraceptive options to consider that don't hijack a woman's biochemistry. Explore all of your options; don't settle for an easy answer. **In short, reproductive function is one of the most miraculous, individualized, and complex multivariate signatures of the human body, so we need to approach it with the attention, gratitude, and respect it deserves.**

THE HEALTH OF THE OVARIES IS INDICATIVE OF WHOLE BODY HEALTH

Ovaries bear a likeness to two grapes, and though they are small, they are one of the most significant and mighty organs in the entire body and one of the keys that distinguish females from males. **Ovaries are mainly**

---

6 Fehring et al., "Variability in the Phases of the Menstrual Cycle."

responsible for producing eggs and secreting sex hormones that promote fertility—what's interesting is, they're also *the first organ to age in
the human body*.

An ovary is composed of many different cell types and structures, and
through every menstrual cycle these complex little organs undergo dynamic
remodeling in a way that doesn't happen in other tissues. **In fact they age at
two times the rate of the rest of the organs.** That means when a healthy
woman is in her late twenties and her body is functioning at peak performance, her ovaries are already showing overt signs of aging—a fact that
many young women are surprised to learn when they try to get pregnant.
That's why—long before menopause—there is a strong connection between
reproductive function and overall health.

Even in young women, if there is underlying dysfunction in the reproductive organs, it dramatically affects other parts of the body. For example,
women with polycystic ovarian syndrome (PCOS) are prone to metabolic
diseases later in life. **So it's clear that studying ovarian health could unlock revolutionary and far-reaching discoveries about aging in other
human tissues and how we might reverse or slow its progression in
both women and men.**

By now you must be asking: **How is it possible that we don't know
how these fundamental aspects of women's health work already?** Consider these two big culprits:

- *Lack of research funding.* Research on women's health overall is grossly
  underfunded considering we are talking about half the population. In
  2021, the National Institutes of Health spent 11.9 percent of the total
  budget on women's health. And of that, less than 0.1 percent went to
  study reproductive aging in women.
- *Lack of data.* Female physiology has been woefully understudied and
  purposefully excluded from research for decades because ovulatory cycles
  are considered confounding "noisy" variables. It was not until 2016 that
  the National Institutes of Health required grant recipients to include
  both sexes in animal studies!

MENOPAUSE IS NOT A BIOLOGICAL IMPERATIVE

So here's what we do know: **Menopause is an unusual reproductive strategy that flies in the face of evolutionary theory. Why do women outlive fertility? We humans are in the extreme minority in the animal kingdom; the only other creatures that go through menopause are a few species of whale.**[7] **Some monkeys have hormonal patterns comparable to humans but they continue to cycle very close to the age when they die.**[8] The reality is, while there are several theories (like the popular "grandmother hypothesis") no one knows exactly why women's ovaries shut down the processes of menstruation and ovulation—otherwise known as menopause—and this is a key piece of the puzzle we need to extend both reproductive span and healthspan.[9]

Now let's consider a scenario where women are not constrained in their reproductive choices by a limited and immutable biological clock, a world where women are not subject to the detrimental health effects of reduced sex hormone levels. . . .

The **Buck Institute for Research on Aging**, in partnership with the Bia-Echo Foundation, recently launched a moonshot effort to tackle female reproductive aging.

We are funding research and building the ecosystem to support discovery and innovation around reproductive longevity. We are accelerating development of products and therapies to positively impact women's lives, from cellular targets like egg mitochondria to ovarian inflammation. Some of the scientists we've funded are redefining diagnostics to tell women where they are in their individual reproductive span, while others are developing novel therapeutics to extend reproductive longevity. Along the way we think understanding why ovaries age prematurely will provide important clues about how aging works in the rest of the body. Quite frankly, we intend to change the world, after all—the future of humanity literally depends on it.

---

7 Ellis et al., "Analyses of Ovarian Activity Reveal Repeated Evolution of Post-Reproductive Lifespans in Toothed Whales."

8 Walker and Herndon, "Menopause in Nonhuman Primates."

9 Powledge, "The Origin of Menopause: Why Do Women Outlive Fertility?"

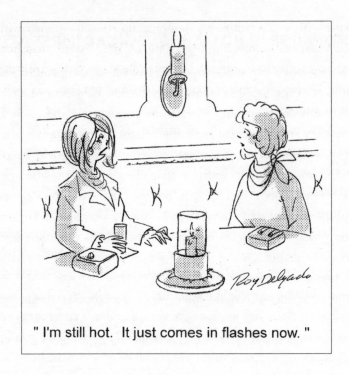

" I'm still hot. It just comes in flashes now. "

THERAPIES AVAILABLE NOW

"Because each has her own unique fertility trajectory, the current standard of care is not right for every woman—we need to tailor therapies to individuals."

—LIZELLEN LA FOLLETTE, MD

While we wait for those important scientific discoveries around the root cause of ovarian aging, **there are some excellent solutions available now to address health and fertility as a woman ages**. It should be noted that the ancient maxim "Know Thyself" is powerful and relevant advice here. Tune into the inherent wisdom of your body and listen to the signals it is sending you each month. **Gather as much baseline data about YOUR BODY and YOUR UNIQUE CYCLE** as possible so that you know what your "normal" is. Remember that the American Congress of Obstetricians and Gynecologists advocates "using the menstrual cycle as a vital sign" and multiple apps (MyFLO, Clue, Ovia, Period Tracker, Glow) can assist with measuring your physiology changes throughout the four phases of your period. New companies are popping up to help women with real-time individualized monitoring over time. (A single static snapshot is not sufficient to capture meaningful information about a woman's dynamic, fluctuating hormonal cycles, so capture as much information as possible over several months.)

If you are facing any issues like an inability to conceive, fibroids, endometriosis, painful periods, or any other condition that interferes with your cycle or quality of life, **ASSEMBLE A TEAM OF DIVERSE HEALTHCARE SPECIALISTS** to help you make sense of the data you collect. **Think of your symptoms as valuable information, signals your body is sending, and just like we've been recommending all along, get more than one opinion.** You might consult a family doctor, nurse practitioner, OB-GYN, endocrinologist, fertility specialist, osteopath, naturopath, midwife, and/or traditional Chinese medicine practitioner. **Remember that you get to decide what options you want to pursue and what's right for you.** If you aren't satisfied with the options being presented to you, don't give up, consult someone else! **You might have the kindest doctor in the world, but if you're facing something that is not within their area of expertise, we encourage you to find a doctor whose expertise best supports you and your vital health. Let's look at four solutions for your hormonal health, sexual function, fertility, and overall well-being. . . .**

1. *Commonsense healthy lifestyle choices:* **We know ovarian aging can be accelerated by many factors including environmental stressors, the food we eat or don't eat, exercise, sleep, toxin load, medically induced agents like chemotherapy or radiation, and a myriad of other conditions.** Quick fixes and magic elixirs may grab marketing dollars, but the truth is that making sound, intuitive lifestyle choices can dramatically affect every aspect of health and well-being, and this includes hormonal regulation and the menstrual experience. Hear how Amanda Laird, holistic nutritionist and author of *Heavy Flow*, explains the circuit:

> Our hormones are very sensitive to stress and nutrition, which means that a high-stress lifestyle and poor diet are going to adversely affect our hormonal health and, ultimately, our periods. Stress suppresses

ovulation, and we need to ovulate in order to get the benefits of progesterone. If we're not making enough progesterone, estrogen can
skyrocket without the counter-balance of progesterone, which contributes to period problems. And in a bizarre twist, higher levels of
estrogen lead to higher levels of cortisol, a hormone that regulates our
stress response—which in turn is going to affect our ability to ovulate.
And so, the cycle goes on and on. The good news, however, is . . . that
means that making some changes to what we eat, how we move, and
the thoughts that we think can have a positive impact on our hormonal health and in turn, our menstrual cycles.

**Be kind to your body. Appreciate its gifts. Sleep. Move. Don't consume
overly processed foods. Eat your greens. Choose organic when you
can. Rest and digest.** For heaven's sake don't smoke. Limit or eliminate
alcohol. Limit or eliminate stress. Know that if you choose to ingest dairy
products from cow's milk, you're choosing to ingest hormones and common
allergens. Drink plenty of water. Keep your blood sugar balanced. Steer
clear of artificial sweeteners. Get rid of the toxins in cleaning products,
detergents, body care, and personal items like aluminum deodorants and
aerosol sprays. Be mindful. Breathe! We know you know these things, we
all know these things, but a friendly reminder never hurt since we're often
pulled in so many directions that we're not actually doing the basics consistently. **(And the basics are so important!)**

Supplements can provide incredible relief and stability, and help support
the body throughout a women's cycle. We know that calcium supplements
may slow the loss of bone density[10] associated with menopause. **Iodine is an
essential trace element necessary for the production of all hormones
in the body and plays a vital role in supporting a woman's thyroid.
B-complex vitamins and zinc help replenish nutrient supplies (that
hormonal contraceptives are known to deplete). Magnesium** is key in
supporting the nervous system, and it also works as a muscle relaxant to

---

10 Bailey et al., "Calcium Supplement Use Is Associated with Less Bone Mineral
    Density Loss, But Does Not Lessen the Risk of Bone Fracture Across the
    Menopause Transition."

help calm those uterine cramps. **Vitamin E** has been shown to reduce period pain, too. This is another area to explore and do your research. Open dialogue with your healthcare team. Communicate with your providers so that they can help tailor their recommendations and therapies to you as an individual—they don't know what you're experiencing unless you tell them.

2. *Hormone replacement therapy (HRT):* The brain controls all aspects of female reproduction, ruling not as a dictator, but by constantly listening to and integrating feedback. There is a dynamic, ongoing conversation between the brain and reproductive organs that determines what happens in the system. **The language of neuronal communication is mediated by chemicals (aka hormones) that travel back and forth conveying mes-**

HRT can reduce the overall health risks associated which menopause and can also ease the symptoms that so dramatically impact a woman's quality of life.

---

sages between the brain, ovaries, and uterus. While we know some of the key words in this conversation, which include steroid hormones (estrogen, progesterone, and testosterone) and neuropeptides (oxytocin, GnRH, and kisspeptin), the full lexicon has yet to be defined. How these pieces fit into the complex network of communication to drive fertility and aging is a puzzle we are still working to solve. **When a woman runs out of eggs and her ovaries stop functioning, that chemical conversation with the brain shuts down, leading to the negative downstream effects of menopause. Hormone replacement therapy (HRT) is a way to replace some of those missing chemical signals that decline during perimenopause and vanish in menopause.**

HRT can reduce the overall health risks associated with menopause and can also ease the symptoms that so dramatically impact a woman's quality of life. Having said that, **there are nuances of HRT** that require careful consideration of risks and benefits in consultation with an OB-GYN. Every individual woman should discuss these risks, including family history of breast cancer, with her doctor to decide whether HRT is the right fit for her.

HRT is not perfect, but at times it has suffered unfairly from a bad reputation. In 2002, a randomized clinical trial made news when it suggested that HRT might increase risk of breast cancer and doctors began shying away from prescribing it. <u>Unfortunately, the study had design flaws that led to incorrect conclusions about HRT, and those misperceptions were amplified and widely reported by the media, leading to widespread misinformation.</u> There has been a lot written on this topic elsewhere, but in short—the age of the patient cohort and the administration of hormones were deemed flawed, and the widely repeated conclusions of **this study did not actually reach statistical significance.** <u>Since then, multiple studies have found that HRT lowered risk of atherosclerosis and heart attack in thousands of women between the ages of 35 and 55.</u>

More recent studies also show that **the age at which a woman begins hormone replacement therapy is critically important.** Not only is HRT

Multiple studies have found that HRT lowered risk of atherosclerosis and heart attack in thousands of women between the ages of 35 and 55.

---

more effective when started closer to menopause, **there was no benefit shown to starting HRT in women who were already ten years past menopause,** and even some evidence that it could be harmful if started too late. In addition, the method of HRT delivery is important to consider, with transdermal patches or topical creams preferred over oral delivery because of a small increase in risk of blood clots associated with metabolism in the liver when ingested orally. **These seemingly disparate results point to a key component of endocrine health and reproductive hormonal signaling—it's complicated.** There's a sweet spot of timing, specific hormone or hormone-like molecule combinations, and individual biology required to derive benefits from HRT. It's also not recommended for everyone, particularly women with a familial risk of cancer—a careful analysis of individual risks and benefits with your physician is important! One of the most exciting developments on this front is personalized telemedicine companies like Evernow that are combining detailed patient histories with novel HRT preparations to customize and democratize HRT on a personal level.

3. *Thermal and radiofrequency-based laser treatment:* Lasers emit heat energy that is absorbed by water in the targeted tissues. The heat emitted causes microscopic damage that triggers wound healing, which in turn encourages tissue remodeling. In dermatology, **this translates into skin tissue structure restoration.** The same principles apply to vaginal tissue. Although lasers have been used safely by dermatologists, surgeons, and medspas for years, laser treatments have not yet been approved by the FDA specifically to treat symptoms related to female health and sexual function.[11] **Many physicians, including Dr. Carolyn DeLucia and Dr. Lizellen La Follette, offer these treatments to their patients off-label because they have observed firsthand that laser therapies can be useful to address symptoms of urinary incontinence, vaginal atrophy (inflammation of vaginal walls that may cause pain, usually after menopause), pain during intercourse, and lack of sexual satisfaction.** There are studies supporting the efficacy of laser technology for these purposes, and we believe them to be a key solution in the near and evolving future.

4. *Platelet Rich Plasma (PRP) treatment:* When a blood sample is drawn from a patient's arm and spun for several minutes (centrifuged), then separated to remove red blood cells, what is left is a concentrate of **platelet-rich plasma (PRP). This plasma, which is rich in high concentrations of cytokines, growth factors, and other bioactive compounds, is then injected back into the patient's tissue, initiating angiogenesis (development of new blood vessels) and stimulating cell regeneration and repair.** There have been multiple studies showing PRP is effective when used in dental surgery, and it has been FDA-approved to treat osteoarthritis and sports injuries. **Preliminary work shows that PRP may be effective**

---

11 Karcher and Sadick, "Vaginal Rejuvenation Using Energy-Based Devices."

in improving uterine lining thickness and treating vaginismus (painful spasmodic contractions), endometritis (inflammation), vaginal dryness, pelvic floor damage, and incontinence but further studies are needed.

THE POWER OF LASER
By Dr. Carolyn DeLucia

Vaginal issues are undoubtedly a very sensitive and personal experience, though many women encounter such problems with hormonal changes, the onset of menopause, after the birthing process, or on account of medical conditions that can cause changes in vaginal tissue structure and mucosal secretions, all of which can have a negative impact on their quality of life.

I have witnessed firsthand the healing treatments like PRP and radiofrequency lasers are capable of. Just as one example, a 42-year-old woman came into my office with urinary incontinence and primary anorgasmia (inability to orgasm). Though she had been suffering for several years, she hadn't shared her challenges with anyone, not even her husband. It was decided to use the **FemiLift laser** to treat the full length of the vaginal canal to increase collagen vasculature. **The heat also improves flow in vaginal blood vessels, which provides the tissues with essential nourishment and stimulates nerve regeneration and mucosal secretion.** It was decided that this patient would further benefit from the use of platelet-rich plasma in the anterior wall of the vagina. <u>**This was all accomplished completely pain-free and she now experiences sexual satisfaction.**</u>

More studies are needed before the FDA will approve these treatments for these indications. **Again, we come back to the imperative that more basic scientific research into female-specific areas of need must proliferate. But think about the impact that just these four solutions can have on improving the quality of life for so many women right now.** We're excited for what the future holds and the promise of it arriving straightaway. Remember, it is important that you always work with your team of doctors and health care specialists to determine the best possible solutions for you.

QUESTIONS WOMEN CAN ASK THEIR DOCTORS

1. Does HRT make sense for me (if I don't have a history of breast cancer)?
2. I am suffering with hot flashes and night sweats. What are my options to deal with them?
3. I am not sleeping at night. Other than sleep medication, what steps can I take to improve the quality of my sleep?
4. When should I get a baseline bone density scan?
5. Are there any features of my menstrual cycle that foreshadow future issues I might have with fertility?
6. I've been on the birth control pill for years and at this stage of my life, I'm starting to think about family planning and getting pregnant; are there steps I could take now to support preconception?
7. I have lost all my desire for sex. Do I just have to accept this?
8. Intercourse is so painful, it is almost impossible. What are my options?
9. I lose urine with a cough, sneeze, or laugh. What can be done?
10. What can you tell me about (FDA-approved) thermography as a valuable tool in my breast health portfolio?
11. After having my children, I feel less pleasure when being intimate with my partner. Are there treatments available for this?
12. My emotions are all over the place. I have mood swings from rage to great sadness. What could be contributing to this, and what are some solutions?
13. My weight is getting more and more difficult to manage. Can we talk about what might be better choices for me at this stage?

HORMONAL CONTRACEPTIVES
By Dr. Carolyn DeLucia, M.D., FACOG

As an advocate for women's health and empowerment, I certainly believe all women should have access to birth control, and while the birth control pill is certainly effective in preventing pregnancy and is often a short-term necessity during fertility treatment cycles, I am always a proponent of educating and informing women about all benefits and possible side effects of any medication they consider taking. I believe in informed consent, that is, full disclosure of risks and benefits. The benefits are well known—improved cycle control, less bleeding and cramps, and ovarian cancer protection.[12]

It may seem strange for me, an OB/GYN for nearly 30 years, not to brim with praise for long-term use of synthetic hormonal contraceptives. What's true about the pill, the patch, ring, implant, injection, IUD, et. al, is that they suppress your body's natural production of estrogen, progesterone, and free testosterone. When we look at the hormonal profile of a woman on hormonal contraceptives, it resembles that of a woman in menopause, because in the words of hormone specialist Alisa Vitti, in her book *In The Flo*, "synthetic birth control does not correct hormonal imbalances; it merely suppresses your own hormonal function."

While there are advantages that many women appreciate about the pill, there are also some side effects to consider, which can include headaches, depression, bloating, weight gain, fatigue, loss of libido, and increased risk of breast cancer[1], just to name a few. Something many women are not aware of is that taking hormonal contraceptives can also increase your risk of thrombosis (blood clots), anywhere from four

---

12 Huber et al., "Use of Oral Contraceptives in BRCA Mutation Carriers and Risk for Ovarian and Breast Cancer."

to seven times your normal risk.[13] The pill is also associated with risk of increasing gallbladder disease, high blood pressure, and strokes.[14]

There are many resources, including *The Fifth Vital Sign* by Lisa Hendrickson-Jack, that are full of research to consider before you make decisions that will affect your body, sexual satisfaction, and fertility while you choose to use hormonal contraceptives, and sometimes even years after you stop. I feel compelled to include this information here because it affects the vital life force of so many women. I encourage you—as I encourage all my patients—to look at the possible risks along with the benefits and make informed decisions after working with your doctor and health care team to consider all options and alternatives.

In Summary . . .

While there is certainly a unique complexity to a woman's biochemistry and an individuality in each experience of her cycle of life, the female body, no matter what age, size, shape, or color, is its own magnificent masterpiece. Some women have the amazing ability to foster new life through birth, if they choose to do so. The female body is an extraordinary mechanism for this phenomenon. The intent of this chapter is simply to provide some additional choices at different stages of the journey. This book is dedicated overall to tools and insights that can powerfully enhance the quality of life *for all*.

All right, dear reader, we're coming around to the last section of this book—Section Four, where we are tackling the "big six"—heart disease, cancer, strokes, autoimmune disease, obesity and diabetes, and Alzheimer's. These chapters will go in depth to show you the latest insights on what you can do to prevent these diseases, what you can currently do to treat them if you or someone you love is impacted, and what's coming soon!

Let's begin . . .

---

13 Helmerhorst et al., "The Venous Thrombotic Risk of Oral Contraceptives, Effects of Oestrogen Dose and Progestogen Type."

14 Etminan et al., "Oral Contraceptives and the Risk of Gallbladder Disease."

TACKLING THE TOP 6 KILLERS

The latest scientific breakthroughs available to help you prevent, treat, and potentially heal some of the most dreaded diseases, including . . .

- Heart Disease: How to Mend a Broken Heart

- Your Brain: Treating Strokes

- How to Win the War on Cancer

- Conquering Inflammation and Autoimmune Disease: Bringing Peace to the Body

- The Double Threat of Diabetes and Obesity: Defeating a Double Threat

- Alzheimer's Disease: Eradicating the Beast

CHAPTER 17

HOW TO MEND A BROKEN HEART

New Tools for the Protection and Restoration of the Most Important Organ in the Body

"There's something about life and also the human heart that wants to renew itself."

—JACK KORNFIELD, PhD,
author of *A Path with Heart*

We take the beating of our heart for granted. Every day, twenty-four hours a day, while we're sleeping and while we're awake, this muscular, ten-ounce workhorse is continuously pumping the equivalent of liquid gold—our blood, the source of life—through 60,000 miles of blood vessels to nourish every cell in our body. To give you some perspective, these arteries, veins, and capillaries, laid end to end, would wrap around the earth more than twice at the equator. That's the power that we were born with—and the power we take for granted.

The heart will continue to do its critical work, dependably delivering this life force to us over and over, beating about 35 million times each year, until finally, one day, it stops. It has become so weakened by lifestyle, by arteries that have become so clogged that the blood flow can't make it through, by disease, or by old age that the heart finally fails. And at that moment, when it stops beating, nothing else matters. An ambulance is summoned and paramedics arrive, to attempt to coax the heart into resuming beating, shock it into submission to keep oxygen flowing. Because without oxygen, you're a goner. Brain cells begin to die within minutes of being deprived of oxygen. For those who survive resuscitation, life is radically altered.

What can you do in thirty-six seconds? That's probably about how long it took you to read the two previous paragraphs. **Well, one American dies** *every thirty-six seconds* **from cardiovascular disease. It's the number one killer of Americans, accounting for one out of four deaths. But that doesn't even begin to convey the scale of this destruction. Globally, <u>one out of five people will die of heart disease, more than any other disease on the planet.</u> It accounts for about 18 million deaths per year. In other words, it kills almost 50,000 people** *every day***.**

Let's step back for a moment and think about what those numbers mean. Because the truth is, they aren't just numbers, are they? What we're talking about here are priceless human lives—people like you and me, our parents, our partners, our closest friends, and possibly our children. So you and I both know what's at stake here. We understand—*intellectually*, *emotionally*, and *viscerally*—the urgent need to protect ourselves and those we love from this devastating threat.

As you'll soon learn, **this is a war that we're increasingly well equipped to fight and win, thanks to an awe-inspiring wave of technological advances that focus on prevention and regeneration.** But before we get to that, I'd like to share with you a little-known aspect of the heart. You're probably unaware of the fact that your heart has its own "brain"—its own intelligence. The heart emits hormones that impact how the brain functions. Your heart was your original guiding intelligence. In the final chapter of this book, we'll talk about the intelligence of the heart and how to use the brain and heart together to make better decisions for a better quality of life—emotionally, physically, financially, spiritually, and, of course, as relates to your health as well.

For now, let me emphasize a simple truth that I hope you'll never forget: You have the power to influence your heart health through factors that you—yes, YOU!—can control. That includes choosing the right foods to eat and avoid, maintaining a healthy body weight, limiting your alcohol intake, not smoking, getting sufficient sleep, and exercising regularly. We've already discussed these simple, preventative actions you can take, in case you missed them, in Chapters 12 through 14.

It's hugely empowering to realize that even the most basic shifts in your behavior can save, extend, and invigorate your life. As we

mentioned in Chapter 14 "Strength, Fitness, and Performance," a major study from the U.K. showed that simply walking twenty to thirty minutes per day can cut the risk of dying from a heart attack in half! So even a modest commitment like deciding to exercise consistently for say 150 minutes each week (twenty to thirty minutes per day, five or six days a week) can transform your health, radically reducing your risk of many chronic illnesses, including cardiovascular disease.

If that doesn't convince you, how about the fact that exercise also increases the blood flow to your brain, improving your cognitive function?

Now, unless you've been living under a rock for your entire life, you're probably not *that* surprised to hear that regular exercise does wonders for your health and vitality. Similarly, you know already that your heart and brain will serve you better if you eat healthily—for example, by consuming more fruits, vegetables, and whole grains while also limiting fatty foods, refined carbs, and sugary drinks. So why am I bothering to remind you of these basic rules of the road?

Because prevention is the single best defense against heart disease and many other life-threatening illnesses. I want you to take care of yourself and stay alive, so you can benefit from all of the incredible technologies coming to fruition over the next few years. But while this book gives you plenty of fundamental tools to help you revitalize your entire body, including your heart, the focus of this chapter is the power of regenerative medicine. As you probably know by now, regenerative medicine is different than other types of therapies because its goal is to cure or reverse underlying injuries, instead of merely treating the symptoms temporarily.

Let's dig into the scientific breakthroughs that can both help prevent this disease and also help a person recover. I'm writing this book for you, number one, to make sure you know what to do to take care of yourselves so you can have that incredible life force pulsing through you. But also so that if you or someone you love has a problem, you can know all about the latest regenerative medicine technologies to help you reclaim your health or perhaps emerge even better than you were in the first place. My hope is to also get you excited about the future, to prepare yourself for a longer and even more enjoyable life than you had been planning for!

At this point, you may be wondering if these technologies are all just pie in the sky—a futuristic fantasy! **But let me tell you, this revolution is happening *right now*.** New tools, treatments, and therapies are becoming available as I write, and the pace of progress is so fast that we expect a cascade of game-changing solutions to be available in the next twelve to thirty-six months. The last game-changer in the world of heart failure was the ventricular assist device, which pumps when the heart can't do so on its own. It's been shown to prolong life and improve its quality for those awaiting heart transplants.[1] But where the future revolution truly lies is in bioengineering and regenerative medicine. In many cases, animal or human trials are already under way, fueling realistic expectations of a brighter and healthier future. You'll be in the know once these technologies are rolled out, so you can improve your quality of life and help others, too. In other words, if you take care to maintain your current level of health, in short order regenerative medicine will unleash an array of truly miraculous tools to help you live better and live longer.

We're about to introduce you to an elite cohort of scientific pioneers and **five tools, technologies, and treatments that will blow your mind.** For example:

- **You'll encounter a company called Caladrius Biosciences, that is using stem cells to overhaul circulation, helping the heart regenerate. And you'll meet other companies harnessing stem cell and other alternative technology to enable heart attack survivors to do everything from generate new heart muscle cells to grow new blood vessels.**
- **You'll meet scientists at Elevian who are injecting naturally occurring molecules and observing the miraculous repair and regeneration of the heart and reversal of stroke symptoms.**
- **You'll encounter a brilliant scientist who has pioneered discoveries from Duke to the Texas Heart Institute, where she figured out how to build "ghost hearts" in the laboratory, providing a new template for organ transplants.**

---

1 Stanford Health Care, "Left Ventricular Assist Device."

- **You'll also meet a Harvard-incubated biotech company using gene therapy to help man's best friend outlast heart failure, paving the way to similar treatments for us, their non-canine buddies.**

Now, you know as well as I do that many people see the future through a lens of fear and worry. I get it. For one thing, it's easy to become discouraged when you're exposed to a daily drumbeat of pessimistic news coverage. You start to believe that the world is going to hell in a hand basket and to focus on everything that could conceivably go wrong. You start to forget that the media thrives on tales of misery and woe because that's what sells! We all know the term "click bait," but as you'll see here, there are so many reasons to be optimistic about the future—and nothing gives me more hope than the spectacular progress that scientists are making in the prevention and treatment of cardiovascular disease. **These advances alone could save** *millions* **of lives. So read on, my friend, and take heart!**

TOOL #1: THE POWER TO REVERSE SCARS

You've already learned a lot about stem cells and exosomes and their amazing power to heal. Caladrius Biosciences is channeling stem cells' incredible versatility and doing something really amazing. Dr. Doug Losordo, the company's global head of research and development and chief medical officer, **is banking on so-called CD34+ stem cells to repair damaged tissue. Losordo witnessed the transformative power of these stem cells to reconstitute mature blood cells in cancer patients who've undergone chemotherapy and radiation.** Losordo started wondering how he could train these stem cells to work their magic in other ways. He knew that **CD34+ cells can also stimulate growth of new blood vessels, including the smaller blood vessels that make up the body's microcirculation.** (Think about the circulatory system as a map. Sure, highways carry the heaviest load. But it's the side roads—the microvessels—that are far more numerous.)

Rather than concentrate on fixing major arterial blockages, Losordo is laser-focused on using CD34+ cells to strengthen circulation, the essence of your body's life force. Would they be effective? No one can really say. But it turns out that **a single dose of these repair cells resulted in normalization of circulation in patients with coronary microvascular dysfunction—a condition in which the heart's microcirculation is compromised.** When circulation is impaired, the tissue doesn't get enough oxygenated blood, which can lead to heart attacks and heart failure. So Losordo's work with CD34+ cells can potentially save many lives.

Now, you might be thinking, "Tony, this sounds like something that would play out twenty years from now." But I'm here to tell you that the timeline is much quicker than you would think.

You see, Losordo began this research at **Tufts University** before he joined **Northwestern University as director of the program in cardiovascular regenerative medicine at Northwestern Memorial Hospital**. He subsequently joined Baxter to oversee the company's regenerative medicine portfolio. Now, at Caladrius Biosciences, **Losordo is optimistic about a Phase 3 trial (this is the final step before FDA approval) injecting CD34+ cells into patients with critical limb ischemia, a chronic condition in which blood supply to the lower extremities is so severely restricted that the tissue starts to break down.** If he's successful, this could be the key to improving circulation in a wide variety of other conditions, strengthening that life force of healthy oxygenated blood.

The trial is taking place in Japan, which is extremely bullish on regenerative medicine since **Kyoto University's Dr. Shinya Yamanaka won the 2012 Nobel Prize for Physiology or Medicine for his discovery—along with James Thomson**, a biologist we'll hear more about soon—that induced pluripotent stem cells can be reprogrammed to become any type of cell line in the body.

Keep in mind that Phase 1 examines safety and Phase 2 looks at efficacy; Losordo has already passed those tests. Phase 3 is efficacy at scale, and after obtaining FDA approval, the next step is widespread distribution of this lifesaving treatment.

Losordo anticipates that the first cell therapy approval for treatment of cardiovascular disease will involve CD34+ cells. Given their awesome ability to jump-start the growth of new blood vessels, he believes these cells would be a "suitable candidate" for any sort of degenerative cardiac condition. **Could they fortify the circulatory system after a heart attack?**

"Caladrius," the name of Losordo's company, provides a clue. In ancient Roman mythology, the caladrius was a mythical bird with the power to make people's illnesses vanish. Today, Caladrius Biosciences is attempting a similar feat of magic, hoping to vanquish the damage caused by a heart attack.

TOOL #2: MAKING OLD HEARTS YOUNG AGAIN

Consider an inspiring vision of a future in which older hearts and brains could become young again. Does that sound far-fetched? That's exactly what's unfolding at a company called **Elevian**, introduced to me by my coauthor Peter (we're both investors), and cofounded by Dr. Mark Allen, MD, with a team of leading-edge scientists that includes stars like **Amy Wagers and Lee Rubin (both professors of stem cell and regenerative biology at Harvard) and Brock Reeve (executive director of the Harvard Stem Cell Institute).**

Elevian, which develops medicines designed to restore the body's regenerative capacity, is using a naturally occurring molecule called **growth differentiation factor 11 (GDF11)** to reproduce the rejuvenating effects of "young blood." Aged mice that received an injection of GDF11 saw a reduction in age-related cardiac hypertrophy—an enlarged or thickened heart, which is a hallmark of cardiac aging.[2] **GDF11 also boosted brain function, improved skeletal muscle repair, and increased exercise capacity.** On its own or in conjunction with other molecules, **GDF11 could prompt the human body to rev up its capacity for regeneration**. Ultimately, technologies like this can be expected to help revitalize your body, including your heart and brain.

Elevian's lead drug candidate, recombinant human GDF11, has shown efficacy in preclinical models of heart failure and stroke, plus Alzheimer's disease and type 2 diabetes. Could this mean that aging hearts and brains are a thing of the past? Time—and painstaking research—will tell. As I write this, Elevian is moving toward an early Phase 1 trial to establish that its approach is safe for human beings.

---

2 Loffredo FS, Wagers AJ, Lee RT. *Cell*, 2013.

TOOL #3: A STEM CELL PATCH FOR HEART VESSELS

Stem cells are also playing a starring role in a recently FDA-approved patch for repair and reconstruction of vessels, even ones that have been severely affected by cholesterol buildup. CorMatrix Cardiovascular has invented a scaffold that allows the patient's *own stem cells* to regenerate tissue. **Already used in more than 100,000 patients worldwide,[3] the exceptionally strong, pliable, and thin material is stitched by surgeons onto the heart, achieving permanent repair. Since it uses your own cells to heal, it isn't seen as a foreign substance the body needs to attack, which makes it vastly superior to current surgical patches.**

As amazing as this development is, the patch still requires surgery to be applied. But there's actually another therapy that might bypass the need for surgery altogether. As we've mentioned before, after someone suffers from a heart attack, the heart experiences permanent structural damage. **Now Ventrix, a company spun out of the University of California, San Diego, is fine-tuning VentriGel, a hydrogel that can be injected via catheter to heal areas heavy in scar formation.** In 2019, Ventrix finished its first in-humans clinical trial, which showed that the gel is both safe and feasible.[4] **Now the company is seeing if VentriGel can reach areas of the heart that the typical surgical approach—coronary artery bypass graft—can't access.** Researchers hope that this could soon replace the need for one of the most invasive cardiac surgeries.

TOOL #4: BUILDING NEW HEARTS

"I was betting the farm that I could regenerate a monkey's heart."

—CHUCK MURRY

After reading the beginning of this chapter, you know already that cardiovascular disease is the number one killer in the U.S. and worldwide. You

---

3 Diagnostic and International Cardiology, "FDA Clears CorMatrix ECM for Vascular Repair."

4 Traverse et al., "First-in-Man Study of a Cardiac Extracellular Matrix Hydrogel in Early and Late Myocardial Infarction Patients."

may even have known that before reading this chapter. After all, it's pretty common knowledge. **But did you ever wonder why?**

"Cardiovascular disease is the number one killer because the heart is the least regenerative organ," says Dr. Chuck Murry, director of the University of Washington's heart regeneration program and chair of the university's Institute for Stem Cell and Regenerative Medicine. "Maybe the brain is almost as bad, but there's at least bona fide stem cells in the brain and spinal cord that can make new nerves. The best evidence is that there are no stem cells in the heart." **In other words, the heart can't heal itself on its own after an injury like a heart attack.**

Here's the problem with that: If you're not taking care of your body, exercising and eating healthy foods, you can suffer gradual heart failure or a sudden heart attack. Consider that **the heart contains 6 or 7 billion heart muscle cells. If you have a serious heart attack and are fortunate enough to survive, you can lose more than 1 billion of those cells. The heart doesn't replace them, so it never replaces their ability to contract either.** The heart's attempt to heal itself results in scars, which interfere with heart conduction, making it even more prone to attacks, like arrhythmias. After that, it's often a slow downward spiral; when the heart can't adequately pump blood through the body, heart failure ensues. The prognosis is worse than for many forms of cancer, which is why it's the world's leading cause of death.

If only we could figure out how to make the heart regenerate, we could cure many kinds of heart disease. That realization took root in Murry's mind in the 1990s; he has been obsessed with it ever since.

The idea first occurred to him as he sat working on a self-proclaimed "crappy paper" that he'd left unfinished as he worked toward his PhD. A postdoctoral fellow at the time, Murry was training in the biology of blood vessels. **He started trying to reprogram scar cells**—fibroblasts—into cardiac muscle cells. Exciting work, except Murry failed abysmally. **"I spent lots of money and had people seriously worried about whether I could be a viable scientist," he recalls.** "My department chair was tapping at his watch."

Murry wasn't sure where to turn next. But his next steps became clear when he and the entire world witnessed a scientific breakthrough. In 1998, a legendary biologist named James Thomson derived the first human embryonic stem cell line. (He later notched the

same accomplishment with human induced pluripotent stem cells, genetically programmed to resemble embryonic stem cells that have the ability to become any specialized cell in the body.) **The embryonic stem cells could turn into any of the 200 cell types in the human body.** Murry's lab was lucky enough to be the first at the University of Washington to get them and start culturing them. "**We began to see little clumps of beating embryonic heart cells—a heart in a dish—beat spontaneously,**" says Murry. "**It was a great joy to watch it.**"

While the study Murry conducted below is not one that I personally support, because I don't support the use of monkeys for research, I still feel compelled to share it with you, because it did create a breakthrough that has generated promising results for those suffering from damaged hearts.

"We began to see little clumps of beating embryonic heart cells—a heart in a dish—beat spontaneously."

Now that Murry had the cells he needed for his research, he set about using them to build new heart muscle. **He induced heart attacks in mice and rats, inserted embryonic cardiac stem cells, and watched them multiply over time and remuscularize part of the heart wall.** "That was cool," he says. **Then he did a study using slightly bigger animals—guinea pigs—and showed that cardiac cells injected into a damaged heart region would engraft, multiply, and improve function.** This sounds like sci-fi, but it's real. **Murry was actually creating brand-new heart muscle.**

Progress was steady but slooooow. "I would always say we're five years from the clinic," says Murry. "I started to feel that if I looked at my death certificate, it would say 'incrementalism.' So **I took the best heart muscle cells I had and decided to put them into a macaque monkey, which could best predict human response. I blew my rainy day account on this experiment. I was betting the farm that I could regenerate a monkey's heart.**"

In went the cells, human heart muscle infiltrating damaged regions of a monkey's heart. For contrast, Murry's team had popped in a variant of a jellyfish gene that flashed green with every heartbeat. "**We could see the cells beating and at what rate and rhythm,**" he says. "**They were in beautiful** synchrony with the heart in which they resided. It was one of the most beautiful days in my life as a scientist."

In 2018, in a paper that generated no small amount of buzz, Murry showed that monkeys who had been given heart attacks and then received injections of human cardiac muscle cells into the wall of their heart, had achieved normal ejection fraction—the amount of blood squeezed out with each heartbeat—within three months after treatment. <u>The injected cells generated new heart muscle cells, which helped the heart resume vigorous pumping, restoring function.</u>

Decades after Murry started his work, it's finally time to see if the promising results achieved in monkeys can be replicated in humans. <u>The goal: transplanting stem cells into heart attack survivors to prevent heart failure.</u> Once again, this sounds like a script from a Hollywood sci-fi flick, doesn't it? Perhaps Murry's dream might come true fifty years from now.

But you won't have to wait nearly that long. A recent clinical trial done in 2015 by University of Texas Health Science Center and the Na-

---

Murry aims to be injecting stem cells into human hearts by 2023. This will be one of the biggest revolutions in heart repair in the history of medicine.

---

tional Heart, Lung, and Blood Institute injected a combination of mesenchymal and cardiac stem cells as regenerative therapy for patients with severe heart failure.[5] This is one of the first clinical trials to introduce engineered cardiac stem cells into patients. It's only a matter of time before we start to see even more of these innovations pass through clinical trials.

Back in Seattle, Murry's team recently shifted its research to a local cell engineering company, Sana Biotechnology, where Murry is the head of cardiac cell therapy. **Ever the optimist, Murry thinks—hopes—he'll be injecting stem cells into human hearts by 2023.** It's working in animals, and if it works similarly in humans, **this will be one of the biggest**

---

5 Davis, "Combination of Mesenchymal and C-kit+ Cardiac Stem Cells as Regenerative Therapy for Heart Failure."

revolutions in heart repair in the history of medicine. "It's complicated and exhausting work," he says. Without a touch of irony, he observes: "This stuff isn't for the fainthearted."

As a quick reminder of another extraordinary cardiac regenerative technology we learned about back in Chapter 8, "Gene Therapy and CRISPR," Dr. Deepak Srivastava, a cardiologist and the president of Gladstone Institutes, learned to control the fate of cardiac fibroblast cells (connective tissue), reprogramming them so they could perform an entirely *different* function within the heart. Srivastava used gene therapy to change the fate of the fibroblast cells, turning them into beating heart cells. **He was able to create brand-new muscle in a failing heart by convincing fibroblast cells already in the heart to change jobs!**

TOOL #5: CREATING GHOST HEARTS

"I took a deep breath and listened to the old bray
of my heart. I am. I am. I am."

—SYLVIA PLATH

While Murry is working on *remuscularizing* a heart, one of his colleagues, **Doris Taylor, PhD,** is focusing on *decellularizing* one. **It's called a *ghost heart.*** What the heck is that? Well, **in 1998, Taylor's team at Duke University was the first to transplant a type of animal cell into the heart of an animal and show improved function after a heart attack.**[6, 7] **The amazing thing is that some of the cells survived and went on to mimic heart cells.** Close to ten years later, though, she hadn't made significant progress. She began to doubt that she'd ever succeed in turning a thin leathery scar from a heart attack back into healthy functioning heart cells. It was time for a completely new strategy. She turned to her trainee, Harald Ott, and said, "Wouldn't it be cool if we could do this a different way?"

---

6 Taylor et al., "Regenerating Functional Myocardium: Improved Performance After Skeletal Myoblast Transplantation."

7 Ott et al., "Perfusion-Decellularized Matrix: Using Nature's Platform to Engineer a Bioartificial Heart."

And that's how the ghost heart came to be.

Their team took a rat heart, stripped it of its cells, then introduced immature rat heart cells to build a beating heart. The process has evolved since those early days, and Taylor has succeeded in doing the same thing with a cadaver heart, using salt to break down the structure and a detergent to wash away the cells. **Ta-da! A decellularized heart, ghostly opaque because it's devoid of its blood and cells, consisting only of the essential scaffolding, the branches that supply blood to the body. As Taylor puts it, "We just hang a heart in a lab while we wait for it to decellularize."**

If anything, the next step sounds even more strange. <u>It entails re-cellularizing the ghost heart by infusing it with millions of immature heart cells made from human stem cells, connecting the entire contraption to a pump, and waiting as the heart regenerates and starts beating.</u> This sounds like a scene out of a mad scientist script, right? <u>But Taylor, who is now an independent scientist, actually grew more than 100 of these hearts at the Texas Heart Institute,</u> where she was the director of regenerative medicine research.

As we discussed in Chapter 5, on organ regeneration, this is just one of many ways that a new generation of replacement organs are being created.

Remember that regenerative medicine is critical for the heart because heart cells don't divide. <u>Heart cells lost to a heart attack are gone forever.</u> There's little room for failure. **"The heart is one organ that really has to work perfectly when you put it in,"** says Taylor. "You don't have two hearts like you have two kidneys or two lungs or multiple liver lobes."

Remember, regenerative medicine is different than other types of therapies because its goal isn't to treat symptoms; it's to cure the underlying injury. "Our responsibility is greater," says Taylor. "It's not like a drug where the therapy goes away in days or weeks. We hope that this therapy is there to stay."

<u>Where Murry is trying to fix a broken heart—one that has suffered a heart attack—Taylor is creating new hearts that could potentially be transplanted into people suffering heart failure or other heart conditions. "Our ultimate goal is to automate the production of human hearts," says Taylor. "I believe we will do that within the next two years."</u>

Taylor attributes her success in part to her gender. "As a woman, I see relationships between ideas that not everyone does," she says. "The reason we're going to succeed is because we're regenerating the heart at the emotional, spiritual, mental, and physical level."

In the early days of trying to build the original recellularized hearts, Taylor was worried that they might not be able to be sustained for very long, that their heartbeats wouldn't hit a regular cadence. "Did you love it enough?" a lab technician asked her. He was joking. Nonetheless, says Taylor, "I think he had a point."

Here's what's really amazing: **Taylor has also used these ghost hearts as a source for a cardiac patch, cutting out a piece of decellularized heart and grafting it to a damaged heart.** And in what sounds like a page from *Frankenstein*, she's experimented with grinding up a ghost heart into a powder that forms the basis for a gel that's injected into a scarred heart. How's *that* for out-of-the-box thinking?

Much of her recent work has focused on building pediatric-sized humanized hearts. "These hearts respond to drugs," says Taylor. "They have electrical signals. <u>We hope to convince the world we've created the first intact heart from human induced pluripotent stem cells.</u>"

Large animal studies, then clinical trials in humans, are next in line. "I'm confident," says Taylor. "You know how you get to a point and you know, 'This is it; we are there'? That's how I feel about this. I credit my team with making this work. **Science is a team sport. And we've reached a critical juncture."**

Indeed, I hope that's one of the key lessons you draw from this chapter: *We've reached a critical juncture.* That's to say, we've arrived at a moment in time where the research is so sophisticated that it's sometimes difficult to distinguish between science and science fiction. **All of this progress toward regenerating the human heart is truly cause for awe and wonder.**

Meanwhile, **Dr. Harald Ott**—Taylor's trainee from many years ago—is also blazing a trail with this historic work of organ regeneration. **His efforts are concentrated primarily on engineering a bioartificial heart for patients who need heart transplants.** "We are all dreamers in this field," says Ott, **a thoracic surgeon at Massachusetts General Hospital (where he also directs the Center for Organ Engineering) and an associate**

professor in surgery at Harvard Medical School. "Regenerating organs, creating living tissue from living tissue, is one of the next big hurdles," he adds. **"We have to come up with a way for us to not die from one organ failing."**

On the academic side, Ott's work revolves around engineering hearts and lungs. But with financial backing from investors like Peter and I, he's also spun out a company, **Iviva Medical. It uses biological scaffolds to create replacement kidneys and pancreases—organs that aren't as complex as hearts.** He's creating personalized organ grafts by stripping an organ of its cells, then reseeding it with cells from the intended donor, which can eliminate one of the biggest threats that accompany organ transplants—the potential for the donor's body to reject foreign tissue.

It's more daunting to work with hearts than kidneys. "You can't just replace a little bit of heart function and get away with it," says Ott. **By contrast, you need just 10 to 15 percent of kidney function to get off dialysis. But his research into kidneys and pancreases can provide useful insights that will also help in his efforts to regenerate the heart.** "If we focus on simpler tissues," says Ott, "we can learn a lot that we can apply to more complex tissues, which can help us get to clinical applications faster." With so many lives at stake, the sense of urgency is palpable.

I hope by now that you have a keen appreciation for some of the radical ways in which regenerative medicine is beginning to heal the human heart. **Just think for a moment about a few of the remarkable advances we've discussed. For example, we've talked about infusing patients with CD34+ cells to restore their circulation, about using stem cells to build new heart muscle in the wake of a heart attack, and about bioengineering artificial hearts for use in transplants.**

When you think about what these innovations represent, **you begin to realize that this scientific revolution challenges some fundamental assumptions that have held true for as long as humans have walked the Earth. After all, what could be more fundamental than the assumption that, as we age, our bodies must inevitably and inexorably deteriorate? Regenerative medicine brings new hope that this process of decline can be reversed—that rejuvenation is a practical option.**

But we're not willing to stop there, are we? We humans want it all! So perhaps it should be no surprise to discover that some of the smartest scientists in the field are now striving to apply the same kind of breakthrough technology to extend the lives of our pets as well. For example, the canine-crazy cofounders of Rejuvenate Bio, a company based in San Diego, are working to advance a gene therapy technology to increase dogs' health span and cure age-related diseases. If you have a beloved pet, be sure to sit up and pay attention because there are some breakthroughs geared toward our furry friends as well.

What's the inspiration behind this work? Bear, a 100-pound German shepherd who belongs to **Rejuvenate Bio's cofounder and chief science officer, Noah Davidsohn**. He became Bear's owner six months into his postdoctoral fellowship in the Harvard Medical School lab of renowned genetics professor **George Church.** Rejuvenate Bio traces its roots to this lab, where researchers used a combination **gene therapy** to treat obesity, type 2 diabetes, kidney failure, and heart failure in mice.[13] **The therapy is given as a onetime intravenous injection. But what's really interesting about it is that it doesn't change the existing DNA of the mice, so there are no concerns about passing along permanent genetic changes to future generations.**

Even more interesting, mice bred with these gene mutations—these "designer creatures" are called transgenic mice—**had their lifespans increased up to 30 percent. Dan Oliver, the CEO and cofounder of Rejuvenate Bio, remarks, "Due to these transgenic mouse experiments, we have three-plus years of safety data showing that the major side effect of this treatment is that the mice live longer."** For pet lovers like me, that sounds like reason to celebrate.

Rejuvenate Bio is now studying whether this technology can address mitral valve disease, the leading type of canine heart failure. **Between 5 to 7 million dogs in the U.S. suffer from this condition. Just imagine your pet being miraculously healed and living longer!** "What everyone is interested in is improving healthspan—increasing health and increasing the number of years of health," says Oliver. "Dogs share our environment and get a number of the same age-related conditions. So, if we want to move into humans, it will be easier. The data ports over nicely."

In other words, figuring out how to help dogs live longer, healthier lives could lead to similar breakthroughs for their owners, which would be an incredible feat. This prospect adds a whole new dimension to the phrase "man's best friend."

I certainly wish this technology had been around to help my 85-pound best friend, Buddha, a pit bull who was the sweetest thing you could ever imagine. He'd climb up on me like he was a little terrier, put his front legs around me, and try to get a hug. He seemed so strong and powerful—the embodiment of health. But he died of a heart attack when he was only three years old. We were devastated. With this type of gene therapy technology, he could still be alive today.

Thanks to the scientists you've met in this chapter, that vision of rejuvenation—for dogs *and* humans—is rapidly becoming a reality.

> *"The only thing greater than the power of the*
> *mind is the courage of the heart."*
>
> —JOHN NASH

I can't emphasize enough the little things you can do that can keep you from needing most of these therapies in the first place. So please take this entire book in for your benefit and for those you love. If you'll take care of yourself today and encourage those you love—mothers, fathers, brothers, sisters, dear friends, family, extended family—to do the same. If they do, technology that can heal one of the most important organs in our bodies and address the number one cause of death on earth. Take care of yourself, because the technology is coming faster than you can imagine. Soon we'll be able to tap into the power of stem cells, gene therapy, and the literal building of new hearts, ghost hearts, to ensure a future that shines brighter than we ever thought possible. Take care of yourself, my dear friend, and celebrate a long, healthy, vital, strong life filled with life force driven by this beautiful magnificent gift from our creator, the heart.

In our next chapter, we'll learn revolutionary techniques and technology that are helping to prevent and treat the fifth leading cause of death in the United State—strokes. . . .

BONUS BREAKTHROUGH: A TWICE-A-YEAR INJECTION TO FIGHT HIGH CHOLESTEROL

Gene silencing technology is a new biotechnology that enables you to **prevent the expression of certain genes. The genes are still present; they've just been muted.** This kind of breakthrough advancement has been around for twenty years. Until now, most treatments using this technology were used to treat rare genetic diseases. But that's about to change.

The U.K.'s National Health Service has recently approved inclisiran, a cholesterol-lowering injection that needs to be administered only twice a year. It's meant for those who suffer from a genetic condition leading to high cholesterol, who have suffered a heart attack or stroke, or who haven't responded well to mainstay treatments like Lipitor. **This new treatment will be prescribed to 300,000 people over the next three years.**

There's a protein, PCSK9, that regulates cholesterol in our bodies. But it's present *in excess* in people with high levels of LDL—the bad cholesterol. But what if we could prevent PCSK9 from being produced in the first place?

If you remember, mRNA is the type of RNA that is responsible for encoding proteins. It turns out a different version of RNA, siRNA (small interfering RNA) has an important role in **targeting mRNA and "interfering with" or destroying it. Inclisiran is an siRNA that targets the mRNA that encodes PCSK9.** It's been heavily modified to withstand degradation in the blood and is able to specifically target liver cells. So there are minimal side effects.

Inclisiran is the first use of gene silencing in such a common disease. Lipitor not cutting it? At high risk for a cardiac event due to high cholesterol? According to the experts, just two jabs a year and you're set. This might be worth checking out with your doctor if you have genetically high LDL cholesterol.

CHAPTER 18

YOUR BRAIN: TREATING STROKES

Revolutionary Techniques Will Increasingly Prevent, Treat, and Vanquish the Fifth Leading Cause of Death in the U.S.: Stroke

"The human brain has 100 billion neurons, each neuron connected to up to 10,000 other neurons. Sitting on your shoulders is the most complicated object in the known universe."

—MICHIO KAKU, professor of theoretical physics in the City College of New York and CUNY Graduate Center

When most people think about someone having a stroke, the image that pops into their head is of someone gray-haired, in their 70s or 80s. They don't picture the dynamic young woman—let's call her Susan—who happens to be one of my own assistants and gave us permission to share her story. Susan was just 32 the day she found herself in a meeting, suddenly unable to say certain words. When she tried to take a sip of water, the liquid dribbled out of her mouth and her left eye was rolling inward toward her nose. Susan wasn't working for me then, and her boss at the time was confused. "He thought I was joking because I was always joking around at work," she recalls. "He said, 'Stop it or I'm going to call 911.'" Luckily for Susan, he proceeded to do exactly that.

In the ambulance, the paramedics were pretty sure she'd suffered a stroke, despite being so young. In fact, rates of stroke among younger adults are on the rise, in part due to increasing stroke risk factors in younger people, such as obesity and/or high blood pressure. Strokes are usually caused when a blood clot blocks a vessel in the brain; they can also be caused by a rupture. The key to boosting the chances of recovering from a stroke caused by a clot is something called **tissue plasminogen activator, or tPA. It's the only FDA-approved treatment for strokes caused by clots, and it gets busy dissolving the clot. But small communities and rural hospitals don't always have a stroke team to quickly evaluate a patient and decide to administer the drug.** To make matters worse, there's a very small window of time during which tPA can be effectively administered—between three to four and a half hours of a person suffering a stroke. You can imagine that this isn't always possible to achieve, especially because **many people experiencing a stroke don't recognize what's happening and don't head to the hospital.**

Because her boss sprang into action, Susan was fortunate; she got tPA and had a thrombectomy, where a thin catheter was threaded through an artery in her groin all the way to the artery in her brain that was blocked. A tiny mesh tube fanned open to trap the clot, then it was pulled back out of her body. Susan had received a new lease on life, thanks to the right hospital, the right experts—and the right mindset. **In rehab, if she applied herself and worked harder than she'd ever worked before, her therapists promised her she'd be able to return to her former self.** Sure enough, within a few weeks she was walking down the hall of the rehab facility in high heels. That positive psychology helped Susan recover completely. Four years later, she is back to her former self.

It will come as no surprise that lots of very smart people are focused on stroke prevention and treatment; after all, your brain is your body's command center. **It has about 100 billion neurons packed into a wrinkly three-pound gray sponge, and it controls your ability to talk, feel, see, hear, blink, form memories, put one foot in front of another—and, of course, think.** We take all this for granted, but it's truly wondrous, isn't it? Think of it like this: You're essentially lugging around the world's most sophisticated supercomputer inside your own head!

So when something goes wrong, the functioning of that sophisticated supercomputer is at stake. Stroke is the fifth leading cause of death in the U.S., killing nearly 150,000 Americans each year. <u>Every forty seconds, someone, somewhere in the U.S., suffers a stroke. More than 50 percent of stroke survivors age 65 or older suffer impaired</u>

<u>mobility.</u>[1] That's heartbreaking for a survivor and equally heartbreaking for their family members, who feel helpless watching a formerly capable person struggle to open a jar of pasta sauce or pop open a can of soda. This chapter is all about bringing hope to what can feel like a hopeless situation. **But the hope is real and tangible because there are regenerative medical solutions that are already here and others that are coming down the pike that can make a huge difference—solutions that don't just attack symptoms but actually reverse injury.**

Of course, prevention is king, with stroke and all kinds of degenerative disease. So make sure to exercise regularly, eat plenty of fruits and vegetables, avoid smoking, and maintain a healthy weight to maximize your body's circulation. Throughout this book, you'll also learn about other breakthroughs that will influence how people cope with strokes and reclaim their lives. I've told you more about how you can access the most efficient, most advanced ways to get a full-body workout in **Chapter 14, "Strength, Fitness, and Performance."** But in this chapter, we're laser-focused on groundbreaking technologies that are helping stroke survivors like Susan—and those who are decades older—not just survive but thrive, now and in the future. I'm going to share with you four incredible developments that are already in play. For example:

1. **You're about to meet some ingenious researchers who are using robotic gloves to help stroke survivors regain motion, giving them new hope for recovery.**
2. **You'll discover how virtual reality headsets, high-tech sensors, and video games that harness hand-eye coordination are now being deployed to improve stroke survivors' dexterity and mobility.**
3. **You'll also learn how scientists are injecting exosomes released from stem cells into pigs in a remarkably promising quest to lessen the impact of strokes on people's everyday functioning.**
4. **You'll learn how those scientists at Elevian, whom you met in the last chapter, are using their GDF11 molecule and seeing the miraculous repair and reversal of ischemic stroke symptoms.**

---

1 CDC, "Stroke Facts."

5. You'll meet the brilliant Dr. Mary Lou Jepsen, whose company, Openwater, is using red laser light and holography to measure the brain blood flow of a patient, in the ambulance, during that first critical three- to four-hour window to determine if tPA therapy is required and to diagnose every stroke.

BREAKTHROUGH #1: A TREATMENT THAT FITS LIKE A GLOVE

"The chief function of the body is to carry the brain around."
—THOMAS EDISON

Have you heard about the gloves that can teach you to play the piano in less time than it takes to do a load of laundry? This isn't some hare-brained idea; it actually works! **What's more, these magical gloves are also being used for a more noble purpose: to restore function in stroke survivors.** I was sitting across from a true genius, **Thad Starner, professor at Georgia Tech's School of Interactive Computing,** eager to hear about his otherworldly creations.

Professor Starner is no stranger to wearable technology. He just may have been the first person to go about his everyday business *wearing* a computer. You see, he helped to pioneer the field of wearable computing and served as a technical lead in the development of **Google Glass,** those futuristic augmented reality glasses that generated tons of buzz but were too ahead of their time to catch on with consumers. But I was there to talk to him about a completely different kind of wearable, a truly miraculous discovery that came about after he suggested to one of his graduate students that he make a glove—picture a fingerless cycling glove or a fingertipless golf glove—and embed it with tiny vibrating motors.

The goal? To see if the pattern of vibrations in the glove could teach wearers to play the piano without a lick of practice. That may sound ridiculous. But it turns out that the untapped potential of human beings runs even deeper than you might imagine. The gloves vibrate, tapping the finger associated with each note as they mimic the finger pattern of a piano song. **As you wear the gloves, you get on with your day—folding that load of laundry, going for a run, scrolling through emails—while your brain is passively trained in the background.**[2] **The theory is that the brain starts to memorize the sequence of stimuli, just as you memorize movements when practicing.**

Thad could see I was still somewhat skeptical. "Tony," he said, "let me show you a video." I could hardly believe what I was seeing: **a TV weatherman with no musical background was able to play "Ode to Joy" live on CNN after wearing the gloves. The reporter on set was astonished** as was I. Even Thad was blown away. What does this have to do with stroke recovery? Well, gloves that passively teach you how to play a song equate to a pretty impressive party trick. But Thad told me a story about something these gloves can do that's even more impressive.

Thad has a friend named **Deborah Backus** who was the **associate director of spinal cord injury research at Atlanta's Shepherd Center**, which is one of the nation's leading hospitals for rehabilitation. Backus helps people with multiple sclerosis and spinal cord injuries. She wondered if Thad's vibrating gloves might improve her patients' dexterity. Thad recalls: "She came by and said, **'I want your piano stuff for my paralyzed patients.' I thought she was joking. She said, 'You don't understand.' She told me that her intuition was that the brain would recruit more neurons. My jaw dropped to the floor and I said, 'Let's get started.'"**

Sure enough, these haptic gloves—"haptics" is a field of technology that involves the sense of touch—worked with these patients, too. **A PhD student showed that people with partial spinal cord injuries displayed a marked improvement in sensation in their disabled hand, helping them to perform critical everyday tasks such as buttoning a shirt.**[3]

Thad was thrilled. His mother was a geriatric nurse, and he had tagged along with her to nursing homes as a boy. "When I was ten," he says, "most of my friends were over eighty." That background helped him to recognize

---

2 Georgia Tech, "Good Vibrations: Passive Haptic Learning Could be a Key to Rehabilitation."

3 Georgia Tech, "Passive Haptic Learning: Learn to Type or Play Piano Without Attention Using Wearables."

that haptic gloves, which had started out as little more than an amusing novelty, had untold implications for helping people live better lives.

That hunch was further confirmed when another PhD student, **Caitlyn Seim, used the same haptic technology to fit blind people with gloves. The vibrations were able to teach them to type and read Braille in _four hours_, instead of the _four months_ that it typically takes.**[4] It's a beautiful reminder that we are capable of so much more than many people can even conceive.

These unexpected successes raised an intriguing question: What if the same technology could be harnessed to help stroke patients? The stakes could hardly be higher, given that stroke is the leading cause of long-term disability in the U.S. Clenched fists are one of the most debilitating aftereffects; a stroke can curl a hand into a claw, making it impossible to carry out mundane but essential tasks of daily living like grasping a fork, wielding a toothbrush, or turning a door handle.

The vibrations were able to teach them to type and read Braille in four hours, instead of the four months that it typically takes.

People who haven't had a stroke take the flexibility of their hands for granted, blissfully unaware that the brain and spinal cord are effortlessly sending signals back and forth to keep the muscles in equilibrium. But in stroke survivors, the signals that cue the muscles to open the hand are disrupted, while the muscles that close the hand become dominant, which results in the hand clenching into a fist.

---

4 Georgia Institute of Technology, "Wearable Computing Gloves Can Teach Braille, Even if You're Not Paying Attention."

BREAKTHROUGH #2:
HAPTIC TECHNOLOGY

Haptic technology provided a crucial breakthrough. The same principles employed in the piano exercise were used to spark improvement in stroke survivors: As the brain is triggered to react to signals, it fires off patterns in neurons and attracts more neurons. That increases sensation, which of course leads to improved dexterity over time. In other words, wearing the gloves seems to make the muscles in the hand wake up.

How stroke impacts survivors depends on which part of the brain has died. **Stroke, after all, results in oxygen starvation of a piece of brain tissue and brain death. One of the biggest challenges that stroke survivors must overcome is that their body no longer does what they want it to do. What do I mean by that? I mean that joints may flex involuntarily; a hand might grab a cup but be unable to release it due to increased muscle tightness.** Imagine the frustration of not having control of your hands—to grasp something, to touch something, to simply feel where you are. What if there was a way to unclench those fists for good? Well, there is!

Up until a few decades ago, scientists were convinced that when brain cells died, they could never be restored. But thanks to decades of research, **we know the brain has plasticity;** it has the ability **to adapt, meaning that patients who have suffered strokes are capable of dramatic recoveries. "The brain can change itself,"** says Dr. Seim, now a postdoctoral fellow at Stanford University. **"So there's a lot of potential for recovery."**

As part of her research, Dr. Seim asked stroke survivors to wear haptic gloves for three hours daily over the course of two months. Tactile stimulation through passive haptic learning—**wearing the computerized gloves preprogrammed to vibrate at specific settings—led to significant improvements in sensation, range of motion, and muscle tone, along with a decrease in muscle tightness.**

How gratifying is that? Dr. Seim says that one of her most satisfying moments came during a meeting with a stroke patient and his wife. When she asked the woman if she'd noticed any improvement in her husband's hands, the wife lovingly kneaded his age-spotted hands and replied: "I can move his fingers. Before, they were in a grip. It was real hard to even get them straight to even get the glove on. But now I see a lot more flexibility. And when we're walking, I can actually hold his hand."

Ultimately, Dr. Seim hopes that haptic gloves could be approved as a long-term and lasting treatment for stroke patients. To that end, she's teamed up with Starner and another of his former graduate students to create a company called **Stimulus Labs**, which is working to bring gloves to market by 2023 for the benefit of stroke survivors. Whatever happens, we now know that hands which were once immobilized can be taught to move again by a boldly imaginative technology that, until recently, wasn't on anybody's radar. What an amazing way to literally reshape someone's life.

BREAKTHROUGH #3: VIRTUAL REALITY MADE REAL

I'm sure you've heard plenty about virtual reality—how you can enter a fantasy world that feels so real, your heart begins to beat faster. Whether you're falling or flying, it feels so real that it induces the same kind of fear or excitement that you'd experience in real life. Now imagine how cool it would be if we could use VR to retrain the nervous system to function again.

That's exactly what's unfolding in a virtual reality world that was conceived in the real-world city of Alameda, California. **In this fantasy world, stroke patients are gamifying the decidedly un-fun process of rehab with the help of a VR headset, some sensors, and a tablet. This game is actually an FDA-approved therapeutic tool known as the REAL System**, developed by an Alameda-based company called **Penumbra**.

Let me tell you about one woman, Deb Shaw of Los Gatos, California, a stroke survivor who has helped develop the REAL System. She tests out the VR exercises and gives feedback to Penumbra under the watchful eye of her occupational therapist, Lisa Calloway. **Shaw was 55 when she suffered an initial stroke in 2016. It happened in her sleep. When she awoke and tried to get out of bed, she was confused to find that she couldn't move her arm. Her husband took her to the ER, where a scan showed that she'd had a stroke.**

Shaw started rehab with traditional therapy, which she hated. She wasn't doing the exercises enough to make progress. **Then her husband heard**

about the REAL System from one of the original developers, who invited Shaw and her husband to visit their offices and try it out. **"It was like night and day," says Shaw. "It immediately took my therapy to the next level."**

Penumbra's software engineers asked her: "What's one of your favorite things to do?" Shaw replied, "Bird-watching!" She suggested the engineers create a game in which a little bird would land in her hand, and then she would have to place it back in its nest. VR transformed this tedious rehab reaching exercise that engages her shoulders, hands, and fingers into entertainment. Shaw dons the VR headset, straps on six sensors, and disappears into an alternate animated universe called **Happy Valley**, with its colorful birds, verdant hills, and a smiling sun. **"You're transported to another world where anything is possible," she says. "It changes the way patients see therapy."**

The tablet collects data about every movement Shaw makes during the course of a treatment session, allowing Calloway to see clearly the areas where Shaw is improving and those where she needs additional attention. Shaw is always motivated to beat her previous score, so her progress is much quicker than when she was just running through exercises with Calloway.

Shaw is no stranger to stroke therapies. She's tried everything: physical therapy from the waist down, occupational therapy from the waist up, cranial acupuncture, acupressure, a hyperbaric oxygen chamber, and hydrotherapy. Her conclusion? **"VR amplifies all of those."**

When we last spoke with the folks at Penumbra, they had started shipping their VR product to market. They anticipate that it will soon be available at many hospitals, inpatient rehab facilities, and outpatient centers—anywhere a therapist might work with a stroke survivor. What a beautiful way for someone to regain skills one little game, one little step, at a time.

BREAKTHROUGH #4: GDF11, THE POWER TO HEAL STROKES

Consider an inspiring vision of a future in which older brains and hearts could become young again. Does that sound far-fetched? That's exactly what's unfolding at **Elevian**, the company **run by Dr. Mark Allen, MD,** whom we met in our last chapter, working with a team of leading-edge scientists that includes stars like **Amy Wagers, Richard Lee, and Lee Rubin (all professors of stem cell and regenerative biology at Harvard).**

As we've learned, Elevian has developed a naturally occurring protein called growth differentiation factor 11 (GDF11) with powerful regenerative properties. Aged mice that received an injection of GDF11 saw a reduction in age-related cardiac hypertrophy—an enlarged or thickened heart, which is a hallmark of cardiac aging. GDF11 also boosted brain function, improved skeletal muscle repair, and increased exercise capacity.[5] On its own or in conjunction with other molecules, GDF11 could prompt the human body to rev up its capacity for regeneration. Ultimately, technologies like this can be expected to help revitalize your body, including your brain and heart.

Whereas the gold standard treatment of ischemic strokes needs to be delivered within a narrow four-hour window, GDF11 can act up to one week later. The scientific data from their preclinical studies looks encouraging for both prevention and recovery, although more research is needed. As I write this, Elevian is moving toward a Phase 1 trial with the aim of treating acute ischemic strokes by early 2023.

A potential treatment that can work *up to a week* after the ischemic stroke would drastically change the face of stroke medicine. But Elevian has set their sights even higher. Their next target is hemorrhagic strokes, which are strokes caused by a brain bleed. Because GDF11 has also been found to play a role in glucose metabolism, insulin sensitivity, and fat reduction, they are hoping to expand to cardiovascular and metabolic diseases such as diabetes and obesity. Who thought a molecule could be so powerful?

While efforts are pouring into treatments for *acute* strokes, let's now turn our attention to another company that is going to drastically change the lives of *chronic* stroke patients and their families.

---

5 Loffredo FS, Wagers AJ, Lee RT. *Cell*, 2013.

BREAKTHROUGH #5: SERAYA MEDICAL: THE GOLD STANDARD FOR BRAIN STIMULATION

There is no effective, approved treatment for the chronic brain damage caused by strokes. Even the treatments for acute strokes do nothing to heal the damage to brain tissue, leaving patients permanently disabled. **Six million U.S. stroke survivors have been abandoned to suffer: Their ongoing disease has neither treatment nor cure.**

But there is now hope for a breakthrough treatment. After a decade of research and development, Seraya Medical recently demonstrated a revolutionary new noninvasive brain stimulation technology, transcranial rotating permanent magnetic stimulation (TRPMS). In a Phase 1/ Phase 2a trial, **TRPMS restored functional activity to damaged brain tissue—up to sixteen years after stroke.**[6] Consisting of a lightweight wearable cap controlled via a smartphone app, the device enables self-treatment at home by patients with **no risk of side effects**. Future trials are planned to demonstrate that by healing the brain, TRPMS can help patients regain the **use of their limbs or other functions—the Holy Grail of stroke medicine**.

Like most medical breakthroughs, TRPMS required someone to recognize its potential early on. That's where **Leeam Lowin and Seraya Medical** came in. Back in 2012, founder and investor Leeam Lowin was involved with stuttering research, seeking to stimulate songbird brains. The only device available for use at the time was a 300-pound transcranial magnetic stimulation machine meant for human brains—much too large to focus on these smaller bird brains. **To solve this problem, the team invented a new miniature magnetic stimulator, consisting of a barely eight-ounce wearable cap with six stimulators targeting separately programmed areas.**

Lowin had long believed that many brain-based neurological disorders resulted from faulty connectivity between brain regions. He realized that

---

6 Chiu et al., "Multifocal Transcranial Stimulation in Chronic Ischemic Stroke: A Phase 1/2a Randomized Trial."

this new, smaller, wearable device might offer a never-before-available tool to recalibrate such disturbed connectivity. Combining a portfolio of his own brain stimulation patients with a license to the new invention, Lowin formed Seraya Medical as the first step in building an entirely new brain treatment therapy platform.

As its initial target, Seraya Medical chose stroke, the most difficult candidate to treat with any therapy. **It would be the first-ever treatment of damaged brain tissue, restoring functionality previously thought to have been "permanently" lost.** The researchers hope that by treating stroke patients, TRPMS will quickly become the gold standard for brain stimulation as a service across other brain disorder targets, such as OCD, PTSD, stuttering, and refractory depression. In fact, as I'm writing this, **Seraya is already collaborating with research labs around the country to test TRPMS in addiction, stuttering, and multiple sclerosis.** The possibilities with this technology are endless.

It would be the first-ever treatment of damaged brain tissue, restoring functionality previously thought to have been "permanently" lost.

BREAKTHROUGH #6: EYES WIDE OPEN

"The most beautiful thing we can experience is the mysterious. It is the source of all true art and all science. He to whom this emotion is a stranger, who can no longer pause to wonder and stand rapt in awe, is as good as dead: his eyes are closed."

—ALBERT EINSTEIN

About **thirty years ago, when he was seven years old, Dr. John-Ross Rizzo noticed that he was having trouble seeing at night.** He couldn't navigate between rows in a darkened movie theater. When he played hide-and-seek with his friends in the evening, he stuck close to home base because he couldn't see anything. **"It was like staring into a black hole at midnight,"** he recalls. It took another seven years for him to be diagnosed with something called choroideremia, a rare genetic disorder that results in problems with peripheral vision, night vision, and cataracts.

In medical school, Dr. Rizzo learned about the field of disability medicine. Motivated by his personal experience, he decided to specialize in rehabilitation. There was no better place to do it than New York University, where Howard Rusk, considered the father of rehabilitation medicine, had launched the field and where Dr. Rizzo did his medical residency. Today, Dr. Rizzo is director of the high-tech Visuomotor Integration Laboratory, which is part of Rusk Rehabilitation at the NYU School of Medicine. Inspired by his own vision problems, Dr. Rizzo is particularly interested in how people use vision to help with motor control—how the eye focuses on an object and how that eye movement then communicates to the hands to pick up the object.

Did you know that the average person makes 11,000 eye movements per hour? It turns out that stroke survivors make many *more* eye movements; they have to exert more effort to do the same thing. It's exhausting, and the more complex the task, the more draining it becomes. Think about trying to pat your head and rub your belly at the same time. "It's that same kind of idea, but amplified with the eye and hand," says Dr. Rizzo. **"As soon as you have a stroke and try to do eye-hand task coordination, it becomes very difficult."**

In a study focused on restoring eye-hand coordination, Dr. Rizzo used a system that resembles a computer game to give feedback and correct reaching errors.[7] He used a headset equipped with cameras to track participants' eye movements and an index-finger sensor to track hand movements. Then he and his team tested a biofeedback-based technique that aims to focus on both the hand and the eye. You know what they learned when they assessed a group of stroke survivors and an unaffected control group? They discovered that hand and eye movements are not coordinated in stroke patients as they are in unaffected people. "We are the only place in the country, maybe the world, that is trying to understand this mechanism," says Dr. Rizzo. "There's no playbook on this because no one else is doing it."

The focus on stroke patients' eyes is important. Dr. Rizzo believes it could be the key to better understanding the struggles they face when trying to pick up objects, and that understanding could lead

to therapeutic applications that can accelerate the pace of recovery. In the works: tablet- and game-based technology and artificial intelligence and VR rehab systems that are building eye-tracking into their programs. "We think we're on to something quite strong," says Dr. Rizzo. "It holds a lot of promise and we're trying to get out the message so others can start to investigate the links between the eye and hand."

BREAKTHROUGH #7: THE POWER OF EXOSOMES TO HELP STROKE RECOVERY

"I am fond of pigs. Dogs look up to us. Cats look down on us. Pigs treat us as equals."

—WINSTON CHURCHILL

Remember how lucky my assistant Susan was to be whisked to a hospital where she received the only FDA-approved treatment for those strokes caused by clots, which account for more than 85 percent of strokes in the U.S.? This drug, called tPA, isn't always available in smaller or rural hospitals. It doesn't repair tissue that's already been damaged. And it has to be administered very quickly because it's effective only within a few hours of a stroke's onset. It works by breaking down the clot and restoring blood flow, like pharmacological Drano for the brain.

But what if there were a treatment that could work up to two full days after a stroke, a treatment that encouraged full recovery within a matter of weeks? That would be revolutionary. And it's happening in Athens, Georgia.

This dream is being turned into reality by **MD/PhD student Samantha Spellicy**, who has been doing research in a laboratory run by **Steven Stice at the University of Georgia's Regenerative Bioscience Center.** Stice's lab studies swine. As it turns out, pig brains and human brains have similarities. In fact, the neuroanatomy of pigs—their gray and white matter—more closely resembles that of humans than of mice, which are more typically the subjects of animal research. But rodents have less than 10 percent white matter compared to humans and pigs, which each have more than 60 percent. And rodent brains are also 650 times smaller than a human brain, while a pig brain is just 7.5 times smaller, making it a more helpful model when trying to figure out the right dose for a drug. **Altogether, this makes a compelling case for using swine to study stroke.**

Stice's lab developed an alternative approach to creating therapeutic uses for neural stem cells—here we are again, marveling at the magic of stem cell therapy! **It involves harnessing the beneficial effects of neural exosomes derived from the "bath" in which stem cells are grown. Exosomes are nanoscale-sized vesicles that carry the key growth factors involved in cell-to-cell communication. Growth factors that are thought to be key to rejuvenation and cell repair. Exosomes are created and shed by all cells, especially stem cells.** There are even exosomes in beer and bread due to yeast cells sloughing them off.

Within four weeks of exosome treatment, the exosome group was walking normally while the untreated group was still experiencing difficulty!

I personally used exosomes along with stem cells to address a variety of challenges I experienced as a result of the work I had done on my shoulder that I told you about in Chapter 2, "The Power of Stem Cells." "The cool thing about these vesicles is that they contain some nucleic acid or protein component from the cell they were secreted from," says Spellicy. "Maybe just by giving exosomes instead of giving the complete stem cell, we can get the benefit of stem cells while avoiding the downsides." Here's another cool thing about exosomes: They can be frozen for months on end. **So a hospital can keep batches of exosomes in a freezer and thaw them on demand whenever a patient needs them, whereas stem cells must be individually cultured, which takes time.**

Here's what Spellicy and her colleagues learned: **In an early study, MRI showed that pigs that had received an exosome treatment after suffering a stroke had less impacted brain volume, less swelling, and better-preserved white matter than those that hadn't received exosomes. Even more impressive, within four weeks of exosome treatment, the** exosome group was walking normally while the untreated group was still experiencing difficulty! Spellicy remarks, "It's pretty striking to see how well the treated animals recovered."

Remarkably, the treated pigs also had significantly higher survival rates—and the idea is that this incredible outcome can be translated to humans. "If we extrapolate to clinical use, if you're a patient who comes in with a really bad stroke and we give you exosomes, you aren't destined to have a bad outcome or poor survival," says Spellicy. "The severity of a stroke can be mediated by the exosomes, which is really exciting to see. This is telling us that there is hope for people who have really bad strokes."

Stice has cofounded a company, **Aruna Bio**, which is moving into the realm of testing exosome therapy in human clinical trials. He's looking to use **proprietary neural exosomes** to **target and repair diseased cells, providing a new way to treat stroke and other neurodegenerative disorders**. As you know, there's a desperate need for more effective stroke treatments, considering **that the drug tPA has a very short window of time when it can be an effective clot-buster. By contrast, exosomes appear to work in experiments that Spellicy has conducted with pigs up to forty-eight hours after a stroke.**

BREAKTHROUGH #8: DETECTING STROKES ON THE WAY TO THE HOSPITAL

Best of all, diagnostic technologies are improving all the time, becoming cheaper, more accurate and compact. One of the heroes in the diagnostic arena is **Mary Lou Jepsen, PhD,** who is the founder and CEO of a startup called **Openwater**. They are developing a new approach to medical imaging. **Jepsen, a former executive at Facebook and Google who has been named one of the 100 most influential people in the world by** *Time* magazine, says her goal is to "lower the cost of high-quality MRI-like medical imaging one-thousand-fold."

A quarter century ago, when Jepsen was studying for her PhD in optical physics at Brown, an MRI revealed that she had a brain tumor. "Everybody I knew was mortified," she says. **"But I hadn't been feeling myself for some time and I didn't know why. When I finally got my** diagnosis, I was thrilled because, with a diagnosis, you can fix it. You can find a neurosurgeon to do surgery." Years later, she's now running a company that is delivering on her vision of a portable device that delivers MRI-quality imaging that is a thousand times cheaper, with a machine that is a thousand times smaller. To do so, she's combining technologies such as solid-state lasers, ultrasound pings, machine learning, and the latest camera chips. Riding on top of the tsunami of exponential change, Jepsen is on the leading edge of dematerializing, demonetizing, and democratizing the field of imagine. "There's no reason that the device itself has to cost more than a cell phone," Jepsen says.

And where is Openwater planning to apply this new technology? They are planning to use this technology to examine brain blood flow in an ambulance, to detect a stroke on the ride to the hospital. As of mid-2020, Openwater has been in human studies with stroke patients in the neuro ICU, and in early 2022 they will scale up to a multicenter trial.

As we discussed earlier, there's a precious two-hour time window to diagnose a severe stroke before it means having a debilitating handicap the rest of your life. Today 55 percent of severe stroke (large vessel blockage) patients die or are severely disabled. During that two-hour window, if you have a large vessel blockage, getting the clot removed gives you a 90 percent chance of a good outcome with no deficit.

According to Jepsen, Openwater's portable MRI can be used in ambulances to quickly diagnose a stroke so the proper treatment can be given safely. No more waiting hours to get to the hospital and have a brain MRI done. Worried that a portable device won't be as good as the multimillion-dollar hospital equipment? Don't be! According to Jepsen, Openwater's blood flow detection is already two hundred times better than ultrasound or MRI!

And where does this technology go beyond the ambulance? This is Peter Diamandis's vision for the future as we move healthcare out of the hospital and into the home: "Imagine Openwater's technology, in combination with artificial intelligence, built into your bed or office, passively scanning you on a regular basis in the privacy of your home," says Peter. "This would allow you (and your AI) to find any problem at the earliest moment when it is most easily fixable." If so, then millions of people like you and me will detect problems early—when the probability of fixing them is highest. How many lives could that save? Peter and I are so passionate about this, we've invested in Openwater to help make this available faster.

Of course, <u>there are also many ways to prevent stroke that are within your control. Regular exercise to increase circulation, like we discussed in Chapter 14, can reduce your risk significantly.</u> In other words, **this entire book contains valuable insights about additional tools that can boost circulation and help prevent stroke.** But now you also know that if someone does suffer a stroke, there is a clear and powerful path to recovery. Whether it's learning to open your hands again with the help of haptic gloves, exploring a fantasy virtual reality world where rehab is all fun and games, trying to boost hand-eye coordination, or using exosomes to coax the brain to self-repair, there is new hope emerging when it comes to treatments for stroke.

Thanks to all these breakthroughs, this is a great time to be alive. Please take care of yourself, and if you know someone who's had a stroke, they might want to consider these amazing tools and technologies. As always, you can find out more details at Lifeforce.com.

Now, let's move on to our next chapter, about a scary subject that no one likes talking about, **cancer. Turn the page, and let's learn how we are winning the war on this dreaded disease. . . .**

REIMAGINING HOW WE DIAGNOSE AND TREAT THE BRAIN

REACT Neuro is a digital health company reimagining how we diagnose and treat the brain. They've successfully **digitized the entire neurological exam.**

It all started when the head coach of the New England Patriots, Bill Belichick, noticed that the medical exam (neurological assessment) that followed a head injury on the field looked very old-school. Basically, the doctor said, "Follow my finger," moving it up and down, left and right. **"It looked like the doctor was signing the holy cross on the field," said Belichick.**

REACT Neuro came out of that observation, asking the question "How do we take all of these vital tests and put them into one device that someone can use on the field, or in the comfort of their home?" The answer turned out to be using virtual reality (VR) technology with built-in sensors to track eye movements, record voice, and capture body movements, as a one-stop solution. **Today REACT's technology takes them less than a minute to run a full brain health diagnostic and figure out someone's attention, memory, and mood.** REACT has developed the most comprehensive brain health platform, with **twenty-plus digital exams**. REACT has a wide range of applications, from tracking healthy aging and performance to monitoring diseases like Alzheimer's.

They've even made a dent in the therapeutic space. In addition to assessing brain health, REACT has **created digital experiences that provide therapy for people who've suffered from a concussion or stroke.** These digital therapeutics are gamelike experiences that are customized to someone's ability in real time; they maximize engagement while gradually increasing the difficulty of the tasks.

REACT's sleek product headset is already being used in senior living homes, the military, and concierge health systems. They are well on their way to achieving their **mission to democratize access to the highest-quality brain medical care from the comfort of your own home.**

CHAPTER 19

HOW TO WIN THE WAR ON CANCER

New Tests, New Drugs, and New Technologies Are Transforming How We Treat Cancer—and, Most Significantly, How We Can Prevent It in the First Place

"Cancer didn't bring me to my knees. It brought me to my feet."

—MICHAEL DOUGLAS, actor and cancer survivor

Everyone knows someone who has been diagnosed with the "Big C"—cancer. This scourge, which is the second leading cause of death in the United States, has probably touched a member of your family. Maybe a friend. Maybe a colleague. Maybe you.

But even though cancer affects millions of people each year, this is one club that nobody wants to join. Along with heart disease and dementia, cancer rounds out the list of killers that cut our life short and steal our golden years with our families. **Each year in the United States alone 1.8 million people are newly diagnosed with cancer. More than a third of that number die from cancer annually. That's 1,600 people a day: 1,600 husbands and wives, mothers and fathers and children, brothers and sisters, billionaires and paupers, scientists and artists.** Globally, there are about 9.5 million cancer-related deaths each year.

What's truly shocking is how likely we are to get cancer. **Almost 40 percent of Americans are expected to develop cancer during the course of their lifetimes.** The cost to families of losing a loved one can't be measured. The cost of care is almost as startling: In 2018, nearly $151 billion went toward cancer care in the U.S.[1] That's such an immense figure that it's hard

---

1 National Cancer Institute, "Cancer Statistics."

to fathom what it means in personal terms. Let me give it a try: **The average cost of a cancer patient's treatment is estimated at $250,000, and the bill often balloons to *millions* of dollars.**[2] In countries like the U.S., the burden of these costs will only increase as the population grows older. Remember: For the most part, cancer is a disease of aging.

As I mentioned earlier, I used to be terrified that cancer was coming for me, and that I'd die slowly and painfully at a young age. My fear was irrational, but not entirely unfounded. I'd watched my mother's dear friend succumb to cancer. I watched the CEO of one of my companies lose his wife to cancer. It was excruciating. I then watched a business partner and close friend and a coworker pass. **Fortunately, with new technology,**

It's when our immune system fails us that cancer takes hold, so it makes sense that a high-performing immune system is one of the most important ways to defend against cancer, and virtually all diseases.

---

last year one of my friends who was told she was terminal tried a new form of treatment that included stem cells; one year later, she is cancer-free!

It is now widely understood that the immune system normally provides protection against cancers.[3] Did you know that we are always developing cancers in our bodies? It's just that our immune system finds them at the very beginning and defeats them. **It's when our immune system fails us that cancer takes hold, so it makes sense that a high-performing immune system is one of the most important ways to defend against cancer, and virtually all diseases.**

What stood out to me then, and now, is how the traditional treatment— the chemotherapy and radiation required to improve their chances of

---

2 Moore, "The High Cost of Cancer Treatment."

3 Pandya, "The Immune System in Cancer Pathogenesis: Potential Therapeutic Approaches."

survival—ended up ravaging them, body and soul. And after they went through hell, that brutal treatment wasn't even successful. I'm an empath. My ability to relate deeply to others enables me to help them. But that same depth of empathy made me feel like I was going through this grueling disease right alongside my friends. Their pain left an indelible impression— and a passionate desire to see progress in the war on cancer, so that millions of others could be spared this suffering.

We all have a stake in this war. So **I'm thrilled to report that the future of cancer detection and treatment has never looked more promising. As you'll learn in this chapter, the technological tide is finally turning in ways that once seemed inconceivable.** That's a stunning achievement and a massive relief because the truth is, **we're long overdue for a revolution in how we approach this disease.** We need to break its frightening grip on our bodies and our minds.

In recent years, we've seen slow but steady progress in the fight against cancer. Between 2001 and 2017, the rate of men's cancer deaths fell by 1.8 percent and the rate for women dropped by 1.4 percent. That's partly because smoking, which dramatically raises the risk of cancer, has lost some of its allure. As treatments become more sophisticated and early detection increases, this declining trend in the death rate is likely to continue. **In 2019, the U.S. had nearly 17 million cancer survivors. By 2030, that number is expected to exceed 22 million. That's a great start. But it's nothing compared to what we're about to see.**

Why am I—along with my co-authors, Peter and Bob, and many leading cancer experts—so optimistic? Because science is now advancing at exponential rates to deliver an unprecedented bounty of breakthrough technologies. In this chapter, we're going to introduce you to **a range of tools aimed at prevention and early detection, which consistently provides a less invasive and more effective approach to healing. And finally, a series of cutting-edge therapies, cures, and treatments that can supercharge our own immune systems to battle and stop cancer,** including, to name a couple, a daily pill that disables cancer's deadly mechanisms and an infusion that vanquished President Jimmy Carter's aggressive melanoma, saving his life.

This wide array of groundbreaking innovations that can help you avoid the debilitating journey of cancer and radiation treatments includes:

1. In the diagnostics chapter, we shared with you a simple blood test that can detect up to fifty kinds of cancer at their earliest and most treatable stage. Here we'll go deeper in our understanding on this, and how a full-body MRI may soon be moving from the hospital to the comfort of your home. Remember, early detection is key to survival!

2. A natural ingredient that thousands of studies have shown can significantly reduce your risk of cancer, and has even been shown to reduce breast cancer cells by 80 percent.

3. An innovative procedure for prostate cancer, the most common cancer among men, that ingeniously sidesteps the common side effects of incontinence and loss of sexual function—and can be performed safely in a doctor's office, without radiation or hospitalization.

4. Four personalized therapies that can augment and supercharge your own immune system to attack cancer. You've already learned about CAR T cells. But as you'll soon see, related cellular therapies involving immune cells and their by-products such as natural killer (NK) cells—along with personalized cancer vaccines and tumor-infiltrating lymphocytes—are at long last making it possible to defeat even those cancers that have been considered incurable. There are even immune boosters called checkpoint inhibitors that have turned around within weeks the prognosis of people with Stage 3 cancer!

5. Remember exosomes, those minute "bags" of molecules or signaling factors that all cells in your body release? It turns out they can be reprogrammed to attack cancer.

This bonanza of new technologies should give us all tremendous hope. Every day, we're getting better at detecting cancer early—long before it becomes life-threatening—and treating it with leading-edge techniques that will eventually make radiation and chemotherapy seem as primitive as leeching.

This subject is so important, and this chapter is a little longer than most of the others in this book. But if you want to make sure that you're armed with the latest breakthroughs for you or someone that you love, this chapter is a must-read.

The first part of this chapter will focus on ways to prevent cancer. The second part will share the newest breakthroughs that are occurring if you or someone you know has already developed cancer to give you what's available today as well as what's coming so that you have choices in how to attack, and ideally win, the war on this disease.

These new developments are *so creative, so imaginative, so transformative*, that talk of vanquishing cancer is no longer a pipe dream. It's real and could change the course of your life. So let's dive in.

THE BEST TREATMENT OF ALL: PREVENTION

"An ounce of prevention is worth a pound of cure."

—BENJAMIN FRANKLIN

What could be better than curing cancer? Preventing it! To state the obvious, the single best way to tackle cancer is *never to develop it in the first place.* In short, there's no treatment as good as prevention, and that's where our most fervent hope lies.

I'm so bullish about the power of prevention. And one of the reasons that I joined forces with Dr. Bob Hariri, Dr. Peter Diamandis, and Dr. Bill Kapp in forming the company Fountain Life, which we introduced in Chapter 2, was to encourage more people to take advantage of the *precision diagnostic testing* that we, our families, and many of our closest friends undergo regularly as a way to detect diseases in their earliest and most treatable stages. Remember, our company's goal is to be a trusted source for people's health and well-being, curating the best solutions to optimize their vitality, improve their healthspan, and extend their lifespan.

If you want to stay healthy and head off trouble, there's no better

diagnostic tool than the newest forms of whole-body MRI. As Dr. Bill Kapp says, "The whole-body MRI is the most useful test right now to find any aberration. Of course, you can also find abnormalities in your genome sequencing and your blood chemistry. But the majority of all the immediate and emergent life-threatening diseases are found in your MRI scans."

What does a whole-body MRI scan entail? You lie still inside a noisy machine that costs millions of dollars, and it takes about 15,000 images of your body, using radio waves and powerful magnets. But the diagnostic data you derive from this test can be absolutely priceless. **Among other things, the MRI can detect solid tumors of the neck, chest, abdomen, pelvis, and brain—along with other life-endangering problems like cardiac disease, aneurysms, and neurodegenerative diseases such as Alzheimer's and Parkinson's.**

Why bother with seeking out all this information? Isn't it better to live in blissful ignorance, hoping blindly for the best? I understand why some people feel that way. **But if you read Chapter 3 on Diagnostic Power, you know that early detection vastly improves your odds of successfully treating countless illnesses, including a wide range of potentially lethal cancers.** I'm guessing you know of people who were diagnosed with Stage 3 or Stage 4 cancer, meaning that it was relatively advanced and extremely challenging to treat. **How much better would it have been to detect that cancer in Stage Zero when it was still small and in one place and hadn't yet spread to nearby tissues, lymph nodes, or other parts of the body?**

During Peter's August 2020 Abundance Platinum trip to San Francisco and San Diego, he arranged for all participants to undergo a battery of the most sophisticated diagnostic tests. This assessment included whole genome sequencing (a breathtakingly complex test that can reveal cancer-causing genetic mutations), a CT scan (to determine the condition of their arteries and gauge their risk of a heart attack), advanced blood work, and a whole-body MRI scan.

As you can imagine, some of these folks felt pretty nervous at the prospect of what this barrage of tests might reveal. Speaking at dinner the night before the testing began, Peter reassured them that these granular insights about their health would enable them to live with a whole new level of confidence and clarity. He remarked, "Most of us are optimists about our health. We all walk around saying, 'Oh, things are great, I feel fine!' Until you don't. And that's the challenge. We know more about what's going on inside our car or refrigerator than we do with our body! The problem is, it's often too late by the time we find something. The smarter alternative is to use high-resolution imaging to scan ourselves every year, find any problem at the very beginning, and take care of it immediately."

As Peter explained, there's one overarching question that we're looking to answer with all of this next-generation diagnostic testing: **"*Is there anything going on inside your body that you need to know about now?* And if you find something, the answer is not 'Oh my God.' It's 'Okay, I'm going to crush it!' So when people say to me, 'I don't want to know,' I say, 'Bullshit! Of course, you want to know. You want to know as soon as possible when you can *do* something about it.'"** Put simply, it's all about empowerment.

One of the guest speakers at Peter's dinner that evening was our very own Dr. Bill Kapp, the CEO of Fountain Life. As mentioned earlier, Dr. Kapp became disillusioned with his profession's entrenched emphasis on **"sick care," which involves waiting until you start to fall apart before trying to put the patient back together, and doing this at a cost that's liable to wipe you out. His driving passion is to promote healthcare that *prevents* the problem in the first place.**

"We can do an amazing job of keeping you alive and can even help patients recover from Stage 3 or Stage 4 cancer," explains Dr. Kapp. **"But wouldn't it be wonderful if you knew you were going to get cancer *before* it happened?"**

That's precisely why Bill Kapp, Peter, Bob, and I are so excited about making this type of precision diagnostic testing more widely available. <u>**What we're talking about here is a radical change of mindset, shifting the focus from sick care to *well care*, from reactive medicine to *proactive medicine*, from fighting disease to *preventing disease.*** After all, do you have any doubt that prevention is the best option of all?</u>

Our friend and partner Dr. David Karow, president of Human Longevity, Inc., and an MD/PhD who is a leading expert in advanced body imaging and genomic analytics, has seen countless lives saved because these diagnostic tests detected cancer an early stage—long before it

escalated and became catastrophic. Dr. Karow points out that there are also massive cost savings associated with early diagnosis. For example, using immunotherapy to treat Stage 3 or Stage 4 renal cancer can cost hundreds of thousands of dollars. But if you detect that same cancer at Stage 1, you can often treat it almost effortlessly by heating or freezing the tumor to destroy the cancer cells—a safe and inexpensive solution that's typically an outpatient procedure.

If you ask me, the choice isn't difficult. I'd much prefer to undergo regular diagnostic testing and catch a problem like this in its infancy than wait until it grows into Godzilla.

Also, once you know what's going on inside your body, you have the option of making smart adjustments to optimize your health and vitality. For

---

Using immunotherapy to treat Stage 3 or Stage 4 renal cancer can cost hundreds of thousands of dollars. But if you detect that same cancer at Stage 1, you can often treat it almost effortlessly by heating or freezing the tumor to destroy the cancer cells—a safe and inexpensive solution that's typically an outpatient procedure.

---

example, the diagnostic tests we use at Fountain Life give you a clear picture of how much inflammation there is in your body. Why does that matter? Because **scientists regard inflammation as a key culprit in aging and specifically in cancer. Having determined your inflammatory age, we can optimize you by giving you tools such as peptides, which, you'll remember from Chapter 10, "Your Ultimate Vitality Pharmacy," are smaller versions of proteins that fight inflammation and aging.** And that's just one way to reduce your risk of cancer.

Dr. Kapp, who also has a master's in immunology and genetics, explains it like this: **"As you age, you lose the ability to stimulate the immune system as robustly as when you were a child. We use peptides to boost immunity by boosting T cells. T cells and their progeny, natural killer cells—which are also known as NK cells—circulate looking for tumor**

cells." We'll return to this subject later because T cells and NK cells are such important allies in the fight against cancer. **But for now, the simple point is that it's good to have more T cells and NK cells in your body because these immune cells help to defend you against cancer.[4] They guard against marauding invaders.**

Another critical aspect of all this diagnostic testing involves accurately measuring your body composition. For one thing, you're able to discover precisely how much visceral fat is secretly stored within your abdominal cavity. **As you may know, excessive visceral fat raises the risk of a wide array of nasty illnesses that you'll be delighted to avoid, including colorectal cancer, breast cancer, heart disease, and type 2 diabetes.** Our tests also measure your ratio of fat to muscle to assess your risk of metabolic syndrome.

> **"The higher the muscle mass, the higher the immune function, the longer you live," says Dr. Kapp. "There's almost a direct correlation with longevity. Strength training can also arrest cognitive decline.**

The point is, once you know exactly where you stand, you can *do* something about it. That includes making informed lifestyle choices about nutrition, sleep, and exercise —all of which play a pivotal role in reducing the risk of various types of cancer—as discussed in Chapters 12, 13, and 14. As you might remember, the most effective things you can do to avoid illness and enhance your vitality is to sleep eight hours per night, minimize your sugar intake, and exercise regularly, with a special emphasis on building muscle strength.

This isn't about looking buff and beautiful on the beach, though there's nothing wrong with that. **The fact is, muscle is the largest endocrine organ in the body, and people with enough muscle mass have a significantly lower incidence of cancer (and other illnesses). "The higher the muscle mass, the higher the immune function, the longer you live,"**

---

4 Eissmann, "Natural Killer Cells."

says Dr. Kapp. "There's almost a direct correlation with longevity. Strength training can also arrest cognitive decline.[5] So getting your muscle mass up is critical." Yet the truth is, most people have no idea how critically important it is to do muscle training—both for their healthspan and lifespan.

I hope you're starting to see a new pattern—a more informed and proactive way of thinking that makes us far from powerless in the war on cancer. **Advanced diagnostic testing enables us to get way ahead of the curve, identifying problems before it's too late.** And the precision data we collect about our bodies empowers us to adjust our behavior in ways that sharply lower the risk of illness. It's a whole different attitude, isn't it? **We're not waiting passively for disaster to strike. We're proactively maximizing the probability of a long, healthy, vibrant life.**

INVENTING THE HOLY GRAIL: FINDING CANCER EARLY

"Heroism doesn't always happen in a burst of glory. Sometimes small triumphs and large hearts change the course of history."

—MARY ROACH, author of *Grunt: The Curious Science of Humans at War*

One of the biggest challenges with detecting cancer is that so few preventive tests exist. The best known are mammography to find breast cancer, colonoscopy to identify colon cancer, and Pap tests for cervical cancer. **Yet, the majority of cancers are found only at an advanced stage, once symptoms emerge.** And as you already know, it can be too late by then. That's why we mentioned to you in Chapter 3, the diagnostics chapter, the power of a new blood test for cancers called **GRAIL**.

In one of the most promising diagnostic breakthroughs in decades, GRAIL has developed a liquid biopsy—a simple blood test that is able to detect most major types of cancer at an early stage when they're significantly easier to treat. Jeff Huber, GRAIL's founding CEO and vice

---

5 Gregory et al., "Physical Activity, Cognitive Function, and Brain Health: What Is the Role of Exercise Training in the Prevention of Dementia?"

chairman, sees this innovation as a way of "shifting the playing field" by **finding cancer "when the odds are in your favor."**

If cancer is detected at Stage 1 or Stage 2, says Huber, "there's about an 80 percent chance that you'll be cured and can continue on with your life." If it's detected at Stage 3 or 4, "there's an 80 percent chance that you're *not* going to like the outcome." In fact, "the five-year survival rate when cancer is detected early is almost 90 percent." That rate sinks to *just 21 percent* when it's detected late. Sadly, "about 80 percent of cancers are diagnosed late—at Stage 3 and Stage 4."[6]

Before launching GRAIL in 2016, Huber was a heavy hitter at Google. During his thirteen years there, he built some of the company's biggest systems, including Google Maps, where he ran a team of more than 5,000 people. As a cofounder of Google X, the company's "moon shot factory," he'd just begun to explore ways of applying genome technology to drive future breakthroughs in life sciences. Then he received a fateful call from Illumina, a leader in genomic sequencing, inviting him to join its board.

At one of his first board meetings, Huber reviewed the progress of a new R&D project inspired by an accidental discovery in pregnant women. Illumina had acquired a company that was doing noninvasive prenatal testing. The test involved taking a blood sample from an expectant mother and analyzing it for traces of fetal DNA that could indicate anomalies such as Down syndrome. While conducting thousands of tests, the researchers discovered some baffling results that didn't correlate with any fetal conditions. Strangely, they correlated with something else entirely: cancer. When the researchers followed up, it turned out that these expectant mothers had undiagnosed cases of Stage 3 and Stage 4 cancers—and the blood test had somehow detected the disease.

"That lit the lightbulb," says Huber. "Here's a test that was developed for an entirely different purpose. But clearly **there's a signal there in the blood that we could use for detecting cancer.**" This unintentional finding spawned a new initiative. **What if the blood test could be fine-tuned, making it sensitive enough to pick up a whole range of cancers "at that *early* stage when interventions would make a difference to outcomes"?**

6 Howlader et al., "SEER Cancer Statistics Review, 1975–2018."

Over the next few months, the research went well. Actually, everything in Huber's life seemed to be going well. **But then disaster struck. It started when his wife, Laura, who was "forty-five years old, super-healthy, super-fit," began to feel "more tired than usual" and had "some hip pain, joint pains—things that were unusual but vague."** Seeing nothing to worry about, her doctor said, "Welcome to pre-menopause. You'll get better." But the symptoms didn't go away, and Laura soon developed gastrointestinal issues, too.

Eventually, she had a colonoscopy and an endoscopy, which revealed a two-centimeter tumor in her colon. At first, says Huber, it seemed like cause for celebration. They'd found the cancer early enough to treat it effectively. But a CT scan and an MRI scan later showed that **"what appeared to be a small colon tumor had actually very aggressively metastasized through her lymph system to her liver and ultimately to her lung."**

Laura underwent an aggressive campaign of chemotherapy. But in November 2015, after eighteen months of treatment, she died. "We had access to the best experts in the world, the best testing possible," says Huber. "But it was evident that for all the work that has been done, we're so far from understanding cancer and how to actually treat it."

One week before Laura's death, Illumina decided to spin out a new company that would focus on developing its blood-based test for cancer. A month or so later, a grieving Huber was offered the job of leading this startup, which would be called GRAIL. The timing was terrible, and Illumina's board kindly suggested installing an interim CEO until Huber felt ready. But the more he thought about it, the more he knew that he *had* to be ready. Laura would have wanted him to be ready. In truth, there was no choice, says Huber, calling GRAIL "a moral and ethical imperative because of the impact it could have" on so many lives. **If its blood test "had been available three or four or five years earlier, it could have fundamentally changed the outcome for Laura" and "many, many others."**

Fueled by an irresistible sense of urgency, Huber took the reins at GRAIL in 2016, hired forty people in a single day, rapidly raised $1 billion for clinical studies, and enrolled 15,000 people in the company's first study. As he says, "We were shot out of a cannon."

That first study involved 10,000 people who had recently been diagnosed with cancer, along with a control group of 5,000 healthy people.[7] The goal? To construct an enormous database of everything we know about cancer that can be measured in the blood. **Building on that research, GRAIL developed a blood-based screening test called Galleri, which could detect more than fifty types of cancer.** How does it work? The test searches for tiny fragments of DNA and RNA that have been released into the bloodstream by a tumor and that reflect the tumor's genomic features. **GRAIL's technology is so sensitive that it can detect even a faint signal that an early tumor exists.**

To put this breakthrough in context, you need to understand just how limited our capacity to screen for cancer has been—until now. Hubert points out that **"80 percent of cancers don't have any screening mechanism. And many of those cancers are ones that have developed a reputation as being deadly—for example, pancreatic cancer and ovarian cancer. But the reason they're so deadly is because they're so frequently detected late. . . . In the rare cases where they're detected early, the prognosis is actually pretty good."**

If you've been tested for a disease like breast, colorectal, lung, or cervical cancer, you know firsthand that the screening mechanisms we rely on now are valuable but far from perfect. For example, plenty of women shy away from the discomfort of having their breasts mashed between metal plates. Likewise, a colonoscopy is nobody's idea of fun. Tests for diseases like prostate cancer have also run into serious problems with high rates of false negatives and false positives, adding another layer of uncertainty and stress.

Enter GRAIL. **Its ultimate mission is to offer one test that can *simultaneously* scan for *every* type of cancer.** Huber, who has a talent for thinking big, says, **"Instead of going in for a colonoscopy or a Pap smear or a mammography for breast cancer, what would it be like if we could, with a single test, effectively detect *all* cancer types?"**

GRAIL launched its Galleri blood test commercially in the U.S. in

---

7 Liu et al., "Sensitive and Specific Multi-Cancer Detection and Localization Using Methylation Signatures in Cell-Free DNA."

2021. For now, it isn't designed to replace the existing tests for cancer, but to complement them. It promises to improve detection of the 20 percent of cancers for which we already have a screening mechanism, while also providing a new way to screen for the other 80 percent.

Like many medical innovations, it's likely to take a while for GRAIL's test to become widely available. Galleri costs $949, which might sound pricy for a regular annual test. But just think about the colossal treatment costs and needless human suffering that could be avoided if a test like this becomes routine. **And in fact, Huber's vision is that you'll actually be able to access this test whenever you visit your doctor for an annual physical exam—in much the same way that you'd expect to have your cholesterol and glucose levels checked. And like all technology, the cost should drop significantly.** In fact, starting in 2021, the UK's National Health Service will offer the test to 140,000 people over the age of 50 with no signs of cancer and 25,000 people age 40 and above who are suspected of having cancer. If all goes well, the test could be adopted in the UK for routine use.[8]

After his wife, Laura, passed away, Huber calculated how much her eighteen months of agonizing late-stage cancer treatment had cost: "It was $2.7 million that was ultimately spent in futility." You didn't read that wrong: the cost of one person's treatment was $2.7 million. Not only did it not work; treatment was an agonizing process at that stage. By contrast, an early diagnosis could have led to a simple $10,000 surgical intervention that might well have produced a positive outcome.

The fact is, we need to start thinking about preventive care in a more pragmatic way. It's a bit like visiting a dentist for a regular cleaning and checkup to stave off a dreaded (and expensive) root canal. But when it comes to cancer, we're talking about life and death.

Meanwhile, the future looks bright for GRAIL. In 2020, the company that incubated GRAIL as a start-up, Illumina, announced its plan to fully acquire GRAIL in a deal valued at $8 billion. That hefty price tag should give you a sense of just how much excitement this technology is

---

8 Faulconbridge, "Britain Begins World's Largest Trial of Blood Test for 50 Types of Cancer."

generating. But you won't be surprised to hear that GRAIL isn't the only genetic diagnostics company pursuing this wide-open market of liquid biopsies. In the fall of 2020, a company called **Freenome** announced $270 million in Series C financing to advance a clinical trial for its own blood test to screen for colorectal cancer, as well as additional blood tests for a variety of other cancers.

Freenome's cofounder, Charles Roberts, points out that early diagnosis is especially critical in the battle against colorectal cancer. If you detect the cancer when it's still localized, the "five-year survival rate is 92 percent," says Roberts, "versus 14 percent when there's any spread at all." If you detect it at Stage 1 or earlier, "it's actually almost 100 percent survival. Given that colorectal cancer is the second most deadly cancer worldwide—lung cancer is first—that's a lot of lives saved."[9]

If everything goes according to plan, Freenome will launch its test in 2022. It's administered every three years and is expected to cost $500. That sounds like a bargain to me. If you've ever had a colonoscopy, you'll never forget the experience of choking down a gallon of sickly sweet, viscous laxative and spending hours on the porcelain throne! I'd never discourage anyone from doing a colonoscopy, because it can truly save your life. But is it any wonder that 45 million Americans aren't up to date on their colonoscopy screening? If Freenome can provide an easy, affordable, laxative-free test for colorectal cancer, sign me up!

AN OUNCE OF PREVENTION IS WORTH A POUND OF CURE

While screening is critically important, wouldn't it be amazing to nourish yourself with a core ingredient that thousands of studies have shown can reduce your risk of cancer, and has even been shown to reduce breast cancer cells by up to 80 percent?[10] The lowly broccoli sprout is a superfood that contains sky-high levels of **glucoraphanin, a precursor to the cancer-**

---

9 World Health Organization, "Cancer."

10 Mokhtari et al., "The Role of Sulforaphane in Cancer Chemoprevention and Health Benefits: A Mini-Review."

busting phytochemical sulforaphane—one of the most powerful food-derived molecules. In fact, broccoli sprouts are up to fifty times more potent than broccoli alone.[11]

Thousands of studies on sulforaphane show that 80 percent of the phytochemical you take in makes its way into your body's cells. And research has also identified sulforaphane as cancer-protective because it revs up antioxidants and detoxification enzymes that guard against the disease. **The sulforaphane in broccoli sprouts can slam the brakes on tumor growth and play an important role in the regulation of hundreds of genes.**

So maybe it's time to take up a new hobby: sprouting broccoli seeds or other cruciferous seeds including radish, cabbage, and arugula! Of course, you can also buy these sprouts at many grocery stores or natural foods

---

The sulforaphane in broccoli sprouts can slam the brakes on tumor growth and play an important role in the regulation of hundreds of genes.

---

stores. (Even if you don't eat sprouts, make sure to keep veggies like cauliflower and brussels sprouts on the menu; along with broccoli, they're chock-full of sulforaphane.) **Keep in mind that the cancer-fighting chemicals in sprouts are at their most robust levels at Day 3, so that's when you'll want to harvest them.** There are many capsule options, though I personally prefer to get fresh sprouts, sprinkled on my salads or blended into my green drinks. They cost pennies and yet their prevention capacity is extraordinary.

---

11 Fahey et al., "Broccoli Sprouts: An Exceptionally Rich Source of Inducers of Enzymes that Protect Against Chemical Carcinogens."

READY, AIM, FIRE: SENDING THE IMMUNE SYSTEM INTO BATTLE

"The harder the conflict, the greater the triumph."

—GEORGE WASHINGTON

Armed with these incredible technologies like liquid biopsies, whole genome sequencing, and whole-body MRIs, and even doing something simple like eating broccoli sprouts—we stand a better chance than ever of putting the brakes on cancer by preventing the problem in the first place. But you know as well as I do that this isn't always feasible. In millions of cases each year, we miss the opportunity to intervene early. And that makes us overly dependent on treatments that leave a lot to be desired.

Did you know that only a few chemotherapy drugs produce an enduring remission, let alone a cure? In the majority of cases, any given

---

Of seventy-one chemotherapy drugs for solid tumors, the median survival edge is an abysmal 2.1 months.

---

drug conveys mere *months* of increased survival or time before the tumor grows or spreads.[12] Of thirty-six cancer drugs approved by the FDA between 2008 and 2012, only five were shown to improve survival compared with existing treatments or—shockingly—compared to *no treatment at all*.[13] And if we're being honest, "improvement" is a generous word for what we're describing here. OF SEVENTY-ONE CHEMOTHERAPY DRUGS FOR SOLID TUMORS, THE MEDIAN SURVIVAL EDGE IS AN ABYSMAL 2.1 MONTHS.

What about radiation therapy, which uses high doses of radiation

---

12 Kummel et al., "Can Contemporary Trials of Chemotherapy for HER2-negative Metastatic Breast Cancer Detect Overall Survival Benefit?" See Table 2.

13 Prasad, "Do Cancer Drugs Improve Survival or Quality of Life?"

to kill cancer cells and shrink tumors? The trouble is, it also kills *normal* tissue, which is why side effects like nausea, vomiting, hair loss, fatigue, and diarrhea are inevitable. To make matters worse, radiation can't treat cancer cells that have spread. Why not? Because whole-body radiation intense enough to cure you would kill you before it could benefit you. And then of course there's the fact that radiation itself can also cause *new* cancers.

It's high time we had some better options. And you know what? We do! Now, for the first time in history, medicine's brutal anti-cancer armamentarium—cut (surgery), poison (chemotherapy), and burn (radiation therapy)—has a fourth weapon: marshaling for battle the body's own natural anti-cancer forces.

There are many different varieties of cancer immunotherapy. But they're all built on the same earth-shaking idea: The immune system can eliminate cancer. It's hard to overstate how jaw-dropping this is.

We've already discussed the spectacular promise of CAR T-cell therapies, which are a hybrid of immunotherapy and gene therapy. As you learned in Chapter 6, a trailblazing scientist named Dr. Carl June has devised a patented technique to modify T cells (which are our immune system's infantry) to defend against cancer. Now I want to tell you a little more about T cells, as well as 7 other forms of therapy, including:

1. Checkpoint inhibitors
2. Personalized cancer vaccines
3. Natural killer cells that are harvested from human placentas and engineered to attack cancer
4. Tumor-infiltrating lymphocytes that multiply a patient's T cells to fight solid tumors
5. Cancer-fighting exosomes that are showing promising results in combating one of the most lethal cancers of all—pancreatic cancer
6. A new technology that is helping to treat prostate cancer without the debilitating side effects
7. A pathway to healing that uses a single small-molecule drug to attack six different cancers

It all sounds mind-blowingly futuristic, doesn't it? And it is. What we're witnessing here is an unprecedented wave of innovation that is stirring new hope that cancer can be cured.

Tool #1: Checkpoint Inhibitors

How did the immune system come to play this central role in the crusade to cure cancer? The obvious place to start that story is by going back a few years to a game-changing breakthrough: the development of immunotherapy drugs called **"checkpoint inhibitors."**

Sharon Belvin was only 22 when she was diagnosed in 2002 with metastatic melanoma. The cancer had already spread to her lungs and brain. Belvin, a tough Jersey girl who had been studying to become a teacher, braved her way through a barrage of different treatments: gamma knife surgery; three kinds of chemotherapy; and infusions of interleukin-2, a protein made by white blood cells that is supposed to sic the immune system on cancer. **Nothing worked. Other patients with Stage 4 melanoma usually died within months, so Belvin figured she would soon become one of the 10,000 people in the U.S. who would succumb to melanoma that year.** A couple of years after her diagnosis, she had clumps of tumors throughout her chest and was struggling to breathe. **"It left me feeling like death warmed over,"** she recalls. **"And now we were out of options."**

Then, in 2005, Belvin's oncologist at Memorial Sloan Kettering Cancer Center in New York threw her a lifeline. "There's this new, experimental cancer drug that works by unleashing your immune system on your tumors," he told her. "Would you like to enter the study that's testing it?" With nothing to lose, Belvin agreed to sign up. That fall, she had a total of four infusions of this new drug, **ipilimumab**, three weeks apart. **"After two or three treatments, I started to feel better." For the first time in months, she even had the strength to walk her dog. Still, she says, "I didn't let myself hope yet."**

After her final infusion, Belvin had a CT scan. **The radiologist at Sloan Kettering asked her doctor if there could have been a mix-up.** *Surely, this couldn't be the scan of a patient who'd been riddled with tumors just weeks before?* **It was. Belvin's tumors had disappeared—destroyed by** her own white blood cells, the warriors of the immune system that had been unleashed by ipilimumab.

Coincidentally, on the very same day that Belvin's doctor told her she was cancer-free, he also mentioned nonchalantly that **James Allison—the scientist who invented ipilimumab—happened to be in the building. Would she like to meet him?** "He came to the room where I was," says Belvin. "I gave him a giant hug, and we both cried." **It was the first time that Jim Allison had ever met a patient whose life his discovery had saved.**

Belvin's tumors had disappeared—destroyed by her own white blood cells, the warriors of the immune system that had been unleashed by ipilimumab.

You may never have heard of him. But believe me, <u>Dr. Allison—who won the Nobel Prize in Physiology or Medicine in 2018—is a legend among cancer biologists. His breakthrough has saved hundreds of thousands of lives and revolutionized cancer medicine.</u> A Texas native, his career initially took him to California and New York. But he returned to the Lone Star state as the preeminent scientist at the **MD Anderson Cancer Center in Houston.** As with so many of the stories you've heard about scientists whose life's work led to breakthroughs, **<u>Allison's motivation was profoundly personal, not just professional: He lost one uncle to lung cancer, another to melanoma, and a brother to prostate cancer. He's also had invasive melanoma and prostate cancer himself.</u>**[14] **<u>So it seems fitting that he was the person who made these immune cells cure cancer.</u>**

Allison is a "T cell whisperer." Back in the 1980s, he learned more about T cells than had ever been known. He discovered one molecule on their surface that recognizes foreign invaders. It's called the *T-cell receptor.* **He discovered another molecule (CD28) that revs up T cells' attack on**

---

14 Benson, "The Iconoclast"; Haney, *Breakthrough* (film).

invaders. **He discovered a third (CTLA-4) that acts like a T-cell brake, which must be *disengaged* for the T cell to be deployed into battle.**

All of this research led Allison to a revelatory idea: Maybe tumors have a fiendish mechanism for keeping the CTLA-4 brake engaged for those T cells in their neighborhood. In 1994, he and a junior colleague conducted a groundbreaking experiment. They introduced a molecule able to block tumor cells from interfering with a T cell's CTLA-4 braking mechanism. **When they gave this same molecule to mice that had been injected with human cancer cells, the animals' T cells swarmed and destroyed the tumors. Dr. Allison had unleashed the animal's own immune system against cancer. That molecule, ipilimumab, is what saved Sharon Belvin's life.**

Approved by the FDA in 2011, ipilimumab was the first in a new class of cancer immunotherapies known as "<u>checkpoint inhibitors</u>." The name comes from the fact that they block (or inhibit) the brakes (or checkpoints) that tumors use to fend off T cells. Since Allison's breakthrough, other scientists have discovered other checkpoints—yes, tumor cells have more than one way to keep T cells at bay—and invented other drugs with the power to disable them.

One of the best known of these drugs is **Keytruda**, which is used to treat a multitude of cancers, including melanoma, stomach cancer, bladder cancer, urinary tract cancer, and esophageal cancer. **Keytruda blocks a checkpoint called PD-1. But you may know it simply as "<u>the Jimmy Carter drug</u>." When the former president was diagnosed with metastatic melanoma that had spread to his brain, this is the immunotherapy that eradicated all signs of his cancer, giving him a new lease on life back when he was 91 years old, and now awarding him the distinction of being the United States' longest-living president.** Other PD-1 checkpoint blockers include **Opdivo** (used to treat melanoma and other cancers) and **Tencentriq** (used to treat small cell lung cancer).

<u>**By clearing a path for T cells to attack cancer, immunotherapies like these make it possible to survive cancers that used to be a surefire death sentence.**</u> **But for reasons that aren't yet clear, checkpoint inhibitors cure only about a quarter of the patients who receive them.** One reason may be that some patients don't have enough T cells, or T cells with

enough energy, to penetrate and kill tumor cells, a concept called **immune exhaustion**. So preventing tumors from stepping on the T cells' breaks, as checkpoint drugs do, doesn't make any difference.

Thankfully, there's a new wave of cell-based therapies that might prove even more powerful. Known as "adoptive cell transfer" treatments, these therapies use naturally occurring or genetically enhanced immune cells to treat cancer.[15] As I stated earlier, the immune system can eliminate cancer. But "can" doesn't mean "always does." These new-wave therapies seek to make it happen more often, generally by giving immune cells a helping hand. **Dr. Elizabeth Jaffee**, deputy director of the Johns

---

By clearing a path for T cells to attack cancer, immunotherapies like these make it possible to survive cancers that used to be a surefire death sentence.

Hopkins Sidney Kimmel Comprehensive Cancer Center in Baltimore, told a reporter from STAT News, **"The hope is that we can turn cancers from ones that don't attract immune cells into those that do."**

In Chapter 6, I told you about CAR T-cell therapy and its awesome ability to vanquish blood cancers like leukemia. **Scientists create CAR T cells by slipping a new gene into billions of a patient's T cells, which have been removed by a simple blood draw.** Once the genetically engineered T cells are returned to the patient, they make a beeline for the tumor cells and morph, Transformers-style, into a lethal fighting machine. Better still, the CAR T cells replicate themselves. **As a result, a whole army of T cells directed against the cancerous invader courses through the body—and, as far as scientists can tell, does so forever! Yes, a single treatment—not weeks of chemotherapy or radiation— could be a *forever* cure.**

---

15 "Developing Neoantigen-targeted T Cell–Based Treatments for Solid Tumors."

Tool #2: Personalized Cancer Vaccines

While CAR T cells are the first cellular therapies for cancer, they certainly won't be the last. Hard on their heels are **personalized cancer vaccines**. Here's how they work: If you look closely at the surface of a tumor cell, you'll see that it's bristling with antigens, typically a unique protein that the **CAR T-cell therapies are able to detect and attach themselves to.**

But what if T cells could be engineered to find and attack *dozens* of tumor antigens at once? With more targets on their back, tumor cells would have a harder time escaping the T cells that scientists unleash on them. And the T cells that hunt down those tumors wouldn't destroy healthy cells that should be left in peace.

That's the reasoning behind **neoantigen cancer vaccines**. *Neoantigen* means that the antigens are new, the result of mutations found only in tumor cells. A *vaccine*, of course, **refers to a mechanism that sends your immune system into battle—in this case, not to prevent a disease** (as vaccines for flu and COVID-19 do) **but to attack it. Part of the challenge is that no two patients' tumor neoantigens are alike.** So a neoantigen vaccine must be uniquely personalized, crafted to find the neoantigens on an individual patient's tumor.

How is this possible? Scientists start by sequencing tiny bits of the tumor obtained via biopsy, looking for mutations that produce neoantigens. They then select the thirty or so "best" neoantigens—those found in abundance and most likely to attract T cells. Those neoantigens are synthesized in the lab and packed into a vaccine. **Over several months, patients receive injections containing millions of these neoantigens, which are designed to trigger the immune system to produce T cells that will attack the neoantigens and the tumor.** Pretty ingenious, right? **By 2020, clinical trials were underway or on the drawing board for a slew of neoantigen vaccines developed to combat illnesses like glioblastoma, triple-negative breast cancer, advanced melanoma, and non-small-cell lung cancer.**

Tool #3: Natural Killer Cells

Meanwhile, another major front in the war on cancer is also opening up. In this case, the cancer-fighting battalion consists of natural killer (NK) cells. Yes, that's their real name, and there's good reason to think that these brawnier, higher-endurance cousins of T cells can be made to live up to their billing. One advantage of NK cells is that they don't incite the sometimes disastrous immune response that CAR T-cells can fuel. Also, NK cells don't even have to come from the patient they're going to treat: Blood from a single donor or banked umbilical cord blood can supply NK cells for countless patients.

Dr. Bob Hariri, my coauthor, is one of the pioneers in using NK cells to combat cancer. His company, Celularity, mentioned in Chapter 2, harvests NK cells from human placentas. The placenta is often regarded as a throwaway organ, but it's packed with stem cells as well as NK cells—and they're more youthful than those found in the bone marrow of adults or even children. Xiaokui Zhang, Celularity's founding chief scientific officer, calls them "Day Zero" cells because they're newborns with "this intrinsic attribute of persisting longer." Tests in lab dishes and mice suggest that these placental NK cells may last twice as long as ordinary NK cells. That's invaluable because ordinary NK cells "hang around for about two weeks and then they're gone," says Zhang. "So we asked, how can we make NK cells into a cancer-fighting product that can last longer?"

Zhang says the placental NK cells also secrete higher levels of enzymes that break apart tumor cells, along with a toxic brew of proteins called cytokines that also kills tumor cells. Plus, the placental NK cells bristle with more receptors—the surface molecules that sniff out targets like "the strange antigens on tumor cells." Just like detectives have a better chance of tracking down a fleeing suspect if they sic more bloodhounds on the trail, so NK cells with their profusion of receptors have a better chance of tracking down tumor cells.

In short, there's mounting evidence that placental NK cells can be used to patrol the bloodstream on a seek-and-destroy mission against cancer. But Celularity isn't planning to send NK cells into battle with only their natural weapons. The company also selects for those with high levels of a receptor that increases NK cells' kill power, and it's genetically engineering them to be more resilient. NK cells also appear to be effective against solid tumors. **"For today's CAR T-cells, solid tumors are the graveyard where they go to die," says Zhang. "We think NK cells can overcome what limits CAR Ts."**

Celularity's experimental NK-cell therapy, **Taniraleucel**, has shown considerable promise in lab mice that had been injected with cells from human glioblastoma multiforme—a fatal form of brain cancer that took the lives of two prominent U.S. senators, Edward Kennedy and John McCain. **After Celularity's specially formulated NK cells were injected in the mice's brains, the cancer cells either vanished entirely or were drastically reduced in number. Celularity has since launched a human clinical study of its NK cells.**[16]

Tool #4: Tumor-Infiltrating Lymphocytes

Yet another battalion in the T-cell army is composed of **tumor-infiltrating lymphocytes** (TILs), which are white blood cells that have already burrowed into a tumor. TILs are a potpourri of cells, packed with different receptors. They can be used to target an array of different tumor antigens, so they have a better chance of attacking every tumor cell. Still, the TILs have infiltrated enemy territory, are heavily outnumbered, and need urgent reinforcements. Fortunately, **Dr. Steven Rosenberg of the National Cancer Institute** has figured out a way to send in more troops to assist them in completing their mission.

So far, his results have been extraordinary. <u>**Just over half of patients with advanced melanoma have benefitted from his TILs, their disease remaining in remission.**</u>[17] After more than three years of follow-up, only one of twenty-four patients who'd had a "complete response" (with their melanoma becoming undetectable) had suffered a recurrence. **In small studies, Rosenberg's TILs have also cured patients with advanced bile duct**

---

16 Awadalla, "Natural Killer Cell (CYNK-001) IV Infusion or IT Administration in Adults with Recurrent GBM (CYNK001GBM01).

17 Goff et al., "Randomized, Prospective Evaluation Comparing Intensity of Lymphodepletion Before Adoptive Transfer of Tumor-Infiltrating Lymphocytes for Patients With Metastatic Melanoma."

cancer, breast cancer, colon cancer, and cervical cancer. A biotech startup, **Iovance Biotherapeutics**, is testing TILs in multiple varieties of cancer, hoping to replicate Rosenberg's remarkable success on a much larger scale.

From the look of things, TILs might have two advantages that the current generation of CAR Ts lack. **They're able to lay waste to solid tumors, as Rosenberg has found. And they might beat back cancer longer than CAR Ts do—possibly even permanently.**

> **Just over half of patients with advanced melanoma have benefitted from his TILs, their disease remaining in remission.**

Tool #5: Exosomes

There's finally even hope of defeating one of the most fearsome enemies of all: pancreatic cancer. At the moment, it has a truly dismal prognosis. Only 20 percent of patients survive for a single year after diagnosis; only 7 percent survive for five years.[18] Enter Dr. Raghu Kalluri of MD Anderson, who is developing cancer-fighting exosomes.

As mentioned in previous chapters, Exosomes are minute bags (or "vesicles") excreted by cells, containing growth factors to stimulate repair and rejuvenation. Their contents range from DNA and proteins to fatty molecules called lipids. While typically we consider exosomes produced by stem cells to be pro-regenerative, exosomes produced by cancer cells are believed to play an important role in the spread of cancer, bursting out of tumor cells, fusing with healthy cells, and turning them malignant. This ability to enter other cells and alter their fate may sound scary, but it could also prove to be fantastically helpful. **"We want to see if we can exploit the capacity of exosomes to enter specific cells by providing them with cargo that has anti-cancer effects,"** says Kalluri. **"We want to use exosomes like a Trojan horse"—but to deliver a _beneficial_ payload, not a _lethal_ one.**

---

18 Hirshberg Foundation for Pancreatic Cancer, "Prognosis."

To achieve that, Kalluri is engineering exosomes to deliver anti-cancer genetic material to tumors. His "iExosomes" are engineered to contain tiny bits of a DNA relative called siRNA, for "short interfering RNA." These siRNAs interfere with a cancer-causing protein called KRAS, which is the result of a mutation found in 80 percent of people with pancreatic cancer.[19] "We incorporate the siRNA into isolated and purified exosomes—trillions of them," says Kalluri. **First developed in pancreatic cancer cells growing in lab dishes and then injected into mice with pancreatic tumors, <u>his iExosomes seemed to cluster around the pancreas, where they shrank the tumors, stopped the cancer from spreading, and extended the animals' survival</u>.**[20]

Granted, scientists have cured cancer in countless mice using therapies that failed when tested in human beings. **So we shouldn't let our expectations run wild when it comes to experimental treatments.** But when we touched base with Kalluri, his hopes were justifiably high as he prepared to test his iExosomes in a human study. Best of all, he believes that exosome-based therapy won't be limited to patients with pancreatic cancer.

His iExosomes seemed to cluster around the pancreas, where they shrank the tumors, stopped the cancer from spreading, and extended the animals' survival.

Tool #6: Focalyx Technology for Prostate Cancer

"Time goes on. So, whatever you're going to do, do it. Do it now. Don't wait."

—ROBERT DE NIRO, actor and prostate cancer survivor

Before we move on, I also want to tell you briefly about another important breakthrough in cancer treatment that's available *right now*. **It's an innovative solution for prostate cancer—the single most common form of cancer among men in the U.S., other than skin cancer. About one in**

---

19 Kalluri, "Exomes in Cancer Therapy."

20 Bradley, "iExosomes Target the 'Undruggable.'"

eight men are diagnosed with prostate cancer during their lifetime, a disease that kills more than 34,000 men each year.[21] So you ought to be aware of this highly effective treatment that might help you or someone close to you.

As you may know, one problem with the traditional approach to treating prostate cancer is that it can have a disastrous effect on your quality of life. In many cases, a surgeon saves the patient by removing his entire prostate gland but robs him of his sexual potency and leaves him incontinent. It's a brutal price to pay. We desperately needed another option, and we've found one, thanks to a urologist in Florida, **Dr. Fernando Bianco**. I was introduced to him because my prostate had enlarged, forcing me to get up multiple times each night to urinate—a common issue as men age.

As I soon discovered, Dr. Bianco has created an ingenious technology called **Focalyx** that works brilliantly for many men with enlarged prostates or prostate cancer. He begins by doing a specialized MRI to detect malignant and benign tumors in the prostate gland. Then, instead of a standard rectal biopsy, **he's figured out a fast and painless way of gathering tumor samples by going through the perineal skin—a less invasive approach that vastly reduces the risk of infection.** Having located any suspicious lesions with GPS-like accuracy, Dr. Bianco then destroys the cancerous cells with intense cold or heat, **preserving the healthy prostate tissue and its function.**

What's great about this ultra-targeted treatment is that it's so much less disruptive than the standard surgical approach. <u>With Dr. Bianco's patented methodology, there's no surgery, no radiation, no hospitalization. The whole procedure is done in a doctor's office. Best of all, his low-key approach lets the patient preserve his prostate function so he doesn't have to live in fear of incontinence and impotence.</u>

When I sat down with Dr. Bianco to discuss his breakthrough, he told me about the personal crisis that had inspired it. For years, he'd performed radically invasive surgery in the traditional manner, sincerely believing that he was making a difference in his patients' lives. **Then a twelve-year study revealed in 2012 that the standard approach was often worse than**

---

21 American Cancer Society, "About Prostate Cancer."

the disease itself![22] Dr. Bianco was stunned. As he told me, "It threw me into a deep depression, but then it turned into a drive to find a new way that would not put men at risk of suffering from incontinence and impotence." The "new way" that Dr. Bianco pioneered offers a safe and precise alternative—"an intervention that is *not* a quality-of-life-changing event." I utilize his services myself and even invested in the company.

It's important to note that in most cases, the disease will not cause harm to the majority of men who have it, and most men tend to outlive the disease.[23] **So it's important not to do treatments that are unnecessary,** but when they are, it's certainly nice to have an option that can be done in a doctor's office versus in a hospital, and one that doesn't leave a man incontinent or impotent. To learn more about how to access his technology, visit focalyx.com.

Tool #7: The Pathway to Restoration

"Just take a daily pill and you are cancer-free."

—OSMAN KIBAR

So far, we've talked primarily about two transformative approaches in the campaign against cancer: the development of diagnostic tests that detect the disease earlier than ever and an array of innovative therapies that harness the power of our own immune system. But there's one other breakthrough that I also want to mention briefly. **Imagine if cancer could be stopped in its tracks and turned into a chronic, manageable disease. Of course, nothing beats preventing or curing cancer. But this is the next best thing.**

In Chapter 9, I introduced you to **Osman Kibar**, the founder of Samumed, now known as **Biosplice**, a biotech company that's attempting to totally revamp the way we heal our bodies from disease. Biosplice is developing targeted treatments to tackle a number of scourges, including cancer. **The**

---

22 Blanding, "The Prostate Cancer Predicament."

23 Bill-Axelson et al., "Radical Prostatectomy or Watchful Waiting in Prostate Cancer—29-Year Follow-Up."

company is leading the way in what Kibar calls "restorative medicine," including drugs that will stop solid tumors (such as lung or breast cancers) and liquid tumors (such as leukemias) from multiplying out of control.

One way to think of these drugs is that they function like a release valve, making it possible to let out toxic air from cancerous tires. The key is the Wnt signaling pathway that dictates to cells how to differentiate into various cell types and regulates how they divide. As we age, this pathway deteriorates, giving rise to problems that can lead to cancer. The solution? Create drugs that rejuvenate the pathway so that cell division doesn't stray off course. Essentially, cancer is the result of cell division gone wild. So restoring the Wnt pathway to its youthful glory can reestablish the body's healthy equilibrium.

The secret probably lies in your kinases. *Huh? What?* As Kibar explains, there are more than 500 types of specialized proteins in the body called kinases. They are master regulators, molecular taskmasters that oversee fundamental biological processes. Biosplice has discovered a sub-branch of kinase that plays a crucial role in translating genes into various proteins. The company capitalized on that discovery by inventing the chemistry to safely and effectively nudge those kinases in the right direction, ensuring that the right composition of proteins is generated within a cell. "Once you do that, the cell is healthy again," says Kibar, speaking as if this biological wizardry is no big deal!

It helps to think of protein production like a factory. If the assembly line gets off-kilter, the product comes out wrong. "In cancer, some switch is faulty, so the assembly line for that production goes to a different path and gives you a different protein," says Kibar. "Our small-molecule drugs can intervene at the right point in that assembly line to channel the production away from those bad faulty proteins and back towards healthy proteins."

There are many different mutations that can cause cancer. But rather than develop different drugs for each of these situations, Biosplice's revolutionary game plan is to fix the problem at the source— the pathway. Just think. You wouldn't need numerous different drugs to treat numerous different cancers. Instead, Biosplice is using a single small-molecule drug to attack *six different cancers* that it expects to respond well: prostate cancer, triple negative breast cancer, non-small-cell lung cancer, ovarian cancer, endometrial cancer, and colorectal cancer.

Biosplice is also fine-tuning that drug compound and splitting it into four additional compounds that are even more targeted. "We're going for exquisite selectivity," says Kibar. "Laser precision." The more precise, the fewer unwanted off-target effects.

Meanwhile, to participate in its clinical trials Biosplice has been recruiting patients who are considered terminal. These are people who are expected to survive a few months at most, whose prospects could hardly be worse. But listen to this: In Biosplice's Phase 1 clinical trial, several such patients have remained stable for up to twelve months.

One molecule that Biosplice is studying actually penetrates the blood-brain barrier, depositing a high percentage of the biologically active therapy into the brain. **Why is that such an important breakthrough? Because cancer that spreads to the brain can be a death sentence, with few available treatment options.** "We're hopeful that this molecule treats both the primary and metastatic tumors," says Kibar. "We believe we should be able to improve the survival of these patients."

Even more incredible, Biosplice's cancer-busting molecule can be delivered in the form of a daily pill. Listen to Kibar explain: **"The idea is if you have cancer, and your cancer-causing mutation matches one of our target indications, then you start taking the pill. The pill doesn't fix the mutation. But as long as you're taking it, the mutation doesn't translate into a cancer."** How amazing is that?

Once again, for scientists at the forefront of innovation such as Kibar, this quest is deeply personal. His father died of cancer, and that prompted Kibar to consider questions he hadn't thought about much. *Why are we here on Earth? What's our purpose?* "By the time you hear the news that you have terminal cancer, you lose the ability to take a step back and take stock of what you've done in life and what you didn't get a chance to do in life," he says. "You're just worried about dying and not dying, and you're off balance with respect to all your feelings and emotions."

Like me, like you, like all of us, Kibar wants to win this war on cancer once and for all, so that nobody has to suffer in this way—so that we can restore health and happiness to millions of families. **His ultimate vision is "to turn cancer into a manageable chronic condition where you just take a daily pill to remain cancer-free." Pop a pill a day to crush cancer? That might just be the greatest prescription ever!**

As I hope you can see, this cascade of stacking technological breakthroughs is creating a nearly unstoppable momentum. And with passionately driven, brilliantly accomplished pioneers like Jeff Huber, Mary Lou Jepsen, Dr. Jim Allison, Dr. Bob Hariri, Dr. Steven Rosenberg, Dr. Raghu Kalluri, and Osman Kibar on the case, we've never had so much reason for optimism.

So please, based on what you've learned here, don't wait; take action. **Get yourself tested, ideally with a full-body MRI and the GRAIL blood test.** Find a location near you, or you're welcome to contact Fountain Life to schedule a test, or arrange one through your own doctor. **In this chapter you've discovered that a multitude of approaches that harness your personal immune system, such as individualized cancer vaccines and NK cells, are helping scores of people treat—and beat— cancers that used to be terminal. And also the power of broccoli sprouts, my favorite prevention technique, which are full of cancer-busting phytochemicals. There are so many options to combat cancer that you no longer have to settle for traditional methods alone, such as chemotherapy and radiation, which for some can feel as bad as the disease itself.**

Most importantly, remember that cancer is an equal-opportunity scourge: Nobody thinks it's going to strike them, and yet cancer will impact 40 percent of the population. The tools you've learned about in this chapter can help you prevent it, catch it when it's small and very treatable, or take advantage of treatments that could be great alternatives and are far less toxic and, in many cases, far more effective than the standard options. I hope that this intensive chapter has inspired you and helped you to perhaps reduce the fear that so many have of this disease.

All right, our next chapter is on an immensely important subject that impacts an astonishing **50 million people in the U.S.—autoimmune disease. Let's turn the page to learn about how inflammation leads to dangerous mutations throughout your body and the latest breakthroughs that are treating it at the source. . . .**

CHAPTER 20

CONQUERING INFLAMMATION AND AUTOIMMUNE DISEASE: BRINGING PEACE TO THE BODY

The Latest Research on Treating Crohn's Disease, Multiple Sclerosis, Rheumatoid Arthritis, and Psoriasis

In this chapter, you'll learn about real healing and relief for people who once had no hope. They're fighting autoimmune disease, an onslaught that strikes tens of millions of people. But it's also the arena for many of the most exciting and imaginative advances in regenerative medicine. <u>Here are some of the new ideas we'll be covering:</u>

- A breakthrough treatment that can obliterate the pain and suffering of Crohn's disease and rheumatoid arthritis with precision electrical stimulation.
- A new approach using the power of stem cells to treat rheumatoid arthritis in children and help adults with late-stage heart failure or agonizing lower back pain.
- A leap in treating type 1 diabetes by replacing missing "beta cells," which once seemed impossible.
- The basis of autoimmune disease (and many other diseases) is inflammation, which leads to dangerous mutations. It's how the body breaks down. You'll learn about new therapies to stop inflammation in its tracks, including one that removes inflammatory factors from blood plasma.

- **We'll also share with you simple ways to modify what you eat and follow an anti-inflammatory diet.**

Before we begin, let's take a step back for a moment. What do we mean by autoimmune disease? **In essence, it's a cellular civil war, and the destruction is brutal.** Peter Diamandis calls it a "breakdown of homeostasis," the delicate balance between letting infections run wild (which would kill you in a New York minute) and ambushing our own cells. Our fine-tuned immune system gets derailed and dysregulated. Instead of following genetic orders to terminate hostile microbes, our white blood cells defect to the dark side. They begin raiding our own tissues and the organs they're supposed to protect. **Friend becomes foe. The result? Relentless pain, soul-killing exhaustion, a severe loss of function, and—in severe cases—reduced life expectancy.**[1]

Quick quiz: What's the most common class of chronic illnesses in the United States? If you're like most people—or like me, before I had the opportunity to do research for this book—you might have guessed **heart disease, or diabetes, or cancer.** But like me, you'd be wrong. <u>**The most prevalent threats to our energy and well-being are autoimmune diseases, more than a hundred in all.**</u>

- **In Crohn's disease, the immune system mauls the cells of the large or small intestines.**
- **In rheumatoid arthritis, it wrecks the membranes that line our fingers and toes, ankles and wrists.**
- **In type 1 diabetes, it destroys the insulin-producing cells of the pancreas.**
- **In multiple sclerosis, it shorts out the wiring of our central nervous system.**
- **In lupus, the invasion is global, tearing into kidneys, lungs, skin, heart, and brain.**
- **Autoimmunity may even be linked to autism.**[2]

---

1 Esposito and Schroeder, "How Autoimmune Diseases Affect Life Expectancy."
2 Velasquez-Manoff, "An Immune Disorder at the Root of Autism."

The leading national organization in the field estimates that *50 million people* **in the U.S. are challenged by autoimmunity**[3]—**nearly double the total diagnosed with heart disease,**[4] **more than twice the number living with cancer.**[5] **It hits women hardest of all, at three or four times the overall rate for men.**[6] (Among them: singers Selena Gomez and Toni Braxton, and my friend Kim Kardashian.[7]) **Autoimmune disease is one of the top ten leading causes of death in female children and women in all age groups up to age 64.**[8] What's more, it's getting more common each year. **Over the last half century, studies show that the incidence of common autoimmune diseases has doubled and even tripled.**[9] **Rates among children are skyrocketing. It's the closest thing in the Western world to a 21st-century plague.**

Does this sound like a national health crisis to you? It does to me, too. Yet to this day, autoimmune diseases are underdiagnosed, undertreated, underreported, understudied, and underfunded. Primary care doctors commonly miss them. Frontline specialists—rheumatologists, gastroenterologists, neurologists—often fail to connect the dots. Federal funding for autoimmune disease research has stalled at an amount equivalent to 15 percent of how much ($7.17 billion) is allotted for studying cancer. **It's hard to fathom that a condition afflicting one of seven Americans could fly under the radar, but there it is.**

3 American Autoimmune Related Diseases Association, "Autoimmune Facts."

4 Centers for Disease Control and Prevention, "Heart Disease Facts."

5 American Cancer Society, "Cancer Prevalence."

6 Angum et al., "The Prevalence of Autoimmune Disorders in Women: A Narrative Review."

7 Anarchy and Autoimmunity, "Flourishing in the Face of Autoimmunity."

8 AARDA, "Autoimmune Facts."

9 Nakazawa, *The Autoimmune Epidemic.*

SO WHERE DOES AUTOIMMUNE
DISEASE COME FROM?

"It is a colossal task for the immune system to maintain tolerance to self and yet be ready to react to everything in the world around us."

—BRUCE BEUTLER, Nobel Prize–winning immunologist and geneticist

With the help of whole genome sequencing, we know that some people are predisposed to autoimmune disease from birth. But heredity isn't the whole story—far from it. **Identical twin studies suggest that our genes account for maybe one-third of our risk, or even less.**[10] **So genetics alone can't explain why these disorders are snowballing.** It's safe to say the human genome has not changed over the past fifty years.

So where does autoimmune disease come from? The usual suspects include infections, toxic chemicals in the environment, heavy metals, and ultraviolet radiation. **(In one study, researchers found 287 industrial toxins** *in fetal cord blood*, **passed to newborns by their mothers before birth.**[11]**)** But while scientists may differ about the specific triggers for autoimmunity, **it's now widely accepted that the root cause of autoimmune disease is inflammation.**

What's really happening when your sprained ankle turns an angry red and swells to twice its size? Why do we feel so much pain? The answer is **inflammation, your body's natural response for healing**—an ancient survival mechanism to fight off infection and repair damaged tissue. The problem is that **the wrong kind of inflammation—and too much of it—takes a mighty toll on your body.**

There are **two main types of inflammation: acute and chronic. Acute inflammation is painful but generally positive, because it starts the healing process.** In the first few minutes after an injury, the damaged tissue sends off an SOS alarm throughout your entire body. By making your blood vessels leaky (hence the swelling), acute inflammation enables immune cells to quickly enter the affected area and start immediate repairs.

---

10 Boston Children's Hospital, "Autoimmune Diseases."

11 Nakazawa, *The Autoimmune Epidemic*.

But what if that original insult to the body never gets fixed, or keeps getting repeated? The result can be chronic inflammation, which activates your immune system into a state of wartime readiness for months or years at a time. Chronic inflammation can lead to epigenetic DNA damage and diseases ranging from rheumatoid arthritis to cancer.[12] Most autoimmune patients get trapped in an inflammatory loop, a lifetime of pain and addictive painkillers. They desperately need a fresh approach, a way to restore their *balance* and get back to their body's natural immune set point.

So what's the solution? Once it's lost, can homeostasis be recovered? A number of emerging therapies suggest that it can. You're going to be so glad you read this chapter. If you know anybody who has lupus or rheumatoid arthritis or Crohn's disease, I strongly encourage you to keep reading. Because we're about to address one of the greatest advances in the fight against autoimmune disease: the exciting field of bioelectronics. Let's start with the story of a brave girl who was at her wit's end with the torment of autoimmunity, for whom nothing seemed to help . . . but who wouldn't take no for an answer.

STORY OF KELLY OWENS

"We have met the enemy and he is us."

—WALT KELLY, creator of the comic strip *Pogo*

At age 13, Kelly Owens was healthy and physically active, like any other normal kid. She was tap-dancing in her New Jersey school play when she seemed to sprain her ankle—no big deal, right? She figured she'd be back to normal in a week or two.

But the swelling refused to go down. The injury sent "a toxic wave" through her body, as Kelly told us. Over the next several months, the pain radiated up the teenager's legs, then her arms . . . until it landed in her gut with a vengeance! Kelly found herself running to the bathroom twenty times a day, like she had the world's worst case of food poisoning. Except it

---

12 National Cancer Institute, "Chronic Inflammation."

didn't go away. Scans showed extensive inflammation in both her small and large intestines—the signature of Crohn's disease, one of the better-known autoimmune diseases.

Crohn's disease is a painful and potentially fatal condition that torments nearly 800,000 people in the U.S. alone. Twenty thousand more are diagnosed each year. (About the same number suffer from ulcerative colitis, a related inflammatory bowel disease.) **Crohn's strikes people in their prime, usually before they turn 35. It causes unimaginable abdominal pain and cramping, diarrhea so severe you feel like you're turning inside out, weight loss and fatigue so crushing that getting out of bed feels like climbing the Himalayas. People with Crohn's run a higher risk of colon cancer, as well as dangerous bowel obstructions. Seventy to ninety percent wind up in surgery, which often winds up failing within ten years.** Large portions of their bowels may end up having to be removed, leaving them forever dependent on an ostomy bag to eliminate waste from their body.

Here's the grim kicker: There's been no definitive cure for Crohn's, or for autoimmune disease in general. When Kelly's GI tract went on strike, nearly twenty years ago, standard treatments were a roll of the dice—at best. At a time of life when her friends were stressing over prom or their next algebra test, Kelly was shuttling in and out of emergency rooms with flare-ups so excruciating she thought she would die.

In spite of everything, Kelly excelled in school and became a high school teacher in Hawaii. Then she turned 25 and her whole body went on tilt. Just as aging is really one disease with many faces, autoimmune disorders are a subset of aging with the same trip wires. Once you develop one of them, you're a lot more likely to get two or three others.

Kelly's knees and ankles swelled up like balloons. Walking became agony, to the point where her husband, Sean, had to carry her from room to room. This all-too-common complication of Crohn's is inflammatory arthritis. It strikes young adults, children, even infants.[13]

---

13 The more common form of arthritis, osteoarthritis, comes from wear and tear on the joints, with no immune system involvement. It develops more slowly, and is more common when we get past 65.

Kelly was forced to quit her teaching job. She lost 32 pounds. There were days, she'd say, when she felt like a 90-year-old woman. She pushed herself to crisscross the country in search of a better treatment option, some new medicine that just might help. Aspirin and ibuprofen, the standard anti-inflammatory drugs, can be GI irritants for people with Crohn's or colitis. Methotrexate, a lower-dose version of a cancer chemo-therapy drug, made Kelly nauseous without easing her symptoms.

For the moment, the gold standard treatment for Crohn's is a group of cellular medicines called *biologics*. **They're genetically engineered proteins derived from human cells,** and you'll be hearing more about them later. **Biologics have benefitted millions of patients and have coaxed some into remission. They don't help everyone, however, and they didn't help Kelly.** Her doctors had nothing else to offer but high-dose prednisone, a corticosteroid—great for quick symptomatic relief, but useless for slowing the disease's progress. **Worse yet, steroids mount a scorched-earth assault on our immune system. Prednisone can lead to glaucoma, diabetes, tuberculosis, and lymphoma, a cancer of our white blood cells.** By her mid-20s, Kelly was diagnosed with osteoporosis, a thin-ning of the bones linked to long-term steroid use. **"Nothing worked," she said, "but I sure got the side effects."**

TOOL #1: TREATING CROHN'S WITH BIOELECTRONICS

"If you're going through hell, keep going."

—WINSTON CHURCHILL, British prime minister during World War II

Though her future looked bleak, Kelly was unsinkable. She refused to give in or give up. She sustained her fighting spirit with an outlook I'd recommend to everyone. **Kelly allowed that Crohn's was her** *now*, **but flat-out refused to accept it as her** *forever*.

Her story turned when she found a trailblazing neurosurgeon on Long Island, an out-of-the-box inventor with a fresh idea for what ailed her. **This game-changing therapy isn't a magic pill or potion or protein. It doesn't mess with our genes. It's totally nontoxic. It taps into the** fundamental force that already runs our nervous system and has a big impact on our immune system, too.

What was the inventor's secret? As you may have guessed, a budding hope for people with Crohn's—and lots of other problems—**is based on electricity.** It's an area with immense potential; **Google's Verily Life Sciences and GlaxoSmithKline have invested more than $715 million into it since 2015.**[14] **Bioelectronics is a prime example of how brilliant minds are working to replenish our natural life force. The most promising potential cures are miracles just waiting to be unleashed from *within* us—in this case, from the electricity that crackles up and down the longest nerve in our body.**

As Kelly Owens will tell you, "If you're going to be stuck with a terrible disease, this is the best century to be stuck with one."

KEVIN TRACEY, BIOELECTRONICS PIONEER

"When you have exhausted all possibilities, remember this: you haven't."

—THOMAS EDISON, iconic American inventor

When Kevin Tracey was a neurosurgical resident at New York–Presbyterian Hospital, an 11-month-old named Janice came in with burns over three-quarters of her body: an accident with a pot of boiling pasta water. Somehow the medical team stabilized her. Three weeks later, with the relieved family smiling on, Tracey celebrated Janice's first birthday in a room decked with streamers and balloons. The baby couldn't have been more cheerful. One day after that, her organs shut down.[15] Her blood pressure plunged through the floor. Janice succumbed to the lethal immune response known as septic shock. Her body flooded with an inflammatory substance called tumor necrosis factor, or TNF. She died in the young surgeon's arms.

Tracey had lost patients before, but he couldn't let this one go. TNF is

---

14 Hirschler, "GSK and Google Parent Forge $715 Million Bioelectronic Medicines Firm."

15 Behar, "Can the Nervous System Be Hacked?"

a *cytokine*, a chemical messenger that promotes pain, swelling, warmth, and redness, the telltale components of inflammation. When it first senses an infection, our immune system deploys cytokines to signal other immune cells to enlist for a limited tour of duty. **Once the infection is under control, the body switches up its immune response by generating *anti-inflammatory* cytokines and getting back to home base.**

But *Janice never had an infection*. It just didn't add up. Why did the baby's white blood cells secrete so much TNF? What pushed her immune system off the rails?

Putting a promising surgical career on hold, Tracey detoured to the field of immunology and endless mice studies. His research led him to challenge a medical gospel: the germ theory of disease, which went back to the 1860s and the French chemist Louis Pasteur. Based on experiments with spoiled food, Pasteur concluded that sickness came from microorganisms outside our body. It followed that our immune system worked to keep us well—that it played a purely positive, protective role.

THE BREAKTHROUGH IN AUTOIMMUNE DISEASE: UNDERSTANDING THE POWER OF THE VAGUS NERVE

When Dr. Kevin Tracey first spotted the hole in the germ theory, he started looking for answers. What could be causing the immune system to attack the body instead of protecting it? He found a clue in some mid-1990s animal research that focused on the power of the *vagus nerve*.

What is it? The vagus nerve runs from the base of the brain—roughly parallel to your ears—through the neck, chest, and abdomen, and then to literally every major organ via bundles of thousands of fibers. **It controls breathing, swallowing, and speech. It also connects the brain to the gut, our "second brain."** Have you ever had a "gut feeling" or "butterflies" in your stomach? Have you ever taken a deep breath to calm down? Whether you know it or not, your vagus nerve was controlling your emotional state.

And Tracey wondered: Could the vagus nerve be the missing link in

chronic inflammation? Could we treat disease by hacking into the nervous system? And here's the breakthrough: Could electrical impulses help a sick person recover?

In 1998, he tested his hypothesis with anesthetized lab rats. Using a handheld surgical tool, he touched the rats' vagus nerve with a live wire. **The animal's inflammatory cytokines were scaled back to a healthy, harmless level. That was a huge eureka moment for Tracey. It led to what he called "the birth of bioelectronic medicine."**

WHAT IS BIOELECTRIC MEDICINE?

"Electroceuticals" have been with us since ancient Egyptians soothed their joint pain by standing on electric catfish. (I'd ask you to not to try this at home—those fish can generate up to 450 volts!) Some better-known examples of bioelectric medicine include the cardiac pacemaker and cochlear implants. I'm sure you've heard of deep brain stimulation, where electrodes are implanted to reduce tremor in Parkinson's patients. In 1997, the FDA approved vagus nerve stimulation for treating epilepsy, and a few years later for depression—among the most dramatic breakthroughs in modern medicine.

But before Dr. Tracey, no one had shown that the nervous system talked to the immune system. In fact, the idea was heresy. Besides, nerves were fixed within tissues. How could they communicate with free-floating white blood cells? Yet the animal experiments proved that those signals were being received, loud and clear. **They pointed to a time when electricity will mobilize the body's own machinery to manage all sorts of illnesses.** (Talk about *future shock*!)

Over the next eleven years, as head of the Feinstein Institute and cofounder of SetPoint Medical, Tracey worked with his team to better understand the nervous-immune pathway—or **the *Inflammatory Reflex*,** as he named it. As it turns out, the human body is one big circuit board, with neurons winding in and out of organs to regulate their immune response. **The vagus nerve is tuned to recognize excess inflammation and send alerts to the brain. Then it carries the brain's electrical response to our spleen, a truck stop for white blood cells.**

<u>We have Tracey to credit for the "cytokine theory of disease," which</u>

clarified the concept of autoimmunity. The germ theory wasn't wrong, but it was incomplete. With due respect to Pasteur, some of the biggest threats to our health come from *within*.

Thanks to Tracey and other trailblazing scientists, we're finding out that some of the best solutions come from the same place.

"We are stronger in the places we have been broken."

—ERNEST HEMINGWAY

Back in the 1980s, Tracey played a big role in developing biologics, those heavily marketed, cell-based medicines like **Humira** and **Rituxan. Now he wants to make them obsolete.** As Tracey sees it, biologics are too broad a brush. Though safer and more targeted than steroids or chemotherapies, **they're lifetime drugs that still weaken the immune system in its fight against pneumonia, diabetes, high blood pressure, and lymphoma.** And as Tracey pointed out, **biologics "don't even work in about half the patients who take them."**

The beauty of bioelectronics is that it takes aim at a specific bundle of nerve fibers. It targets the tissues or organs where the immune system has run amok, but nowhere else. The therapy calms inflammation by depressing cytokine levels across the board, but stops short of wiping out any one of them. **The immune system stays intact to fight another day: gain without pain.**

**One woman came in unable to hold a pencil
and was soon bicycling ten miles.**

In 2011, Tracey launched a proof-of-concept trial for patients with **rheumatoid arthritis,** a rampant, stubborn **disorder that shortens the lives of more than 1.3 million Americans.**[16] **The first results were astound-**

---

16 According to a 2018 study at Washington University School of Medicine, people with rheumatoid arthritis are more than twice as likely to develop heart disease.

ing. Within two weeks of receiving vagus nerve stimulation, subjects reported less pain. Their swelling went down—and MRIs revealed that bone erosion had actually been *reversed*. Six of eight patients saw their disease ebb away. One woman came in unable to hold a pencil and was soon bicycling ten miles.

In 2017, Kelly Owens ran across a notice for another early bioelectronics trial—for Crohn's disease—on clinicaltrials.gov. (As an aside, let me recommend that resource to anyone saddled with a disease with no effective treatment. Experimental therapies come with no guarantees. But you give yourself a shot by enrolling in a legitimate trial, and clinicaltrials.gov is the best place to find one.)

The study was being run by Kevin Tracey's associates in Amsterdam. Did a little thing like moving to Europe stop Kelly? Not a chance. She and her husband, Sean, sold their car "and everything in our house that wasn't nailed to the floor," she says. They raised money from friends and family and GoFundMe. With Kelly's cane and wheelchair in tow, they moved to Holland for five months.

In a forty-five-minute procedure, a surgeon implanted into Kelly's chest a device the size of a thumb drive, a "microregulator" that spoke the vagus nerve's language: a pattern of electrical impulses, dished out in tiny milliamp doses. The device was activated by a small magnet that Kelly held over her chest four times a day, one minute at a time. The results were almost instantaneous. Going to sleep the night after the surgery, she realized she didn't need her pain meds. Two weeks later, running late for a doctor's appointment, she sprinted up two flights of stairs without thinking twice—and then looked down at her husband, still at the bottom, standing there slack-jawed.

The trial enrolled sixteen Crohn's patients, none of whom had responded to conventional therapies. While the number of subjects in this trial was small, the results were impressive. <u>With bioelectronics, eight made dramatic progress: markedly less inflammation, greater mobility, fewer hospital admissions. Four of those eight made it all the way to remission, with little or no residual disease—and no side effects.</u>

Kelly is one of those four. Her inflamed colon has healed. She eats salads without a second thought. **The swelling in her joints is gone. She works out on an elliptical these days, and hikes for miles**—when she can spare the time, that is, from her full-time job as director of education and outreach at the Feinstein Institute in Manhasset, New York. **Three years[17] after her trip to the Netherlands, she has no symptoms, no pain. She's off all her meds. Kelly has reset her immune system to where it was at age 12,** before she began fighting her fifteen-year war.

Kevin Tracey is the first to acknowledge that bioelectronics isn't a panacea for autoimmune disease, not yet at least. The search for optimal "dosing" is still a work in progress. Some subjects have shown little improvement. Tracey suspects that **different Crohn's patients might benefit from pulses aimed at different bundles of nerve fibers, just as various types of breast cancer respond to diverse biologics.**

In a prime example of Moore's Law, SetPoint's second-generation implant is the size of a pencil eraser, fastened directly to the vagus nerve. **An integrated battery has a ten-year-plus lifespan and is recharged with a wireless collar.** Doctors control the electrical doses with an iPad app. As the technology advances and the science moves through larger trials, **bioelectronic medicine is poised to help millions of patients.** Tracey believes it could someday replace both chemical drugs and biologics, with less risk and lower costs. <u>**The technology's potential for eliminating pain—not only in your back, but throughout your body—is breathtaking.**</u> (Remember we covered multiple solutions for living pain free in Chapter 11.)

To show her gratitude for "the person who gave me back my life," Kelly Owens sent Tracey a gift: her pink cane. It's proudly displayed in the scientist's office, among his framed diplomas and plaques and piles of papers on his world-shaking discovery.

Kelly's sure she'll never need the cane again.

Now let's turn to a second powerful tool that's showing even more near-term promise for treating the most difficult autoimmune diseases.

---

17 As of mid-2020.

TOOL #2: USING STEM CELLS TO
TREAT AUTOIMMUNE DISEASE

"These tiny cells (stem cells) may have the potential to help us understand,
and possibly cure, some of our most devastating diseases and conditions."

—BARACK OBAMA, 44th President of the United States

While bioelectronics is still in a relatively early stage of testing on various autoimmune diseases, there's another therapy that's already well into advanced FDA trials.[18] It was pioneered by Dr. Silviu Itescu, whom I had the great pleasure of meeting at the Vatican's Unite to Cure conference. As CEO of Mesoblast and former chief of transplantation immunology at Columbia University Medical Center, Dr. Itescu found that your body—your bone marrow—contains a homegrown pantry of non-steroidal, anti-inflammatory medicines. We know them as stem cells. In the fight against autoimmune disease, early evidence suggests that all these cells may need is some reinforcement.

The native stem cells are also known as *mesenchymal precursor cells*, some of the body's most versatile and potent building blocks. They differentiate into bone, cartilage, muscle, or fat—whatever we need. **After an injury, they're crucial on two counts. They keep inflammation within normal, healthy bounds, plus they repair damaged tissue. The problem, as you know by now, is that stem cells grow scarcer with age,** especially in people with chronic problems like rheumatoid arthritis. **As our stem cell army gets exhausted, Itescu explained, there comes "a tipping point where the immune disease is rip-roaring away and you don't have enough of your own stem cells to control the immune response."**

Mesoblast's solution is to replenish the body. A highly concentrated dose of stem cells goes to just the right spots, whether it's the bloodstream or the knees or the heart muscle. The company collects the cells from healthy adult donors, cultures and expands them at industrial scale, and injects them into a patient. Though different cell subtypes are matched to a

---

18 Mesoblast, "Biologic Refractory Rheumatoid Arthritis."

disease's inflammatory "signature," the two-step therapy stays essentially the same—what Itescu calls "a package of goodies" from "living delivery vehicles."

When the injected stem cells sniff out signals from injured tissue, they go into action mode and release a first wave of anti-inflammatory cytokines. Then comes the second wave, the recovery phase, where the stem cells secrete growth factor cocktails **to build new blood vessels and improve circulation and oxygen supply. As I described to you in Chapter 2, this is just the way stem cells solved my rotator cuff tear and the stenosis in my spine—without surgery. They removed the inflammation and stimulated my body to heal itself.**

While the stem cells leave the body after just a month or two, the secreted growth factors may circulate for a year or more. Those anti-inflammatory molecules are Mesoblast's secret sauce. **They recalibrate the body's immune thermostat to its natural setting.** And since they don't suppress the immune system, there's no added risk of infection or malignancy.

As a bonus, Mesoblast's proprietary medicines can be administered off the shelf. Our immune system doesn't mark these cells as "foreign." As a result, donors and recipients don't need to be matched.

"In a Phase 3 trial, after a single Mesoblast injection into the problem disc, 60 percent of patients reported minimal to no pain after twelve months."

Again, this is exactly what happened with me!

In advanced trials, Mesoblast is hitting triples, not singles. The company's first approved product has made remarkable headway in combating what Itescu calls **"the mother of all inflammation": graft-versus-host-disease. GVHD** is a dangerous complication of bone marrow transplants after blood cancer chemotherapy. **Most of these transplant patients are children. Even with steroids as a buffer, half of them get attacked by the donor marrow. The immune response is so violent that their mortality rate runs as high as 90 percent.** As of mid-2020, there were no approved therapies in the U.S. for children under 12.

Mesoblast's completed Phase 3 trial involved four weekly IV infusions of a product called Remestemcel-L. It was tried on children who'd failed to respond to steroids—who were at death's door—and yet 69 percent reached the six-month survival point. The stem cells pushed them into remission.[19] Just like that, the playing field for GVHD changed.

Other Mesoblast therapies have also shown dramatic promise in recent studies and are close to FDA approval. Here are just a few:

1. **Rheumatoid arthritis:** In a placebo-controlled Phase 2 trial with rheumatoid arthritis patients who'd failed to respond to biologics, **36 percent showed significant clinical improvement after one stem cell infusion, versus none in the placebo group.**[20]

2. **End-stage heart failure:** These patients face a one-year mortality rate of more than 50 percent, meaning half die within a year. In the past, these people have had only two options: heart transplants, where demand far exceeds supply, and mechanical pumping devices, which often send patients back into the hospital with gastrointestinal bleeding. Itescu believes that late-stage heart failure is "all about inflammation" and out-of-control inflammatory cytokines. **In another Phase 2 trial, a Mesoblast cellular medicine called Revascor, injected into patients' heart muscles, resulted in 76 percent fewer GI bleeding events and 65 percent fewer hospitalizations.**[21]

3. **Back pain:** More than 3 million people in the U.S. suffer from persistent low back pain, a chronic condition that accounts for more than half of all opioid prescriptions. **Many are lured into invasive and costly spinal fusion surgery, which fails at least half the time.**[22] While the typ-

---

19 Mesoblast Limited, "Children Treated with Remestemcel-L Continue to Have Strong Survival Outcomes at Six Months in Mesoblast's Phase 3 Trial for Acute Graft Versus Host Disease."

20 Reuters, "Mesoblast Cell Treatment Shows Promise in Rheumatoid Arthritis."

21 Mesoblast Limited, "FDA Provides Guidance on Clinical Pathway to Marketing Application for Revascor in End-Stage Heart Failure Patients With an LVAD."

22 Greene, "Health Insurers Look for Ways to Cut Costs for Back Surgery."

ical diagnosis is "degenerative disc disease," **Itescu is convinced that the root of this agony is inflammation**—specifically, an autoimmune response involving ingrown nerves and blood vessels.

In a Phase 3 trial, after a single Mesoblast injection into the problem disc, <u>60 percent of patients reported minimal to no pain after twelve months and 54 percent after twenty-four months.</u>[23] This therapy has already received conditional approval in Japan, where it's being fast-tracked to market. **Instead of fusing or removing the problem disc, regenerative medicine is healing it.** According to Hyun Bae, a professor of surgery at the Cedars-Sinai Spine Center, **"We are fast approaching [an] inflection point in the treatment of low back pain."**[24]

As I write this, there's no single approved cure for any of the hundreds of autoimmune diseases. But there's plenty of grounds for optimism, as you've seen in this chapter. We're at the stage where breakthrough interventions may be closer than most people think. **Like Kevin Tracey's bioelectronics and Dr. Itescu's mesenchymal stem cells, these innovative solutions aim to help our system self-correct—to** *reset* **our immune response, not suppress it.**

In fact, for those with type 1 diabetes, a disease that's widely believed to be manageable but not curable, **Harvard's Dr. Douglas Melton is transplanting lab-grown, insulin-producing beta cells—and hiding them from hostile immune cells by modifying the epigenome. His goal is nothing less than a cure.**[25]

Here's another example, a CAR T-cell cancer therapy spinoff. Scientists are extracting immune cells that have slacked off on the job. They get reengineered to do their duty, then reinjected into the patient.[26]

---

23 Anson, "Promising Results for Stem Cell Treatment of Degenerative Disc Disease."

24 Mesoblast Limited, "Durable Three-Year Outcomes in Degenerative Disc Disease After a Single Injection of Mesoblast's Cell Therapy."

25 Lau, "Epidemic of Autoimmune Diseases Calls for Action."

26 Tenspolde et al., "Regulatory T Cells Engineered with a Novel Insulin-Specific Chimeric Antigen Receptor as a Candidate Immunotherapy for Type 1 Diabetes."

Finally, **Cedars-Sinai Medical Center in Los Angeles is using virtual reality "distraction" therapy to alleviate chronic, severe pain, one of the most demoralizing aspects of autoimmune disease.** In a recent study there, patients using VR headsets for thirty minutes a day reported significantly less pain than a control group. How does VR work? The answer is that human beings are bad at multitasking—it wasn't on our evolutionary agenda. **An immersive, 3D experience floods the brain with so much multisensory input that pain can't get through.**[27]

TOOL #3: BLOOD BOYS AND THE POWER OF BLOOD PLASMA

Our next approach is the power of "young blood," a technology we mentioned briefly in Chapters 17 and 18 on heart disease and stroke. Have you heard of "parabiosis"? Let me explain it this way: If you splice together the circulatory systems of a young mouse with an old mouse, the old mouse gets biologically younger! The concept was satirized in the HBO series *Silicon Valley*, where a tech billionaire pays a young man to be his "blood boy" and transfuse his plasma as a longevity booster.

Setting moral issues aside, at least where the mice were concerned, **the rejuvenation impact was shocking. The old mouse's tissues and organs—even its fur—regained the characteristics of a far younger, healthier animal.** Follow-up studies both confirmed this finding and showed the reverse also held true. **Transfuse younger mice with blood from older ones and the biological clock spins forward, accelerating decrepitude and aging.**[28]

So how exactly does parabiosis work? There's no shortage of theories. Elevian, the Harvard team, is focusing on a protein called GDF11, a "young blood" factor that gets depleted in your blood serum as you get older. They are using it to treat heart disease and stroke. Another idea is that aging generates so many pro-inflammatory molecules that it shifts the body to an "always-on" alert mode and throws the immune system into overdrive. Over

---

27 Brody, "Virtual Reality as Therapy for Pain."

28 Wein, "Senescent Cells Tied to Health and Longevity in Mice."

time, this hyper state makes the body more prone to strokes, heart attacks, and neurodegenerative disease—in people as well as mice.

This is where blood plasma comes in. **What is plasma?** It's the liquid component of blood that contains no blood cells but is rich in hundreds of different proteins—plus, in people with autoimmune problems, disease-causing auto-antibodies. **The concept—at least in theory—is simple:** If we can flush out pro-inflammatory molecules, we can delay or even block the aging process, right? **That's the question that Irina and Michael Conboy, a dream team of bioengineers at the University of California, Berkeley, sought to answer.**

In their seminal 2005 study,[29] they connected the circulatory systems of two inbred, genetically identical mice—one old, one young. **For the older mouse, it was like the ultimate spa weekend. <u>Within _five weeks_, its dormant, aged stem cells began dividing again, repairing its muscle and liver cells. Its inflammation subsided. On a cellular level, the older mouse became absolutely younger and the younger mouse got objectively older</u>.**

Now, thanks to a new twist, we may be able to get these rejuvenating benefits without the vampire element or needing our own blood boy. Researchers are exploring a concept called **therapeutic plasma exchange, or TPE**, to replicate the Conboys' results and **slow the effects of aging in humans**. Therapeutic plasma exchange separates out the aging plasma and reinfuses the person with their old blood cells plus a plasma replacement fluid composed mostly of fresh albumin (the major protein in plasma) and saline. In this fashion, the inflammatory blood factors are winnowed out. **TPE has already been proven to help patients with autoimmune diseases like myasthenia gravis and Guillain-Barre syndrome, or those with relapses of multiple sclerosis.**[30] More recently, the remarkable AMBAR study showed that <u>**TPE slowed the cognitive decline of Alzheimer's patients by 66 percent.**</u>[31]

---

29 Conboy et al., "Rejuvenation of Aged Progenitor Cells by Exposure to a Young Systemic Environment."

30 National Multiple Sclerosis Society, "Plasmapheresis."

31 Loeffler, "AMBAR, an Encouraging Alzheimer's Trial that Raises Questions."

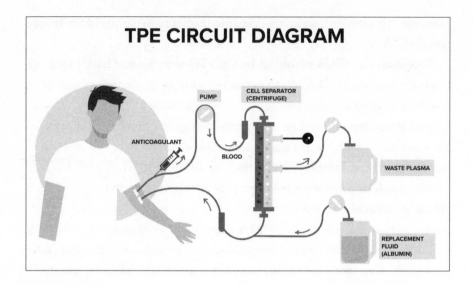

TPE CIRCUIT DIAGRAM

While the jury is still out on exactly how TPE does what it does, the therapy's combination of rapid-fire results, a strong safety profile, and profound regenerative effects could land it a starring role in the future of regenerative medicine.

TOOL #4: NEUTROLIS IS DISSOLVING NETS: A POTENTIAL CURE FOR AUTOIMMUNE DISEASE

Our next breakthrough technology could change the face of autoimmune disease, inflammation—and COVID-19! That's right, I said COVID. You're probably wondering what they all have in common. It involves the most prevalent white blood cell in our immune system, the **neutrophil**. When neutrophils are helping to repair a wound after you damage your skin, they actually release the DNA from the nucleus, like Spider-Man spinning a web to entrap his enemy. This mass of DNA, called **neutrophil extracellular traps, or NETs, sticks and helps to close and heal a wound**—a sort of **biological bandage**. The problems start when neutrophils are signaled to release their NETs at the wrong time or in the wrong place.

Problem #1: The NETs appear to be one of the fundamental causes of autoimmune diseases throughout the body—lupus, Crohn's disease, psoriasis, rheumatoid arthritis—because neutrophils improperly release their NETs.

Problem #2: NETs activated by COVID are causing blood clots. In the early days of the COVID-19 pandemic a sinister side effect of the infection was a blood-clotting problem where victims of COVID were getting clots in their smaller blood vessels for unknown reasons. Now we know that the cause was these NETs, which were trapping clusters of red blood cells into large clumps, blocking flow through blood vessels.[32]

So how does your body rid itself of these dangerous NETs? Is there a solution that could possibly impact this pervasive underlying ailment called inflammation? As it turns out, a brilliant Boston-based biotech company called **Neutrolis (Peter and I are both investors) has created several promising therapies, including one ongoing clinical trial in COVID.**[33]

Led by a pair of young immunologists out of the **Max Planck Institute and Harvard Medical School,** the company has invented a technology— a molecular scissors that cuts up free-floating DNA—to chop NETs (composed of DNA) into small pieces. Once the NETs are slashed, their fragments get cleared from the body. **The bottom line? Significantly lower inflammation, and an end to dangerous clumping in COVID patients.**

TOOL #5: AN ANTI-INFLAMMATORY DIET

"Tell me what you eat and I will tell you what you are."

—JEAN ANTHELME BRILLAT-SAVARIN,
19th-century French lawyer and essayist, and the
father of the low-carbohydrate diet

The second-best way to deal with autoimmune disease is to leverage the most powerful diagnostics and therapies on tap. **But the best way is to avoid getting sick in the first place. In either case, enemy number one**

---

32 Zuo et al., "Neutrophil Extracellular Traps in COVID-19."

33 LABline, "Neutrolis Announces Development of Enzyme for Severe COVID-19."

is chronic inflammation—which isn't altogether bad news. We can't do much about our genome, but there's a lot we can do to block inflammatory toxins that wreak havoc on our bodies.

It takes some planning and effort, but we can all take affirmative steps to shield our immune systems. You might begin with stress management: Stressful events are associated with an increased risk of having MS relapses, and periods of high stress are linked to the onset and worsening of rheumatoid arthritis.[34] We'll address this issue more fully in the context of mindfulness, in our concluding chapter.

One especially powerful tool to contain or prevent autoimmunity is an anti-inflammatory diet. Nutritional research counts on self-reported data and is generally less than reliable, especially when it tries to link diet and disease. Studies on certain foods, including dairy products and red meat, are all over the map. Even so, there's a fairly strong consensus over the following two lists, as cited by the **Harvard Women's Health Watch:**

Foods that cause inflammation	Foods that fight inflammation
Refined carbohydrates, white bread, and pastries	Olive oil
	Green leafy vegetables
Soda and other sweetened beverages	Brightly colored vegetables
Processed meat (hot dogs, sausage)	Fatty fish (wild salmon, mackerel)
French fries and fried food in general	Most fruits
Margarine and shortening	Nuts and seeds
	Green tea

Taken altogether, I'm sure you can see how these five latest breakthroughs on autoimmune disease can be invaluable in fighting this debilitating disease. Though many of these advances are in relatively early stages, the returns so far are strongly encouraging. **If you or anyone you care about is battling one of these conditions, you now have real answers you can discuss with your doctor. By controlling our stress and diet, we can go a long way toward alleviating and even preventing this 21st-century scourge.**

---

34 Nakazawa, *The Autoimmune Epidemic.*

Now that we know how to deal with inflammation, our next chapter examines a pair of challenges that impact a dramatic number of people both in the United States and worldwide. Where the root problems—and some of the most promising solutions—are all about lifestyle: obesity and type 2 diabetes.

MEASURING YOUR INFLAMMATORY AGE

To control and alleviate chronic inflammation, we first need to learn how to measure it. Edifice Health has created the world's first diagnostic test to reveal a person's "inflammatory age," or "iAge." It's built on data from Stanford's 1000 Immunomes Project, which uses AI and machine learning to home in on the most significant blood biomarkers. Their conclusion? The best gauges of our inflammation level—and our inflammatory age—are about 7,500 proteins. Edifice has condensed this large set to a core panel of five protein biomarkers—and **their predictive power is startling. They can foretell frailty seven years before it happens. They can predict cardiovascular aging—arterial stiffness and heart thickness—even in currently healthy people. The Edifice blood test and iAge metric is also able to pinpoint people with undiagnosed autoimmune diseases.**

This technology is up and running today, and should be commercially available by mid-2022. It costs $250 per test, or you can get a subscription service for $60 per month. But Edifice isn't stopping there. **Once you know your iAge, what can you do to *improve* your outlook?** Beyond lifestyle guidance, Edifice Health will also offer personalized supplements—currently under study by an Institutional Review Board—to improve a client's inflammatory profile.

CHAPTER 21

DIABETES AND OBESITY: DEFEATING A DOUBLE THREAT

How to Conquer the Twin Epidemics Hiding in Plain Sight

"The 'diabesity' epidemic is likely to be the biggest epidemic in human history."
—PAUL ZIMMET, MD, PhD

Diabetes and obesity are dangerous twins that are combining to produce one of the worst epidemics the world has ever seen. The "diabesity" epidemic is running rampant in wealthier parts of the world and has also begun to infect many developing nations as they adopt aspects of our unhealthy Western lifestyle. So let me ask you some direct questions. **Are you or is anyone you really care about overweight or obese? Are you frustrated with a lack of progress in achieving the level of fitness and energy that you desire and deserve? Are you or any of your family members currently dealing with the modern scourge of diabetes?**

Let me be clear. **This isn't about your appearance.** What I'm focused on here is enhancing your health and optimizing your life force, so that you feel joyously alive. With that in mind, this chapter will bring you up to date on where we are as a society and how we got here. Why? **Because we need to understand what's gone wrong in order to fix and avoid those mistakes.**

Most important, we're going to give you some simple yet highly effective tools that can change everything, helping you lose weight and prevent—or even reverse—diabetes. Many people, including plenty of doctors, have come to believe that diabetes is just something to accommodate and adjust to—a grim inevitability. But the best experts in

this field have shown how to turn it around. We'll share with you their proven strategies for success.

The solutions you'll encounter in this chapter are surprisingly straightforward—although, like most things in life, getting where you want to be requires knowledge, motivation, and determination. Bottom line? We've got you covered, whatever your situation. In this chapter here are some of the key tools and insights you will learn:

- **The diverse range of diseases accelerated by obesity and the difference between type 1 and type 2 diabetes, and what is meant by being prediabetic and why it matters.**
- **How if you're average weight or slightly overweight, reducing your daily caloric intake by just 300 calories (about one bagel per day) can offer a striking improvement in your cardio-metabolic health.**
- Our challenge with obesity isn't in our genes, or the failure of our willpower. **You'll learn that real culprit is *our food environment*, and what to do about it.**
- **That type 2 diabetes is actually reversible, and your pancreatic insulin-producing islet cells can come back to life and function.**
- **Finally, I'll show you two cutting-edge weight-loss medications that can radically change your life: an all-natural pill called <u>Plenity</u> that's been cleared by the FDA as a new tool for appetite and weight management and shown an average weight loss of 22 pounds. Plus a remarkable weight-loss drug called <u>Wegovy</u> that hit the market in June 2021.**

But first, let's start by simply acknowledging the severity and urgency of our situation. . . .

UNDERSTANDING THE DATA ON OBESITY

As much as we *say* we want to be in shape, more people today are obese than ever before. "An escalating global epidemic of overweight and obesity—'globesity'—is taking over many parts of the world," warns the World Health Organization (WHO). "If immediate action is not taken, millions will suffer from an array of serious health disorders." Globesity has almost tripled since 1975, according to the WHO. **Nearly 40 percent of the world's adults are now overweight and more than 13 percent are obese.** And as if that weren't bad enough, **more than 340 million children and adolescents ages five to 19 are obese or overweight**.

The U.S. tops the list of high-income countries with obesity and maintains the dubious distinction of having some of the fastest-growing obesity rates in the world. **In 2018, adult obesity in the U.S. surpassed 42 percent, up from 30 percent since 2000,** according to the Centers for Disease Control and Prevention. **About 74 percent of Americans age 20 and older are now either overweight or obese.** It's worth pausing for a moment of stunned silence to let that sink in.

To give you a sense of how important your weight can be, let's just take COVID-19 as an example. The number one factor for someone dying from COVID in 2020–2021 was age (the average age was 80). The second biggest factor was obesity. **Studies have shown that 78 percent of those who died from COVID were overweight or obese.**[1] Obesity stresses your immune system and your heart, and it leads to diabetes, so it's no surprise that obesity radically increases the risk of dying from COVID.

HOW TO TELL IF YOU'RE OBESE

Body mass index (BMI) is calculated by dividing your weight in kilograms by the square of your height in meters. But it's important to recognize that BMI—which was invented by a mathematician in the 1830s—isn't an ideal measure, to say the least. According to researchers from the University of Pennsylvania, BMI doesn't take into account muscle mass, bone density, overall body composition, or differences in race and gender. You could be a bodybuilder, with 1 percent body fat, but your weight might well mean that you'd be labeled as morbidly obese!

---

1 Kompaniyets et al., "Body Mass Index and Risk for COVID-19."

What I'm about to share with you isn't precisely accurate, but it should give you a sense. Most of us know if we're overweight if we're conscious about our own bodies. So, for example, if you're an average male at 5 feet 9 inches, overweight would be approximately 170 to 190 pounds, obese would be approximately 200 to 260 pounds, and severely obese would be 270 pounds or more.

If you're an average female at 5 feet 4 inches, overweight would be approximately 150 to 160 pounds, obese would be approximately 180 to 230 pounds, and severely obese would be 240 pounds or more. Again, these are not precise because the way BMI is calculated, hold on to your hat for this one and see if you can read the next sentence without going into a deep mathematical trance.

Body mass index (BMI) is calculated by dividing your weight in kilograms by the square of your height in meters. A healthy BMI is defined as 18.5 to 25, while a BMI of 25 to 30, is considered overweight. Obesity is defined as having a BMI of 30 to 34. Severe or morbid obesity is defined by a BMI over 40.1.

There are many other ways to measure how your weight contributes to your health, such as waist circumference, waist-to-hip ratio, skinfold thickness, and DEXA scans for bone density. This isn't to say that we need to get rid of the BMI altogether. It's still a useful way to track your progress. But I just want to stress that it's only a single data point among many and that it doesn't give you the whole picture.

And with three-quarters of Americans overweight or obese, the prognosis for this country's health is only getting worse. A leading team of medical scientists has predicted that, by 2030, *nearly half of all adults* in the U.S. will be obese. Nearly one in four will have what the CDC calls "moderate" obesity—a higher level of obesity that is just one step away from "severe" obesity. That report, published in the *New*

England Journal of Medicine, reveals in stark relief a country that is *dangerously* overweight and becoming more so every day.

How can you tell if you're obese? Well, obesity is defined in medical terms as having a body mass index of 30 to 34. **According to the CDC, moderate obesity is defined as a BMI of 35 to 39, while severe obesity is defined as a BMI of 40 or above. To put this in less technical terms, severe obesity corresponds to about 100 pounds of excess body weight.** Another shocking development is that more children are obese than ever before. **Since 1990, obesity rates have more than doubled among kids ages two to five and nearly *tripled* in kids over the age of six, according to the CDC. More than 20 percent of adolescents in the U.S. are now obese.**[2] **It's crazy, right? More than one in five of our kids face the perils of obesity! Why should we care that our kids are fat?**

In a meta-analysis of twenty-one studies involving more than 300,000 people, obese participants had an 81 percent higher risk of developing coronary artery disease.

Unfortunately, it turns out that obesity is the number one predictor of type 2 diabetes,[3] **which has also skyrocketed in recent decades.** Type 2 diabetes occurs when your body doesn't respond properly to insulin. **It now ranks as the seventh leading disease-related cause of death in the U.S. Besides being the top contributor to type 2 diabetes, obesity is associated with all of the leading causes of death, including heart disease, cancer, and stroke.**[4] **Overall, obesity is the second leading risk factor of premature death in North America and Europe, second only to smoking, according to the WHO.**

---

2 National Institute of Diabetes and Digestive and Kidney Diseases, "Overweight and Obesity Statistics."

3 Davies, "Type 2 Diabetes and Obesity: The Link."

4 CDC, "Adult Obesity Causes and Consequences."

In fact, it's hard to overstate how broadly damaging to your health it is to be obese. According to the Harvard T. H. Chan School of Public Health, **"excess weight, especially obesity, diminishes almost every aspect of health, from reproductive and respiratory function to memory and mood."[5] For example, in a meta-analysis of twenty-one studies involving more than 300,000 people, obese participants had an *81 percent higher risk of developing coronary artery disease* than those whose weight was categorized as normal. The Harvard T.H. Chan School also cites studies showing that obesity raises the risk of multiple diseases:**

- **Ischemic stroke risk is raised by 64 percent.**
- **Asthma risk is raised by 50 percent.**
- **Alzheimer's disease risk is raised by 42 percent.**

Obesity has direct associations with many types of cancer, including cancers of the breast, uterus, gallbladder, colon, esophagus, pancreas, liver, thyroid, and kidney.

And finally, obesity has direct associations with many types of cancer, including cancers of the breast, uterus, gallbladder, colon, esophagus, pancreas, liver, thyroid, and kidney.[6]

So what do you do? How do you begin? For starters, you need to know right now that obesity is preventable—if not 100 percent, pretty darn close. The same goes for type 2 diabetes. And for those of us who are already suffering, the science surrounding what we can do to help ourselves (and each other) has never been clearer.

Most exciting of all, there's emerging evidence from the UK that type 2 diabetes is potentially reversible. That's right, *reversible*.

---

5 Harvard T.H. Chan School of Public Health, "Obesity Prevention Source: Health Risks."

6 Massetti et al., "Excessive Weight Gain, Obesity, and Cancer."

Groundbreaking studies are shattering the widely held belief that type 2 diabetes is a lifelong disease that worsens over time.

This research shows that our bodies have an immense capacity for regeneration—that our bodies actually *want* to rejuvenate and restore. It's what we're programmed to do. **Specifically, losing weight rejuvenates critical insulin-producing cells in the pancreas known as *beta cells*. And regenerating those cells can actually put type 2 diabetes into remission.**

So when it comes to lessening the burden of obesity and diabetes, in many ways it's about regenerating our pancreatic or beta cells. And where do we begin on this journey of regeneration and repair? With food of course. **To a great degree, we are what we eat.**

THE SEDUCTIVE DANGERS OF
OUR FOOD ENVIRONMENT

"Sugar is now the most ubiquitous foodstuff worldwide, and has been added to virtually every processed food, limiting consumer choice and the ability to avoid it. Approximately 80 percent of the 6 million consumer packaged foods in the U.S. have added caloric sweeteners."

—ROBERT LUSTIG, MD

Is our challenge with obesity in our genes, or the failure of our willpower, or even a lack of exercise (if anything, exercise rates have gone up over the last couple of decades)? *No,* **say the experts.** The real culprit? *Our food environment.* Food is everywhere, all the time. **"The food environment is a powerful predictor of how we eat,"** says **Scott Kahan, MD,** director of the National Center for Weight and Wellness. **"And in America, the unhealthiest foods are the tastiest foods, the cheapest foods, the largest-portion foods, the most available foods, the most fun foods."**

As you've probably noticed, food now shows up in places where it never used to be: gas stations, toy stores, drugstores, and even bookstores. The array of foods and drinks available to us is dizzying, and the vast majority are highly processed. **To make matters worse, a growing number are *ultra-processed*.**

These food categories have recently been identified as risk factors for obesity as well as for diseases like type 2 diabetes, cardiovascular disease, and cancer.

Many of these products also contain added sugars or other sweeteners like high-fructose corn syrup—substances associated with obesity, type 2 diabetes, and nonalcoholic fatty liver disease. **Researchers have found that fructose can also disrupt healthy functioning of the immune system by causing inflammation.**[7] Meanwhile, these ingredients even show up in foods billed as healthy, such as granola bars, yogurt, and fruit drinks.

Yup, many of the foods and drinks that masquerade as being healthy are part of the problem, not the solution. **Why? Because low-fat often means high-sugar.** As I mentioned in Chapter 1, you really need to appoint yourself as the CEO of your own health, educating yourself to make informed and independent decisions while always retaining a great deal of healthy skepticism.

Another challenge is that we eat out a lot and people typically consume 20 to 40 percent more calories when they eat at a restaurant. In 2015, for the first time on record, Americans spent more money in restaurants than in grocery stores—meaning we're cooking less.[8] And this means we're consuming more calories than ever. By some estimates, <u>the average American now packs in more than 3,600 calories a day—a 24 percent increase from 1961</u>, when the average was about 2,880 calories. How many calories should we be consuming? Well the 2015–2020 U.S. Dietary Guidelines specify that women should consume about 2,000 calories daily and men about 2,500, although the requirements can vary depending on factors like age, height, and exercise status.

<u>What's even crazier is that restaurant meals today are *four times larger* than in the 1950s, according to the CDC.</u> Here are some examples:

- **In 1995, the average bagel measured three inches across and contained 140 calories; by 2015, just two decades later, it had more**

---

7 Jones et al., "Fructose Reprograms Glutamine-Dependent Oxidative Metabolism to Support LPS-Induced Inflammation."

8 National Restaurant Association, "Restaurant Sales Surpassed Grocery Store Sales for the First Time."

than doubled in size and calories, according to the National Institutes of Health.

- The average cheeseburger expanded from 333 to 590 calories.
- The average soda ballooned from 6.5 ounces and 82 calories to 20 ounces and 250 calories!

We've supersized everything—including ourselves!

That last example—the average soda size, not just in the U.S. but worldwide—points to one of the biggest problems of all: the seductive taste of liquid sugar.

The single largest contributor to calories and added sugar in the American diet now comes from sugary drinks, also known as sugar-sweetened beverages (SSBs), which include everything from soda and fruit drinks to sports and energy drinks. On average, SSBs add 200 calories a day to American diets. And when you drink SSBs, you absorb that sugar into your bloodstream in a matter of minutes. It is like mainlining a drug.

Sure enough, <u>studies show that people who drink one to two sugar-sweetened beverages a day have a 26 percent greater risk of developing type 2 diabetes than those who drink less than one sugar-sweetened beverage a month</u>![9] **I encourage you to create a habit that I adopted in my early 20s—no more soda. Try drinking water with lemon. It's one of the simplest things you can do to transform your health. And after a while, you don't even miss it.**

And while eliminating soda from your diet is one of the quickest and simplest ways to protect your health, *please don't replace it with juice*. Juice can contain as much or more sugar and calorie content, and the same goes for sports and energy drinks. Besides being packed with calories and sweeteners, many contain substances that haven't been evaluated by the FDA, not to mention high doses of caffeine. **These drinks have been shown to cause a dangerously rapid rise in blood pressure.**[10]

Okay, let's now turn our attention to the next food culprit: ***ultra-processed***

---

9 Harvard School of Public Health, "Sugary Drinks."

10 Wassef, "Effects of Energy Drinks on the Cardiovascular System."

foods. These contain ingredients common in industrial food manufacturing, like hydrogenated oils, high-fructose corn syrup, flavoring agents, and emulsifiers.

Researchers now associate ultra-processed foods—often loaded with sugar, salt, fat, and calories—with an increased risk of type 2 diabetes, hypertension, and cardiovascular disease. How tasty does that sound to you?

A 2018 study in the *British Medical Journal* also found that every 10 percent increase in the consumption of ultra-processed foods correlated with a 12 percent increased risk of cancer! As you'd expect, ultra-processed foods have been engineered to be as irresistible as possible. "Food companies do vast amounts of research to determine the optimal level of saltiness, the optimal level of sweetness, and what's the best mouthfeel," observed longtime nutrition scientist **Walter Willett, MD,** during a Harvard T.H. Chan School of Public Health discussion entitled Why We Overeat: The Toxic Food Environment and Obesity.

But you know what? **When it comes to food, your knowledge can set you free.** Let's say you're racing out to a morning meeting or to drop off your kid at school, so you grab a granola bar for a quick and convenient breakfast. It's healthy, isn't it? After all, it has *granola* in it, and that's good, right? *Wrong!* **Even with words like "nutri-grain" and "oats" emblazoned on the wrapper, that ultra-processed granola bar is packed with sugar, corn syrup, and preservatives. But once you know what's going on, it's easier to avoid these sneaky traps.**

A better solution: a bowl of oatmeal with a little milk and fresh fruit. It may not sound exciting; it requires a bit more effort than a granola bar; and you can't gobble it down in the car. *But that's the point!* These tiny changes—like swapping out a breakfast bar for a bowl of whole-grain oats or grabbing an apple—may seem too trivial to make a difference. Yet they add up in astonishing ways.

As you'll soon discover, changing what you eat for breakfast is just one of several simple tweaks—including a short "no-sugar challenge," brisk walks, and a minor increase in fiber consumption—that can help you shed pounds, boost your energy, and escape the dire threat of diabetes.

Equally important, you can also upgrade your own food environment

so that it actually *supports* your efforts to improve the way you eat. <u>For a start, what if you were to clean out all the unhealthy foods (and drinks) in your home that don't serve you? Have a healthy meal before you go shopping for food so you're not hungry when you're walking the isles, and stock up on things like fresh fruit, vegetables, and whole-grain bread instead of white bread.</u> Having reasonably healthy food options in your home when you're hungry or craving a snack makes a huge difference in your fight against obesity!

But first we need to talk a little more about why these subtle changes matter *so much more* than most of us realize.

DIABETES + OBESITY = DIABESITY

"The risk of type 2 diabetes increases geometrically with increasing body mass index."

—SCOTT KAHAN, MD, director of the National
Center for Weight and Wellness

The number of Americans diagnosed with type 2 diabetes has exploded in recent decades, almost doubling between 1980 and 2014. According to the CDC, **"more than 34 million Americans have diabetes (about one in ten), and approximately 90–95 percent of them have type 2 diabetes."** That figure is expected to swell to almost 40 million by 2030 . . . and to more than 60 million by 2060.

Before we go any further, I want to make sure that we're clear about some important distinctions between the different forms of diabetes. Type 1 diabetes, formerly known as juvenile diabetes, is an autoimmune disease in which the pancreas doesn't make enough insulin—a hormone that regulates many metabolic processes and allows your body's cells to receive the energy they need from glucose. This disease accounts for 5–10 percent of diabetes cases in the U.S., so it's much less common. According to the Juvenile Diabetes Research Foundation, about 64,000 new cases are diagnosed each year.

By contrast, type 2 diabetes, formerly known as adult-onset diabetes, accounts for 90–95 percent of all diabetes cases in the U.S. It's characterized by insulin resistance, high blood sugar, and a relative lack of insulin. It's also defined by a decline in the functioning of beta cells, whose primary role is to keep blood glucose levels in check by producing and releasing insulin.

I'm guessing that you've also heard the term *prediabetes*—**and there's even a good chance that you or a relative or close friend already have it. How come? Because an estimated 88 million adults in the U.S.—that's more than one in three people—have prediabetes.** What is it? Well, prediabetes is characterized by blood sugar levels that are higher than normal due to insulin resistance, but the levels aren't yet high enough to qualify as diabetes.

While prediabetes usually leads to type 2 diabetes—especially in people who are also obese or even overweight—about 85 percent of those with prediabetes don't know they have it. The fact that prediabetes frequently flies under the radar is all the more troubling because it's also a risk for other serious health issues, including heart disease and stroke. What should you do? **A simple blood sugar test can tell you if you have prediabetes,** so it's a smart precaution to ask your doctor if you should be tested.

YOUR FIRST BREAKTHROUGH: A TINY CHANGE IN CALORIES OVER TIME WILL TRANSFORM YOUR ENERGY, VITALITY, AND YOUR HEALTH

> *"To accomplish everything we did with caloric restriction, you'd need five drugs."*
>
> —WILLIAM E. KRAUS, MD, professor, Department of Medicine and Cardiology at Duke University

During the two-year investigation published in the *Lancet,* **people who reduced their daily caloric intake by an average of 12 percent—just 300 calories—showed striking improvements in cardiometabolic health among study subjects who were of average weight, or slightly overweight, and healthy. That's less than the number of calories in a bagel or a Starbucks scone or a power bar or a sweet-topped coffee.**

Avoiding just 300 calories per day allowed individuals to lose weight and body fat; their cholesterol levels and triglycerides improved, their

<u>blood pressure fell, and they had better blood sugar control and less</u> <u>inflammation.</u> This, my friend, is fabulous news! What other minor intervention can produce such massive changes for the better with so little effort?

"There isn't one drug that does all that," says William E. Kraus, MD, lead author of the study and a professor of medicine in the Division of Cardiology at the Duke Molecular Physiology Institute. "To accomplish everything we did with caloric restriction, you'd need five drugs."

Just 300 calories a day. It's incredible, right? Simply skipping that mid-morning donut or that afternoon Frappuccino or that evening bag of chips in front of the TV boosts all of your metabolic markers. And if that's not enough, check this out: It'll make you feel better, too. <u>Study subjects who succeeded in cutting 300 calories a day reported</u> <u>improvements in various measures of quality of life, such as increased</u> <u>energy, better sleep, and enhanced mood. In other words, this minor</u> <u>shift in lifestyle delivers *huge* gains in terms of life force!</u>

Study subjects who succeeded in cutting 300 calories a day reported improvements in various measures of quality of life, such as increased energy, better sleep, and enhanced mood. In other words, this minor shift in lifestyle delivers huge gains in terms of life force!

I love this finding because it doesn't take a massive amount of effort or willpower to cut 300 calories a day. Yet this one move brings disproportionate rewards in so many areas of your life! That's one of the key lessons I learned in interviewing billionaire investors for my book *Money: Master the Game*. One thing that sets them apart is that they're always looking for asymmetrical bets where the downside is small and the upside is enormous. This idea of moderately reducing your daily calorie intake is a winning bet that can yield really impressive benefits for your health.

What about people who are overweight and at risk of developing type 2 diabetes? **It turns out that losing weight—even amounts that may** seem relatively trivial—can dramatically benefit overweight people with insulin resistance or prediabetes. "Fortunately, even extremely small weight losses improve glycemic control—and moderate weight loss often prevents or ameliorates type 2 diabetes," says Dr. Kahan. "Weight loss of as little as 3–5 percent of body weight begins to improve insulin action and glycemic control."

In fact, the landmark NIH study known as the Diabetes Prevention Program found that overweight adults with impaired glucose tolerance who lost just 5–7 percent of their body weight—about 10–14 pounds in a 200-pound person—and logged 150 minutes a week of moderately intense exercise (like brisk walking for twenty minutes or so a day), reduced their risk of developing type 2 diabetes by *58 percent*.[11] Again, this is a simple solution with an outsized benefit. And while lifestyle changes and treatment with metformin (a popular diabetes medication) *both* reduced the incidence of diabetes in people at high risk, the lifestyle intervention was "significantly more effective than metformin."

The program proved so effective that other structured lifestyle intervention programs based on it are now offered in many communities for those at a high risk of type 2 diabetes. To find a center near you, Dietary carbohydrate is the major determinant of postprandial glucose levels, and several clinical studies have shown that low-carbohydrate diets improve glycemic control. In this study, we tested the hypothesis that a diet lower in carbohydrate would lead to greater improvement in glycemic control over a 24-week period in patients with obesity and type 2 diabetes. To find out more, visit their website at cdc.gov/diabetes/prevention/index.html.

---

11 The Diabetes Prevention Program Research Group, "The Diabetes Prevention Program: Description of Lifestyle Intervention."

DIABETES PREVENTION PROGRAM DETAILS

Research design and methods

Eighty-four community volunteers with obesity and type 2 diabetes were randomized to either a low-carbohydrate, ketogenic diet (<20 g of carbohydrate daily; LCKD) or a low-glycemic, reduced-calorie diet (500 kcal/day deficit from weight maintenance diet; LGID). Both groups received group meetings, nutritional supplementation, and an exercise recommendation. The main outcome was glycemic control, measured by hemoglobin A1c.

Results

Forty-nine (58.3%) participants completed the study. Both interventions led to improvements in hemoglobin A1c, fasting glucose, fasting insulin, and weight loss. The LCKD group had greater improvements in hemoglobin A1c (-1.5% vs. -0.5%, p = 0.03), body weight (-11.1 kg vs. -6.9 kg, p = 0.008), and high density lipoprotein cholesterol (+5.6 mg/dL vs. 0 mg/dL, p <0.001) compared to the LGID group. Diabetes medications were reduced or eliminated in 95.2% of LCKD vs. 62% of LGID participants (p <.01).

Conclusion

Dietary modification led to improvements in glycemic control and medication reduction/elimination in motivated volunteers with type 2 diabetes. The diet lower in carbohydrate led to greater improvements in glycemic control, and more frequent medication reduction/elimination than the low glycemic index diet. Lifestyle modification using low carbohydrate interventions is effective for improving and reversing type 2 diabetes.

LOSING WEIGHT CAN REGENERATE ISLET CELLS

"Type 2 diabetes is a reversible condition, and remission can be achieved and sustained."

—ROY TAYLOR, MD

A lifelong disease. A chronic condition. A progressive disease. Those have been the prevailing views of type 2 diabetes among doctors and patients for as long as anyone can remember. But researchers in the UK are now demonstrating that it really *doesn't* have to be that way.

The latest findings from the Diabetes Remission Clinical Trial (DiRECT), published in the *Lancet* and showcased at the American Diabetes Association's 2019 scientific session, are nothing short of remarkable. **In a nutshell, <u>losing a substantial amount of weight in a relatively short period of time can actually *reverse* type 2 diabetes</u>. "<u>People with type 2 diabetes now have a choice rather than a life sentence</u>," says Roy Taylor, MD, senior author of the study and professor of medicine and metabolism at the University of Newcastle in England.**

And that's not all. Not only did investigators demonstrate that reversal is possible, they also determined that it involves what is fast becoming **the Holy Grail in the treatment of diabetes—*the restoration of beta cells*—those insulin-producing cells in your pancreas.** Indeed, the trial's findings challenge and upend two of the most basic and widely held beliefs about type 2 diabetes: that the condition can't be reversed and that beta cells damaged during the diabetes disease process are lost forever.

For the longest time, everyone assumed that once beta cells were damaged due to obesity, they were *done.* Lost forever. Kaput. Well, guess what? **Dr. Taylor and his colleagues have shown that the beta cells are still there—they're just unable to perform because of excess fat in the liver and pancreas.** "These beta cells are not dead," says Taylor. "They've gone into a survival mode under the metabolic stress of excessive nutrition"— a polite term for too much food and fat.

Bottom line, when you take away the fat, the beta cells regenerate. They start producing insulin. And the diabetes disappears. And you've slashed your risk of a whole host of devastating complications, like

cardiovascular disease, kidney failure, Alzheimer's, amputations, impotence, depression, and blindness. I don't know what the scientific term is for a simple intervention that can heal your body in so many vitally important ways. But here's mine: magnificent!

So how much weight did people need to lose to send their type 2 diabetes into remission? The minimum magic number was about 22 pounds. But most of those who achieved remission lost even more—at least 33 pounds.

The impact of that weight loss was quite amazing. **For example, says Dr. Taylor, the risk of cardiovascular disease plummeted when participants lost around 33 pounds.** What's more, he adds, in a two-year follow-up with the patients in the DiRECT study, "there were no new cancers" among the 149 patients in the "weight-loss group." That's an exceptional result.

Bottom line? **"If people lose twenty-two pounds," says Taylor, "and keep it off for two years, there's a two-thirds chance they'll escape from type 2 diabetes."**

Now, if the truth be told, DiRECT's weight management program may sound pretty brutal, but Dr. Taylor was pleased to discover that **the participants in his study found this diet regimen "very acceptable" and that their hunger disappeared "after the first thirty-six hours."** It involved caloric restriction in the form of a milkshake diet totaling about 825 calories a day for about twelve weeks, followed by a gradual reintroduction of solid foods over another six weeks.

Let's take the example of Allan Tutty, who entered the study at the age of 52. **He'd been diagnosed with type 2 diabetes about a year earlier when he visited his doctor for a routine physical exam.** He remembers his shock when the doctor broke the news to him. "Are you sure?" asked Tutty. "Is this a mistake?" After all, he was just living a normal life, working and raising a family. Sure, he'd gained weight over the years, but nothing extreme. "I was feeling okay," he recalls.

At the local diabetes clinic he heard the same message, recalls Tutty. **"It was like the doctor said, 'You've got diabetes, deal with it. You've got it for life. There's no cure. There's no hope.'"**

Tutty, who lives in Sunderland, England, was still feeling angry and upset when he heard about the DiRECT clinical trial in nearby Newcastle. **But his attitude soon changed from *Why me?* To *Why not me?* Upset turned to hope—along with a healthy dose of resolve. When he told a doctor at the local diabetes clinic about the trial, the doctor remarked, "Well, good luck with that. You'll probably fail."** But Tutty was determined to prove him wrong.

When Tutty began the weight management program, he weighed 216 pounds. At a height of 5'10" this meant that he had a BMI of 31, putting him just over the line of obese. The diet was difficult at first, but he quickly adjusted. He made it through Christmas and New Year's without eating (or drinking) outside the daily regimen. **And by the end of the program he weighed 187 pounds, down a total of 29 pounds. It was a triumph!**

<u>**The effect on his health was spectacular. His fasting blood sugar level dropped into the normal range. Six months out he continued to be diabetes-free. And that's *still* the case more than seven years later.**</u> **While Tutty acknowledges that he hasn't kept off *all* the weight, he's kept off enough to remain free of diabetes.**

What's the secret of his continuing success? Tutty says he now eats meals at regular times and has taken to waking up early. "I like to get into work around half past seven in the morning, so I'm up at five, I take the dog for a walk, come home, and I religiously now have a bowl of porridge oats with milk and some nuts or fresh fruit." At lunch it's bean soup, and around 6 p.m. an early dinner of chicken or fish with vegetables.

To access the diet used in the DiRECT trial as well as several do-it-yourself versions, visit www.directclinicaltrial.org.uk. Click on **"Remission Resources"** for a preview of different eating plans. Before undertaking any such intervention, you should always check first with your doctor. You can also check out Dr. Taylor's recent book, *Life Without Diabetes*, which offers more of his detailed advice on how to reverse type 2 diabetes with dietary changes.

WHAT REALLY MAKES YOU GAIN
WEIGHT: CARBS OR FAT?

*"In every decade since 1950, people have been eating more fat, sugar,
meat, and calories—an average of 67 percent more fat, 37 percent more
sugar, 57 pounds more meat, and 800 more calories per person."*

—DEAN ORNISH, MD

We can't go any further without drilling down a little deeper into the all-important subject of *what **not** to eat.* The answer? *Refined carbohydrates*—which also happen to be the main ingredient in many of the low-fat so-called "health food" products that have become ubiquitous in recent decades, and which have contributed mightily to the epidemics of obesity and diabetes.

What's the problem with carbs? They cause spikes in blood sugar that raise insulin levels. And high levels of insulin—aka "the fat-storage hormone"—push the body to store calories as fat.

For now, one vitally important point to remember is that highly processed or refined carbs—for example, white flour, white bread, and pasta—are not your friends, however much you like them. The truth is, they behave almost like sugar in the body.

"Refined carbs are the hidden sugar," warns **Dariush Mozaffarian, MD**, dean of the Friedman School of Nutrition Science and Policy at Tufts University. "The weight gain associated with Skittles is exactly the same weight gain that's associated with Corn Flakes or white bread or a bagel," he adds.

A PRACTICAL GAME PLAN TO CRUSH DIABESITY

*"Highly processed carbohydrates are among the lowest-quality
components of the food supply, accounting for the majority
of diet-related disease in the United States today."*

—DAVID LUDWIG, MD, PhD

Before we wrap up this chapter, I want to leave you with two simple but powerful solutions that can help you to triumph over the double threat of obesity and diabetes. Please also remember to go back to review

Chapter 12, "The Longevity Lifestyle and Diet," to get additional motivation and insights on the extraordinary benefits of combining a plant-based diet with regular exercise and intermittent fasting.

Solution #1: Radically Reduce Your Intake of Sugar.

My coauthor and dear friend Peter Diamandis doesn't mince words. He declares simply that "sugar is a poison." Not convinced? Then check out Dr. Lustig's talks at youtube.com/c/RobertLustigMD. **If you're going to watch one video to improve your health and understand the devastating impact of sugar on our bodies, I highly recommend listening to Dr. Lustig's TEDx talk.**

Gary Taubes, author of *The Case Against Sugar*, concludes that "enough evidence exists for us to consider sugar very likely to be a toxic substance, and to make an informed decision about how best to balance the likely risks with the benefits. To know what those benefits are, though, it helps to see how life feels without sugar." That's exactly what Peter decided to do.

He and about two dozen of his Abundance members and my Platinum Partner Group teamed up in 2020 and created a WhatsApp group to complete a twenty-two-day "no-sugar challenge," which meant that they could eat no added sugar and very limited carbs during this sugar detox period. The challenge was guided by Guillermo Rodriguez Navarrete, PhD, a global thought leader on the effects of sugar addiction.

How did it pan out? Peter, whose sister, niece, and various staff members also took part, says, "It's been one of the most impactful things I've done. I had more energy, significantly reduced my need for blood pressure meds, and lost about five pounds."

What made it easy and possible? Doing it with other people and checking in with every meal. "The two-dozen people in the WhatsApp group would text each other photos of their meals, their weight loss, and we'd cheer each other on. The group support made it easy and fun," says Peter.

If you have a significant issue with weight, why not start by eliminating this single element from your diet for twenty-two days? Having done this myself, I can tell you that you'll see a radical shift in your energy and strength. Why not commit today? If you'd like more details about how to do this twenty-two-day challenge, visit lifeforce.com. But please make sure that you consult with your doctor before you do the challenge, to confirm that it's suitable for you.

Solution #2: Shift Your Diet to High-Quality Foods.

We've talked a lot about what *not* to eat. But what *should* you eat? **One core principle from experts like Dr. Ludwig is that we need to emphasize high-quality foods. That applies to carbs *and* fats. It might seem counterintuitive, but healthy fats can actually help to stabilize your blood sugar.** In his bestselling book *Always Hungry*, Ludwig declares, "The fastest way to lower insulin levels is to substitute fat for processed carbohydrates." **What fats? Consider olive oil, avocados, nuts, fatty fish (like wild salmon, arctic char, Atlantic mackerel, and sardines), and maybe even some full-fat dairy products (such as unsweetened yogurt). "Foods rich in fat will help you feel satiated, and they won't trigger the insulin high and crash that most processed carbs do,"** Ludwig writes. "Without insulin highs and lows, your blood sugar will be more stable and your body can access the fuel it's storing in your fat cells."

For carbs, consider non-starchy vegetables; any and all greens, including fresh salad greens; and beans, legumes, fruits, and whole grains. **Sometimes known as "slow carbs," whole grains can be a key component of a healthy diet, in part because they take longer to digest than refined grains and cause a relatively gradual rise in blood sugar.**

Think about replacing low-quality "white grains" with high-quality "whole grains"—for example, brown rice, quinoa, farro, and steel-cut oats (so, oatmeal for breakfast instead of sugar-sweetened cereal from a box). If you want to take it one step further, go for ancient grains like buckwheat, barley, wild rice, and spelt, which are even more nutritious.

Here's another valuable insight that's so simple and practical! Whole grains offer an added benefit: fiber, which some nutritionists call an overlooked superfood.

A meta-analysis in the *Journal of Diabetes and Its Complications* found that cereal fiber (that's to say, from whole grains) protects against type 2 diabetes. **A review of forty years of research by the WHO found critical health benefits associated with consuming at least 25–29 grams of fiber daily,** such as a reduced risk of type 2 diabetes, stroke, coronary heart disease, and colorectal cancer.

TWO BREAKTHROUGH
TECHNOLOGIES FOR OBESITY

Now that you understand the basic principles about what to eat and what *not* to eat, you're in a strong position to avoid or undo the many damaging effects of being overweight or obese. **But I also want to make sure that you know about two ingenious technological breakthroughs, which, when combined with smart lifestyle choices, can offer you powerful new weapons in the war on diabetes and obesity.**

First of all, <u>Gelesis</u>, a biotech company based in Boston, has created an all-natural pill called **Plenity** that takes the edge off your appetite by filling you up right before you eat. How does it work? Plenity is a superabsorbent hydrogel made from cellulose (which is derived from plants and vegetables, specifically cucumber) that is bound together with citric acid (also derived from plants). Plenity takes its cues from nature, basically mimicking the effect of eating raw vegetables like cucumbers. **As a result, there are minimal to none of the dangerous side effects and toxicities that we've come to expect from many other diet-related pills.**

Twenty to thirty minutes before lunch and dinner, you simply swallow three Plenity capsules along with two glasses of water. **The tiny hydrogel particles in these capsules expand by about one hundred times inside your stomach as they absorb the water around them. The result? You feel fuller and less inclined to overeat.**

Plenity, which has been cleared by the FDA as a weight management tool, is available by prescription for overweight or obese adults with a BMI of 25 to 40—a total of about 150 million people in the U.S.

How effective is Plenity? In a clinical trial involving 436 adults who were overweight or obese, the results were impressive.[12] Patients took

---

12 Greenway et al., "A Randomized, Double-Blind, Placebo-Controlled Study of Gelesis100: A Novel Nonsystemic Oral Hydrogel for Weight Loss."

three capsules twice a day in conjunction with a sensible diet and moderate exercise for about thirty minutes a day. **Over six months, 59 percent of the group that took Plenity lost an average of 10 percent of their body weight—about 22 pounds!** Patients in the group that took a placebo lost weight, too, thanks to the benefits of diet and exercise. But the results were significantly better for the Plenity group.

Even though it's natural and safe, you'll still need to talk to a healthcare provider, who can prescribe Plenity and have it shipped directly to your door. I also can't stress enough how effective Plenity was when used **in conjunction with exercise and diet—in other words, as part of an overall healthy lifestyle, not as a quick fix**. To learn more, visit MyPlenity.com.

Wegovy is the second technological breakthrough I'm excited for you to learn about. **A recently FDA-approved medication,** Wegovy has the potential to change the trajectory of your life or the life of someone you love. That may sound like hyperbole, but it's precisely what happened to Jeffrey Huang.

For many people who are struggling in vain with their weight, there's nothing more frustrating than walking into a doctor's office and being told that they need to control their diet in order to lower their HbA1c, a measure of glucose that's used to diagnose diabetes. This was exactly the case for Huang, who had reached the point where he could no longer bear to visit a doctor in person and resorted instead to conducting his medical appointments over the phone.

How come? Well, he weighed 380 pounds and felt ashamed of his weight. He was terrified of walking into a doctor's waiting room and finding that he couldn't fit in any of the chairs. He was sick of sitting in a doctor's office and listening to the same old lecture about eating healthier foods. It's not that he wasn't trying.

Huang felt like he was in a downward spiral with no way out. He'd been fired from his job, his marriage fell apart, and now his two daughters were living with their mother. At 43, Huang found himself alone, unemployed, and depressed.

In January 2021, a doctor warned that Huang's HbA1c level was at 11.6 percent. A cutoff of 6.5 percent is an indication of diabetes. He was already so far beyond this boundary that his doctor thought it was inevitable that Huang would end up in the hospital with perilous, life-threatening complications from diabetes.

Huang was skeptical when his doctors told him there was a new drug option called **semaglutide** (sold under the brand name **Ozempic**). **The doctor had seen some astounding results from this new drug, including a 50 percent drop in HbA1c levels and a weight loss of as much as 50 pounds. What's more, these dramatic improvements could happen quickly—sometimes within a couple of months.**

Huang's doctor mailed him some Ozempic pens, which he would use to inject himself with this groundbreaking drug once a week. He started on a low dose, which was then slowly increased. In the past, Huang had experienced almost every side effect under the sun from his medications. But you know what? With Ozempic, he experienced no side effects at all.

Six months later, when Huang heard his new HbA1c level, he was speechless. He asked if he'd been given the wrong patient's lab results. But they were his! His HbA1c level had dropped to 7.5 percent, and his glucose was now well-controlled. Incredibly, he had lost 65 pounds! Once his weight started to plunge, Huang could feel the bounce in his step again. His motivation and ability to exercise returned. He was a new person.

Leaving the doctor's office that day, Huang vowed that he'd win his family back and show them that they still had a husband and father worth fighting for. He was determined to prove that he could take care of himself and turn his life around.

Curiously, Ozempic wasn't originally intended to be a weight-loss drug. In fact, it's still better known as a treatment for type 2 diabetes. But initial studies showed how effective it could also be for adults who are overweight or obese. **In one study, people who took a once-weekly dose of Ozempic for nearly eighteen months lost an average of 15 percent of their body weight. Even more impressive, one-third of all participants lost 20 percent of their body weight.[13] That's comparable to what you**

---

13 Wilding et al., "Once-Weekly Semaglutide in Adults with Overweight or Obesity."

might expect from undergoing bariatric weight-loss surgery—a much more risky and invasive intervention.

The results were so striking that, in June 2021, **Novo Nordisk**—the giant Danish pharmaceutical company—was granted FDA approval for semaglutide as a weight-loss drug. **It's now marketed under the name Wegovy as a prescription medicine for adults who are obese or for adults who are overweight and have at least one weight-related ailment (such as hypertension).**

How does Wegovy work? It mimics a hormone, GLP-1, that helps to lower blood sugar levels after you've eaten a meal. It slows down how fast your stomach empties food. And by blocking a hormone that causes your liver to release sugar, it makes you feel less hungry.

Before taking this drug, you'll obviously need to discuss all the risks and benefits with your doctor. It's also worth emphasizing that this isn't a magic bullet that will somehow free you from the critical need to eat well and exercise regularly! **Like Plenity, Wegovy is designed for use as an adjunct to smart lifestyle choices such as a healthy diet and regular exercise.**

I hope by now that you're feeling excited and empowered! As you can see, there's so much you can do to take control of your weight and turn your health around, whether you're overweight, obese, or simply concerned that you might be letting things slide. **And what's so important to recognize is that little changes can make for big rewards. Remember? If you consistently remove 300 calories a day—that one muffin!—the effect over time can be transformative. Imagine if you did a bit more?**

But the best news of all is that we now know beyond any shadow of a doubt that type 2 diabetes is not a life sentence. We have the choice, the knowledge, the power, to *prevent* it and even *reverse* it, so that it's gone from our lives completely and never has to return.

Now let's turn our attention to a very different but equally urgent challenge: the quest to preserve—and even enhance—our cognitive powers and mental energy as we age. **Let's explore the newest breakthroughs in the war to combat Alzheimer's disease and dementia.**

CHAPTER 22

ALZHEIMER'S DISEASE: ERADICATING THE BEAST

"To put it simply, our brain span should match our lifespan."

—MERYL COMER, author of *Slow Dancing with a Stranger*,

a chronicle of her husband's war against Alzheimer's

Of all the gargantuan challenges in this section of our book, none is more daunting than Alzheimer's disease, the dominant form of dementia, with close to 6 million cases in the United States alone and at least 50 million worldwide.[1] Other degenerative ailments are ruthless, robbing people of their independence, their dignity, their zest for life. But Alzheimer's takes grand larceny a terrible step further. It steals our ability to plan or to follow an argument. It destroys language and memory and logical thought. **It robs people of their very *identity*, of all they are and everything they've been. If we lose our capacity to think clearly, who are we?**

Alzheimer's kills more Americans than breast and prostate cancer combined, and now ranks as the sixth-leading cause of death in the U.S. Pneumonia is a common cause of death in people with Alzheimer's because the loss of ability to swallow means that food and beverages can enter the lungs and cause infection. Other common causes of death among people with Alzheimer's include dehydration and malnutrition. It's a brutal way to die.

Alzheimer's strikes roughly 10 percent of people over 65. In the

---

1 World Health Organization, "Dementia Fact Sheet."

85-and-up set, it's more than one in three.[2] The toll is enormous—for patients, their loved ones, and society as a whole.

But today, there is tremendous reason for optimism! As you'll see in this chapter, **a new generation of medical pioneers is refusing to let Alzheimer's continue its devastating march through humanity.** They're leaving the beaten path and testing new clinical modalities, such as molecular pharmacology, immunology, neurosurgery, and even gene therapy, that may be widely available within the next five years or less. **If even one or two of these approaches find the success they're expecting,** *everything* **changes. Dementia could soon lose its awful power.**

What's more, all of us can take concrete steps *today***, from simple lifestyle changes to cognitive training, to greatly improve our odds of staying sharp through the years. We'll have a much better chance of dodging the gray twilight of Alzheimer's—for which there is only one recently FDA-approved medicine—as well as the less severe but more common disorder called** *mild cognitive impairment* **(MCI). In short, there is legitimate hope that dementia won't be scripted into our future. Leading scientists now believe that in the coming new normal, we'll preserve—and even** *enhance***—our mental energy as we age.**

Currently there are five[3] **FDA-approved drugs that manage these symptoms and just one**—Biogen's Aducanumab—that targets disease modification. Aducanumab was fast-tracked in 2021, with efficacy to be shown by 2030, causing no shortage of controversy.

But there's a high-beam halogen light at the end of this long, twisting, agonizing tunnel.

In this chapter, we'll introduce you to amazing original thinkers who are picking up the gauntlet against dementia. They're junking old assumptions and looking for upstream factors—like **neuroinflammation—that might be fueling the buildup of two very specific proteins that cause plaque in the brain, amyloid and tau. Best of all, they're not satisfied**

---

2 *The Economist*, "As Humanity Ages, The Numbers of People with Dementia Will Surge."

3 National Institute on Aging, "Alzheimer's Disease Medication Fact Sheet."

<u>with slowing people's descent into the oblivion of Alzheimer's—they're
seeking an outright cure.</u>

We'll share with you their exciting new scientific developments and
a few approaches that you can actively use yourself, including some
noninvasive options that have nothing to do with drugs, *period*. Because for the first time ever, legitimate breakthrough solutions are on
the horizon. They include:

- A simple **blood test that can predict Alzheimer's**—years before
  symptoms—with up to 96 percent accuracy,[4] enabling people to take
  protective measures to supplement protein levels and keep amyloid levels
  low, which some experts believe can prevent Alzheimer's.
- New drug discovery platforms that have identified **more than fifty
  drugs that prevent dangerous proteins from taking root** and a company called Marvel Biome that is **harnessing the power of the microbiome to fight neurodegeneration**.
- **A new system intended to clear toxins from the brain** that has been
  shown to improve cognition in older **mice when they received plasma
  infusions from younger mice**.
- An **Alzheimer's vaccine in late-stage clinical trials that has slowed
  disease progression with *few unwanted side effects***. Just one shot from
  Vaxxinity's vaccine every three to six months may train your immune system to fight Alzheimer's, reduces the number of brain amyloid deposits,
  and enhances mental functioning.
- Believe it or not, a blend of **psychedelic mushrooms that trains fungi's
  healing effects on neurodegenerative diseases like Alzheimer's**.
  Lion's Mane mushrooms have induced cognitive improvements in dementia patients—and they taste like lobster!
- **Simple but effective measures you can take to boost brain health**—
  everything from getting enough sleep (which naturally purges amyloid)
  to social interaction (which cuts Alzheimer's risk by twofold) to exercise
  (I'll explain why **a brisk walk is even better than a hardcore gym
  workout** when it comes to decreasing the risk of dementia).

---

4 *The Economist*, "The Search for a Cure for Dementia is Not Going Well."

- And an emerging treatment that has perhaps the greatest promise of all. The common belief has been that once a person's brain begins to deteriorate, memories and cognitive function are lost forever. And yet new research from USCF studying animals has demonstrated the brain does NOT permanently lose essential cognitive capacities and memories as previously thought. Rather, these resources have become trapped and blocked, and by reconnecting the communication between parts of the brain, they can be restored! We're going to look at thirteen cutting-edge approaches to tackling Alzheimer's that potentially can put us on the path of eradicating the beast.

ERASING ALZHEIMER'S

"I don't say 'curing' Alzheimer's. I talk about eradicating it."

—DR. RUDY TANZI

One of the leading scientists and pioneers in the world of Alzheimer's Disease is **Dr. Rudy Tanzi**, director of the Genetics and Aging Research Unit at Massachusetts General Hospital and vice chair of neurology and codirector of the McCance Center for Brain Health. Much of what we know about the elusive Alzheimer's disease is founded on his research, and he is the chair of the Cure Alzheimer's Fund Research Leadership Group. **Early in his career, he discovered the Alzheimer's gene, the beta-amyloid gene. He then played a key role in discovering subsequent genes that cause early onset familial Alzheimer's.** And the list goes on. He is a man of many hats, **as he is now both directing the Alzheimer's Genome Project and searching for the exact microbes (bacterial, viral, fungal) that populate an Alzheimer's brain and trigger amyloidosis, a hallmark of the disease.**

Rudy was born in Cranston, a suburb of Providence, Rhode Island, to parents of Italian descent. When he looked around him, he saw that most kids his age didn't go on to college. But Rudy always dreamed big. While he was tempted to pursue his passion for music, he decided to follow his interest in science. He majored in microbiology at the University of Rochester and entered the Henry Tabor Lab, where his career took off.

When other college students in his major were taking introductory biology classes, Rudy was devouring nature and science papers on the latest DNA mechanisms and molecular genetics. **He liked to think of himself as a visionary, not allowing himself to be locked into existing rules and formulas and unafraid to take science where it hadn't been before.** In the Tabor Lab he worked on genetic mapping of bacteria, where he soaked up knowledge like a sponge, surrounded by other pioneers of molecular biology.

Before he applied for graduate school, Rudy worked as a technician in Dr. James Gusella's lab. At that time, it was rare for a technician to be given their own project. But again, rules didn't mean much to Rudy. After asking Dr. Gusella for a small project to work on that could be his own, he was tasked with building the first **full genetic map of chromosome 21**, implicated in Down syndrome. **Rudy soon realized that people with Down syndrome have a high propensity for Alzheimer's. He told Dr. Gusella that he was going after the Alzheimer's disease gene, beta-amyloid.** His optimistic and driven mindset set him up for success, as you'll soon see.

In graduate school at Harvard, Rudy set off in hot pursuit of the amyloid gene. It was an ambitious, almost impossible goal. **People told him and his adviser that they were crazy and were going to waste years chasing a gene that was nonexistent, since amyloid is just the garbage in the brain.** But there was no doubt in Rudy's mind. **It took years of experiments, but he successfully cloned the gene and discovered the amyloid precursor (APP) gene.**

Rudy continued his passion for molecular genetics and neuroscience by staying at Harvard and **becoming a professor at Harvard Medical School and eventually the director of the genetics and aging unit at MGH.** There, he cemented his reputation as a leader at the forefront of Alzheimer's research and **co-discovered the first two early-onset familial Alzheimer's genes, PSEN1 and 2.**

So let's take a look at 13 possible solutions—tools for taming this beast that you can consider for yourself or those you love who might be facing a future of dementia or a current form of dementia or Alzheimer's.

Tool #1: Gamma-Secretase Modulators

For the last twenty years, Rudy has been working on drugs called gamma-secretase modulators. You can think of them this way: What Lipitor does for high cholesterol, gamma-secretase does for the brain. In Alzheimer's, neuroinflammation leads to loss of brain function and health. As the "housekeeping" cells in the brain, microglia are implicated in neuroinflammation. For thousands of years, they've been programmed to clear out toxic, foreign substances. The problem is they still assume your lifespan is thirty-five years. Nerve cells die as they form plaques and tangles, so the microglia get the signal to wipe out this part of the brain to "protect" you.

But how does this cause the loss of memory, mental sharpness, and personality we're all afraid of in Alzheimer's? The massive degradation of the brain from the microglia's overzealous housekeeping results in neuroinflammation that leads to cognitive decline. The only Alzheimer's drugs on the market remove the amyloid plaques in the brain. The catch is that this doesn't restore your cognition. It's like putting out a fire that has already destroyed the entire forest. But understanding the role of these plaques in Alzheimer's has opened up a golden age for drug development.

Tool #2: A New Way to Test Drugs That's 100 Times Faster and 100 Times Cheaper

What's equally amazing is that Rudy has also invented a way to test these drug candidates. He calls it "Alzheimer's in a dish": an index card–sized 96-well plate with a brain. According to the *New York Times*, it's going to "make drug discovery 10 times faster and 10 times cheaper." In practice, according to Rudy, it made drug discovery 100 times faster and 100 times cheaper. In these dishes, they've grown neurons and glial cells in a gel-like matrix that acts like the brain. Only four weeks after inserting the Alzheimer's genes, a classic plaque forms. A few weeks later, the amyloid causes the classic tangles to form. Now they have a platform to screen every drug and test each against both amyloid and tangle formation.

As a result, they have already identified fifty-one drugs that exist in

safe and natural products that stop amyloid production. Rudy has now brought forth a leading gamma-secretase modulator clinical trial candidate. **These are safer alternatives for reduction of the toxic amyloid protein in the brain.** These modulators cut gamma-secretase, which is responsible for forming the amyloid beta-peptide (APP) precursor to Alzheimer's; they prevent the dangerous proteins from forming in the first place. **Rudy's team has also identified several genes that are responsible for amyloid clearance.** They are planning to take these gamma-secretase modulators into clinical trials as I'm writing this chapter.

Tool #3: Testing Brain Amyloids as Part of a Routine Screening Could Allow You to Take Action Today

Remember how Rudy said he doesn't think of curing Alzheimer's, but eradicating it? He envisions a future where everyone is tested for brain amyloid levels as part of routine health screening. A simple blood test can tell you your amyloid levels and other biomarkers that are either protective or may predispose you to developing Alzheimer's. **Knowing your levels allows you to take the necessary supplements to either boost protective proteins you're missing or keep your amyloid levels low. In such a world, the vast majority of the population won't need some insanely expensive drug to reverse the damage that amyloid buildup has already wreaked on their brain. All you'll have to do is take a daily low dose of a drug—like Lipitor for cholesterol—to maintain your brain health.**

Tool #4: The Power of Microbiomes

But Rudy isn't stopping there. He has helped start another company, **Marvel Biome**, that sits at another game-changing intersection: the power of microbes in targeting neurodegenerative diseases. There are roughly 8,000 strains of bacteria in your gut and hundreds of billions of bacteria. Marvel Biome discovered that the relationship between the brain and gut is a two-way street. **In patients with Alzheimer's, the gut microbiome gets out of whack. When they altered the diets of mice in a study, they found a dramatic reduction in amyloid and neuroinflammation.** Specifically, they found six kinds of bacteria that prevent oxidative stress. The idea is to take these bacteria, figure out which metabolites within them are helpful, and make them available to people. **They are currently in clinical trials and hope to bring this easy fix to the world soon.**

Tool #5: Taming Microglia with CD33

Want to hear something unbelievable? **Based on autopsy studies, about 30 percent[31] of older adults have brains loaded with enough amyloid or tau—or both—to indicate an Alzheimer's diagnosis, despite not showing so much as a hint of the disease before their deaths.** Remember the classic line in the New York deli scene from *When Harry Met Sally* when Meg Ryan proves a point to Billy Crystal by loudly faking an orgasm, prompting an older woman at another table to say, "I'll have what she's having"? **There are scientists who believe we could all avoid Alzheimer's— plaque or no plaque—if they could only give the rest of us whatever is protecting the resilient brains in that 30 percent. "You can have abundant plaques and tangles without having Alzheimer's disease," says Rudy.** "The challenge is to figure out how."

In 2019, one of Tanzi's colleagues reported[32] the strange case of a woman from Medellin, Colombia. She had a genetic mutation that was known to generate astronomical levels of amyloid and—in every other such individual known to science—early-onset Alzheimer's. Yet this resilient woman has stayed dementia-free. **What was her secret? It may have been an ultra-rare form of the gene APOE3, which stops tau from spreading through the brain.**

Similarly, Tanzi discovered that a mutant form of the gene CD33 can protect people from Alzheimer's. It stops the brain's palace guard immune cells, called *microglia*, from going rogue. Microglia are normally protective, clearing out dead cells and other brain debris. But without warning they can turn into assassins, kindling a wildfire of neuroinflammation that Tanzi says "kills ten times more neurons than plaques and tangles do." **Most anti-inflammatories either can't reach the brain or involve too many risks**—from ulcers to strokes—**to be used long-term. But AZTherapies, a Boston-based startup Tanzi cofounded, is concluding a Phase 3 trial to tame the microglia. It tested more than 600 early-stage Alzheimer's patients with reengineered versions of two common and well-tolerated medications: ibuprofen and cromolyn, an asthma drug. AZTherapies'**

cocktail has the potential to slow the progression of Alzheimer's, and—if given to healthy people at the first hints of pathology—it might actually prevent the disease.

Tool #6: Lifestyle Changes

In the meantime, Rudy cannot stress enough how much your lifestyle choices can help improve your brain health and prevent the onset of Alzheimer's. Here are six that he recommends, and he uses the acronym SHIELD to remember them:

1. **SLEEP:** For one, **getting enough sleep** is of vital importance. Rudy calls sleep "mental floss" because sleep clears amyloid out naturally.
2. **HANDLE STRESS: Reducing stress** is also key because stress causes release of cortisol in the body, which causes neuroinflammation and kills neurons.
3. **INTERACTION: Social interaction**, especially in the elderly, is critical since it **lowers Alzheimer's risk by twofold.**
4. **EXERCISE: Exercise** is one of the most important and most studied ways to improve brain health. **Recent studies have shown that exercise actually induces neurogenesis, the birth of new neurons.**
5. **LEARNING:** Learning new things—a language, an instrument— stimulates neuron growth. **Intellectual stimulation** can actually cause new synapses to form in your brain.
6. **DIET:** A low-sugar diet is important for health. Sugar causes inflammation.

Tool #7: Arethusta: Clearing Toxins from the Brain

When trying to understand what goes wrong in Alzheimer's, neurobiologist Doug Ethell believes it's helpful to think of this deadly disease as a *plumbing* problem. When the aging brain is unable to drain away the protein sludge that accumulates over time, billions of neurons die. The cerebral cortex—home to awareness, memory, language, and consciousness— wastes away. Think of it this way: There's lots of unpleasant stuff in your bathroom's pipes all the time, just as all brains contain amyloid and tau. But it becomes a problem only when the pipes get stopped up.

According to Ethell, who founded Leucadia Therapeutics in 2017 after leaving a promising career in academia, the solution is a neurosurgical Roto-Rooter, a low-risk procedure to get things flowing again.

In most of the body, waste materials—dead cells, inflammatory molecules, globs of problem proteins—get swept away by our lymphatic disposal system. But the brain, buffered by the blood-brain barrier, relies on a different sanitation service: cerebrospinal fluid. This natural cleanser percolates through the interstitial spaces of the cortex and works its way outward to the medial temporal lobe and hippocampus, the seat of memory, where telltale signs of Alzheimer's are found early on. In a healthy brain, the fluid sweeps amyloid plaque and tau tangles down to a porous, bony, dime-sized plate between our eyes. Once it passes through this cribriform plate, the debris exits harmlessly through our nasal cavity.

Leucadia's CT scan studies show that the cribriform plate thickens with age. In some cases, a bony veil may cover the plate's pores entirely. With no place to go, Ethell says, the protein debris accumulates in the brain like dead, matted leaves in a dried-out creek. (He believes the process may be accelerated by head injuries and even a broken nose, which helps explain why ex-boxers and football players get "punch-drunk.") In an experiment with ferrets, the ideal animal model for human Alzheimer's, Leucadia showed that blocking the cribriform plate killed 40 percent of neurons in nearby brain regions. Five months later, the blocked animals were much slower in navigating a maze than untouched control ferrets. "That told us we were on the right track," Ethell says.

Leucadia has engineered a specialized CT scan to determine whether a person's cribriform plate is so obstructed that the brain is at risk for mild cognitive impairment or—if that ship has already sailed—and become Alzheimer's disease. "By looking at the clearance capacity of the cerebrospinal fluid and combining that with memory testing, we think we can predict who will get Alzheimer's and when, years before cognitive impairment sets in," Ethell told us. By itself, though, this predictive test wouldn't be all that helpful. Ethell's goal is "to *do* something about it: not just tell someone they're likely to develop Alzheimer's disease in eight or ten years, but offer them a solution."

Enter Arethusta, a new experimental technology to restore

cerebrospinal flow and clear toxins from the brain. Named after a nymph in Greek mythology who fled a lustful river god by turning into an underground stream, Arethusta is intended to be a safe and simple shunt that can be implanted through the nose in a twilight-anesthesia procedure that will create a "hidden stream that allows people to escape Alzheimer's even if they have MCI, mild cognitive impairment." Next steps include clinical trials and the FDA approval process, stepping stones on the way to what Ethell foresees as a way to reverse MCI and stop Alzheimer's in its tracks.

Tool #8: Blood Plasma Treatments

Meanwhile, small pilot studies have indicated that blood plasma just might be an effective way to mitigate symptoms of Alzheimer's. It's not terribly surprising considering the connection between the circulatory system and the brain, through which more than 1,000 liters of blood course every single day.

Therapeutic plasma exchange swaps a person's blood plasma—the yellowish liquid that transports proteins and nutrients—with donated blood products to strain out toxins.

In animal studies, when plasma from young, healthy mice was infused into mice bred to have Alzheimer's, the ailing mice experienced an improvement in cognition.[5] And when 322 patients with Alzheimer's got multiple infusions of enriched plasma, their cognitive decline slowed down. Could elderly folks benefit from having their plasma replaced? Time will tell.

Tool #9: ISRIB: Is It Possible to Restore Memories?

At the University of California, San Francisco, researchers have found that an experimental drug can improve memory and mental flexibility in mice.[6] Older mice regained cognitive abilities more typical of younger mice when treated with several doses of ISRIB. Researchers suggest an extraordinary possibility—that "the aged brain has

---

5 Imbimbo et al., "Perspective: Is Therapeutic Plasma Exchange a Viable Option for Treating Alzheimer's Disease?"

6 Weiler, "Drug Reverses Age-Related Mental Decline Within Days."

**not permanently lost essential cognitive capacities, as was commonly
assumed, but rather that these cognitive resources are still there but
have been somehow blocked, trapped by a vicious cycle of cellular
stress," explains Dr. Peter Walter, a professor in the University of California San Francisco (UCSF) Department of Biochemistry and Biophysics.** His lab discovered ISRIB in 2013.

In a 2020 study, scientists found that older mice who got small doses of
ISRIB during a three-day training designed to teach them how to escape
from a watery maze performed as well as younger mice and significantly
outperformed mice their own age who hadn't gotten the drug. Calico, a Bay
Area company working to unlock the biology of aging, has licensed ISRIB.
There's reason to think the drug could be effective against dementia and
Alzheimer's, as well as age-related cognitive decline. For now, it's **essentially
a rodent's version of the fountain of youth, but in time, it could translate to humans as well.**

Tool #10: Vaxxinity—Creating a Vaccine to Treat Alzheimer's

*"We know the right target, and we know intervening
earlier in the disease is better. So a vaccine proposition
makes much more sense now than ever before."*[7]

—MEI MEI HU, cofounder and CEO, Vaxxinity

When *Time* magazine named **Mei Mei Hu to its 2019 "100 Next" list,
it gave her the highest praise:** that "you don't need a PhD to make a
breakthrough" in entrepreneurial science. A Harvard-trained lawyer, Mei
Mei excelled at an elite New York law firm and as a management consultant
at McKinsey before returning to the family business: cutting-edge medical research. Hu's mother, **Chang Yi Wang**, is a legendary biochemist and
immunologist who studied and developed a game-changing technology
under three Nobel laureates, and then cofounded **United Biomedical.
She's best known for her immune-based therapies for both people
and livestock—including a vaccine to make male pigs healthier (and
tastier) by suppressing their testosterone.** Mei Mei and her husband,

---

7 *Time*, "*TIME* 100 Next: Mei Mei Hu."

Lou Reese—now the company's executive chairman—have since spun off a subsidiary, **Vaxxinity, in which my coauthor Peter is a cofounder and vice chairman**. I'm so impressed with their work that I became one of the early investors in the company. They've leveraged Chang Yi's platform technology, Mei Mei told us, for a very specific purpose: "to develop vaccines that harness the power of people's own immune systems to treat and prevent major diseases such as Alzheimer's and Parkinson's."

As I was wrapping up this book, Vaxxinity's Alzheimer's vaccine, code-named UB-311, was about to **enter a large-scale efficacy trial (Phase 2/3) trial, after demonstrating it was safe and effective** at harnessing the body's immune system to manufacture antibodies that target and remove those ill-formed amyloid proteins. <u>**According to Mei Mei, Vaxxinity's early clinical data suggests a slowing of disease progression by up to 50 percent compared to placebo in all four cognitive and functional measures tested.**</u>[8] In addition, through state-of-the-art functional MRI and PET (positron emission tomorography) imaging, **"UB-311 was seen to increase brain connectivity and reduce amyloid deposits in all eight brain regions tested." Moreover, the safety profile appears to be excellent, with no cases of the drug-induced brain swelling that has been seen in other monoclonal antibody treatments** and can result in serious side effects like confusion, changes in mental state, and even coma.[9]

Just as vaccines against measles or COVID-19 stir the immune system to produce antibodies against a particular virus, UB-311 enlists antibodies against clumps of amyloid, empowering your own body to generate antibodies against a similar target to the one the FDA just approved for Biogen's Aduhelm (aducanumab). The difference is that UB-311 appears to be safer, more effective, and far more convenient than Aducanamab.

Vaxxinity is pursuing a radically new angle of attack. First of all, they're focused on warding off Alzheimer's *as early as possible, ultimately long before* **symptoms surface. Second, they're taking a more**

---

8 https://www.sec.gov/Archives/edgar/data/1851657/000119312521295612/ d142511ds1.htm

9 14th International Conference on Alzheimer's and Parkinson's Diseases (AD/PD) in Lisbon, Portugal, from March 26–31, 2019.

selective "Goldilocks" approach to the amyloid cascade hypothesis. The Vaxxinity team argues that mainstream science took a wrong turn by targeting the wrong *kinds* of amyloid: either the full-blown sticky plaques first observed by Alois Alzheimer, or single molecules that hadn't clumped together.

The "just right" target, according to some experts, is in between: small amyloid oligomeric clusters ranging from two to eight molecules. "These are the forms of amyloid that kill neurons," Lou Reese told us. They're the ones the vaccine trains the immune system to destroy.

Vaxxinity's treatment is delivered through a simple intramuscular injection, similar to a flu shot. It contains specially engineered antigens, amyloid impersonators that wake up the immune system. As with any good vaccine, Mei Mei says, "this vaccine trains the body to fight disease."

In testing so far, PET and MRI scans show that Vaxxinity's Alzheimer's vaccine has reduced the quantity of brain amyloid deposits. Most important, it has resulted in real-world improvement in patients' cognitive and everyday mental functioning scores. It's passed its safety tests with flying colors.[10]

In fact, according to Mei Mei, if all goes well, soon after the time of this publication, Vaxxinity's gamechanger could soon be approaching Phase 3 trials. Their plan is to administer it quarterly to anyone with Alzheimer's and once or perhaps twice a year to anyone whose brain scan shows preliminary signs of amyloid buildup. In a stark departure from typical big pharma and biotech pricing structures for life-changing medicines, Mei Mei said she feels a "moral obligation" to make the Alzheimer's vaccine more affordable than aducanumab's $56,000 annual price tag. "We can manufacture millions of doses a year at a few dollars per dose," she said. The goal is to price at a fraction of the monoclonal antibodies and make it accessible to everyone who needs it.

It's worth also pointing out that Vaxxinity's vaccine platform goes way beyond only Alzheimer's treatment. "Our goal is to use the Vaxxinity platform to transform the treatment of many chronic diseases," says Lou Reese,

---

10 Ibid.

listing targets like Parkinson's, migraines, allergies, bone loss (osteopenia), muscle loss (sarcopenia), and most recently, a vaccine against COVID-19. **"We are building Vaxxinity to be more like a tech company such as Apple or Tesla than a pharma company,"** continues Reese. "Our goal is to pioneer the next biologic revolution and expansively disrupt the chronic disease area, treating diseases with a technology that is orders of magnitude cheaper and easier."

Vaxxinity's vaccines against migraines and hypercholesteremia are now entering early Phase 1 clinical trials, while its vaccine against Parkinson's is entering Phase 2 trials with strong support from the Michael J. Fox Foundation.

I haven't talked about this publicly before now, but my biological father had Alzheimer's. He didn't know who I was at the end; it was an excruciating experience for me and our whole family. That's when I promised myself to do all I could to find an answer for this disease—so that I'd never be a burden to others and could enjoy my own family forever. That's the reason I became one of the earliest investors in Vaxxinity.[11] I wanted to help provide capital to push these breakthroughs forward and make them available to all those who need them around the world. For me, this fight is personal.

Tool #11: Believe it or Not—Phenomenal Fungi: The Power of Mushrooms

When it comes to the most unexpected of candidates for neurogenesis, mushrooms might take the cake. One of the most elusive and overlooked regenerators in nature, **fungi comprise their own kingdom, with over 1.5 million species—six times more than plants—and extraordinary network intelligence. Fungi's root network, called a** *mycelium*, **has more networks than our brains have neural pathways and sends signals in much the same way, using electrolytes.** Unlike our brains, however, a mycelium can live forever, as long as it has food to grow *into*. In fact, the oldest

---

11 As of this writing, in February 2021, Vaxxinity had entered a Phase 2 trial for a highly promising COVID-19 vaccine, based on them mini-proteins known as peptides.

and largest organism on planet Earth is a fungus, spanning thousands of acres and thriving for thousands of years. **As a potent natural regenerative force, fungi have given rise to everything from life-saving penicillin, to novel pesticides and insecticides, to compounds that regrow nerves in the brain.** Yet we've barely even scratched the surface of the fungal genome.

But what does this have to do with brain health? Let me introduce you to **Paul Stamets**, one of the world's foremost mycology experts and pioneers. An unlikely hero, Paul first began to uncover the medicinal and ecological secrets of mushrooms in 1974. Working as a logger, he was intimately familiar with the woods, although not from studying their ecology; rather, from cutting them down. But during an impromptu visit to Paul's workplace in Darrington, Washington, his brother, John, began pointing out clusters of mushrooms that inhabited the woods—a phenomenon Paul had never noticed. **Forty-five publications, twenty-six patents, and twenty-nine patent applications later, Paul's fascination with fungi has never stopped. (In fact, there's a fascinating documentary called *The Power of Funghi* on Netflix that you might find it very interesting and fascinating to watch.)**

Paul's latest launch, **MycoMedica Life Sciences**, promotes **"Stamets Stack,"** a blend of neuroregeneration-inducing ingredients, including lion's mane mushroom, psilocybin, and niacin (nicotinic acid, the flushing form of vitamin B3). **Stamets Stack may have diverse indications, including for Alzheimer's and dementia, neuroinflammation, Parkinson's, traumatic brain injury (TBI), depression, anxiety, pain, and addiction.**

Let's start with its first mushroom: **lion's mane, which tastes like lobster or shrimp when cooked and was discovered to stimulate nerve regrowth by Japanese biochemist Dr. Hirokazu Kawagishi.** In 1993, he realized it induced the synthesis of nerve growth factors (NGF), proteins that promote the survival and proliferation of nerves. <u>**Small-scale clinical trials found that lion's mane soup led to physical and cognitive improvements in dementia patients.**</u> This mushroom has continued to show promise in Alzheimer's ever since.

The second key ingredient in the Stamets Stack? Psilocybin. While psychedelics were at the vanguard of psychiatric research in the 1950s and '60s—helping alcoholic patients maintain sobriety and treating end-of-life anxiety and depression in late-stage cancer patients, among other therapeutic applications—funding was promptly shut off with Nixon's declaration of the war on drugs. **Today, however, psilocybin is seeing a powerful renaissance; in 2013, it was the experimental ingredient in an animal model study, in which mice treated with psilocybin were found to overcome fear-conditioned stimulus responses by growing new neurological pathways.**

Ever since, psilocybin has proved an extraordinary ingredient through the microdosing data generated by Paul's Microdose.me, the largest psychedelic medicine data set, collected from more than 14,000 participants. In addition to statistically significant reductions in anxiety and depression, microdosing has now shown groundbreaking outcomes for restoring fine motor ability in patients with Alzheimer's, Parkinson's, and mild cognitive impairment.

Stamets Stack is now on a clear path to becoming a legalized drug for treatment of depression and similar indications, which Paul predicts will pave the way for fungi's magical healing properties to extend to other neurodegenerative diseases, including Alzheimer's.

HOW A PSYCHEDELIC MOLECULE COULD POTENTIALLY TRANSFORM MENTAL HEALTH

One thing we can always be certain about is that humanity will rise to overcome adversity. The COVID-19 pandemic has fueled a second crisis. A mental health crisis. According to *"The Lancet,* **about one-third of COVID-19 survivors will go on to develop anxiety or depression."**[12] There has also been a rise in substance abuse and suicide attempts. We have all seen Big Pharma scramble to develop COVID-19 vaccines, but one start-up that I'm an early investor in has been scrambling to revolutionize how mental health disorders such as these are treated.

---

12 Taquet et al., "6-Month Neurological and Psychiatric Outcomes in 236,379 Survivors of COVID-19: A Retrospective Cohort Study Using Electronic Health Records."

Cybin, a biopharmaceutical company focused on progressing "Psychedelics to Therapeutics," released pre-clinical findings that demonstrate multiple advantages for its newly developed novel deuterated psilocybin formula (a modified molecule) over oral psilocybin for the treatment of mental health.

As we revealed earlier, breakthrough research at Johns Hopkins University has indicated oral psilocybin to be very effective in the treatment of mental health disorders, but with significant limitations, specifically: **slow onset of action, extended duration of effect, and a variability in response among patients.**

Cybin's proprietary molecular advancements offer positive benefits and address the challenges and limitations of oral psilocybin. In multi-species pre-clinical studies, the Company's CYB003 program has demonstrated:

- **A 50 percent reduction in variability compared to oral psilocybin; indicates potential for more accurate dosing in patients with MDD (clinical depression) and AUD (those with heightened risk to depression).**

- **A 50 percent reduction in dose compared to oral psilocybin; indicates potential to maintain equivalent efficacy while reducing side effects, such as nausea.**

- **A 50 percent shorter time to onset when compared to oral psilocybin; indicates potential for shorter duration of treatment, lower inter-subject variability, better therapeutic control and safety, leading to a better patient experience, with lower cost and scalability.**

- **Nearly double brain penetration when compared to oral psilocybin; indicates potential for a less variable treatment response, a lower dose therapeutic effect, and reduced patient side effects.**[13]

---

13 Davs et al., "Effects of Psilocybin-Assisted Therapy on Major Depressive Disorder A Randomized Clinical Trial. JAMA."

The deuterated psilocybin analog in CYB003 has the potential to reduce time and resource burden on patients, providers, and payers, and possibly improving scalability and accessibility from the following conclusions:

- Faster onset of action equates to less down time in the clinic before effects begin;

- Half the duration of effect translates to shorter clinic days or more patients per day;

- More predictable dose effects create a safer and more effective patient response;

- Lowered peripheral exposure diminishes the risk of nausea; and

- Better brain penetration suggests lower overall dose needed to achieve clinical efficacy.

Doug explains, "While we are all encouraged by the benefits of psilocybin, we need to transparently and openly discuss its limitations if we are to translate psychedelics to therapeutics for patients in need. The majority of current clinical studies are based on psilocybin. We have taken the necessary steps to potentially unlock the powerful benefits of psychedelics and engineer a superior molecule as demonstrated by the data."

Tool #12: Preserving Your Hearing

One of the most powerful things you can do to head off dementia is to use a hearing aid, if you need one. Trust me, this is huge! I've been leading events for 45 years, since I was 17 years old. Forty-five years in stadiums with music blasting like a rock concert—not for two or three hours, but twelve hours a day, five or more days a week, multiple times each month. Some years back, I developed a case of tinnitus, a ringing in my ears. I could barely hear people talk in restaurants or crowded rooms. It got more and more frustrating, but I certainly didn't want to wear a hearing aid at 59 years old—that was for old people, right?

But then I studied more about the neurological impact of hearing loss. **When your ears aren't processing information at the level they used**

to, your brain doesn't process the same way, either. That can be a one-way street to impaired cognition; functional MRIs show that the brain will overwork to compensate for hearing loss.[14] I changed my tune. I got tested by an audiologist, Stacy O'Brien, who confirmed the issue. "It's not the hearing loss alone that drives the link to developing dementia," she told me. "It's if the hearing loss is NOT treated."

It was easy to put my vanity aside when I found some hearing devices that are literally invisible and built with AI technology. When someone is speaking, they translate the language in real time within my ears—it's pretty wild. **Not only can I hear people better and use my iPhone without those white cords, but my tinnitus calmed down, too.** So do yourself a favor: If you think you might have a problem, get it checked out and then get the technology you need. There are some very cool components out there—you might find yourself eavesdropping without even trying!

Here are the dozen things that you can change or try to avoid—that could actually stave off a full 40 percent of dementia cases according to the Lancet Commission on Dementia Prevention, Intervention, and Care.[15] In order of significance, they are:

1. Hearing loss: 8.2 percent of cases
2. Low education levels (in youth): 7.1 percent
3. Smoking: 5.2 percent
4. Depression: 3.9 percent
5. Social isolation: 3.5 percent
6. Traumatic brain injury: 3.4 percent
7. Air pollution (including secondhand smoke and wood-burning fire-places): 2.3 percent

---

14 Campbell and Sharma, "Compensatory Changes in Cortical Resource Allocation in Adults with Hearing Loss."

15 Hughes, "Twelve Risk Factors Linked to 40% of the World's Dementia Cases."

8. Hypertension (systolic blood pressure higher than 130): 1.9 percent

9. Physical inactivity: 1.6 percent

10. Diabetes: 1.1 percent

11. Excessive alcohol consumption (more than three drinks per day): 0.8 percent

12. Obesity (a body mass index greater than 30): 0.7 percent

Tool #13: Mental Fitness and Video Games for Brain Health

If you want to be even more proactive in keeping your wits about you for a lifetime, we can recommend one more option: consistent, systematic workouts for your brain. Not all mental exercise is equally useful, however. **Data suggests that crossword puzzles and Sudoku don't do much to ward off mild cognitive impairment or Alzheimer's, but learning a new language or practicing the piano, on the other hand, seems to confer real benefits.**[16] Are you a gamer? Well, you're in luck. **Some of the most effective anti-dementia tools around may be specialized video games devised by elite neuroscientists.** Beyond inhibiting cognitive decline, they've shown potential to help healthy people stay sharp and become even *sharper*.

The basis of video "brain training" is *neuroplasticity*, which offers a world of hope in the war against Alzheimer's. In a nutshell, it means that **the adult brain is a work in progress. It never stops evolving.** The "gray matter" in our prefrontal cortex, the site where decisions are made and problems are solved, can expand over time. **We can grow new neurons and revamp our mental circuitry into our 70s and 80s and beyond.** "Neuroplasticity is evident through older adulthood," says[19] neuroscientist Adam Gazzaley of the UCSF, a leader in the field.

One of Gazzaley's early discoveries was that **circuits that handle spatial attention (spotting objects in a visually cluttered scene) overlap with those for short-term working memory.**[21] **Work on one and you boost the other.** When a mixed-age group of adults was trained over several

---

16 Mills, "Does Music Benefit the Brain?"

days to press an iPad button whenever a pre-specified target flashed on the screen, **they improved their working memory by 20 percent. Even more impressive, the 70-year-olds held their own against the 25-year-olds. The older people's underlying neural circuitry was intact. It just needed some high-intensity activity to snap back into shape.**

In collaboration with LucasArts, the UCSF team subsequently developed a 3D video game to improve "cognitive control,"[23] the ability to switch from one focus of attention to another within microseconds. **People's capacity for multitasking declines steadily after age 20. But after twelve one-hour sessions of Gazzley's NeuroRacer, where players use a joystick to navigate a virtual car while at the same time watching for road signs, people from 60 to 85 multitasked as well as untrained 20-year-olds. It was the first evidence that a customized game can be a "powerful tool for cognitive enhancement,"** Gazzley told us. An updated NeuroRacer is under study as a diagnostic for Alzheimer's and **a therapy for vascular dementia, depression, and autism. In 2020, the FDA approved the game as a treatment for children with attention deficit hyperactivity disorder.**[17] **These young people can now "play their medicine" instead of taking drugs like Adderall!**

They improved their working memory by 20 percent. Even more impressive, the 70-year-olds held their own against the 25-year-olds. The older people's underlying neural circuitry was intact. It just needed some high-intensity activity to snap back into shape.

The best brain training programs, according to an independent analysis,[24] target spatial attention and "speed of processing," or how quickly our circuits pass signals from one neuron to the next. **One outfit that stands head and shoulders above the rest, the experts say, is Posit Science, the creator of BrainHQ. Their app is offered free by some Medicare**

---

17 Kurtzman, "FDA Approves Video Game Based on UCSF Brain Research as ADHD Therapy for Kids."

Advantage plans and also by subscription. "Cognitive training works," says Posit CEO Henry Mahncke, "and it's time to put it to use."

But can brain training <u>reduce the risk of Alzheimer's?</u> In a ten-year study led by Jerri Edwards, a neurobiologist at the University of South Florida, healthy older adults (average age 74) were divided into a control group and three intervention arms. In a course of ten sessions over six weeks, plus some booster sessions one and three years later, one subgroup learned memory strategies. Another received instruction on reasoning strategies. The third subgroup got computerized brain training "designed to improve the speed and accuracy of visual attention, including both divided and selective attention exercises."[18] At the end of the ten years, among subjects who'd completed fifteen or more one-hour sessions, there were nearly as many people with dementia in the memory and reasoning groups as in the control group— the ones who'd done nothing at all. **But people in the brain training group reduced their dementia risk by a whopping 45 percent—for an investment of less than twenty hours of their time.** Imagine the possibilities if people trained their brains as frequently as they hopped on a treadmill!

HYPERBARIC OXYGEN THERAPY
A Powerful Epigenetic Treatment Whose Time Has Arrived

By Dr. Paul G. Harch, M.D., clinical professor of medicine, Department of Medicine, Section of Emergency Medicine and Hyperbaric Medicine, former director, LSU Hyperbaric Medicine Fellowship, former director, Department of Hyperbaric Medicine, University Medical Center, New Orleans

Hyperbaric oxygen therapy (HBOT), which has been misunderstood and maligned for 359 years, has now become understood as the most pervasive epigenetic therapy known to man. Applied to more than 130 medical diagnoses, HBOT has confused and confounded the medical profession since its debut in 1662.[19] Dramatic healing effects have been

18 Meketa, "Intervention Becomes First to Successfully Reduce Risk of Dementia."
19 Trimble, *The Uncertain Miracle*.

documented along with what have been considered wildly exaggerated claims. Physicians, determined to know the mechanism of action of a therapy before referring patients for any treatment, have been unable to elucidate the mechanisms of action of HBOT . . . until now.

Known as a treatment for diver's disease, inflammation, and wound conditions, HBOT heals wounds by growing new tissue. To grow new tissue, the nucleus of every cell must be stimulated to divide and multiply. In 2008, Dr. Godman took the most reactive cells in the human body, the cells that line all of the tiniest blood vessels, subjected them to a single HBOT, and measured the activity of all 19,000 protein-coding genes in the 46 chromosomes of these human cells.[20] At the end of 24 hours 8,101 (40 percent) of our 19,000 genes were turned on or off by a single HBOT session. The largest groups of genes turned on: the growth and repair hormone genes and the anti-inflammatory genes. The largest groups of genes temporarily turned off: the pro-inflammatory genes and genes that code for cell death. For 359 years, every time a patient went into a hyperbaric chamber they were inhibiting inflammation, stimulating tissue growth, and stopping cell death, and did so not by changing the DNA code but by affecting the proteins that are the gatekeepers for the genes. Essentially, HBOT was an epigenetic therapy and the net result was healing.

In addition to its epigenetic effects, HBOT heals wounds through wide-ranging effects on stem cells. HBOT has been shown to stimulate proliferation of stem cells in our bone marrow, release of bone marrow stem cells into our circulation, maturation of released stem cells, homing to, implantation, and maturation of stem cells at sites of injury, and proliferation, migration, and maturation of stem cells within the brain to sites of brain injury. Realizing the combination of stem cell and HBOT's gene modulatory effects on wounds and inflammation, HBOT

---

20 Robin, "Hyperbaric Oxygen, a Therapy in Search of Diseases"; Godman et al., "Hyperbaric Oxygen Induces a Cytoprotective and Angiogenic Response in Human Microvascular Endothelial Cells."

can now be appreciated as a treatment for wounds in any location in the body and of any duration.

Traditionally applied to long-standing diabetic foot wounds, radiation wounds in cancer patients, and other extremity wounds, as well as acute wounds like crush injuries and plastic surgery wounds where skin grafts and flaps fail it is obvious that there is no difference between a wound in the arm, face, or leg, and a wound in the liver, bone, or brain.[21] In the past 50 years HBOT has been shown to be the most effective therapy for traumatic brain injury (TBI).

A few HBOT sessions within the first few days after severe TBI has reduced death from TBI by 50 percent, a salvage rate rivaled in the history of mankind only by penicillin.[22] In chronic mild TBI HBOT has been shown since 2012 to be the most effective therapy for patients suffering from persistent concussion symptoms.

Realizing that wounds in the body, especially to the brain, can be caused by such a vast array of insults such as chemicals, trauma, lack of blood flow, lack of oxygen, food additives, pesticides, herbicides (Agent Orange, for example), bubbles in the blood stream, general anesthesia, toxic gases, stress of all types (physical, emotional, psychological, sexual, combat), birth complications, infection, etc. it is now easy to appreciate the rapidly increasing scientific evidence showing that HBOT can treat dementia, mild cognitive decline, and vascular dementia.[23]

Given that our genes are one of the largest targets of HBOT activity, that HBOT is an epigenetic therapy, that aging is rooted in our genes, and HBOT is showing effectiveness in aging of the brain, claims that

21 Weaver, ed., "Hyperbaric Oxygen Therapy Indications."

22 Holback et al., "Reversibilität des Traumatischen Mittelhirnsyndromes bei Anwendung der Hyperbaren Oxygenierung. (Improved Reversibility of the Traumatic Midbrain Syndrome Following the Use of Hyperbaric Oxygenation.)"

23 Cheng-Hwang et al., "The Treatment of Cognitive Dysfunction in Dementia"; Jacobs et al., "Hyperoxygenation Effect on Cognitive Functioning in the Aged"; Hadanny et al., "Cognitive Enhancement of Healthy Older Adults Using Hyperbaric Oxygen."

HBOT may have regenerative anti-aging effects and effects on longevity is understandable.

For HBOT it is a whole new world, and it has been so in my practice for the past 35 years. Initially attempting to identify HBOT-responsive diagnoses in 1989, I have now treated nearly 100 conditions, the majority of which are neurological. In the past 18 years I have found that the success of this therapy is dependent on the dose of oxygen and pressure used, i. e., precision dosing, since different gene clusters are activated by different levels of oxygen and pressure.

While all living organisms are sensitive to changes in atmospheric pressure and oxygen, each patient and their disease are idiosyncratic, and respond to a dose of hyperbaric oxygen and pressure that is right for them. With custom-dosing to a patient's condition, this 359-year-old therapy, hyperbaric oxygen therapy, has become a foundational biological treatment of the future. . . .

Which brings me to the reason I was invited by Tony to write this short segment on hyperbaric oxygen therapy. In 2017, Tony contacted me about a two-year history of memory problems, fatigue, and losing his train of thought. His closest aides and associates were concerned to the point of tears about his health and cognitive abilities. Tony had been diagnosed with mercury poisoning due to a high fish diet and had undergone detox, but problems remained. During these years he had received limited hyperbaric oxygen therapy at eight different facilities in the U.S. and internationally without noticeable benefit.

In April of 2017 I evaluated Tony in New Orleans and custom-dosed him with SPECT brain imaging before and after a single HBOT. The imaging showed a significant increase in brain blood flow at the chosen dose of HBOT. With Tony's being unable to stay in New Orleans for the typical eight weeks of treatment and dosing, my staff flew around the world with Tony, treating him at performance sites in Los Angeles, Fiji, Australia, Panama, New York, and the Netherlands..By the twenty-sixth treatment, he was feeling remarkably better and received a stem cell treatment. After 9 more HBOTs that likely stimulated implantation of the stem cells (see above) Tony was on top of the world again.

Since 2017 my staff and I have continued to treat Tony on a regular basis. Along with the many other therapies he receives, HBOT has rejuvenated Tony and helped facilitate his record-breaking superhuman performance. For more information on HBOT, please visit www .HBOT.com.

MIND OVER MATTER

"I think, therefore I am."

—RENÉ DESCARTES, 17th-century mathematician and philosopher

We've covered *a lot* of ground in this chapter. **We wanted to show you that for one of the most feared and largest challenges in medicine, there are so many solutions being brought to you now or are on the horizon. You now have thirteen cutting-edge developments to look for so that you know ways to prevent Alzheimer's and dementia as well as tools that are coming if you or someone you love is beginning to experience symptoms. I hope you come out of this feeling an air of optimism about what the next few years may bring to prevent, control, and manage Alzheimer's.**

As a quick review, we've learned about a blood test that can predict Alzheimer's before symptoms emerge. We've seen how infusing young people's blood plasma into older folks may put the brakes on their cognitive decline. We've found that a drug discovered in a university lab can boost memory in mice and hopefully in people eventually. And we've seen that an Alzheimer's vaccine in clinical trials has dramatically slowed the disease's progression and so much more.

It goes without saying that a new era is dawning. **I am so grateful to be alive at a time when there are legitimate grounds for hope that you and I will be keeping our wits about us for as long as we walk this earth.**

Now that we're refreshed on ways to keep our minds limber,

youthful, and strong, let's turn to the last section of the book, about
longevity and mindset. Throughout this book, we have learned about
countless incredible tools available to help us live our best lives. In these
final chapters, we'll look at the giant technological wave and what it
means for the future of health. And why taking control of our mindset
matters the most. Mind and emotions shape not only our health, but
the quality of our life.

In the next chapter, I'm going to turn you over to my coauthor
Peter Diamandis, who will share with you all of the exponential breakthroughs that are coming, as well as the forces that may well lead us to
longevity escape velocity, then I'll join you for the final chapter on how
you can create the most extraordinary quality of life by tapping into
the power of your mind and then make a few decisions to transform
the experiences of your life. So let's turn the page and discover the
power of longevity and exponential technologies. . . .

LONGEVITY, MINDSET & FULFILLMENT

The power of longevity, mindset, and the decision that will help you take control of your mind, your body, and your emotions—enhancing your entire quality of life. Discover . . .

- The power of longevity and exponential technologies from my coauthor Peter H. Diamandis.

- The amazing power of placebos and how our mind can heal our bodies, as well as the latest breakthroughs in combatting depression, anxiety, and PTSD.

- The Power of Decision: Learn the most important tool in creating and sustaining an extraordinary life. A life of joy, happiness, gratitude, and true aliveness.

CHAPTER 23

LONGEVITY AND THE POWER OF EXPONENTIAL TECHNOLOGIES (BY PETER H. DIAMANDIS, MD)

How Accelerating Technologies and an Abundance of Capital Are Powering the Quest for Healthy Longevity

> *"I don't want to achieve immortality by being inducted into the Hall of Fame. I want to achieve immortality by not dying."*
>
> —WILLIAM DE MORGAN

It's hard to remember how extraordinary our world is today compared to centuries past, and how far we have come, especially after surviving two waves of the COVID-19 pandemic and living with the constant bombardment of negative news emanating from our TVs, radios, and newspapers.

Perhaps to make you feel a bit better about what we all endured in 2020, history provides some valuable comparisons to remind us how far we've come in handling pandemics. Consider the following:

- Between 1347 and 1351, the bubonic plague, the most fatal pandemic recorded in human history, caused the death of 75 to 200 million people in Eurasia and North Africa, and wiped out some 30 to 50 percent of England. They never found a cure.
- The 1918 influenza pandemic (also known as the Spanish Flu) was the most severe pandemic in recent history. It was caused by an H1N1 virus with genes of avian origin. It's estimated that about

500 million people—one-third of the world's population—became infected with this virus. The number of deaths was estimated to be at least 50 million worldwide, with about 675,000 occurring in the United States. This virus is still with us today, and is the reason for our annual flu shots.

If these were our current headlines, our governments would be paralyzed, our financial markets in ruins, and the problems we have today would look comparatively like a sunny day in California.

We forget how much the world has progressed in just the last century and how today's scientific and technological muscle allowed humanity to emerge from the first COVID-19 pandemic waves relatively quickly, with a fraction of the deaths and economic impact. Technologies like mRNA vaccines, global high-speed data connectivity, supercomputers, and global supply chains allowed science to design, test, and begin distribution of vaccines in under twelve months. At the same time, the convergence of exponential technologies made possible companies like Amazon, Zoom, Google, and Slack, which allowed global business to progress relatively unabated.

Just like these exponential technologies have changed how we detect, prevent, and treat viral pandemics, these same technologies are now giving us the tools to fight the pandemic of aging.

THE BEST WAY TO PREDICT THE FUTURE IS TO CREATE IT YOURSELF

Throughout most of this book we've focused on the topics of vitality, strength, energy, and curing disease. **But what about those of us who are actively seeking healthy longevity, the ability to shoot past the accepted limits of old age into our 100s while preserving our cognition, mobility, and aesthetics? Is it desirable? Is it possible? That's what this chapter is about.** For example, we'll explain:

- Why we are biased to believe that we can only plan for eighty years of healthy life, and why we can probably expect more

- How exponential technologies such as artificial intelligence, sensors, and biotech are transforming today's health-tech revolution
- How a massive amount of investment capital flowing into the field of longevity is accelerating health and longevity-related breakthroughs
- Why longer lives won't lead to overpopulation of Earth, and frankly why longevity is critical to the future of humanity
- And finally, we'll close this chapter with the insights of two of the most brilliant longevity scientists on what type of healthspan you should be shooting for.

Before diving into the details above, I'd like to give you some context on my personal journey that has led me to this point of making longevity-related research, investments, and entrepreneurship my focus for the past decade, and the decade ahead. I'd like to share with you why I'm so excited and why you should be, too.

I'm the son of two Greek immigrants, Harry and Tula, who since my birth wanted me to become a physician (my dad was an obstetrician-gynecologist). But, while medicine was interesting, **I was a child of the Apollo program, born in the 1960s, passionate about space. The Apollo program showed us what humanity could achieve, and that "scientific documentary"** *Star Trek* **showed me where our species was going.**

While I was passionate about space—it was everything to me—I had promised my parents I would go to medical school, which I did, at Harvard. Luckily for me, while Harvard was hard to get into, it was even harder to fail out of! Thank goodness, because during my fourth year of medical school, I was running two space-related companies (a university and a launch company) and barely attending classes.

By the late 1980s I was extremely disappointed by the weak vision of NASA. Adding the space program's glacial speed, and the 1986 *Challenger* Space Shuttle accident, everything ground to a stop. I remember thinking that in order for me to actually experience the space future I desired, I would need to do two things: live longer and help to accelerate the development of human spaceflight.

One of my first space-related efforts was cofounding the International

Space University (ISU), started in a modest 500-square-foot headquarters above a bagel shop in Boston's Kendall Square. It was here, with my cofounders the late Todd Hawley and Bob Richards, that I dreamed great space dreams. **It was also here that I first encountered Murphy's Law, that pessimistic and defeatist proclamation: "If anything can go wrong, it will." Todd had jokingly put the poster up on the wall because he knew how much it bothered me. To counter the mental offense, I wrote on my whiteboard, "If anything can go wrong, fix it!** *(To hell with Murphy!)***" and wrote above it, in all capitals, "PETER'S LAW."**

That began my accumulation of **twenty-eight "Peter's laws,"** some created and some borrowed, that have governed my life, and which interestingly impact my views and efforts in the field of longevity. Laws like:

"The day before something is truly a breakthrough, it's a crazy idea."

"If you can't win, change the rules."

"If you think it is impossible, then it is for you."

"The best way to predict the future is to create it yourself."

While ISU has grown from a 500-square-foot office to a $100 million campus in Strasbourg, France, it was the XPRIZE that really accelerated my dreams of opening the space frontier. Still jaded about my future prospects of spaceflight, in 1993 I read Charles Lindbergh's autobiography, *The Spirit of St. Louis*, and learned that his famous 1927 flight from New York to Paris was inspired by a $25,000 "incentive prize" offered by hotelier Raymond Orteig for the first nonstop flight between his birthplace of France and his new home in New York.

It hit me then that maybe, just maybe, a large cash prize on the order of $10 million might inspire engineers and entrepreneurs to build a spaceship to take the rest of us into space. Not knowing who my benefactor would be (i.e., my Orteig, Pulitzer, or Nobel), I called it the XPRIZE, with the "X" as a stand-in for the eventual sponsor. **With no prize money or any competing teams, I announced the $10 million competition on May 18, 1996, under the Arch in St. Louis.**

Five years later, a visionary entrepreneur, Anousheh Ansari, and her family stepped up to fund the prize purse. **Eventually twenty-six teams from seven nations registered to compete, and on October 4, 2004, a team** called Mojave Aerospace Ventures, funded by Microsoft cofounder Paul Allen and led by the legendary aerospace designer Burt Rutan, flew their vehicle, SpaceShipOne, on two consecutive flights to a 100km altitude to claim the $10 million Ansari XPRIZE. And, as hoped, the fuse was lit, and the commercial spaceflight industry began. Seventeen years later in 2021, we now see the fruits of the XPRIZE as Sir Richard Branson (who licensed the rights of SpaceShipOne for Virgin Galactic) and Jeff Bezos (with Blue Origin) have commercially duplicated those XPRIZE flights to open a tourism marketplace.

Since 2004, the XPRIZE Foundation has gone on to design and launch more than $250 million in prizes, with another $200 million under development, across topics ranging from energy, water, and food to healthcare, oceans, and the environment. To fund these prizes, we've been able to attract an extraordinary group of visionaries, doers, and benefactors—a group we call our Innovation Board. We intentionally choose challenges that can't be fixed overnight. Problems that were stuck, where not enough attention was being paid. Our goal at XPRIZE is simple: to give innovators a target to shoot for, to tackle and conquer. Ultimately to kick the most brilliant minds into high gear.

Every year I take the Innovation Board on an "adventure trip" to explore different topics and brainstorm new prize concepts. In years past our trips have focused on artificial intelligence, 3D printing, VR, and AR. And in 2018, we focused on the twin topics of longevity and regenerative medicine, venturing to Vatican City, piggybacking on a preexisting event called United to Cure, organized by Robin Smith, MD, and hosted by the Pope. It's this visit that Tony recounts in the opening chapter of this book.

THE MORALITY OF IMMORTALITY

The Vatican conference lasted three days and gathered the leading scientists and thinkers from around the world, covering many of the topics you've read about in the previous chapters. But without doubt, my favorite session of the event, and one in which I participated, was titled "The Morality of Immortality."

The discussion was moderated by CNN medical anchor Dr. Sanjay Gupta, and included me, Rabbi Dr. Edward Reichman, Elder Dale Renlund, Reverend Father Dr. Nicancor Austriaco, and NIH director Dr. Francis Collins.

At the start of our panel, Dr. Gupta asked Rabbi Reichman to provide a historical context from the Old Testament about human aging and longevity.

"Adam lived to 930 years old," started Rabbi Reichman. "Methuselah lived to 969 years old. Abraham lived 175 years. . . . Moses died at 120, and it is after Moses that the human lifespan is set at its maximum to 120 years."

Rabbi Reichman continued recounting biblical studies: "At the time of the flood of Noah, God pronounced that [humans] will be 120 years old. That did not occur immediately. [It] took roughly 750 years for the longevity of man to gradually taper down from roughly 900 years old to 120 years old."

Rabbi Reichman cited the work of Nathan Aviezer, a contemporary scientist and physics professor in Israel who writes on the Torah from an Orthodox Jewish perspective. Aviezer's interpretation is that, during this period, a divine intervention introduced specific genes which curtailed longevity, and it took several generations for these genes to proliferate and shorten the human lifespan.

"It could perhaps be that we are attempting to identify those genes that God introduced at that stage of history and now reverse it to achieve that longevity again," explained Reichman.

Whether we accept the biblical interpretation or not, the scientific record on human evolution tells a very different story regarding lifespan, one which does not include longevity.

In the time of early hominids, 1 million years ago, our ancestors would enter puberty at the age of 12 or 13, and, prior to birth control, quickly become pregnant. By the time they were 28, they were grandparents. Because food was always scarce, the best outcome for the perpetuation of the species would be for the grandparents to die early and not take food needed by the newborns. As such, the average age of early humans was only about 28 years old. "Aging is not just a running down of the system," said Dr. Collins at the Vatican. "It is a

programmed process. Evolution probably had an investment in having the lifespan of a particular species not go on forever. You've got to get the old folks out of the way, so the young ones have a chance at the resources."

Fast-forward to the Middle Ages and the average human lifespan had grown to 35. At the turn of the year 1900, the average lifespan increased into the mid-40s. Today, it's approaching 80.

So why do we age and die, and how long should we expect to live? While we've touched on this in a few earlier chapters, that will be the focus of the pages ahead.

NEARING "LONGEVITY ESCAPE VELOCITY"

When I was in medical school in the late 1980s I had little time to watch TV. On occasion I would sneak in an episode of *Star Trek*, but it was rare for me to sit on the couch and zone out. But I distinctly remember one Sunday afternoon when I became intrigued with a documentary on the topic of "long-lived sea life." It turned out bowhead whales from the Arctic could live for more than 200 years, and the Greenland sharks can live to 400 or 500 years.

I remember thinking, *If they can live that long, why can't we?*

As an engineer, I figured it was either a hardware or software problem.

As we have seen earlier in this book, we are just now entering an era where we can correct those hardware and software problems, given our newly created tools to read, write, and edit the software of life, grow organs, and modify the biologic hardware of our bodies.

My dear friend, **Ray Kurzweil**, speaks about a concept called **"longevity escape velocity."** It's an intriguing notion that in the near future, science will be able to extend your life by more than a year for every year you are alive. Once that happens, we can begin to think about true longevity.

Ray's prediction is that we'll reach longevity escape velocity in the next ten to twelve years. Professor George Church of Harvard Medical School echoes that same time frame. "The exponential technologies that have improved the speed and cost of reading, writing, and editing of DNA and gene therapies now apply to the category of aging reversal," said Church on my most recent Longevity Platinum trip. **"Today science is adding one year of life for every four years that we're alive. But I think age-reversal advances could mean that we reach longevity escape velocity within a decade or two, within the range of the next one or two rounds of clinical trials."**

What does that mean? Can we extend the healthy human lifespan past that stated biblical limit of 120? Can humans live indefinitely? **I implore you to think of what *you* would do with an additional thirty years of healthy life.**

As we'll see in this chapter, those exponential technologies that Dr. Church spoke about, **technologies such as AI, CRISPR, gene therapy, DNA reading and writing, robotics, digital manufacturing, sensors, and networks, are accelerating and being focused on health.** While many scientists are conservative in their beliefs about extending the healthy human lifespan, I remain confident that we'll discover a number of longevity-extending (or age-reversing) technologies faster than most believe. If this is true, then all of us need to stay healthy and free of accidents in order to intercept the technology breakthroughs coming our way. **To paraphrase Ray Kurzweil's book on this subject, *Fantastic Voyage*, it means we need to strive to "live long enough to live forever."** This is the reason for you to take advantage of the tools, platforms, and companies highlighted in this book, which can help you to maintain an optimal state of health and detect any disease at its earliest occurrence. Now let's jump into those accelerating technologies that are making the future faster than we've ever imagined.

EXPONENTIAL TECHNOLOGIES DRIVING LONGEVITY

In 2005, futurist and friend Ray Kurzweil wrote the cornerstone book on the topic of exponential or "accelerating" technologies, called *The Singularity Is Near: When Humans Transcend Biology*. As Bill Gates noted, **"Ray Kurzweil is the best person I know at predicting the future of artificial intelligence.** His intriguing new book envisions a future in which information technologies have advanced so far and fast that they enable humanity to transcend its biological limitations—transforming our lives in ways we can't yet imagine."

When I say "exponential tech," what I mean is any technology that **doubles in power while dropping in price on a regular basis.** Moore's Law is the classic example. In 1965, Intel founder Gordon Moore noticed that the number of transistors on an integrated circuit had been doubling every eighteen months. This meant that every year and a half, computers would get twice as powerful, while their cost remained the same.

Moore thought this was pretty amazing and he predicted that this trend might continue. Well, it has for fifty-five years. **Moore's Law is the reason the smartphone in your pocket is a thousand times smaller, a thousand times cheaper, and a million times more powerful than a supercomputer from the 1970s.**

And it's not slowing down!

Despite reports that we are approaching the death of Moore's Law, in 2020 it continued unabated and on schedule. **By 2023 it's projected that the average thousand-dollar laptop will have the same computing power as a human brain (roughly 10^{16} cycles per second). Twenty-five years after that, that same thousand-dollar laptop will have the equivalent computational power to all the human brains currently on Earth.**

More critically, it's not just integrated circuits that are progressing at this rate. **In the 1990s, Ray Kurzweil discovered that once a technology becomes digital, or once it can be programmed in the ones and**

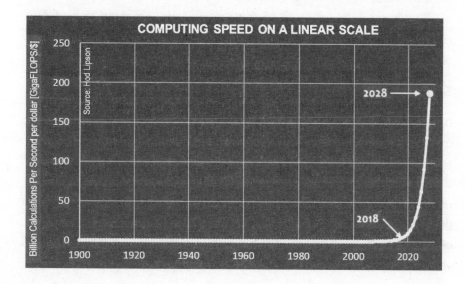

zeroes of computer code, it hops on the back of Moore's Law and begins accelerating exponentially. The technologies now accelerating at this rate include some of the most potent innovations we have yet dreamed up: **quantum computers, artificial intelligence, CRISPR, gene sequencing/ writing, robotics, nanotechnology, material science, networks, sensors, 3D printing, augmented reality, virtual reality, blockchain, and more.**

While these technologies are accelerating before our eyes, it's hard for us to grok what it means, or fathom the speed of change. The reason has to do with how our brains perceive change. Humans evolved 300,000 years ago on the savannas of Africa in a world that was local and linear. Back then, you existed in your own bubble, all within a day's walk from your village. **Nothing changed century to century, or millennium to millennium. And it stayed that way through generations. As a result, our brains evolved to only perceive, intuit, and interact with a linear world. We are all linear thinkers.**

Take thirty linear steps, one . . . two . . . three . . . four . . . five, etc., and you end up about thirty meters (just over ninety-eight feet) down the road. But if I ask you to take thirty exponential steps—where an exponential is a simple doubling . . . one, two, four, eight, sixteen, thirty-two, and so on—you'll end up a *billion* meters away (about 621,000 miles)—put differently, you'll circumnavigate Earth twenty-six times!

Predicting exponential growth is not intuitive.

So why am I discussing all of these numbers in a chapter on longevity? Because the technologies involved in extending healthspan and longevity are exponential, and their impact on our lives is not intuitive. I want you to understand that a lot can happen in just a decade or two.

It's probably worth memorizing the following:

- Double something ten times, you get a **1,000**-fold increase
- Double something twenty times, you get a **million**-fold increase
- Double something thirty times, you get a **billion**-fold increase

Entrepreneurs who understand the power of such exponential growth have developed many of the most successful companies on the planet today: Google, Facebook, Amazon, Apple, Tesla, SpaceX, Tencent, Microsoft, Alibaba, and Netflix just to name a few.

Let's consider a fun experiment. . . . If you have a child, niece, or nephew, consider giving them the following choice:

Option #1: Offer them $1 a day for the next thirty days.

Option #2: Offer them a penny on the first day, two cents on the second day, four cents on the third day, and so on.

Chances are, they take the first option.

Thirty dollars isn't bad for zero work.

But if they took the second offer, what started out with a penny would **result in $10 million on the final day.**

Now we're talking!

And this is the same exponential power that is now driving changes in biotechnology around the world. Let's take a look at just a few examples.

Exponential Growth in Genome Sequencing

Consider the cost and speed of sequencing your genome. **The Human Genome Project, backed by the NIH, took thirteen years and $3 billion to sequence the first genome—all 3.2 billion letters of your life. Today, it's under $1,000 per genome and takes less than one day.** Within two years, with Illumina's newest machines, it could **cost as little as $100 and be completed in one hour.** Incredibly, the cost of genome sequencing has been demonetizing at a rate five times faster than Moore's Law.

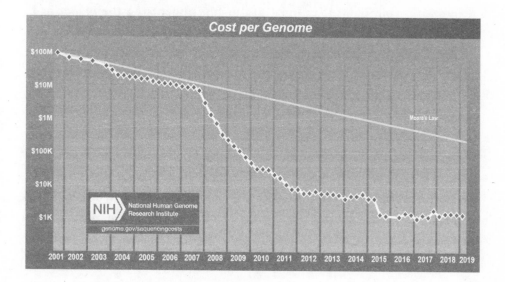

Exponential Growth in Storage

Consider data storage, which is critical for the genomics world today. The 3.2 billion base pairs of your **genome** correspond to about 725 megabytes of data, or 0.75 gigabytes of storage. **In 1981, if you were to store your uncompressed genome, a 1-gigabyte hard drive of storage cost half a million dollars. Today, it's *50 million times cheaper* at under 1 cent per gigabyte.**

Exponential Growth in Computation

How about computation? In 1971, Intel put out its first computer chip, the Intel 4004. **It had 2,300 transistors on it, at $1 each. Intel no longer actually tells you how many transistors are on their chips, but the recent Core i9 had 7 billion transistors at less than a millionth of a penny each.** This represents a **27-billion-fold increase in price performance in forty-five years.**

But it's not slowing down. **In 2021, the Cerebras Wafer Scale Engine-2 set the world record as the largest integrated circuit chip, 8.5 inches to a side, housing a jaw-dropping 2.6 trillion transistors.**

Exponential Growth in Communications

If you have a smartphone, you have access to more computational power in your hand than most of the governments on the planet had just thirty years ago. You also have better access to ubiquitous, low-cost, high-quality communication than the top CEOs and heads of state from thirty years ago. The challenge is we take such computational power and communications for granted, cursing our service provider when the occasional call gets dropped.

Digital Communications has been one of the poster children for exponential growth, showing iconic one-hundred-times growth from generation to generation. For example, when **4G mobile service rolled out its 2009 offering, it offered 100 Mbps speeds. A decade later in 2019, 5G began deployment offering speeds of 10 Gpbs (one hundred times faster).** When 5G first began rolling out in 2019, the number of subscribers was 13 million. By 2025 the 5G user base is expected to have grown to

2.8 billion. But it doesn't stop there. In August 2020, a team from Osaka University and Nanyang Technological University in Singapore **announced the design of a new mobile phone chip that could be the basis for 6G, <u>promising speeds up to one hundred times faster than 5G—fast enough to download 142 hours of Netflix in a second.</u>**

These terrestrial networks promise to connect every person on Earth, all 8 billion of us, in the next five years. They represent a lifeline for health sciences. These high-bandwidth, low-cost connections offer everyone the ability to upload health data or to get support from medical AIs wherever you live.

And it is not just people being connected, it's every device and sensor on the planet, what is referred to as the Internet of Things (or IoT). Already, IoT-connected devices have multiplied at unprecedented rates, reaching 35 billion connected devices this year and projected to exceed 75 billion by 2025. **One hundred and twenty-seven new devices get connected to the internet per second.** In terms of health, every single person will have the ability for real-time monitoring of their health and physiology from sensors in their body and on their body, measuring everything from blood glucose and blood pressure, to microRNAs that might indicate an impending heart

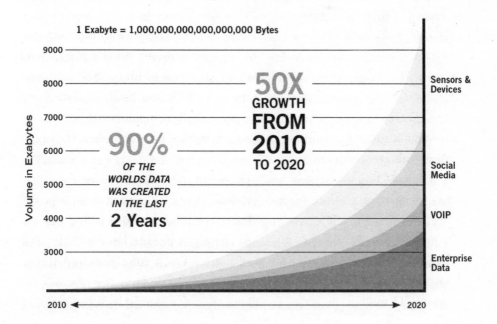

attack, or the quality of their sleep. Ultimately all of this data will be uploaded to an AI that can monitor and advise you on your exact health status.

Today we have Amazon Alexa, Apple Siri, and Google Now; eventually **we will all have a personal AI, a version of J.A.R.V.I.S. from *Iron Man*. These personal AIs will collect and monitor our health data and enable us to ultimately become "the CEOs of our own health."**

ARTIFICIAL INTELLIGENCE, NEURAL NETS, AND PROTEIN FOLDING

"This computational work represents a stunning advance on the protein-folding problem, a fifty-year-old grand challenge in biology. It has occurred decades before many people in the field would have predicted. It will be exciting to see the many ways in which it will fundamentally change biological research."

—PROFESSOR VENKI RAMAKRISHNAN, Nobel
Laureate and president, Royal Society

Perhaps the most important exponential technology transforming our lives this decade is artificial intelligence. **In the world of AI, machine learning emerged first, using algorithms to analyze data and make predictions about the world.** This is how Amazon and Netflix make their suggestions on things you should buy and movies to watch. **Next came neural networks, inspired by the biology of the human brain.** These layered circuits are capable of unsupervised learning from unstructured data. Simply unleash a neural net on the internet and the system will do the rest.

The success of neural nets over the past five years is nothing less than breathtaking. **In March 2016, Google's AlphaGo defeated the world Go champion, Lee Sedol, four games to one. Go has a game tree complexity of 10^{360}—it's chess for superheroes.** A few months after that victory, DeepMind upgraded AlphaGo to a neural net called AlphaGo Zero by updating their training style. **Between 2015 and 2016, AlphaGo had been educated by consuming the data of thousands of games previously played by humans, which taught it the proper move and countermove for every possible position. AlphaGo Zero, on the other hand, <u>learned</u>**

to master the game of Go with *zero* data. Instead, it relies on "reinforcement learning"—it essentially learned by playing itself over and over and over again.

Starting with little more than a few simple rules, in mid-2017, **AlphaGo Zero took only three days to beat its parent, AlphaGo, the same system that beat Lee Sedol. Three weeks later, it trounced the sixty best players in the world. In total, it took forty days for AlphaGo Zero to become the undisputed best Go player on Earth.**

So how does this relate to health and longevity? Enter Alphafold.

Ever since the 1980s, when I was completing my engineering and medical degrees, I've been tracking a particular supercomputing problem that if solved would revolutionize medicine. **Called the grand challenge of biology, the "protein folding problem" asked the following question: "Given an amino acid sequence, can you predict the ultimate three-dimensional protein structure that would result?"**

Why does that matter? Proteins are perhaps the most important class of molecules in the human body, essential to life, supporting practically all its functions. They are macromolecules made up of chains of amino acids, and **what a protein does largely depends on its unique 3D structure.** Once folded, proteins carry out a vast array of functions, ranging from catalyzing metabolic reactions, DNA replication, responding to stimuli, providing structure to cells and organisms, and transporting molecules from one location to another. **Enzymes and antibodies are proteins, as are insulin, collagen, elastin, and keratin.**

If we could accurately predict protein structures from an amino acid sequence, it would open the door to an entire new avenue of low-cost and accurate drug development.

Back in 1994, to monitor progress in this supercomputer protein-folding problem, a biannual competition called the **Critical Assessment of Protein Structure Prediction (CASP)** was created. **Until 2018, success was fairly slow and incremental. But following the success of AlphaGo Zero, the team at DeepMind turned their neural networks loose on protein folding. They called their newest neural net AlphaFold.**

On its first foray into the CASP competition, AlphaFold got twenty-five of the potential forty-three protein-folding problems right. The second-place team managed a meager three! **How accurate was Alpha-Fold's prediction? Incredibly accurate, within the width of an atom (or 0.1 of a nanometer)!**

Arthur D. Levinson, chairman of Apple and CEO of Alphabet's longevity company Calico, had this to say about DeepMind's success: **"AlphaFold is a once-in-a-generation advance, predicting protein structures with incredible speed and precision. This leap forward demonstrates how computational methods are poised to transform research in biology and hold much promise for accelerating the drug discovery process."**

AI AND DRUG DISCOVERY

Beyond predicting the structure of a protein, **what if AI could generate novel drugs to target any disease, overnight, ready for clinical trials? What if it was able to design a drug that was perfect specifically for you? Imagine leveraging machine learning to accomplish with fifty scientists what the pharmaceutical industry can barely do with an army of 5,000?**

This is the promise of using AI for drug discovery. It's a multibillion-dollar opportunity that can help billions of people around the world.

To provide context on how incredible this opportunity really is, let's examine the global pharmaceutical market, one of the slowest, most monolithic industries to adapt, surpassing $1.25 trillion in revenue in 2019. In 2021, the top ten pharmaceutical companies alone are projected to generate over $355 billion. At the same time, **it currently costs more than $2.5 billion (sometimes up to $12 billion) and takes over ten years to bring a new drug to market. And nine out of ten drugs entering Phase I clinical trials will never reach patients.**

But a world of pharmaceutical abundance is already emerging. As artificial intelligence converges with massive data sets in everything from gene expression to blood tests, novel drug discovery **is about to get 100-fold cheaper, 100-fold faster, and more intelligently targeted.**

One of the hottest startups I know in this area that Peter and I have invested in is called **Insilico Medicine**, founded and lead by **CEO Dr. Alex Zhavoronkov**. In 2014, Zhavoronkov started wondering if he could use these massive data sets and AI to significantly speed up the drug discovery process. He'd heard about a new technique in artificial intelligence known as generative adversarial networks (or GANs). **By pitting two neural nets against one another (adversarial), the system can start with minimal instructions and produce novel outcomes (generative).** Researchers had been using GANs to do things like design new objects or create one-of-a-kind, fake human faces, but Zhavoronkov wanted to apply them to pharmacology. He figured GANs would allow researchers to verbally describe drug attributes: **"The compound should inhibit protein X at concentration Y with minimal side effects in humans," and then the AI could construct the molecule from scratch.**

To turn his idea into reality, Zhavoronkov set up Insilico Medicine on the campus of Johns Hopkins University in Baltimore, Maryland, and rolled up his sleeves. "It took us three years of hard work to develop a system that researchers could actually interact with in this way," he explains. **"But we pulled it off, and this has allowed us to reinvent the drug discovery process. The results are an explosion in potential drug targets and a much more efficient testing process,"** says Zhavoronkov. **"AI allows us to do with fifty people what a typical drug company does with five thousand."**

The results have turned what was once a decade-long war into a month-long skirmish. In late 2018, for example, Insilico was generating novel molecules in fewer than forty-six days, and this included not just the initial discovery, but also the synthesis of the drug and its experimental validation in computer simulations.

Right now, they're using the system to hunt down new drugs for cancer, aging, fibrosis, Parkinson's, Alzheimer's, ALS, diabetes, and many others. They're also in the early stages of using AI to predict the outcomes of clinical trials in advance of the trial. If successful, this technique will enable researchers to strip a bundle of time and money out of the traditional testing process.

But even as extraordinary as these AI capabilities are, they might not compare to what's coming this decade in the field of nanotechnology and micro-robots able to course through our bodies to effect repairs.

MICROBOTS AND *FANTASTIC VOYAGE*

The Academy Award–winning 1966 science fiction film *Fantastic Voyage* chronicled the adventures of a submarine crew who were shrunk to microscopic size and placed into the body of an injured scientist to repair damage to his brain.

Exactly six decades later, in 2016, Bionaut Labs was founded in Israel and has turned a version of this concept into science fact, having built and demonstrated remote-controlled microbots, *smaller than a grain of rice*, that travel through the body to deliver drug treatments to precise locations.

Why does this matter? Many of the issues we face in medicine today are local in nature. Take brain, lung, or ovarian cancer. **Unfortunately, we treat these local cancer issues with solutions like chemotherapy that affect the *entire* body, resulting in significant side effects.**

Bionaut Labs first seeks to revolutionize the treatment of central nervous system (CNS) disorders using these microbots less than a millimeter in diameter, called Bionauts, that are remotely controlled by directed magnetic forces to steer their payload. **Once inside the brain tissue, located adjacent to a tumor, for example, the Bionauts are magnetically triggered to release their payload. Their accuracy is on par with surgeons' accuracy, whose standard deviation falls in the single-millimeter range.**

Today, Bionauts can deliver biologics and small-molecule therapeutics with unprecedented precision. Future generations of the devices could provide electrical stimulation, thermal ablation, or radioactive plaque to treat other diseases. And further down the road, as these resident microscopic robots shrink in size toward the nano scale and increase in intelligence, they may lead to the future described by K. Eric Drexler in his pivotal book *Engines of Creation: The Coming Era of Nanotechnology*, **when universal assemblers, tiny machines that can build objects atom by atom, will be used as medicinal robots that help clear capillaries, target cancer, and repair any damage.**

In the nearer term, Bionauts are focused on the early diagnosis and treatment of Alzheimer's disease, Huntington's disease, and gliomas. Bionauts could provide ongoing surveillance to stave off the progression of these and many other diseases, which is why Peter and I invested in this company through BOLD Capital.

THE ACCELERATING SPEED OF ACCELERATING TECHNOLOGIES

So there you have it—**the power of computation, artificial intelligence, sensors, networks, and robotics to transform sick care into healthcare. For most readers, the idea of achieving age reversal or "longevity escape velocity" may sound like science fiction.** But I'd love for you to consider that **it may not be any crazier than some of the other extraordinary advancements we've made in the past few decades . . . flying cars, free global video calls on FaceTime, or AI's ability to accurately predict the folding of proteins, run Google Maps navigation, create "deep fakes," and diagnose patients.** It's perhaps no crazier than Elon Musk and Jeff Bezos taking us to Mars and the Moon in the coming decade. **While our linear human mind is great at making near-term predictions, we vastly underestimate what can be achieved in the longer term.**

Of course the exponential technologies discussed above aren't standing still; we haven't reached humanity's pinnacle of technology. Our speed of innovation is actually accelerating. As I mentioned earlier, the only constant is change.

A decade of progress between 1950 and 1960 is not the same as a decade of progress, say, fifty years later, between 2010 and 2020. The reasons for this are multifold. First, the exponential growth of computing power discussed above, namely Moore's Law. Second is the convergence of accelerating technologies such as the intersection of AI and robotics, or AI and gene therapy. Third is a specific **set of three forces: saved time, demonetization, and capital abundance.** Let's take a quick look at each and why they are important.

The first force is saved time. Innovation needs time and focus, the ability of a researcher or entrepreneur to focus their available time on slaying scientific challenges. **How we spend our time has changed a lot in the past few decades. Our ability to get almost any question we want**

answered instantly on Google is perhaps chief among them. Compare this to the days when you'd need to drive to the library and hope you could find a published book that had the data you needed. Add to this **the saved time resulting from instantaneous global communications, and the ability to find the exact product you need and order it online, having it delivered the very next day.** And of course, as of the Pandemic of 2020, there's **the acceptance of connecting with someone over Zoom, rather than spending an entire day flying from LA to New York for an hour-long meeting.**

All of this has an impact on the rate of innovation. **As this bonanza of extra hours continues to pile up, inventors, entrepreneurs, those proverbial gals and guys in the garage, will get far more time to experiment, fail, pivot, fail again, pivot again, and, eventually, get it right.** Technology has shrunk innovation development timelines and expanded the time innovators can devote to development. **It's a force that accelerates the rate of acceleration—but it's not the only one.**

Our second force is the demonetization of technology and services. While startups and researchers are getting access to more and more cash, the **impact of every dollar is also accelerating. Meaning you can now do much more with a research investment dollar than you could just a decade ago.**

Perhaps there is no better example than the cost of DNA sequencing mentioned earlier in the book. To remind you, <u>the Human Genome Project took about a decade to sequence a single human genome, completed in April of 2003 at an approximate cost of nearly $3 billion. Today Illumina's latest generation sequencer has the potential to sequence your genome in an hour and for $100—or 87,600 times faster and 30 million times cheaper.</u> As a result, if you're working in genomics, then your government research grant or your last financing round now goes much further than ever before, accelerating insights and catalyzing breakthroughs.

And what is true for gene sequencing is true in dozens of fields—everything from access to supercomputers on the cloud, near infinite, no-cost data storage, and free global videoconferencing on Zoom. **Add to this the impact of 3D printing, and research tools such as sensors, cameras,** accelerometers, just to name a few, that have shrunk a thousand-fold in size and a million-fold in price.

Our third and final force is the abundance of capital. Nothing accelerates technological innovation like cash. *Lots* of cash. **More cash translates into more people, equipment, experimenting, failing, and eventually creating breakthroughs.**

There is now more "capital abundance" than any other time ever. As the *Economist* points out, **companies raised more capital in 2020 (in the midst of a pandemic)** *than anytime in human history.* Perhaps the best example of this is the story of venture capital funding, the traditional source of startup capital that has helped to birth household names from Apple and Google to Amazon and Uber. **In 2020, U.S. venture capitalist firms invested $156.2 billion in startups,** *equivalent to about $428 million every day of the year.* This record sum was up from $136.5 billion invested in 2019. And, as one might expect, the biotechnology industry experienced massive year-over-year growth, **from $17.2 billion in 2019 investments to an all-time high of $27.4 billion invested across 998 deals in 2020,** largely driven by medical breakthroughs in vaccine development and COVID-19 therapies.

Any way you slice it, this era of unprecedented capital abundance is massively accelerating innovation and funding crazy ideas and moonshots.

FOLLOW THE MONEY

To reinforce this final point about capital abundance, and to give you **increased confidence that we may yet reach longevity escape velocity in the next decade or two,** it's worth sharing the stories of some of the pioneering venture funds and government programs that are literally pouring billions of dollars into the field every year. Venture funds like BOLD Capital Partners (my own fund), Prime Mover Labs, Khosla Ventures (which Tony and I are investors in), Section32, Kitty Hawk Ventures, Google Ventures, Founders Fund, Arch Ventures, the Longevity Vision Fund, RA Capital, OrbiMed, LUX Capital, and the Hevolution Foundation just to name a few, all of whom, cumulatively, are deploying many billions of dollars per year into this field.

"I am on a mission to positively impact one billion lives by bringing an affordable and accessible version of healthcare and longevity to the world," says Sergey Young, managing partner of the Longevity Vision Fund and author of the book *The Science and Technology of Growing Young*.

Then there's a $3 billion fund by the name of **Prime Mover Labs (PML)**, run by **Dakin Sloss**. Tony Robbins is one of the partners in this fund. "PML invests in breakthrough scientific inventions that transform billions of lives," says Dakin. **"We deploy about $200 million each year in the area of longevity in order to extend the quantity and quality of life for our human family."**

Add to this **Khosla Ventures**, which manages $14 billion under management, and OrbiMed, whose $19 billion is dedicated solely to healthcare.

And it isn't all private money moving this field forward. The Biden administration deserves accolades for their proposed $6.5 billion Advanced Research Projects Agency for Health, referred to as ARPA-H, modeled on the Advanced Research Projects Agency (ARPA) arm of the U.S. Defense Department, which in the 1960s gave America ARPANET, the precursor to today's global internet. It's proposed that ARPA-H would aim to deliver breakthrough treatments for diseases like Alzheimer's, cancer, and diabetes.

Perhaps one of the most extraordinary (and newest) players in the aging field is the Hevolution Foundation, a nonprofit organization headquartered in Riyadh, Saudi Arabia. Hevolution was formed in partnership with leaders of both the Kingdom of Saudi Arabia and the United Arab Emirates, and **endowed with an initial budget that allows them to deploy at least $1 billion per year to fulfill their vision of "extending healthy lifespan for the benefit of all humanity."**

To run the foundation, the leadership tapped a brilliant and visionary veteran in the field, Mehmood Khan, MD, to be its CEO. Mehmood is a powerhouse in the longevity field, having served as PepsiCo's former vice chairman and chief scientific officer, president of global R&D at Takeda Pharmaceuticals, and most recently the CEO of Life Biosciences (one of David Sinclair's companies).

"Every human has the right to flourish throughout their life, regardless of age, geography, or economic circumstance," said Khan. **"We see aging as humanity's greatest opportunity and want to catalyze science to** achieve significant healthspan breakthroughs. To enable this, Hevolution will be underwriting scientific research to accelerate therapeutic approaches to aging, and will be making investments in companies engaged in work aligned to that research."

Any way you cut it, that is a lot of capital accelerating the rate of healthspan and age-reversal technologies. While few would argue that being healthier longer and not suffering in your final years is a good thing, some are concerned about the consequence of more humans on Earth, the specter of overpopulation.

WILL LONGER LIVES CAUSE OVERPOPULATION OF EARTH?

"Earth is going to face a massive population collapse over the next twenty to thirty years. . . . This would be civilization's way of dying with a whimper."

—ELON MUSK, founder, SpaceX and Tesla

In the 1980s, Paul Ehrlich released a book, *The Population Bomb*, that incited a worldwide fear of overpopulation. He said that too many people, packed into too-tight spaces, would take too much from the Earth. Unless humanity cut down its numbers, all of us would face "mass starvation" on "a dying planet." Original estimates by the United Nations had the world's population peaking at **10.9 billion** people by 2100.

To this day, **when I speak publicly about age-reversal and longevity, many express their concerns about overpopulation. But data over the past few decades is painting a very different picture, one where the problem of society may well be** *underpopulation* **later this century.**

In 2021, the *Lancet*, one of the world's most prestigious medical journals, **challenged the UN demographers' forecast, projecting that the global population will peak at 9.7 billion by 2064 and** *decline* **to 8.8 billion by 2100.**

That's four decades earlier and 2 billion fewer people.

As it turns out, globally improving standards of living and declining reproductive rates have done just the opposite of what had been predicted, putting us in potential danger because of underpopulation.

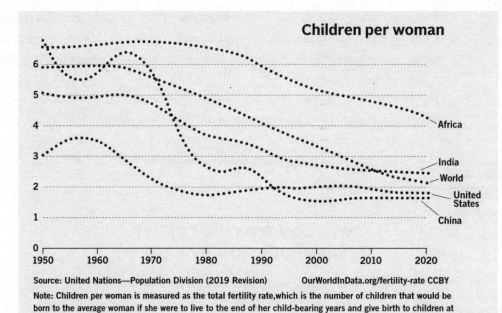

Children per woman

Source: United Nations—Population Division (2019 Revision)   OurWorldInData.org/fertility-rate CCBY

Note: Children per woman is measured as the total fertility rate,which is the number of children that would be
born to the average woman if she were to live to the end of her child-bearing years and give birth to children at
the current age-specific fertility rates.

Fewer people overall mean fewer workers. The population will shift toward the elderly, creating a heavier burden on the younger working population.

Total fertility rate is a metric that demographers use to measure number of children per month. **The population replacement rate, which is the average number of children per family for each generation to *exactly* replace itself, is roughly 2.1.**

The chart above tells a fascinating and hopeful story. **Seventy years ago, the global average fertility rate was 5.05.** Several countries, such as Rwanda, Kenya, and the Philippines, had a fertility rate higher than 7 children per woman. China had a fertility rate just over 6, while India was just below 6. Only *one* country in the world had a fertility rate below 2, and that was the small European nation of Luxembourg. **The United States, in comparison, had a total fertility rate of 3.03 in 1950.**

But *a lot* has changed since then. **Today, roughly 80 percent of the world's population lives in countries with a fertility rate below 3. As of 2020, the global average fertility rate has *more than halved, to 2.44.* Several countries now have a fertility rate that is *significantly below* the** replacement level, **with the U.S. at 1.77,** and women in countries such as Iran and Thailand having just 1.6 children on average.

What is the reason for this unprecedented decline? In short, there are *three major reasons*: the empowerment of women, declining child mortality, and the rising cost of raising children.

And the COVID-19 pandemic seems to have accelerated this trend toward underpopulation. **Historically, there's been a spike in births nine months after disasters, and some people are wondering whether there will be a COVID baby boom.**

But it's more complicated than that.

Many people are now more unsure of their financial safety. Childcare during the pandemic has been difficult. Parents are cut off from extended family, who would have been part of a newborn's upbringing.

And the numbers reflect these trends. **Clinics are reporting an increase in requests for birth control prescriptions. The pandemic has changed the way the world thinks of children—it might even bring the world closer to underpopulation *sooner* than we think.**

Back in April 2021, when **I interviewed Elon Musk for the launch of the $100 million XPRIZE Carbon Removal, I asked him his concern on the topic of population.** He shook his head and said, "Earth is going **to face a massive population collapse over the next twenty to thirty years. . . . This would be civilization's way of dying with a whimper."**

More than ever, we need to *increase our productive and healthy lifespan*. If we don't extend health life and productive healthspan we are likely to face a significant shortage of labor. So, not only will longer healthy lives allow us to spend more time with loved ones and fulfill our bucket list dreams—they also have the potential for *enormous* economic value to society.

In 2021, researchers from Harvard, Oxford, and London Business School have demonstrated just how much increasing healthy lifespan is worth in dollars.

Slowing aging *by only one year* is worth +*$38 trillion* to the global economy.

That is just *one year*. **Imagine the societal benefits and economic value of increasing healthy lifespan by *ten to twenty years*.**

DREAMS OF IMMORTALITY

So, there you have it. A tour de force of the exponential technologies and capital abundance being applied to health and longevity, a set of tools that may allow many reading this book, should they desire it, **to get to the goal of longevity escape velocity**.

How long might you live? Does an age of 120 years mean a wheelchair and drool? What might be possible this decade or the next?

To close out this chapter, I'll highlight the work and predictions of two friends whom you've met earlier in this book, age-reversal experts, both at **Harvard Medical School, Drs. George Church and David Sinclair.**

As we touched on in Chapter 4, in December 2020, **Dr. Sinclair was the principal author on a landmark paper, the cover story of** *Nature* **magazine. The article was titled "Turning Back Time: Reprogramming Retinal Cells Can Reverse Age-Related Vision Loss."**

Dr. Sinclair summarized the significance of the published work as follows: **"The main point of the paper is that we found that there is a backup copy of youthful information in the cell that we can access that gives us the ability to reboot cells, even in a living animal. In the case of the** *Nature* **paper, we found that we could reboot the cells of the mouse eye and rejuvenate them, taking them back in time.** The vision system of the mouse didn't just appear younger, it was literally younger. And the fact that there is this backup copy of youthful information gives me a lot of hope we can do this in other organs and tissues as well.

"The field has come a long way over just the last five years, where we can now openly speak about the idea of aging reversal. Now it's one of the hottest topics to study and hundreds of labs around the world are working on this topic. It's a gold rush to see what tissues and organs we can epigenetically reprogram to make them more youthful."

When asked how age reversal might work in humans, **David describes a scenario where someone, perhaps 60 years old, goes for a treatment that uses three of the four Yamanaka Factors** (Dr. Shinya Yamanaka won the 2012 Nobel Prize in Medicine for describing the use of four factors able to produce induced pluripotent stem cells) **to epigenetically reprogram their body. Following the treatment, everything from their skin, to**

their brain and their liver, would rejuvenate, reversing in age some number of decades. And then when you "age-out" a few decades later, you would go in for another rejuvenation treatment and keep resetting the system. **"We don't know how many times we can reset a person's age,"** continues Sinclair, **"but I would be surprised if it couldn't be done multiple times."**

When asked for a timeline, Dr. Sinclair answers, **"I hope we'll have proof of concept done in the next two to three years. And if that works, we'll go as fast as the FDA allows."**

What tissues are Dr. Sinclair and his colleagues working on reprogramming? He quickly rattles off a list, "Liver, spleen, muscle, kidney, hearing, brain. **And one of my colleagues reprogrammed the hippocampus in mice and those mice regained their memories."**

The other great thinker in the field of age reversal mentioned earlier in this chapter and in the book is the prolific scientist and parallel entrepreneur **Dr. George Church**. His work and predictions, alongside Dr. Sinclair's, have left me in awe and with great optimism about the decades ahead.

"The strategy of aging reversal treatments," began Church, "is to test them against various diseases that have nothing in common other than they happen to be diseases of aging in the same animal. **If a single treatment can reverse a multitude of age-related diseases, then you have an age-reversal treatment. And that's exactly what was demonstrated in mice by one of the post-doc students, Dr. Noah Davidson."**

As we discussed in Chapter 17, Dr. Davidson, alongside Dr. Church, has started a company called **Rejuvenate Bio that is looking to treat six different diseases of aging in dogs. "Early results are very positive, and we hope to have approval for these age reversal treatments in dogs within the next couple of years,"** said Church. "Then if all goes well, we will start human clinical trials a couple of years after that."

When asked about how old humans might be able to live given the progress in rejuvenation science, Dr. Church responded, "I don't think there's an upper limit, I think it's a matter of how quickly we get there. Everything is pointing towards the fact that exponential technology growth is especially effective in biology, which is now an information science. It is quite possible that some of the people alive today will see no upper limit. **And it's quite** possible that some of us in this conversation today will be seeing 150 or 200 years [of age], and at that point our technology will be so advanced that it just keeps going."

Twenty-five years ago, when my dreams of spaceflight seemed to be moving too slowly, it was the $10 million Ansari XPRIZE for spaceflight that helped spark the private spaceflight industry we are now experiencing. For the same reason, leaving nothing to chance, and hoping to accelerate the realm of age-reversal as fast as possible, today I'm working with top scientists (David Sinclair, George Church, and Sergey Young included) to **design and fund a $100 million Age Reversal XPRIZE (as of this writing $55 million has been committed thus far).** Our goal is to inspire as many teams as possible to demonstrate the technology needed to rejuvenate each of us by at least 25 percent of our lifespan. For more information, please visit xprize.org.

So there you have it. A future in which CRISPR, gene therapy, stem cells, replacement organs, AI, and a multitude of other exponential technologies have the potential to extend what society believes to be the typical human healthspan. Will we be able to reach the 120-year age of Moses? It seems likely. But what about Adam at 930 or Methuselah at 969 years old? Many of us reading this book, should science succeed in achieving longevity escape velocity, may just find out.

I, for one, am doing all I can to remain vital and healthy to intercept the next few decades of exponential change coming our way. At a minimum, it includes all of the recommendations made in earlier chapters on diet, exercise, sleep, supplements, and an annual diagnostic upload. But perhaps one of the most important things you can do is to **adopt a longevity mindset. A mindset characterized by a more fulfilling, passionate, and purposeful life.** To guide us through the power of decision, mindset, and how to create an extraordinary quality of life, there is no one better than Tony Robbins. . . .

CHAPTER 24

CREATING AN EXTRAORDINARY QUALITY OF LIFE: THE POWER OF MINDSET

"However vast the darkness, we must supply our own light."

—STANLEY KUBRICK, legendary American filmmaker

If you've stayed with me this far, congratulations! By now you know the score. The thrilling dawn of regenerative medicine is leading us to radically healthier, more vital lives. **The insights and breakthroughs of the healthspan revolution are transforming every facet of medicine, from 3D replacement organs to the living drugs that are conquering cancer with our own modified cells. CRISPR and gene therapy are allowing us to literally redesign how our bodies function. And we're getting closer each day to answering the riddle of why we age, and how we soon might be able to turn back the clock.**

But there are still some critical questions left to answer: **How can we make the most of our expanded healthspan?** Is a longer, more physically vibrant existence an end in itself? And—most of all—**how do we find fulfillment?**

Here's the short answer: **It's not the number of years that matters most.** Let's return to the Vatican conference that opened this book. At a panel on longevity, Peter Diamandis asked the audience: "How many of you would want to live to one hundred twenty if you could?" Peter was astonished by the response. Judging from the show of hands, about two-thirds wanted no part of a 120-year lifespan—and these were people in the rejuvenation business!

Why the lack of enthusiasm? I think it's because most people I know love the *idea* of longevity, but when push comes to shove, we want more than *quantity* of life. We're looking for an extraordinary *quality* of life. Good health is the foundation, no question. But people can be physically healthy and still miss out on the quality of life they desire. Why is that? **Because they haven't yet mastered their own mind.** They haven't learned how to make the most of their time on Earth, however long that may be. As we travel through these last pages together on this long and amazing journey, let's look at one last tool for health, healing, and vitality. It's the most incredibly powerful tool of all.

That's right: It's your mind!

If you were about to die *right now*, if the Grim Reaper were on your doorstep, you'd negotiate if you could, right? Let's say you bargained successfully for one more week of life. **How would you spend that week?** Would you be whining, worrying, complaining, regretting? Would you be frustrated and angry over some ancient disappointment? Would you *suffer* your way to the end?

Or would you choose to leave the world loving and laughing? Would you spend those last hours on the friends and family you love—giving, connecting, sharing your most honest and intimate emotions? **Would you try to squeeze every ounce of exhilaration out of every moment you had left?**

Either way, it would be up to you. We can't predict the number of days we've got left. But we can absolutely control what we get out of them. **That's the subject of these final two chapters of the book—the power of the mind and what it truly takes to be fulfilled.**

PLACEBOS AND THE POWER OF MINDSET

"The mind is powerful, and you have more control than you think."

—SCOTT D. LEWIS, mindfulness practitioner

Here's a fascinating example of your mindset at work: the placebo effect. What are placebos? They're harmless "medicines" or procedures that are used to test a therapy's effectiveness. But if you thought placebos had no real impact, you'd be mistaken.

Many people have heard about patients in Stage 3 or Stage 4 cancer—and suddenly they shift into spontaneous remission and the cancer is gone. Do you remember Ginny, my former girlfriend's mother, the woman given nine weeks to live? **More than forty years later, she is alive and well.** Some people believe that these seeming miracles are the result of prayer; others think a change of diet made all the difference. But here are two things we know for sure:

- Traditional medical science can't explain what happened.
- The mind contains the power to heal the body.

There are countless examples of placebos duplicating—or even surpassing—the impact of the real actual drugs. **By mobilizing the brain's frontal lobe, placebos can have tremendous power over pain, over medicines' side effects—even over degenerative disease.** Let's take a quick walk through the history of this amazing phenomenon to show you just how powerful your mind really is:

- **The placebo effect was discovered during World War II by an anesthesiologist named Dr. Henry Beecher, who'd run out of morphine in the middle of a German bombardment.**[1] Desperate to ease a soldier's pain, Beecher's nurse injected a syringe of salt water but told the wounded man he was getting the powerful painkiller. To Beecher's astonishment, the saline soothed the soldier's agony and kept him from going into shock. After Beecher returned to Harvard Medical School after the war, he pioneered the use of "controlled" clinical studies for new medicines, where some of the test subjects would unknowingly get a placebo. By subtracting the improvement in the placebo control group, researchers could determine whether a drug really worked or not.
- **In a migraine pain study at Harvard Medical School, the placebo was found to be nearly as effective as the actual drug. What made the results even more astounding was that the scientists clearly labeled**

---

1 Silberman, "Placebos are Getting More Effective. Drugmakers Are Desperate to Know Why."

it "PLACEBO"—the patients knew what they weren't getting![2] As the lead researcher noted, "The placebo effect is more than positive thinking. . . . It's about creating **a stronger connection between the brain and body** and how they work together."[3]

- **Not all placebos are equal.** The bigger the "intervention," the more profound the result. **Higher placebo "doses"—bigger pills—boosted the effect.[4] The placebo effect can be strengthened or weakened by the outward qualities of the placebo: Taking more placebo pills generally has a greater effect; capsules do a better job than pills; and injections do better than capsules.[5] An even more powerful example is what's known as placebo "sham" surgery. Meaning the person was put under anesthesia and cut open, but no repair was made. Yet, the patient was made to believe one was.[6]**

- In a Harvard study, one hundred medical students were enlisted to test two drugs: a "super stimulant" red pill and a "super tranquilizer" blue one. Unbeknownst to the students, the drugs were purposely switched—the red was actually a barbiturate, and the blue an amphetamine. **Even so, the subjects who were given a "downer" experienced stimulation because of their expectations, while those who took the "upper" that was actually a barbiturate felt tired.[7]** Talk about the power of the mind! <u>**The subjects' expectations actually overpowered the drug and reversed its impact to the very opposite of what the chemicals normally create.**</u>

- **And I bet this one will amaze you:** A trial at the Houston Veterans Affairs Medical Center enrolled 180 subjects with significant pain from osteoarthritis. Two-thirds underwent arthroscopic knee surgery; the other

---

2 Kam-Hansen et al., "Altered Placebo and Drug Labeling Changes the Outcome of Episodic Migraine Attacks."

3 *Harvard Health Publishing*, "The Power of the Placebo Effect."

4 Meissner and Linde, "Are Blue Pills Better Than Green? How Treatment Features Modulate Placebo Effects."

5 Srivastava and More, "Some Aesthetic Considerations for Over-the-Counter Pharmaceutical Products."

6 Wartolowska et al., "Use of Placebo Controls in the Evaluation of Surgery: Systematic Review."

7 Martin, "The Power of the Placebo Effect."

60 had a fake **"placebo surgery"** procedure. Both groups had the same prep and were cared for overnight by nurses who didn't know who'd had the real operation. The results? **The placebo patients reported just as much pain relief—and functional improvement—as the ones who'd had the real surgery. <u>One year later, the placebo group was doing _better_ at walking and stair-climbing than the surgical patients.</u>**[8] **<u>The results were so profound that the Department of Veterans Affairs told its doctors to stop performing these operations.</u>**[9]

You don't have to pop a sugar pill to get this effect. Simply changing your outlook can add years to your life! According to an Ohio study, <u>**middle-aged subjects with positive attitudes on aging wound up living more than seven years longer on average than those with negative attitudes.**</u>[10] And research out of Yale found that <u>**older people with a positive focus on aging were 44 percent more likely to fully recover from a disabling health problem.**</u>[11]

In a seminal study on the mind-body connection, my friend **Ellen Langer, PhD,** a professor of psychology at Harvard, took a group of older men on an isolated New England retreat—but with a twist. The hotel was retrofitted with every visible cue—magazines, TV shows, movies—from twenty years earlier. The subjects were told to act as if they'd actually traveled back in time.[12] When they discussed "current" events from two decades earlier, they spoke in the present tense. (If you did this today, you'd be dancing to Eminem.) **At the end of the five-day "counterclockwise" experiment, the men showed measurable improvement in memory, hearing,**

---

8 Moseley et al., "A Controlled Trial of Arthroscopic Surgery for Osteoarthritis of the Knee."

9 Kolata, "VA Suggests Halt to Knee Operation / Arthroscopy's Effectiveness Questioned."

10 Pagnini et al., "Ageing as a Mindset: A Study Protocol to Rejuvenate Older Adults with a Counterclockwise Psychological Intervention."

11 Levy et al., "Association Between Positive Age Stereotypes and Recovery From Disability in Older Persons."

12 _Newsweek_, "Can We Reverse Aging by Changing How We Think?"

vision, grip strength, joint flexibility, and posture. Their arthritis eased up. Based on before-and-after photos, they even *looked* younger.[13]

It turns out cultural stereotypes about aging, good or bad, become self-concepts—and self-fulfilling prophecies. **Positive attitudes protect against dementia,** even in people with the high-risk ApoE4 gene.[14] **What's the common thread of these studies? A positive mindset can reverse the aging process!** Remember that saying, *You're only as young as you feel?* The science tells us it's true!

Want one more piece of evidence? In a more recent study by Professor Langer, a group of hotel room cleaners was told that their everyday work met the surgeon general's requirements for an active lifestyle. A control group wasn't given this information. **Four weeks later, the first group had lowered their systolic blood pressure, their body mass index, and their percentage of body fat. The control group showed none of these improvements.**[15] As Professor Langer wrote, **"it is clear that health is significantly affected by mind-set."**[16]

Now that you know that your mind can simulate surgery or drugs, or make you feel a generation younger, the next step is to control it— something very few people do. **And here's the problem: An undirected mind tends to go to fear. We saw this tragically during COVID-19. According to the Centers for Disease Control, the number-two mortality risk factor for people with COVID, just behind obesity, was "anxiety and fear-related disorders."[17] Fear was more deadly for COVID patients than severe diabetes, chronic kidney disease, chronic obstructive pulmonary disease, or heart disease.[18] It sounds crazy, doesn't it? But the CDC science shows it to be true.**

---

13 Pagnini et al., "Aging as a Mindset."

14 Levy et al., "Positive Age Beliefs Protect Against Dementia Even Among Elders with High-Risk Gene."

15 Crum and Langer, "Mind-Set Matters: Exercise and the Placebo Effect."

16 West, "Mind-Set Matters."

17 Kompaniyets et al., "Underlying Medical Conditions and Severe Illness Among 540,667 Adults Hospitalized with COVID-19."

18 Ibid.

As we've noted, we have a two-million-year-old "fight-or-flight" brain that evolved to protect us from saber-toothed tigers. The tigers are long gone, but our brain still overblows every "crisis." It worries what people are thinking about us, or that we don't have enough money. It turns bumps in the road into matters of life and death. But we don't have to play along. We can kill this fear monster before it grows up and destroys our life, family, and community.

> *"Our bodies are apothecaries. We convert our*
> *expectations into chemical reality."*

—NORMAN COUSINS, American author, journalist, and professor

We've seen that our minds can make us healthy, but they can also make us sick as well. And not only that, **they can also create a contagious effect of fear.** One of the earliest heroes in the science of neuroimmunology, the study of how the nervous system and immune system interact, was UCLA professor and bestselling author **Norman Cousins**. He was diagnosed with a rare, autoimmune form of inflammatory arthritis called ankylosing spondylitis. In its advanced stages, the condition can lead to the total fusion of the spine—it's incredibly debilitating and painful.

Instead of sitting at home to suffer, **Cousins decided to cure himself by laughter.** Determined not to let the diagnosis limit his positivity in life, **he found that just ten minutes of deep belly laughter would give him two to three hours of relief from his agony. In place of pills, he would watch funny movies as often as necessary for pain reduction and a good sleep. <u>Many years later, doctors found that his arthritis had been stopped in its tracks, with no progression. Baffled by the results, they decided that Cousins must have been misdiagnosed and the condition had resolved on its own.</u>** Cousins, however, knew that there was something else at work.

This is one of the best-known cases in the science of psychoneuroimmunology, or PNI, the study of how what we think (psycho) changes the brain (neuro) and in turn affects our immune system. Cousins's life and work were so significant that the University of California at Los Angeles now houses the Norman Cousins Center for Psychoneuroimmunology.

I had the privilege of meeting Norman Cousins in my early 20s. He came to one of my events and even walked on fire! In an interview in one of my early PowerTalks, he shared how the mind can make us healthy or ill just as the CDC has found. He retold a story about the power of the mind from his book *Anatomy of an Illness*. During a football game in Los Angeles, a few people came down ill with symptoms of food poisoning. The doctor who treated them ascertained that they'd all had Coca-Cola from one of the two dispensing machines by the stands. He naturally wondered if the soda's syrup had been contaminated or the machines' copper piping had corroded. But before they could pinpoint the cause, he didn't want anyone else to be exposed. So he went on the public address system and described the symptoms of the sick people and warned everyone not to drink any more Coca-Cola.

Within minutes, the whole football stadium became a sea of retching people—including many who hadn't gone to either soda machine. There were five ambulances shuttling back and forth to bring people to a nearby hospital. Later that day, they found out there was nothing poisonous in the Coca-Cola machines. As soon as they got the news, the people in the hospital stopped throwing up. There was nothing wrong with them. Cousins called it "a mass-induced hypnosis," an acute physical reaction caused completely by people's minds.

There's no question that fear can cause a shortness of breath, our temperature to rise, and even make us vomit. So whether you're dealing with COVID, the flu, or going into the hospital for some procedure, mindset is critical. Since we live in a world today where fear is the cultural standard, and we're supposed to avoid risk at all costs, most people let fear take over their lives. But here's the reality: Life is risky. It's so risky, in fact, that none of us are going to get out of it alive! So it's critical that we learn to direct and control our own minds. Once you master your mind, you'll make yourself not only healthier but happier as well. You will transform the absolute quality of your life.

EMOTIONAL HOME & THREE DECISIONS

"I don't want to be at the mercy of my emotions. I want to use them, to enjoy them, and to dominate them."

—OSCAR WILDE, 19th-century Irish poet and playwright

Have you noticed that people in certain parts of the world—including the United States—live in areas where there's a good chance they'll get wiped out by a huge hurricane or tornado every three or four years? You see it on TV and you feel their anguish as they collect what's left of their lives and begin to rebuild—and then it happens again! And again! **And at some point as you watch this, despite your feelings of compassion, you may ask yourself,** *Why don't those people move?* **Why? Because it's their home.** It's what they've always known. They don't want to leave what's familiar—even if it's a disaster waiting to happen.

What's less obvious is that we also have an *emotional* home. **In good times or bad, we keep going back to it. The external environment may be positive or negative, but we'll use it to reach the emotional place we know best. And here's the most important thing to remember: the quality of your life is the quality of your habitual emotions. Where you live emotionally determines what your life is really like.**

If you have three beautiful children and an incredible spouse who adores you, but you're constantly worried and anxious, you'll have a worried and anxious life. If you're a big success at your job but feel inadequate and un-fulfilled, you'll have an insecure life. Heck, if you have $1 billion but your primary habitual emotions are frustration and anger, then your life isn't wealthy—it's poor! It's filled with frustration and anger. As someone who grew up with abuse, I know how negative emotions can become a person's go-to pattern. If we're unaware of these habits, we create an environment that guides us back home to the emotions we've made habitual. Nobody *wants* a sad life, but for a lot of people, it's who they feel they are. **Your emotional pattern follows you like a shadow . . . until you consciously and deliberately draw a line in the sand and change it.**

The power of our emotional homes was made clear to me one day on the Big Island in Hawaii, at a ten-day seminar I used to call Life Mastery. We had people come from all over the world, with translations in 6 languages. We hired some of the creators of Cirque de Soleil to design the opening. It was filled with energy and excitement. There was drum music and confetti and incredible energy, and on the first night with all of this pandemonium I zip-lined over the crowd from a forty-foot ceiling in the back of the house. I'd rehearsed it all week, but when I touched down on the stage, with people going out of their mind, I called an audible. My soul took over my brain and said, **"Living. When do people really start to live?"** I paused and I said, **"When they face death."**

I had no plan to say this or anything like it, but I took a long pause, and then asked, "If you knew this was the last week of your life and you couldn't get off this island, how would you live? What would you give? What would you do? Whom would you call? What would you share with them from your heart and your soul? How would you spend these days? Whom would you thank? Whom would you forgive? Whom would you express your love to? And how much energy would you expend to squeeze every bit of celebration out of every moment you had left?"

We finished the seminar that night around midnight, and by the time I got back to my room, it was 2:30 a.m. Hawaii local time. Half an hour later, just as I was falling asleep, the phone rang and someone said, "Turn on the television. An airplane just hit one of the Twin Towers."

I turned on CNN to see the same scene that everyone alive in the year 2001 remembers. Knowing that more than forty of our seminar participants worked in the World Trade Center, and had friends and coworkers there, I called my team and said we'd get more details in the morning to help address the crisis with that group. I tried to go back to sleep, only to get a second phone call. This time they said, "It has to be a terrorist attack—a second plane just hit the other tower." From that moment on I was riveted to the TV screen. I watched in horror as the South Tower collapsed. I knew that none of us witnessing these images would ever forget them.

By the time the North Tower went down, it was around 4:30 a.m. in Hawaii. I could hear people crying and screaming, and what sounded like fighting outside my room. With thousands of people there for our event from every walk of life, from more than three dozen countries, from every imaginable religion—well, it's safe to say they were all reacting to this extreme situation very differently. As I ventured into the hallway to connect with people, I witnessed every emotion of the human condition. Some people were shaking with fear and others were so angry they could barely speak. And believe it or not, some people were celebrating. I knew that I'd need to bring everyone together that day to align for the greater good in the midst of total insanity. Ironically, the theme for that day's class was supposed to be "emotional mastery." How could I use this opportunity to honor the people lost in this terrible tragedy while also creating a balance and perspective on what we can do to serve others?

Before I share with you what I did, let me take a moment to tell you about a time when I was just 11 years old and living in California. **It was an extremely painful experience, but it also put me on the road to find the answers that ultimately allowed me to help this audience of diverse souls in Hawaii on this critical day of 9/11. . . .**

It was Thanksgiving, I was 11 years old and I was on my fourth father, and he'd lost his job and we were completely broke. All we had for the holiday dinner were Saltine crackers and butter. My mom and dad were fighting, saying the kind of things to each other that you can never take back. My little brother and sister were crying, and I was trying to protect them from the brutal battle between our parents.

Then came a knock on the door. In the midst of all this chaos, I opened it to find a tall stranger standing in front of me and holding two giant bags of groceries. He even had a frozen turkey and an empty pan on the ground beside him. The man asked, "Is your father home?" I said, "Just one moment." I was euphoric and ran back to tell my dad, "There's someone at the door for you!" He said, "Answer it yourself." And I said, "I did, Dad, he needs to speak to you." I held my breath with such excitement to see how happy my father would be. But when he opened the door and saw the groceries, he got furious and shouted, "We don't accept charity!" and tried to slam the door in the man's face. But the guy had leaned in holding the bag of groceries and his foot caused the door to bounce back open. When my dad tried to close the door again, he leaned in even farther and said, "Sir, this is not charity. Someone knows your family is having a tough time, and they want you to have a beautiful Thanksgiving. I'm just the delivery guy." My father looked like he wanted to punch him in the face. He grabbed the groceries and slammed them down on the floor and stormed off.

That was a turning point for me. Why? Because it made me wrestle with the question: **Why wasn't my dad happy? I felt so grateful for the unexpected gift—why wasn't he grateful? I was baffled, and so sad.** It took me a long time to figure it out. Years later I realized that our lives are controlled by **three decisions. You're making these decisions right now even as you're reading this story. And how we make these decisions determines the quality of our life. The first decision we all make is . . .**

DECISION #1: What we decide to FOCUS on

Whatever you focus on, you're going to feel—whether it's true or not— because **focus equals feelings. If you focus on the worst-case scenario, you're going to feel fearful and sick to your stomach. If you focus on the best case, you're going to feel confident. Again, whether it's true or not doesn't matter. What we focus on creates our feelings.** I know what my father was focused on that day because he kept muttering how we didn't take charity, how it wasn't his fault that we didn't have food. He was angry, but most of all he was sad. **His real focus was on how he had failed his family, that was obvious. And as he focused on it, he felt more and more angry with himself and with his life.**

I felt differently, because I focused on something totally different: *We've got food! What a concept! How amazing!* Remember, if you focus on the worst-case scenario, that's what you'll feel. If you're focused on how people might take advantage of you, you'll feel bitter and resentful regardless of what's really going on. Remember, **wherever focus goes, energy flows. Some people constantly focus on what's wrong.** Guess what—**what's wrong is always available, isn't it? But so is what's right!**

DECISION #2: What does this MEAN?

As soon as we focus on something, our brain has to make another decision, and that is: What does this mean? This choice directly controls your quality of life. Because as soon as our brain focuses on something, we give it meaning. And whether that meaning is positive or negative completely shapes our life. **For example, when something happens that's a**

big problem in your life, only *you* can decide what meaning to give to it. Is God punishing me or is God challenging me? Or is this problem a gift from God to make me grow?

In an interaction with another person, you may ask yourself: **Is this person insulting me, coaching me, or loving me? The meaning you choose will radically change how you feel and what you decide to do.** Think of it this way, what if you think it's the end of a relationship versus the beginning? Will you react differently? Of course! If you think it's the end, you're going to treat your partner differently as well!

Here's what's most important to remember: **We are the creators of our own meaning . . . if we take control. Otherwise we let the external world tell us what is good, bad, terrible, or horrific, and it usually isn't a positive meaning, is it? In the end, our life is controlled by what we focus on and the meaning we give it.** In fact, **meaning equals emotion, and your emotions equal the quality of your life.** Or let me put it another way: **We don't experience life. You and I experience what we focus on and the meaning we give to it—so choose well.**

DECISION #3: What am I going to DO?

Every moment we're making those first two decisions: What am I going to focus on, and what does it mean? Again, meaning creates emotions, and our emotions shape the third and most important decision: *__What am I going to do?__* **This is the make-or-break choice that defines your life, the one that leads either to massive action or accepting life as it is.** But remember, actions don't happen in a vacuum. They're shaped by those first two decisions, on focus and meaning. **The emotions that grow out of meaning powerfully affect what action we take. If one person is infuriated by an incident at their job, and someone else is inspired by the very same situation, how do you think they'll respond—the same way, or different ways?** When a major disappointment happens, some people get depressed and the others feel driven to change it; you know these two people are going to accomplish very different things in life. **So these are decisions that we're literally making moment-to-moment. The problem is that most people make them unconsciously, and so our life becomes a habit of failure or success depending on what type of habits we have in this area.**

Years later, I realized that my father and I had radically different experiences that Thanksgiving Day in California. To review: **My father was focused on how he'd failed to take care of his family. The meaning he took from that focus was that he was worthless.** How do I know that's what he thought? Because he'd say it over and over again, under his breath. **And finally, the action he decided to take shortly thereafter was to leave our family. At the time, it was one of the most painful experiences of my life. I loved him as if he was my natural father.**

I focused on the fact that someone brought us food. My father had always said that no one cares about anyone else, and it looked that way from where we lived and that rough part of town. But my experience that day completely changed that belief. Because some stranger, who didn't even want credit, looked out for my family. **The experience that day changed my life. Why? Because I created a very different meaning that day, and it's probably one of the reasons that I'm writing to you in this moment. It shifted my entire trajectory. I came up with a meaning that strangers care, and if they cared about me and my family, then I needed to care about strangers. I made a decision right then and there—that someday I would do the same thing for another family, and find a way to give back.**

So you see, it wasn't the experience that changed my life—it was how I processed it. I could have just accepted the food or expected someone should help us or been appreciative but nothing more. **Instead, I decided I wanted to pay it forward.** So when I was 17, I called a local church. At the time I wasn't very successful in business or financial terms, but with a little bit of savings I accumulated, I certainly had enough money to be able to provide some food for another family at Thanksgiving. So I called a local church and asked if there were two families who really needed food but might be too proud to come get help. Much like my father had been.

I borrowed a friend's van and put on some old jeans and a T-shirt. I went to the grocery store with two baskets and filled them with food for two families. It was the most exciting shopping trip of my life! After loading up the groceries, I wrote two notes that said "This is a gift from a friend. Everyone has tough times. So please enjoy this Thanksgiving with your family. And if you can someday, help another family in some way and pay it forward." And I wrote, "Love, a friend." I also knew where the two families lived was primarily Hispanic, so I had a friend write the same note on the back in Spanish.

I won't bore you with all the details of that day, **but delivering that food completely changed me.** In one of the families, the father had just left them the week before with no money or food. There were four boys, all under the age of ten, and their joy and excitement to see that someone cared for them—it was overwhelming for me.

I was hooked. The next year I decided to feed four families, and the following year it was eight, and then I got my small company and employees involved. **Eventually I was feeding a million people per year, then four million. Today, in my partnership with Feeding America, I've committed to providing a billion meals in the United States, 100 million per year. At this point we've done it for seven straight years, and we're a year and a half ahead of schedule with 850 million meals. In fact, this book is providing 20 million meals as well as the balance being donated to some of the top researchers. Hopefully by the time you're reading this, we'll be close to reaching the billion meal mark!**

Why did I tell you this story? Because if you take control of your mind by making better decisions, **sometimes the worst day of your life can become your best day.** Think about it: If I'd never suffered myself, would I have the same passion for feeding people? Probably not. **But our job in life is to use what life gives us, not to complain or whine or point the finger at those who have done us wrong. The real question that matters most is this: <u>When life gives you pain and suffering, will you just suffer? Or will you find a way to grow and use it to find a way to serve others? My core belief is that life is always happening *for* us, not *to* us, but it's our job to find the benefit in the challenge.</u>**

If you take control of your mind by making better decisions, sometimes the worst day of your life can become your best day.

And remember: Your mind can both heal and/or hurt your body. As the placebo studies prove, the mind can even overcome the impact of drugs and get the body to react in the opposite way—to speed up after you've taken a barbiturate, for example. Again, it's not such a stretch to understand that our mind can change our emotions, and therefore our quality of life.

"Between stimulus and response there is a space. In that space is our power to choose our response. In our response lies our growth and our freedom."

—VIKTOR FRANKL, author, neurologist, psychiatrist,
philosopher, and Holocaust survivor

Let's get back to Hawaii, to the microcosm of humanity I encountered at my hotel on 9/11. As the sun rose that morning and I could hear the screams of shock and disbelief echo down the corridors, **I could see that people's reactions were as different as the people themselves. Sad people got *really* sad. Worried people worried like they'd never worried before. Caretakers tried to comfort those around them. Some people were saying to others that 9/11 was retribution and the beginning of end times.**

I had to make a decision. Would we continue the seminar that morning, when everyone thought we should cancel? The U.S. had shut down its airspace and the phone lines were messed up. I pulled the 2,000 people at the event together in the room and said, **"Listen, we can't get off the island, so let's focus on what we *can* do."** Our first action step was a blood drive. But I also knew that our participants needed to process their feelings, because I was seeing every kind of emotion across the board.

The first thing I did was to ask everyone at the event to write down their answers to these three core decisions that I realize shape my life and everyone else's: What did they *focus* on when they first heard the planes that hit the Twin Towers? What did it *mean* to them? And what did they decide to do? Then I asked people to gather in groups of five or six people with a mix of different nationalities, and both men and women in them. And then I went from group to group as they shared their emotions—**and I got the lesson of a lifetime.** As I approached the first group, I could see one woman with a thick accent who was whipped into a frenzy of rage. As she spoke, she was so intense that spit was flying out of her mouth as she shouted about what had happened. After a few minutes, I interrupted and said, "Ma'am, I see you're angry, and I understand. But can I ask you this question?"

She said, "What is it?"

I said, "I'm just curious, I want to ask you, how often do you get angry?"

"What do you mean?"

I said, "Well, do you get angry once a month, once a week, or multiple times a day?"

And she glared at me and said, "What kind of question is that?"

I said, "The way you're responding tells me you get angry more often than you might realize."

And she said, "Well, I do get angry a lot. I can't help myself." **I asked her what anger meant to her. And she looked at me and started speaking with intensity, and then a small smile crept in at the corner of her mouth and she said, "Well, for me, it's like jet fuel. It gives me energy."**

Hmm. What an interesting response! But it was only one interaction, not enough to see a pattern. So I went to the next group, where a nurse from New York was sobbing uncontrollably. She kept saying, "I feel so guilty. I should be there to help people, and I'm stuck on this island. I just feel so guilty!" After listening for several minutes to hear her out about how guilty she felt, I interrupted and said, "Ma'am, can I ask you a question? How often do you have these feelings of guilt?"

She said, "What do you mean?"

Once again I said, "Is it once a year, once a month, once a week, or multiple times a day?"

The woman paused for a moment and then she said, **"I guess I feel guilty all the time." She felt guilty about working too hard and not having enough time for her kids. She felt guilty about not being there enough for patients. She felt guilty about not being a good enough wife. Just as the first woman went to the anger room, this nurse went to the guilt room.**

After a dozen of these encounters, I began to form one of the most important insights in my life. **Everyone in this room had used 9/11 to go to their own emotional home, to the place they went out of habit.** The attack on the World Trade Center was an extreme external trigger that returned them to their primary emotional pattern. **Regardless of what**

586   TONY ROBBINS: LIFE FORCE

happens in the outside world, we interpret events as a way to get back to what we know emotionally. It's so important for us to realize that our emotions aren't based on our soul, our heart or spirit. They're simply products of patterns and emotional habits. They're no more significant than a physical habit like drumming on a desktop . . . but they certainly have more impact on our lives.

So what did I learn that day? I learned that under stress, angry people got more angry and sad people got sadder. Happy people looked for the good. In the most difficult situation, caring people were focused on helping others. Once we realize that our emotional home shapes our relationships, our careers, our parenting styles, even the level of intimacy we accept or reject, we can actually start to have a different life.

Once we start taking 100 percent responsibility for our experience of life rather than blaming others, we can awaken to a truth that makes all the difference: Whatever life offers us, we get to decide what to focus on what it means and what we're going to do about it. And if we do this consciously and consistently, we can change the quality of our lives forever.

On that transformational morning in Hawaii, I called on another woman from New York whose boyfriend had proposed marriage to her just before she left for our seminar. She told him she couldn't marry him because her previous boyfriend had been kidnapped and killed years before, and she still wasn't over it. He responded in anger, "If you go to that seminar, it's over between us."

As the woman stood before the audience to tell her story, her hand was shaking. You could see the dried tears on her face, the tears she'd been having for hours before the seminar began—since the moment she learned what had happened. She looked at me and said, "I want to play an audio for you. Because last night, after you talked about death, and whom do you love, and what would you share with them, I realized I really loved him. But because it was so late back home, I decided to leave him a message that he'd receive when he got to work, so I wouldn't wake him. In the message, I just told him how much I loved him, and that I wanted to marry him. And that I was sorry for all the difficulties."

And then she took a deep breath and began to cry once again. She went on, "I left a message for him on his voicemail at work, in his office at the top of the World Trade Center. And he called me in the early hours this morning, but I slept through it." And she had a little recorder, and she said, "I'd like to play it for you."

Then we all heard a man saying, "Honey, I can't tell you what your message means to me—to know that you truly love me as much as I love you. But I have bad news to share. There's a fire in the tower here, and it's so big, I can't get out. I'm trapped." His voice cracked, "I'm going to die, honey. But I want you to know that your message made me the happiest man in the world." He paused again, and you could hear the cry in his voice. "Honey, I'm sure you must be wondering: How could God do this to you twice? How could he take away two different people that you loved? I can't answer that question. **But all I want to say to you is that I love you and I hope in the future you won't hold back your love, give it all. I love you for eternity.**"

And as we heard the click that ended the message, the room burst into tears, myself included. But not everyone had the same reaction. A young man named Assad Rezzvi from Pakistan stood up and said, "I'm a Muslim. I wish I could hold your hand and say I'm sorry, but this is retribution." He told people that morning that his only regret was that he was not on one of those planes. He had actually been recruited into an Al Qaeda camp and his father had gotten him out and sent him to the U.S. for college. With his words, "this is retribution," as you can imagine, the room erupted in shock and anger.

The interaction that followed is on video and available if you want to watch it, but for now I'll just give you a summary: A Jewish man stood up whose family lived in the Israeli-occupied territories in Palestine. He'd worked in the World Trade Center, and more than thirty of his dearest friends had died that day. You can only imagine the intensity that passed between these two passionate people. But we took an hour and a half to do a process to get both of them to move beyond the external world and see how much pain there was for everyone. **They both changed their focus from what had been done to them or their people to what they could do to bring them together. They shifted the meaning from being all about themselves to seeing how they could be part of a solution. After almost two hours, they embraced each other as brothers.** Two people from opposite worlds found a way to connect. **Afterward, they gathered** all the Christians, Jews, and Muslims in the room, and began working on a plan to bring more understanding to the Middle East. Later Assad wrote a book called *My Jihad: A Muslim Man's Journey from Hate to Love.* As you see, if we change what we focus on, we can change what things mean to us—and how we act. And that's the only way we can change our lives.

> *"Be the change that you wish to see in the world."*
>
> —GANDHI

We all got the most important lesson of our lives on 9/11—and anyone who was there will never forget it.

However, the three core decisions aren't limited to times of such momentous events. They also determine the little things; let me give you a simple example from daily life. Have you ever had a dinner date with somebody you care about—your husband, wife, boyfriend or girlfriend—and you're supposed to meet at 7 p.m., you get there at seven and they're not there? When that happens, what do you focus on? What do you feel? How do you react? When I've asked this to people in seminars, often they'll say, I'm angry. Or I'm frustrated. Or I'm worried. **Interesting, don't you think? Same scenario, very different reactions.**

Then I say, what if it's 7:30 and the person has still not arrived? And they haven't called or texted—they just haven't shown up. And one person will say, "I'm *really* angry." Or you'll hear someone else say they're really worried and concerned. **Why are two people in the same situation having a very different experience?** Both are waiting for a partner who is thirty minutes late, and has not yet arrived. Well, the angry one is not just focused on the fact that they aren't there, he or she is also giving it a meaning that the other person is *always* late or they "don't care." Or perhaps they picture in their mind that their loved one is screwing around with somebody else. Even if it's not true, that thought will make them crazy angry. Am I right? What are they going to do when the person arrives? Let's just say it won't be a very pleasant dinner.

But what if someone was focused instead on the fact that they're not here, and they start focusing and asking themselves what happened to them? And that the meaning was the possibility that the other person was in an accident—maybe they've been hurt! Their focus translates to feelings of concern and compassion. And when their partner arrives, they'll treat them with compassion and concern.

<u>Notice that it's the same event, identical circumstances, but very different experiences.</u> **All that shifted was the psychological focus and a shift in meaning. What if it wasn't your partner? What if pre-existing patterns within yourself made you angry, worried, stressed or depressed? But remember, there are also patterns that will make you feel grateful, playful, loving, and courageous.** You just need to be open to changing your habits. Maybe it's time to move from one emotional home to another, or maybe upgrade your emotional home to something that's more beautiful, nurturing, and fulfilling.

BEATING DEPRESSION WITHOUT DRUGS

I've understood for a long time that our minds have an incredible ability to change our biochemistry and heal diseases, based on our expectations—hence the power of the placebo, from saline injections to fake surgeries. And as we've shown, our minds can clearly change our bodies to change our emotions. But sometimes we attempt to change something but fail to get the outcome. After a while we can begin to feel that it's unchangeable. We start to believe that there's something wrong with us and that we can't change. And once we have that belief, it becomes self-fulfilling—very little will change.

How many of you know someone who takes antidepressants and is still depressed? I ask that question all the time at my events, and no matter where I am in the world, whether it's a room with 10,000 people or an arena with 30,000, 80 percent or more raise their hands. **How is that possible?** Because antidepressants can be very useful in numbing people's emotions, but they don't deal with the source of the problem. The real causes can be found in people's patterns of focus, meaning, and action. Let me give you an example that **you can test for yourself. Our pattern of focus and meaning powerfully shapes how we live our lives. Take this simple little test that I ask audiences all the time:**

1. **We all have many patterns of focus, but do you tend to focus more on what you HAVE, or on what's MISSING from your life?** Of course,

most of us do both. And it can be healthy to focus on what's missing when you're trying to solve a problem in business or in life. But it's not so healthy when it becomes a habitual pattern. **If you're always focused on what's missing, how can you ever sustain happiness?** You can't! This is why so many people with such abundance are still unhappy.

2. Do you tend to focus on what you CAN or CAN'T control? In my seminars, more people are going to focus on what they *can* control, which is why they've come to us in the first place. They want to take control of their mind, their body, their emotions, their business, their life, their career. But people who are feeling depressed inevitably spend more time focused on what they can't control—and believe me, we all have plenty of things we can't control. If we habitually focus on them, we can feel extremely over-whelmed. And during the recent times of COVID shutdowns, you can only imagine how many people were focusing on what they can't control and experiencing sadness, anger, loneliness, or depression.

3. Do you tend to focus more on the PAST, the PRESENT, or the FUTURE? We all do all three, but where do you spend most of your time? Depressed people often focus on the past, regretting decisions or events that can never be changed. Or they may focus on present challenges and project them into the future. **No matter what drug you're prescribed, as long as you're focused on what's missing, what you can't control, and past regrets or anxiety over the future, you're going to be angry, frustrated, and/or depressed.**

But how can we address these issues? More people than ever are getting diagnosed with depression, **"the second most common cause of disability worldwide after back pain."**[19] Often they're treated with **antidepressants,** heavy-duty drugs that often carry **unfortunate side effects that can trigger anxiety, agitation, insomnia, and aggression. In young adults and teenagers, antidepressants have been shown to increase the risk**

---

19 Briggs, "Depression: 'Second Biggest Cause of Disability' in World."

of suicide, the second-leading cause of death in adolescents.[20] In fact, the pharmaceutical companies are required to put a warning on the side of the box that these **drugs can create suicidal thoughts.** In some cases, the treatment can be worse than the original disease! What's more, for many people, the drugs simply don't work.

According to **Dr. Ariel Ganz, PhD,** a postdoctoral fellow at Stanford University's School of Medicine, metastudies (studies that combine and analyze all discoverable results) show **less than half the people with depression respond to *any* antidepressant drugs, even when they're combined with therapy—barely better results than what you'd get from a placebo.** And even then, as she told us, their symptoms on average were reduced by only around 50 percent: **"This is not people going from depressed to super happy. They're going from depressed to less depressed."** Many people continue these treatments for years, in some cases for decades. Obviously, this is not a great outcome.

The current depression epidemic, which expanded exponentially with the COVID lockdowns, has been pushing some scientists to find other therapeutic options. **In a controlled study at Johns Hopkins, twenty-four patients with severe depression were given two treatments with psilocybin, the psychedelic ingredient in "magic" mushrooms, with supportive psychotherapy for four weeks. A month later, this experimental therapy produced a result never before seen: <u>54 percent were declared to be in remission</u> thirty days later—they were truly depression-free!**[21] According to Dr. Alan Davis, PhD, an adjunct assistant professor of psychology at Johns Hopkins, **<u>"The magnitude of the effect we saw was about four times larger than what clinical trials have shown for traditional antidepressants on the market."</u>**[22]

There's just one challenge. Psilocybin, which is chemically similar to LSD, is classed as a Schedule 1 controlled substance. It's not approved for

---

20 FDA, "Suicidality in Children and Adolescents Being Treated with Antidepressant Medications."

21 Davis et al., "Effects of Psilocybin-Assisted Therapy on Major Depressive Disorder."

22 McMains, "Psychedelic Treatment with Psilocybin Shown to Relieve Major Depression."

treatment, and many people would hesitate to use a hallucinogen to try to change. Still, it holds exciting potential, and scientists and legislators are evaluating how to move forward.

Over the decades, I've helped thousands of people eliminate their depression patterns in a variety of ways. We've done extensive tracking of the impact of our events. **You may have seen the Award-winning Netflix documentary:** *Tony Robbins: I Am Not Your Guru,* in which a film crew followed me over six days and nights as I worked with several people who were suicidal and/or depressed. Or perhaps you've seen some of the training films that have been made with my brilliant partner, the master therapist and author Cloe Madanes, that show the impact of these therapeutic interventions. **Robbins Madanes Training Core 100 and Core 200 are now used in the state of California as accepted continuing education credit for LMFT (Licensed Marriage and Family Therapist), LCSW (Licensed Clinical Social Worker), and LPCC (Licensed Professional Clinical Counselor) licensure. More than one hundred films are now in circulation, including ones used to help train psychologists and psychiatrists.** While I am not a licensed therapist, the interactions and strategies presented in the films provide healthcare professionals valuable "real-world learnings."

With so many researchers now looking for non-drug approaches to depression, our organization was approached two years ago by a research team from Stanford University's school of medicine's Snyder Lab of Genetics. The team was made up of Dr. Ariel Ganz, PhD, Dr. Michael Snyder, and Benjamin Rolnik, PhD, in partnership with Jacob Wilson, PhD, from the Applied Science and Performance Institute, and they conducted a unique experiment on my Date with Destiny event, a 6-day immersion program that I do once a year. Though we've had thousands of successes over the years, they were not studied in a clinical environment and could be called anecdotal. Dr. Ganz wanted to see if there was scientific proof to back up these examples. **Mirroring the structure of the study done with psilocybin, but without drugs, her team assessed a group of forty-five participants, many of whom were clinically depressed, before the seminar and conducted a follow-up thirty days later to measure the results.** A portion of the subjects also formed a control group that didn't attend the event but used a psychology tool known as gratitude journaling for thirty days.

The results were mind-boggling. The gratitude journal group improved their depression, anxiety, and stress levels—for a time. By one month after the experiment started, however, the benefits diminished and the subjects trended back to their depression baseline. **But for the group who'd attended Date with Destiny, benefits persisted. One month following the event, 100 percent of initially depressed participants were in remission (no longer depressed!). Additionally at the beginning of the study, 17 percent of participants experienced suicidal thoughts. One month after Date with Destiny, none of the participants reported suicidal thoughts!**

The study results found double the percentage of people no longer depressed than the previous study done with psilocybin.[23] **Which, as you recall, was four times more impactful than the drugs on the market, and research showed our event was more impactful than that! How is this possible? These people literally changed the pattern of their focus, with corresponding shifts in their beliefs, their values, and most important, what they decided to do. Their meanings had changed, and so had their emotions and actions. Thirty days after the event, with no drugs or side effects, they had a 100 percent remission rate.** As Dr. Ganz put it, the experience **"shifted their underlying framework of beliefs in the way that they see the world."**

> *"I've been doing research for almost twenty years and have published almost three hundred papers, and I've never seen anything like this! The results are absolutely incredible."*
>
> —JACOB WILSON, PhD

The researchers were stunned by the results. As Dr. Ganz told me in a podcast interview after the study was concluded, the impact was beyond anything she could have imagined—far greater than the efficacy for standard-of-care drugs, and even better than the psilocybin success rate. The numbers were so dramatic that she decided to submit her data to blinded teams of external researchers, and the results held up.

---

23 Results from interview with Stanford Genetics Lab Team at www.ScienceOfTony Robbins.com

In fact, the results were so impressive that the **Stanford team collaborated on a second study on my weekend program Unleash the Power Within. They wanted to better understand the physiological, biochemical, and psychological events that underlie the powerful emotional changes that occur at my seminars. This study, now published in the** *Journal of Physiology and Behavior,*[24] divided participants into two different groups. One group participated in my four-day program Unleash the Power Within, and the second group was put into a control condition where they learned the same content in an intensive traditional lecture format that was given by an individual with more than fifteen years of award-winning university teaching experience.

Participants' knowledge of advanced psychological and behavioral principles known to impact emotional states were tested before the event, and at twenty-four hours and thirty days following. The study found **300 percent improvement in participants' ability to cognitively retrain their beliefs and attitudes, reprioritize need states, and increase intrinsic motivation and fulfillment.**

<u>**These results were more than three times greater than the traditional lecture format, and were sustained thirty days later.**</u> The study also found that I was able to radically alter the physiology of participants including more than **2,000 more calories burned and 206 percent greater physiological output than the control condition.** We also saw that participants **increased hormones known to improve learning by 159 percent.** Even more intriguing is that participants **increased their ratio of testosterone to cortisol by 139 percent** following my end-of-event priming session (which I'll share more about with you later). **To experts, this is known as an index of readiness** to perform and is reflective of a signature biochemical marker of achievement.[25]

Beyond studying a live event, the Applied Science and Performance Institute, a laboratory which has studied the greatest performers in

---

24 Wilson et al., "Non-Traditional Immersive Seminar Enhances Learning by Promoting Greater Physiological and Psychological Engagement Compared to a Traditional Lecture Format."

25 Ibid.

the world, including Superbowl and Stanley Cup champions, Olympic athletes, and thousands of subjects across lifespan from all walks of life, also tested my ability to deliver the same impact in a virtual Unleash the Power Within event that I conducted during July 2020 in the midst of COVID. This study examined the impact of a virtual event for up to a year following.

To give you context, when COVID hit and people were trapped in their homes all around the world, I built a state-of-the-art studio in Palm Beach Florida, so that I could reach people when everything was shut down. It has 20-foot-high screens, with the highest level of resolutions possible, 50 feet wide, and surrounding me 180 degrees. And I worked out technology with Zoom and other companies so that I could see and interact with everyone just like a live event.

In this study, they measured my biochemistry, including my levels of cortisol (the stress hormone) and testosterone and my variable heart rate. At the same time, they measured a sampling of people from all over the world, a portion of the more than 25,000 people in ninety different countries who were participating in the program for four days in our Zoom stadium. They were literally experiencing the program in their own homes, and yet, when they took saliva examples throughout the weekend to assess the event's impact on memory and learning, **the biochemical impact on virtual participants attending was the same as when they attended a live in-person event.**

We've talked about how lonely and disconnected people felt during the pandemic. <u>According to this study of our events by the Applied Science and Performance Institute, feelings of anxiety in a control group increased by 28 percent. But ASPI found that people attending our events felt 38 percent *less* anxiety—not just thirty days later, but *eleven months* later!</u>

As ASPI's Jacob Wilson, PhD, told me, "I've been doing research for almost twenty years and have published almost three hundred papers, and I've never seen anything like this! The results are absolutely incredible. Much less for a single event that was held virtually."

Why am I telling you this? I want to bring you back to the basic truth that drives this final chapter of our book: that you have the power to decide on what to focus on, what things mean, and what to do. And when you make these decisions consciously, when you look for empowering focus, empowering meanings, and empowering actions, I can promise that your life will change. **That's not a guarantee that your life will be perfect—that isn't the way life works.** But I *can* guarantee that you'll be offered the opportunity to appreciate life, with all its challenges, and to grow from whatever the world throws at you. **We can't control everything, but we do control the most important thing of all: what things mean to us, our emotions, and our actions.** Yes, we can control what we focus on, what we feel, and what we do. And by doing that, we can absolutely enhance the quality of our life.

So there you have it: Regardless of what happens to us, our minds can make us sick or healthy, miserable or happy, fearful or faithful and grateful. At our events, we don't sugarcoat the threats or obstacles out there in the world. We can't make the world a "safe" place. But we *can* shift people's belief systems and feelings. We can help them change their emotional home and begin to live with the emotions that empower them—**to begin to see what they can control verses what they can't.** There are two games we have to master to have a great life—the external world and the internal world. **We can't control the external world—we can influence it—but we can shape and control our thoughts, feelings, emotions, and actions.** Once people take back control of their own minds and emotions, the dividends are immense.

According to Benjamin Rolnik, Dr. Ganz's Stanford associate, people's experience at Date with Destiny not only brought down their depression levels but also helped them to "max out on gratitude, happiness, well-being, and sexual satisfaction." Talk about a testimonial! (If you'd like to know more about these scientific studies, or watch our interview with the researchers, you can visit us at **ScienceOfTonyRobbins.com**.

I won't tell you I was surprised by these outcomes, because I've been doing these events for forty-four years and have seen their impact more times than I can count. Even so, I was thrilled to have the power of mindset confirmed by such a rigorous, data-based approach. If you'd like to experience it firsthand, come join one of our events; you can get information at TonyRobbins.com. You might start by watching *I'm Not Your Guru* on **Netflix** to get a feel for what is possible. **Now let's turn to our final chapter and the most important tool you have to change your life, and final lesson of our journey. It's called . . . the power of decision.**

CHAPTER 25

THE POWER OF DECISION: THE GIFT OF LIVING IN A BEAUTIFUL STATE

HOW TO TRULY CREATE AND EXPERIENCE AN EXTRAORDINARY QUALITY OF LIFE

If we look at how our lives have turned out, both what we love and what we're not happy with, there are many ways we can view, evaluate, or justify our experience. We often give ourselves credit for all of the good things that have happened, but are quick to blame others for injustices, the "bad" things, and the things that don't match our expectations. In order to do that, we have to ignore the evidence that people's lives are not based on what was done to them, and the fact that **biography is *not* destiny.**

All you have to do is spend a little time reading the autobiographies of some of the most extraordinary human beings in history, world leaders, scientific geniuses, sociologists, and businesspeople. **What you'll discover is that often people who were given everything—all of the love, support, education, money—can often find themselves going in and out of rehab; and then those whom life seems to have hit the hardest, who went through the most injustice, physically, mentally, emotionally, often develop a hunger to break through the limits of their past.**

They don't settle for a life lived in reaction to what's been done to them or what they failed to achieve. Instead, they find a way to use whatever life has given them to move forward, and not only grow

personally, but as they grow and develop, to use the internal strength, skill, and insights to help others along the path. Extraordinary people like Oprah, Nelson Mandela, and Viktor Frankl, who against all odds created life on their terms. What's the difference? I would submit to you that it's *not our conditions*, but our *decisions* that determine the quality of our lives.

If we want to know why we are where we are in our lives, look back on our decisions. If I asked you, can you think of any decision that you've made in the past five to ten years, that, if you look back on it, if you had made a different decision your life would be completely different? Of course you can! Sometimes the decisions were tough, where you had to get beyond your fear or take a risk. Other times, it may have been small decisions that led to something important. Like where to go to school, and then meeting the love of your life. Or you picked up a certain profession which led you in a whole new direction or to living in a different part of the country or the world.

THE GIFT OF EXTREME STRESS

"If you're going through hell, keep going."
—WINSTON CHURCHILL

The illusion that many of us have is that some people are just luckier than others—they don't really have the big challenges that we've faced. But having had the privilege to work with tens of millions of people from 195 countries at my events, and privately coaching the most successful leaders in business, politics, sports, and finance, from moms and dads to the most challenged people in our society—I can tell you that there is one common denominator in all of our lives. In spite of people's beliefs, no matter how smart, attractive, successful in business or financial terms, no matter how good a person you are—everyone will experience extreme stress at some point in their lives. Probably more than once. No one escapes it.

Aren't you glad you read this positive chapter? But it's true. The illusion we have that some people don't go through extreme challenges or we're the only ones who experience injustice—and that's just an egocentric lie. In fact, no matter how much we don't want it to happen, we're going to lose a family member or a relationship that we treasure. **We're going to lose a job, or the government is going to do something that shuts your business down, as was the case with COVID.** You're going to be robbed, or your house might burn down or be struck by a natural disaster. Somebody in your family might be diagnosed with a "terminal illness"—and if they are, maybe there will be answers in this book that can turn it around, as others have done.

I'm speaking to you from experience. I've been told I have a tumor in my brain. Early in my career I was on the verge of bankruptcy and somehow managed to pull things through. I've ended long relationships and had the pain of burying three fathers and a mother. I've had homes burn down and lost things that I thought were irreplaceable. Of course nothing is irreplaceable except your soul and your ability to use whatever life brings you to still create a beautiful life.

So the real key to have an extraordinary quality of life—life on your terms—is not to hope you get lucky and that nothing happens, but to develop the kind of psychological and emotional strength that makes you resilient enough to use whatever life brings you to create something even greater.

Extreme stress is going to be a given in your life. So the real key to have an extraordinary quality of life—life on your terms—is not to hope you get lucky and that nothing happens, but to develop the kind of psychological and emotional strength that makes you resilient enough to use whatever life brings you to create something even greater. So if you can accept that extreme stress is going to happen, then the real key is, **what are you going to decide to do when it hits?**

Winston Churchill famously said, "If you're going through hell, keep going." If you do, I can tell you from experience, having gone through extreme stress many times, **there are three invaluable lessons that only extreme pain can teach—and only if you don't give up. If you push through these times of extreme stress, you'll discover:**

1. You're stronger than you think you are.
2. Who your real friends and family are. Because the fake ones disappear when the going gets rough. An invaluable lesson.
3. Pushing through the pain will build in you a psychological and emotional immunity. Having been through the most stressful times, all the normal challenges of life will seem like nothing by contrast. You'll have become more so you can live life more fully regardless of what's happening in the external world. <u>In other words, you'll use stress; not let stress use you.</u>

So . . . what's a problem?

I would suggest that our biggest problem is that we think we're not supposed to have any. What is a problem anyway? It's all relative. . . .

Say you've left work and you're in bumper-to-bumper traffic and you're late getting home. How do most people respond? They get really stressed. They can't control the traffic, and they're focused on what they can't control. They're focused on what's missing—on whatever they're supposed to be on time for. They think that's a problem, and their emotions may boil.

But what happens if suddenly the car overheats, and you can't restart it and you're stuck in the middle of the freeway? You've got to find a way to get your car off to the shoulder or people will be honking at you. Now *that's* the problem.

Suffering is not in the facts but in the *perception* of the facts.

Now you've got to pull out your cell phone to call for help, and there's no cell service! So you have to walk a mile to the next off-ramp to get to a gas station to find a phone, and as you're walking you trip and break your ankle. *Now* is the traffic a problem? Is the overheated car a problem? No.

You call a car service, and they take you to the hospital, where you get an X-ray and a cast. And then you listen to the messages on your phone. And there's a message from the love of your life, who says, "I'm leaving you." *Now* is the traffic a problem? Is your overheated car a problem? Is your ankle a problem? No.

You finally make it home and find a message from your doctor, saying he needs to discuss your MRI with you. You call and find out you have cancer. *Now* is the traffic a problem? Is your overheated car or your broken ankle or your relationship a problem? *No!*

So here's the challenge in life. **Our "problems" amount to anything different than what we expect. It's all perspective, isn't it? Some are bigger than others, but problems are healthy signs of life.** They're challenges for us to grow mentally, emotionally, and spiritually. We can't get rid of them, but we can become stronger, smarter, and better in dealing with them. **We must learn to *discipline* our disappointment. Some people let disappointment destroy them, while others let it drive them—that's a choice.** Whenever people say they are suffering, or when I start to feel overly stressed or that something is life-or-death, **I try to remind myself that suffering is not in the facts but in the *perception* of the facts.** For example, if you're incredibly sad or depressed because your mother died, of course that would be a natural reaction. **But if you're staying depressed about this years later, you're not sad or depressed because your mother died, you're sad because you believe she shouldn't have.** Remember, it's not the fact that she died, it's your perception of the fact that's creating your suffering.

And as we discussed, we are the meaning makers. We can decide what to focus on and what things mean, and what we're going to do as a result. But if we don't do this consciously, our survival brains will take over and we'll find ourselves stuck in a pattern of frustration, anger, or fear instead of breaking through and finding a way to grow. And we all need to grow, not just for ourselves but so that we can be a vessel of love and strength for those we care about most.

THE TWO MASTER SKILLS FOR AN EXTRAORDINARY QUALITY OF LIFE

So how do we create an extraordinary quality of life? There are two worlds we need to master: the external world and the internal world. I call these the *science* of achievement and the *art* of fulfillment.

The science of achievement is how to turn your dreams into reality. And while that's not the subject of this book, that's what I've spent most of my life teaching people through my books, events, and private coaching. But the second skill I would attest to is even more important, and that's mastering the art of fulfillment. Notice I didn't say the science of fulfillment, because it is truly an art—what fulfills one person is totally different than others. Some people can look at a piece of art that looks like a colored square on a wall and pay $50 million for it, someone else thinks they're insane and finds the same joy in a sunset or their child's smile. Obviously, the easier it is to be fulfilled, the more fulfilled you can be. But there is a secret beyond just your personal style, and that is understanding a lesson that I got from a brilliant man in India one day.

TO SUFFER OR NOT TO SUFFER— THAT IS THE QUESTION

Let me tell you the story of what's changed in my own life. I'm always looking to grow personally, so I'm constantly exploring different ideas about how to reach a whole new level. A couple of years ago, I was in India, visiting a dear friend of mine, Krishnaji, who is equally fascinated by these questions about how to achieve an extraordinary quality of life. As my friend knows, **I've taught for many years that if you want an extraordinary life, you need to live in an extraordinary mental and emotional state. I talk about how being in a peak state creates peak performance. If you keep yourself in a high energy or "energy-rich" state, you'll deal with problems so much more easily and find the solutions more quickly. You're also more enjoyable to be around and find more passion in life and in relationships.** By contrast most of us let ourselves get in the habit of an "energy-poor" state, a lousy state of mind. When that happens, our minds feel sluggish, and even little problems can trigger great frustration, anger, worry, or fear.

Krishnaji shared with me how valuable it had been to learn the tools to change your state quickly, which we do in all my seminars. We don't just talk about it; we train ourselves. But then he asked me a question, "You know how you talk about peak states or energy-rich states? What if we called them *beautiful states?*" Beautiful states include any high-energy state like love, joy, happiness, appreciation, gratitude, playfulness, fun, driven. I said that that works. And then he said, "What if we took all of those low-energy states and called them *suffering?*" I paused for a moment, and smiled. I could see where he was going with this. Those low-energy states would include frustration, anger, sadness, loneliness, depression. Fear and worry.

For a moment I paused. I didn't like the idea of suffering. I pride myself, as you probably do, on being an achiever, and we don't just sit around and "suffer." When things don't work, we fix them, we turn things around, right? But I smiled to myself. Achievers don't ever get fearful, do we? No! We just get "stressed"! "Stress" is the achiever word for "fear." I finally saw where he was going. Yes, I do get frustrated and stressed at times. So by that defini-tion, I suffered, and I didn't like that idea. Which was really good, because it gave me a different standard for thinking about this. It's easy to say, Well, everybody gets frustrated, angry, sad, worried—and that would be true. **But you and I are not everybody.** We want a greater quality of life. What if we disciplined our minds to live in a beautiful state?

I asked him, "Where are you going with this?" He replied, "It's really simple. **I've decided my spiritual vision for my life—the way I want to live every day—is being committed to living in a beautiful state, no matter what happens!** Even if it rains on my parade, even if there's injus-tice, even if things are unfair, even if I was disappointed." He continued, "Tony, you always talk about **disciplining your disappointment**, and that's what I'm talking about." I said, "You know what, that's beautiful. If you live that way every day, it's not to say you wouldn't ever feel these feelings, you just wouldn't stay there—you'd snap yourself out of it." **By consciously choosing and committing to live in a beautiful state, my friend believed that he could not only enjoy so much more of life, but also give so much more to his wife, his child, and to the world at large.**

I turned to him and said, "That's a brilliant spiritual vision, and now I'm going to steal it. He laughed, and responded, "That's okay, I've stolen a lot of your stuff, too," with a big smile. Think about it, what would your life be like if you could commit, no matter what happened, including the inevi-table injustices, challenges, disappointments, and frustrations? **What if you** didn't stay in those states but immediately held yourself to a standard that the greatest gift in my life is staying in a beautiful state?

I used to convince myself that when I get angry or frustrated or upset, my mind gets faster, and I solve problems quicker. And that's true, but I just I realized that when I'm in a beautiful state of mind, I can solve problems faster, too, but I enjoy my life more and I'm much more enjoyable to be around for the people whom I love. I realize it's so true. **We miss so much of life by reacting to what happens in front of us. Life is too short to suffer! Do you agree?**

The challenge, though, is that **many people believe that someday, somehow, someone or something will make them happy. But I've found that the road to "someday" often leads to a town called "nowhere." <u>Even if something happens in the moment that makes you happy, will it last? Not if you'll be unhappy the minute things don't go your way!</u>**

Let me give you an example. Have you ever achieved a goal that you've worked your tail off for years to achieve, and you finally got it, and said, "Is this all there is?" That's almost worse than failing! If we fail, as achievers, most of us will pick ourselves up and keep trying and push until we get there. **But if you succeed and are *still* unhappy, that's what I call "technically screwed"!**

Maybe there's a time in your life when you succeeded, and you were genuinely very happy about it. Can you think of one right now? How long did that feeling of fulfillment last? Five years? One year? Six months? Six weeks? Six days? . . . Six hours? When I ask this at my seminars, 90 percent of people are in the six-hours-to-six-weeks category. Why? It's because **we're not meant to sit at the table of success for too long. We'll get fat and bored. Everything in the universe is beholden to these two fundamental truths: Everything in the universe either grows or it dies . . . and everything in the universe either contributes or it's eliminated by evolution.** These aren't my laws, these are universal truths. Would you agree?

THE MOST IMPORTANT DECISION:
TO LIVE IN A BEAUTIFUL STATE

<u>The most important decision that you can make is to decide that life is too short to suffer and that you're going to appreciate and enjoy this gift of life, no matter what happens.</u> There's simply too much beauty that we're missing because we're so caught up in our minds instead of in our hearts, our souls, and our spirit.

So many people become obsessed with what they're getting, or not getting, and when they don't get what they want, they get upset. I began to realize in my own life that my happiness was pretty cheap. With more than one hundred companies, thousands of employees on multiple continents—what do you think the odds are that right now, somewhere in the world, someone is screwing up? Well, if my definition of them "screwing up" is doing something different than I think they should, it's probably 100 percent that it's happening right now somewhere! (By the way, what I think is incorrect behavior might actually be a breakthrough way to success, but we all have our expectations, don't we!)

<u>So if the only time you're going to be happy is when everyone is acting the way you want them to act, whether it's your kids, your spouse, your coworkers, or even yourself—it's going to be hard to stay in a beautiful, happy, and fulfilled state.</u> If you're not careful, it would be easy to turn into one of those people who spend all of their time on social media attacking people who say or do things they don't like. What an illusion. **Life does not adapt to us—it's our job to adapt to life.** Part of the beauty of humanity is diversity. If you want to know what the universe or God, or whatever you believe, wants, go to the forest and you'll see it. Every tree, leaf, animal, snowflake, it's all different. We have certain things in common, but it's the differences, the diversity, that makes life rich.

So my friend's advice was brilliant. **Decide to live in a beautiful state no matter what happens around you. It simply means to find the beauty, find something to be grateful for, something to appreciate and then solve your problems.** Think about it, what's more rare than a billionaire? Someone who truly lives in a beautiful state every day, even when it doesn't go their way, even when things are unjust.

When I interviewed more than fifty of the most successful billionaire titans of finance on Earth for my book, *Money: Master the Game*, there were only a handful that appeared to be truly consistently happy. And I don't mean fake happy, I mean lived in a state of gratitude, appreciation, and were able to find meaning in problems and challenges.

So I made a decision that has changed my life. I decided that it wasn't enough to achieve or be fulfilled when things worked out. I decided I'm going to live in a beautiful state every day, no matter what. And it's a mental discipline, it's a daily practice that's far from perfect, but it is an incredible standard to hold yourself to, and its rewards are more than I can describe in words. It means that regardless of what happens, your life will have meaning because you find the beauty, and make it all that you want it to be.

> *"Most people are as happy as they make their minds up to be."*
>
> —ABRAHAM LINCOLN

It doesn't matter what problems strike us, if we buy into a belief that **life is always happening *for* us, not *to* us. It is our responsibility to find the good, and we usually can. Can you think of something that's happened in your life that was terrible, and you'd never want to go through it again, or have anyone you care about go through something like it, but when you look back at it, you see the higher purpose? Going through it made you stronger, more compassionate, made you care more, or made you come up with solutions that now allow you to succeed at a higher level? Can you relate?**

So why wait? Why not decide that everything has a higher purpose? What would your life be like if you lived in a beautiful state? **It all starts with a decision that you can make today—right *now*, before you leave this book—that no matter what happens, you're going to find a way to stay in a beautiful state of mind . . . not because things are going your way or everyone is behaving the way you think that they should, but because you can snap out of those negative states in moments and find the good in anything. You can solve any problem that needs to be solved, keep growing, and giving.**

TRADE YOUR EXPECTATION FOR APPRECIATION

So as we come to the end of our journey together, and the beginning of your next journey, consider this: There are few decisions in your life that shape you most powerfully—whom you love and spend time with is certainly one of them, but how you decide you're going to live and be every single day, I would argue, is the most important decision, and it will affect all those you love.

Most people suffer all the time because their expectations aren't met. Technology has made us more and more impatient, and our phones are tools for instant answers and immediate gratification. We ask Google, we search online, and we quickly get what we want. Have you ever seen someone holding their phone, poking it with their fingers aggressively because a text or a website isn't coming through quickly enough? You might even want to yell at the person, "Give it a minute! It's going up to a satellite, for goodness' sake!"

For the last thirty years, up until the pandemic, I used to fly back and forth between America and Australia several times a year. Nowadays I'm privileged to have my own plane, which is a bit like having a high-speed office in the sky. For better or for worse, there's no need to ever disconnect from work! But I vividly remember the dread I used to experience when I'd sit down on a commercial flight to Australia and wonder how I could possibly live without connecting to emails and texts for the next fourteen hours! Plus, when I landed I'd have a whole day's worth of work still waiting ahead of me on top of all of the things that would come in during those fourteen hours!

Then, one magical day, I was sitting on a Qantas Airways flight to Sydney, when the captain proudly announced that the plane had international Internet access. All around me, people started cheering, clapping, and high-fiving one another! It was as if God had descended from on high and entered the plane! I didn't stand up and do a jig, but I have to confess: In my mind, I was clapping, too. People all over the plane whipped out their iPhones, iPads, and laptops and began to respond to their emails, texts, Slacks, and social media!

But then, what do you think happened just nine minutes later? All of the giddy delight disappeared. What happened? You guessed it. We lost Internet access. For how long? For the entire rest of the flight—it's probably still not working after all these years!

So how do you think the passengers reacted? We were crushed! One minute, we're euphoric. The next minute, people were cursing the airline and their terrible technology.

Here's what amazed me most: how quickly our perspective changed. Nine minutes earlier, it was a miracle; now it was already an expectation! All we could think about was that the airline had violated our inalienable right to Internet access—a right that hadn't existed until that very day.

In our outrage, we instantly lost sight of the wonder that we were flying through the air like a bird, crossing the globe in a matter of hours, and watching movies or sleeping as we flew! Why? Because it had become an expectation.

<u>Expectations are what destroy happiness</u>—whether it's in our relationships, with our kids, or with our work. **Expectations are why so many people are so unhappy today, even in a world with so much abundance.** They're also why we have so much intolerance in the world, because we expect everyone to be, think, act, and behave the way we want them to. How do we overcome this? **<u>Trade your *expectations* for *appreciation* and in that moment, your whole life will change.</u>**

Think about it this way: If you ask someone, "How was your day today?," *there are three primary patterns of response:*

- "Oh, it was really good." Why? Because the day went the way they wanted it to go.
- "It was *incredible*, one of the greatest days of my life." Things went better than they'd expected.
- "It was a *terrible* day." You guessed it—things didn't turn out the way they'd hoped for or anticipated.

All three of these responses are based on expectations. Again, if your day met your expectations, it was a good day. If it was better than expected, you were over the moon. If it was worse than you expected, it was a terrible day. **If you stick with these patterns, your life will be an emotional** rollercoaster, completely controlled by the outside world. If our happiness is so weak that it requires the world to meet our expectations, then most people aren't going to stay happy very long, and they're going to miss out on this extraordinary quality of life.

What's the alternative? <u>To find a way to appreciate whatever life gives you.</u> It doesn't mean that you have to just settle for whatever comes. If you don't like the status quo, appreciate what you *do* have and find a way to use it to create something greater. This requires you to believe something simple—that whatever happens, including the toughest challenges and problems, it's meant to serve a purpose. And it's our responsibility to find that higher purpose, and use it.

I encourage you to first make this decision right now for yourself. Second, take a moment and write a note to yourself about why you want to live in a beautiful state no matter what, and why life is too short to suffer. Why wait for someday to feel good, when the journey is what makes life beautiful? Maybe send this letter to someone you respect, someone who can hold you accountable. And third, when you do find yourself in a state of suffering, use my Ninety Second Rule.

When I feel stress is getting the better of me, **I invoke my 90-Second Rule.** I take in a slow, full breath, and then exhale completely and with it let go of the emotion. I allow myself 90 seconds to feel whatever negative

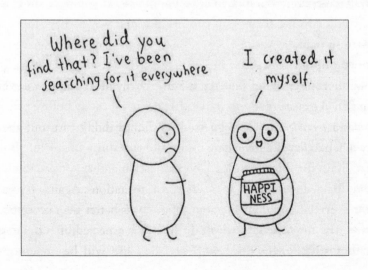

emotion has surfaced and let it go. Then I follow with ninety additional seconds to focus on what's *great* about this situation and how the challenge is going to make me grow. And I focus on what is beautiful in my life already to put things in balance. It makes me look at a situation in a new way—it leads me to find new answers. And when I acknowledge what's not perfect yet, I ask myself, **"What do I need to do to make it better?" In a beautiful state, the answers flow. In a lousy state, the answers are slow or nonexistent.**

Finally, I focus on what I can appreciate or be grateful for in this moment. Because no matter what's happening, you still have people who love you. You still have the gift of life and breath in your lungs. And I let the fog of the negative emotion drift away, and I replace it with the emotions of resourcefulness and resiliency. I let go of the past and decide what to move forward with right now. And the fog disappears. I've made it like a game, and I'm by no means perfect at it. At the beginning I was good at small things but some big ones should have been called the 90-minute or 90-hour game. But I've gotten better as I've practiced more. But the more you play, the better you get and the better your life gets. **After all, happiness is a muscle; the more you use it, the stronger it gets. Finding gratitude and appreciation starts to come naturally once you make it a pattern, and it's one that will transform your life. Think about it. Most people have a highway to stress and a dirt road to happiness. If you develop this new habit, you'll reverse that—you can build a highway to happiness and a dirt road to pain.**

Are you up for this game in your own life? Would you be willing to do this for ten days and just try it out? Or even 21 days to develop a true habit? Are you ready to make this decision today before you close these pages—not only to make yourself healthier, but to find a way to embrace whatever life gives you and find something beautiful about it? You can live a life filled with fear and frustration and anger and sadness, or you can direct those emotions to drive you to find better answers and appreciate everything in your life along the way. **It's not an easy approach, which is why most people won't do it. But it's incredibly effective and powerful for those who do.**

THREE POWERFUL TOOLS TO LIVE
IN A BEAUTIFUL STATE

If you want to live in a beautiful state, we have to be realistic that there will be things that will trigger us. We'll often find ourselves getting triggered by past experiences, pain, or challenges, and go into our survival brain where we start to overreact to things with frustration, fear, anger, sadness, or some combination of emotions that disempower us. There are so many great tools that I teach at my events, but I wanted to mention three here that you might find useful and impactful.

Tool #1: Energy Medicine: A Scientific Antidote To Stress

The first is a tool that works with people even with extreme trauma. **You may have heard of Energy Medicine, a set of EFT (Emotional Freedom Techniques), also known as tapping. It combines ancient Chinese acupressure with modern psychology.** It involves lightly tapping on the endpoints of the meridians of your body, such as your chin or eyebrow or collarbone. At the same time, you're reciting specific meditations that acknowledge your emotions and release them. Oftentimes, even if you think you're over something, the emotion or the energy is still trapped in your body.

While this tool has been around for decades, it's only lately that we've gotten some **rock-solid science to confirm its ability to lower stress levels, quiet the mind for sleep, improve focus and productivity, and strengthen our immune system. In a study published by the American Psychological Association, subjects who tapped for an hour showed a 43 percent decrease in salivary cortisol, your stress hormone.**[1] **In fact, more than 125 studies have found that tapping can effectively treat conditions ranging from anxiety and depression to traumatic stress**

---

1 Stapleton et al., "Reexamining the Effect of Emotional Freedom Techniques on Stress Biochemistry."

and chronic muscle pain.[2] **EFT can even subdue people's cravings for carbohydrates and fast food![3]**

I have a dear friend named Nick Ortner, to whom I taught this technique more than twenty years ago, and he's since gone on to become one of the foremost experts in this, and we've partnered together in the past to help survivors of extreme trauma, including the families of the Sandy Hook shooting, and the Batman shooting in Aurora, Colorado.

We've even built an app together. To experience this transformative technique for yourself, you can download the app for free (or get a special discount on the premium version) by visiting thetappingsolution.com/tony. My portion of the company's profits are all donated to Feeding America, so that while you're making yourself feel better you're actually helping someone else in need.

Tool #2: Priming: Wiring Yourself for a Peak State

The second tool is something that I do every single day to start my morning; it's called **priming**. I won't try to explain it here, but it's a ten-**minute process to supercharge your mind and emotions before you begin your day.** I made it 10 minutes, so there's no reason not to do this. If you don't have 10 minutes, you don't have a life! Don't you agree? If you would like to see how this tool works, you're welcome to go to TonyRobbins.com /Priming. I also have a version of this in our tapping app that I mentioned above.

Tool #3: Incredible Solutions for Those Suffering from Extreme Anxiety or PTSD

For years after his discharge from the U.S. Air Force, Evan Moon was in fight-or-flight mode from morning till night. His heart rate was constantly elevated. He was jumpy and easily startled, as if something terrible could happen any time. As his self-confidence crashed through the floor, he

---

2 Church et al., "App-Based Delivery of Clinical Emotional Freedom Techniques: Cross-Sectional Study of App User Self-Ratings."

3 Peta Stapleton et al., "Online Delivery of Emotional Freedom Techniques for Food Cravings and Weight Management: 2-Year Follow-Up."

avoided seeing friends. Eric couldn't stop thinking about his experiences in Afghanistan. Even his dreams were haunted by the trauma of seeing the lives of his fellow airmen who had perished in battle.

To ease his pain, Eric became dependent on alcohol. As he wrote to me, "I lost interest in most things. Everything seemed bland. The best way I can describe the way I was feeling was that every day seemed like I was waking up inside of a jar of molasses. Even though I may have had moments of escaping the jar, the stickiness never truly washed off."

Did you know that twenty-two U.S. military veterans commit suicide each day?[4] Many are combat vets who served in Iraq, Afghanistan, or Vietnam and came home with posttraumatic stress disorder. PTSD is a chronic, debilitating, life-wrecking condition—and one of the toughest to overcome. The standard approaches include antidepressants, cognitive behavior therapy (to change the patient's thought process) and "exposure" therapy, where people relive the traumatic event that triggered their trauma in the first place. **None are ideal. Their results are unreliable, or they require years of treatment or set off serious side effects—or all of the above.**

I have worked with people like this before. A man who had lost thirty-two of his fellow veterans in multiple tours of Iraq and Afghanistan came to one of my events wearing dark glasses. The PTSD was so bad that light could stimulate it. He was unable to sleep, and night sweats had continued for years. It took me two and a half hours to help him. In fact, he came on CNN and was interviewed, and they showed the before and after over a six-month period. It was extraordinary. While I knew I could help, the challenge is that with twenty-two veterans committing suicide every day, so I committed myself to finding a scalable solution.

The good news is that there's a new and promising therapy for PTSD: simple, safe, and fast-acting injections that have been used effectively for years to relieve nerve pain or circulation problems.[5] **In a recent controlled study at three U.S. military hospitals, one hundred active-duty personnel received a pair of shots two weeks apart into their** *stellate ganglion,* **the nerve tissue on either side of your voice box that**

---

4 Kemp and Bossarte, "Suicide Data Report, 2012."

5 Cleveland Clinic, "Stellate Ganglion Block."

connects to the amygdala,[6] the fight-or-flight center of the brain. It's an outpatient procedure with virtually no side effects aside from some temporary hoarseness.

Eight weeks later, the troops who got the actual block showed twice as much impact as those who'd received a sham placebo treatment. They had relief from depression, distress, anxiety, and pain, and showed marked progress in their physical and mental functioning.[7] The method had an 85 percent success rate,[8] which beats many standard-of-care drugs. I committed to sponsoring 150 veterans through this program, and one of them was . . . was Evan Moon. Here is what he wrote to me about what he calls his "miracle" treatment:

"I'm writing you, Mr. Robbins, to let you know that after the shot everything has changed. Colors are brighter, my nightmares are gone, and life seems so hopeful. I feel as if I am bathing in a warm ocean throughout the day of peace and joy. Going into social situations feels like a breeze, and I love being around new people and learning more about them. Most importantly, I find myself laughing like a child and smiling through my day. I feel present and in the moment. Right after the shot I was able to go back and spend time with my children and my wife. It feels like a different world. This is only the beginning, and I am thrilled to see what happens next."

He wrote me again a year later, and he's now gone out to help other veterans get the help they need through this treatment.

Scientists agree that more long-term studies of this therapy are needed. But thus far it's safe to say that stellate ganglion block gives anyone damaged by trauma new hope for a compelling future—and for a rich and beautiful life. If you know of someone in need, this is something worth searching out. To learn more, please visit TheStellateInstitute.com.

---

6 Cornell Pain Clinic, "Stellate Ganglion Block for PTSD."

7 Olmsted et al., "Effect of Stellate Ganglion Block Treatment on Posttraumatic Stress Disorder Symptoms."

8 TheStellateInstitute.com

THE ULTIMATE PATH TO FREEDOM

"As I walked out the door toward the gate that would lead to my freedom, I knew if I didn't leave my bitterness and hatred behind, I'd still be in prison."

—NELSON MANDELA, South African freedom fighter

I know that staying in a beautiful state can sound like an impossible task, especially when we're going through challenging times. To finish up, let me give you three examples of people who have experienced a level of injustice and pain that would have easily justified their staying angry, sad, or even enraged. But these three individuals instead chose to live in a beautiful state, to find the good in anything, and find a way to use what life gave them to grow and to serve. Victimhood was not for them, so, as a result, they transformed themselves and touched people all over the world.

I had the privilege of meeting **Nelson Mandela** in the early 1990s, not long after he was finally released after twenty-seven years in South African jails and then became president of his country. Having a moment to be with this legend, I wanted to understand how he made it through such challenging times. So I asked him how he survived all that time under such miserable conditions—in a dank and tiny cell with only a straw mat for a bed. **Boy, it was the wrong question to ask. President Mandela literally rose from his chair and glared at me as we got up and said, "I didn't survive. I prepared."**

That led to a conversation that I'll never forget. He told me that when he was in jail, he understood that his life could lead in one of two directions—and that either path was filled with purpose if he chose it. He might die in prison, which would spark a revolution that he thought could change his country for the better. Or he might live, which meant he'd need to let go of his pain and prepare to lead South Africa forward—not just Black people, but the entire country. So Mandela taught himself Afrikaans, the language spoken by his white jailers. He wanted to be able to speak to the people of South Africa in their own language, so they would feel the truth in his voice. In the midst of all of the pain he'd endured, **he found a beautiful state in radical forgiveness.** "I figured I might as well enjoy the guards," he told me. "I might as well enjoy the day." **What an amazing capacity for appreciation! What a beautiful state to live in! Mandela rose above his own plight and focused instead on how he could serve others and something greater than himself.** And the changes that he brought to the country under his leadership were transformative.

You don't have to be a world-famous icon to decide to enjoy your life, no matter what.

Sam Berns was only 17 years old when he told a TED talk audience: **"I have a very happy life. . . . I don't waste energy feeling bad for myself. I surround myself with people I want to be with, and I keep moving forward."**

What made Sam's outlook remarkable was that he was born with *progeria*, **a rare genetic disease that speeds aging by a factor of eight.** Progeria stunts children's growth and makes them biologically old before their time, which is why it's often called Benjamin Button disease. Starting in the first few years of life, it quickly leads to a slew of maladies associated with old age: stiff joints, vision and hearing loss, kidney failure, atherosclerosis. On average, these children die of heart attacks or strokes by age 13.

Against these scary odds, **Sam Berns faced the next day without fear or dread. He didn't squander his energy worrying. He saved it for** *living*. He was a straight-A student at his Massachusetts high school, an aspiring cell biologist, and a standout percussionist with the marching band. After he met and befriended Francis Collins, head of the National Institutes of Health, Sam's unquenchable spirit inspired research that led to a groundbreaking discovery: progeria was triggered by a single devastating typo in the DNA code. That one mutation floods the body with *progerin*, a toxic protein that weakens cell nuclei. In 2012, a clinical trial by Lesley's team found a cancer drug that slowed the onslaught of progeria and extended Sam's life. Their continuing research—adding a second drug, a form of rapamycin—has given the world new insights about cardiovascular disease and the aging process.

Sam offered one last piece of advice at his TED talk: **"Never miss a party if you can help it."** He was thrilled to share his personal philosophy on an international platform. But what he *really* looked forward to was his school's homecoming dance the next night. **Whenever fun was on the agenda, Sam was first in line.**

Sam died a month later—way too soon, but not before showing us the way to a magnificent, extraordinary, meaningful life. He weighed just 50 pounds, but he left a legacy—of living in a beautiful state—the size of a mountain. His TED talk has more than 33 million views on YouTube. Sam refused to let anything spoil the glorious gift of our every day on Earth. He was unshakably committed to live each hour to the utmost. **He kept moving forward, no matter what.**

Not long ago, I was also lucky enough to meet Sam's kindred spirit, a woman named **Alice Herz-Sommer. I interviewed Alice when she was 107 years old—nearly 70 years after the Nazis murdered her mother and put her and her son in a concentration camp.** Alice was a famous concert pianist in Europe, and she was forced to play in the inmate orchestra. She was told that if she didn't look happy, they'd murder her son in front of her. The Nazis actually made films of her playing to try and convince the world that they were treating Jews well. But in real life, the conditions were beyond brutal. Alice slept on a frozen dirt floor and channeled all her energy into trying to keep her son happy, even though they had little to eat.

Yet Alice refused to let pain become her story. She gave more than a hundred concerts, and while she was forced to entertain the Nazis, something beautiful happened. The music echoed through the yard, into the barracks, where the prisoners who were sick and hungry were fed by the sounds. **When Alice was playing, many of them said it was like God was present. The music was an extension of life's beauty in the middle of the most painful situation. Alice told me the prisoners would yearn to listen to it and feel their spirits lifted out of suffering. It was as if someone had transported them out of the hell of the camp and into the heaven of life's most beautiful moments. By serving others, Alice did more than survive the Nazis. She found a way to *appreciate* and *enjoy* her existence.**

Years later she wrote a book, and the title says it all: *A Garden of*

Eden in Hell: The Life of Alice Herz-Sommer. It's a book I highly recommend. But during our interview, I was struck by how *everything* was so beautiful to Alice. She was living on her own at 107, still swimming and playing the piano. People in the building would listen to her play, just as they had in the camps seven decades earlier.

Alice was grateful for everything. She talked about how beautiful life is, and how grateful she was that her son made it through that time. How beautiful it was that she survived cancer at 80 and was now 107! She even remarked how beautiful the microphone was—as well as my wife! **Life is beautiful if we look for the beauty regardless of the external environment.**

ONE FINAL LESSON

So hopefully this reminds you to **get rid of the illusion that so many of us have—that if life was just a certain way, then we'd be happy.** Let me give you one last powerful example. . . .

When I travel around the world and ask people what the best thing that could happen to them in life is, the most common answer is winning the lottery! And if you ask people what's the *worst* thing that could happen, many might say it would be to become a paraplegic. But in a famous study of dozens of major lottery winners and people paralyzed in accidents, **which group would you guess was happier—the lottery winners or the paraplegics?** My bet is that you're thinking it must be the paraplegics—**but you'd be wrong.** So now you'll tell me the lucky lottery winners were the happy ones—and you'll still be wrong.

In fact, the lottery winners were no happier overall than a control group who hadn't won a dime. Sure, they had more money, but they also had people constantly demanding and expecting things from them. **And the paraplegics? They rated *their* happiness above the midpoint on a zero-to-five scale.**[9] **After you're in a terrible accident, your mindset changes. If you relearn to move your fingers, it feels like a miracle.** A reason for joy! You take nothing for granted. When we find a larger

---

9 Brickman et al., "Lottery Winners and Accident Victims: Is Happiness Relative?"

meaning in our lives, we heal mentally, emotionally, and spiritually. **And that is the ultimate gift.**

THE ULTIMATE GIFT

"Live life fully while you're here. Experience everything. Take care of yourself and your friends. Have fun, be crazy, be weird. Go out and screw up! You're going to anyway, so you might as well enjoy the process."

—TONY ROBBINS

Well, we've covered a lot of ground—and a lot of tools—in these 700-plus pages. I hope this book can serve as a field manual, an ultimate resource to enhance your healthspan. A book you can return to any time you face real challenges. **But before you turn the final page, I hope you really take a moment to commit to live in a beautiful state, no matter what happens.**

A beautiful state isn't perfect. It's *better* than perfect. It's messy, playful, full of fun. It's being generous with yourself and others, and not taking yourself too seriously. It's working to keep getting better to foster a life filled with joy and happiness and meaning. It's finding something or someone you want to serve more than yourself. Because that's the true meaning of *grace*— a life well lived—a life of service and a life filled with love.

Finally, will you remember the creative power of your mind and emotions? And that **you're one decision away from changing anything in your life?** If you don't like your body, change it. If you don't like your business or career, change it. If you don't like your relationship, change yourself first, or change it. All actions are fathered or mothered by decision. This chapter is about to end, but on page 649, there is the opportunity for you to make some decisions about what you've learned. I've broken it into a 7-step potential action plan that includes deciding what you want for your body, emotion, and your life, and getting clear about where you are.

The second step is to educate yourself and keep learning about the cutting-edge tools that can increase your energy, strength, and vitality, and hopefully extend both the length and quality of your life. This book has been filled with so many tools, but which ones will you use?

Third, you need to look at your lifestyle. After going through those seven steps in a moment, you'll have an action plan. In the end, information is not what changes your life—action is. You don't need to do everything in this book, just pick a few things that you're going to follow through on and commit to do them immediately.

I've always taught that the key is momentum and to never leave the site of a decision without doing something in that moment that commits you to following through. Make a phone call, send a text or an email, schedule a meeting, but get the ball moving.

And finally, please remember these three decisions that you're making each day, and choose well:

1. Decide what you're going to **focus** on. It will determine what you experience in life.
2. Decide what things **mean.** It will determine what you feel.
3. And decide what you're going to **do.** It will determine your results.

Remember, it's in those moments of decision that your destiny is shaped. So please, choose well. Choose now.

When I began writing this book, I envisioned you reading these final words, because I knew it would mean that you had read the many other pages in this book containing answers that you may have needed for yourself or others in the future. **I want to thank you for taking this journey with me, for having such perseverance and for the gift of your time and attention. These are two of the most valuable things you can share with everyone, and I don't take it lightly.**

It's my heartfelt prayer that this book has touched not just your head, but your heart as well. And that as a result you'll take even better care of yourself and those you love. Perhaps you'll get those tests in advance, or make a list of the things in this book that are worth making new habits out of. So that when a challenging time comes, you're already prepared.

If this book has helped you find less fear and more joy to heal and move forward, then our time together was well spent. So now the real journey begins! I also hope I have the privilege to meet you someday, and that you can tell me the insights that you pulled from this book that have helped you and those you love. So until we meet again, or until our paths cross, I wish for you a long, healthy, passion-filled life with many blessings to you and your family.

—With love and respect,
TONY ROBBINS

NOTES

Chapter 1: Life Force: Our Greatest Gift

1. John J. McCusker, "How Much is That in Real Money? A Historical Price Index for Use as a Deflator of Money Values in the Economy of the United States: Addenda et Corrigenda," *Proceedings of the American Antiquarian Society* 106, Iss. 2 (January 1, 1996), 327–34, https://www.americanantiquarian.org/proceedings/44525121.pdf.

2. Jon Gertner, "Unlocking the Covid Code," *New York Times Magazine*, March 25, 2021, https://www.nytimes.com/interactive/2021/03/25/magazine/genome-sequencing-covid-variants.html.

3. Suzana Herculano-Houzel, "The Human Brain in Numbers: A Linearly Scaled-Up Primate Brain," *Frontiers in Human Neuroscience* 3, no, 31 (November 2009), https://doi.org/10.3389/neuro.09.031.2009.

4. Glenn Rein, Mike Atkinson, and Rollin McCraty, "The Physiological and Psychological Effects of Compassion and Anger," *Journal of Advancement in Medicine* 8, no. 2 (Summer 1995), 87–105, https://www.issuelab.org/resources/3130/3130.pdf.

5. Monica Van Such, Robert Lohr, Thomas Beckman, and James M. Naessens, "Extent of Diagnostic Agreement Among Medical Referrals," *Journal of Evaluation in Clinical Practice* 23, no. 4, 870–74, https://doi.org/10.1111/jep.12747.

6. Elizabeth Zimmermann, "Mayo Clinic Researchers Demonstrate Value of Second Opinions," Mayo Clinic News Network, April 4, 2017, https://newsnetwork.mayoclinic.org/discussion/mayo-clinic-researchers-demonstrate-value-of-second-opinions/.

7. Patrick Radden Keefe, "The Sackler Family's Plan to Keep Its Billions," *New Yorker*, October 4, 2020, https://www.newyorker.com/news/news-desk/the-sackler-familys-plan-to-keep-its-billions.

8. Josh Katz and Margot Sanger-Katz, " 'It's Huge, It's Historic, It's Unheard-Of': Drug Overdose Deaths Spike," *New York Times*, July 14, 2021, https://www.nytimes.com/interactive/2021/07/14/upshot/drug-overdose-deaths.html.

9. Jan Hoffman, "Purdue Pharma Is Dissolved and Sacklers Pay $4.5 Billion to Settle Opioid Claims," *New York Times*, September 17, 2021, https://www.nytimes.com/2021/09/01/health/purdue-sacklers-opioids-settlement.html.

10. Rachel Sandler, "The Sacklers Made More Than $12 Billion in Profit from OxyContin Maker Purdue Pharma, New Report Says," *Forbes*, October 4, 2019, https://www.forbes.com/sites/rachelsandler/2019/10/04/the-sacklers-made-12-to-13-billion-in-profit-from-oxycontin-maker-purdue-pharma-new-report-says/.

11. Jan Hoffman, "Drug Distributors and J&J Reach $26 Billion Deal to End Opioid Lawsuits," *New York Times*, July 21, 2021, https://www.nytimes.com/2021/07/21/health/opioids-distributors-settlement.html.

12. Rita Rubin, "Pfizer Fined $2.3 Billion for Illegal Marketing," *USA Today*, September 3, 2009, https://www.pressreader.com/usa/usa-today-us-edition/20090903/283038345573224.

13. Beth Snyder Bulik, "The Top 10 Ad Spenders in Big Pharma for 2019," *Fierce Pharma*, February 19, 2020, https://www.fiercepharma.com/special-report/top-10-advertisers-big-pharma-for-2019.

14. Ruggero Cadossi, Leo Massari, Jennifer Racine-Avila, and Roy K. Aaron, "Pulsed Electromagnetic Field Stimulation of Bone Healing and Joint Preservation: Cellular Mechanisms of Skeletal Response," *Journal of the AAOS Global Research and Reviews* 4, no. 5 (May 2020), https://dx.doi.org/10.5435%2FJAAOSGlobal-D-19–00155; Food and Drug Administration, "FDA Executive Summary: Prepared for the September 8–9, 2020, Meeting of the Orthopaedic and Rehabilitation Devices Panel: Reclassification of Non-Invasive Bone Growth Stimulators," 2020, https://www.fda.gov/media/141850/download.

15. Daniel Yetman, "What You Need to Know about the Stem Cell Regenerating Gun for Burns," *Healthline*, April 17, 2020, https://www.healthline.com/health/skin-cell-gun.

16. Food and Drug Administration, "What Are the Different Types of Clinical Research?", January 4, 2018, https://www.fda.gov/patients/clinical-trials-what-patients-need-know/what-are-different-types-clinical-research.

Chapter 2: The Power of Stem Cells

1. Devon O'Neil, "No More Knife: The Stem-Cell Shortcut to Injury Recovery," *Outside*, March 10, 2014, https://www.outsideonline.com/health/training-performance/no-more-knife-stem-cell-shortcut-injury-recovery/.

2. Jef Akst, "Donor-Derived iPS Cells Show Promise for Treating Eye Disease," *Scientist*, April 30, 2019, https://www.the-scientist.com/news-opinion/donor-derived-ips-cells-show-promise-for-treating-eye-disease-65817.

3. Kevin McCormack, "Stem Cell Treatment For Spinal Cord Injury Offers Improved Chance of Independent Life for Patients," *Stem Cellar: The Official Blog of CIRM*, July 18, 2018, https://blog.cirm.ca.gov/2018/07/18/stem-cell-treatment-for-spinal-cord-injury-offers-improved-chance-of-independent-life-for-patients/.

4. Charlotte Lozier Institute, "Fact Sheet: Adult Stem Cell Research and Transplants," November 21, 2017, https://lozierinstitute.org/fact-sheet-adult-stem-cell-research-transplants/.

5. Technische Universität Dresden, "Blood Stem Cells Boost Immunity by Keeping a Record of Previous Infections," *ScienceDaily*, 13 March 2020, https://www.sciencedaily.com/releases/2020/03/200313112148.htm.

6. Solveig Ericson (Study Director) for Celularity Incorporated, "A Multi-Center Study to Evaluate the Safety and Efficacy of Intravenous Infusion of Human Placenta-Derived Cells (PDA001) for the Treatment of Adults with Moderate-to-Severe Crohn's Disease," U.S. National Library of Medicine: ClinicalTrials.gov, July 22, 2020, https://clinicaltrials.gov/ct2/show/NCT01155362.

7. Daniel Yetman, "What You Need to Know About the Stem Cell Regenerating Gun for Burns," *Healthline*, April 17, 2020, https://www.healthline.com/health/skin-cell-gun.

8. Food and Drug Administration, "FDA Warns About Stem Cell Therapies," FDA Consumer Updates, September 3, 2019, https://www.fda.gov/consumers/consumer-updates/fda-warns-about-stem-cell-therapies.

9. Trang H. Nguyen, David C. Randolph, James Talmage, Paul Succop, and Russell Travis, "Long-Term Outcomes of Lumbar Fusion Among Workers' Compensation Subjects: A Historical Cohort Study," *Spine* 36, no. 4 (February 15, 2011), 320–31, https://doi.org/10.1097/brs.0b013e3181ccc220.

10. Jiang He, Paul K. Whelton, Brian Vu, et al., "Aspirin and Risk of Hemorrhagic Stroke: A Meta-Analysis of Randomized Controlled Trials," *Journal of the American Medical Association* 280(22), 1998, 1930–35, doi:10.1001/jama.280.22.1930.

Chapter 3: Diagnostic Power: Breakthroughs That Can Save Your Life

1. Hyuk-Jae Chang et al., "Selective Referral Using CCTA Versus Direct Referral for Individuals Referred to Invasive Coronary Angiography for Suspected CAD," *JACC: Cardiovascular Imaging* 12, no. 7 (July 2019), 1303–12, doi: 10.1016/j.jcmg.2018.09.018.

2. Farhad Islami, Elizabeth M. Ward, Hyuna Sing, et al., "Annual Report to the Nation on the Status of Cancer," *JNCI: Journal of the National Cancer Institute*, djab131 (July 8, 2021), https://doi.org/10.1093/jnci/djab131.

3. N. Howlader, A. M. Noone, M. Krapcho, et al., "SEER Cancer Statistics Review, 1975–2018," National Cancer Institute, based on November 2020 SEER data submission, posted April 2021, https://seer.cancer.gov/csr/1975_2018/.

4. Ron Brookmeyer, Nada Abdalla, Claudia H. Kawas, and María M. Corrada, "Forecasting the Prevalence of Preclinical and Clinical Alzheimer's Disease in the United States," *Alzheimer's and Dementia* 14, no. 2 (February 2018), 121–29, https://doi.org/10.1016/j.jalz.2017.10.009.

Chapter 4: Turning Back Time: Will Aging Soon Be Curable?

2. William F. Marshall III, "Can Vitamin D Protect Against the Coronavirus Disease 2019 (COVID-19)?," *Mayo Clinic Expert Answers*, https://www.mayoclinic.org/diseases-conditions/coronavirus/expert-answers/coronavirus-and-vitamin-d/faq-20493088.

3. Jared M. Campbell, Matthew D. Stephenson, Barbora de Courten, Ian Chapman, Susan M. Bellman, and Edoardo Aromataris, "Metformin Use Associated with Reduced Risk of Dementia in Patients with Diabetes: A Systematic Review and Meta-Analysis," *Journal of Alzheimer's Disease* 65, no. 4, 1225–36, https://dx.doi.org/10.3233%2FJAD-180263.

4. George Citroner, "Diabetes Drug Metformin May Help Reverse Serious Heart Condition," *Healthline*, April 21, 2019, https://www.healthline.com/health-news/how-diabetes-drug-metformin-can-reduce-heart-disease-risk; Pouya Saraei, Ilia Asadi, Muhammad Azam Kakar, and Nasroallah Moradi-Kor, "The Beneficial Effects of Metformin on Cancer Prevention and Therapy: A Comprehensive Review of Recent Advances," *Cancer Management and Research* 11 (April 17, 2019), 3295–313, https://dx.doi.org/10.2147%2FCMAR.S200059.

5. Richard D. Semba, Anne R. Cappola, Kai Sun, et al., "Plasma Klotho and Mortality Risk in Older Community-Dwelling Adults," *Journals of Gerontology, Series A, Biological Sciences and Medical Sciences* 66, no. 7 (July 2011), 794–800, https://doi.org/10.1093/gerona/glr058.

6. Laura Kurtzman, "Brain Region Vulnerable to Aging Is Larger in Those with Longevity Gene Variant," *UCSF News*, January 27, 2015, https://www.ucsf.edu/news/2015/01/122761/brain-region-vulnerable-aging-larger-those-longevity-gene-variant.

7. Nuo Sun, Richard J. Youle, and Toren Finkel, "The Mitochondrial Basis of Aging," *Molecular Cell* 61, no. 5 (March 3, 2016), 654–66, https://dx.doi.org/10.1016%2Fj.molcel.2016.01.028.

8. Matthew Conlen, Danielle Ivory, Karen Yourish, et al., "Nearly One-Third of U.S. Coronavirus Deaths Are Linked to Nursing Homes," *New York Times*, June 1, 2021, https://www.nytimes.com/interactive/2020/us/coronavirus-nursing-homes.html.

9. Andrea Peterson, "Final FY21 Appropriations: National Institutes of Health," FYI: Science Policy News from AIP, February 9, 2021, https://www.aip.org/fyi/2021/final-fy21-appropriations-national-institutes-health.

10. Ananya Mandal, "Heart Rate Reserve," *News Medical Life Sciences*, June 4, 2019, https://www.news-medical.net/health/Heart-Rate-Reserve.aspx.

11. Ekaterina Pesheva, "Rewinding the Clock," *Harvard Medical School News and Research*, March 22, 2018, https://hms.harvard.edu/news/rewinding-clock.

12. Alejandro Ocampo, Pradeep Reddy, Paloma Martinez-Redondo, et al., "In Vivo Amelioration of Age-Associated Hallmarks by Partial Reprogramming," *Cell* 167, no. 7 (December 15, 2016), 1719–1733, https://doi.org/10.1016/j.cell.2016.11.052.

13. A. R. Mendelsohn and J. W. Larrick, "Epigenetic Age Reversal by Cell-Extrinsic and Cell-Intrinsic Means," *Rejuvenation Research* 2019, no. 22 (2019), 439–46, https://dx.doi.org/10.1089/rej.2019.2271.

14. Adam Bluestein, "What if Aging Could be Slowed and Health Spans Extended? A Q+A with Nir Barzilai, M.D.," *Medium Life Biosciences*, February 19, 2019. https://medium.com/@lifebiosciences/what-if-aging-could-be-slowed-and-health-spans-extended-bc313443a98

15. Diana C. Lade, "Reaching 100: Survivors of the Century," *South Florida Sun-Sentinel*, July 30, 2001, https://www.sun-sentinel.com/news/fl-xpm-2001-07-30-0107300116-story.html.

16. *The Science of Success Podcast*, "How to Stop and Reverse Aging with Dr. David Sinclair," July 30, 2020, https://www.successpodcast.com/show-notes/2020/7/30/how-to-stop-amp-reverse-aging-with-dr-david-sinclair.

Chapter 5: The Miracle of Organ Regeneration

1. "Wake Forest Physician Reports First Human Recipients of Laboratory-Grown Organs," Atrium Health Wake Forest Baptist news release, April 3, 2006, https://newsroom.wakehealth.edu/News-Releases/2006/04/Wake-Forest-Physician-Reports-First-Human-Recipients-of-LaboratoryGrown-Organs.

2. Kevin Daum, "Celebrate These LGBTQ Business Leaders Who Are Changing the World," *Inc.*, June 14, 2019, https://www.inc.com/kevin-daum/celebrate-these-lgbtq-business-leaders-who-are-changing-world.html.

3. Neely Tucker, "Martine Rothblatt: She Founded SiriusXM, a Religion, and a Biotech.

For Starts," *Washington Post*, December 12, 2014, https://www.washingtonpost.com
/lifestyle/magazine/martine-rothblatt-she-founded-siriusxm-a-religion-and-a-biotech
-for-starters/2014/12/11/.

4. Lisa Miller, "The Trans-Everything CEO," *New York*, September 7, 2014, https://
nymag.com/news/features/martine-rothblatt-transgender-ceo/.

5. Martine Rothblatt, "My Daughter, My Wife, Our Robot, and the Quest for Immortality," *TED Talks*, March 2015, https://www.ted.com/talks/martine_rothblatt_my_
daughter_my_wife_our_robot_and_the_quest_for_immortality.

6. RF Wireless World, "Satellite Orbit Types: Molnya, Tundra, Low Earth Satellite
Orbit," *RF Wireless World Tutorials*, https://www.rfwireless-world.com/Tutorials/satel
lite-orbits.html.

7. SiriusXM, "SiriusXM Reports First Quarter 2020 Results," SiriusXM press release,
April 28, 2020, https://investor.siriusxm.com/investor-overview/press-releases/press
-release-details/2020/SiriusXM-Reports-First-Quarter-2020-Results/default.aspx.

8. United Network for Organ Sharing, "More Deceased-Donor Organ Transplants Than
Ever," October 14, 2021, https://unos.org/data/transplant-trends/.

9. Sarah Zhang, "Genetically Engineering Pigs to Grow Organs for People," *Atlantic*,
August 10, 2017, https://www.theatlantic.com/science/archive/2017/08/pig-organs
-for-humans/536307/.

10. Alice Park, "Why Pig Organs Could Be the Future of Transplants," *Time*, February 15,
2018, https://time.com/5159889/why-pig-organs-could-be-the-future-of-transplants/.

11. Nikola Davis, "Baboon Survives for Six Months After Receiving Pig Heart Transplant," *Guardian*, December 5, 2018, https://www.theguardian.com/science/2018
/dec/05/baboon-survives-pig-heart-organ-transplant-human-trials.

12. Karen Weintraub, "Using Animal Organs in Humans: 'It's Just a Question of When,' "
Guardian, April 3, 2019, https://www.theguardian.com/science/2019/apr/03/animal
-global-organ-shortage-gene-editing-technology-transplant.

13. Karen Weintraub, "A CRISPR Startup is Testing Pig Organs in Monkeys to See If
They're Safe for Us," *MIT Technology Review*, June 12, 2019, https://www.technology
review.com/2019/06/12/239014/crispr-pig-organs-are-being-implanted-in-monkeys
-to-see-if-theyre-safe-for-humans/.

14. Peter Diamandis, "Fireside with Dr. Martine Rothblatt," *Abundance 360 Summit*,
May 19, 2020.

15. Roni Caryn Rabin, "In a First, Surgeons Attached a Pig Kidney to a Human, and It
Worked," *New York Times*, October 19, 2021, https://www.nytimes.com/2021/10/19
/health/kidney-transplant-pig-human.html.

16. Karen Weintraub, "A CRISPR Startup is Testing Pig Organs in Monkeys."

17. Brian Lord, "Bladder Grown from 3D Bioprinted Tissue Continues to Function After
14 Years," *3D Printing Industry*, September 12, 2018, https://3dprintingindustry.com
/news/bladder-grown-from-3d-bioprinted-tissue-continues-to-function-after-14
-years-139631/.

18. Vanesa Listek, "Dr. Anthony Atala Explains the Frontiers of Bioprinting for Regenerative Medicine at Wake Forest," World Stem Cell Summit blog, April 30, 2019, https://
www.worldstemcellsummit.com/2019/04/30/dr-anthony-atala-explains-the-frontiers
-of-bioprinting-for-regenerative-medicine-at-wake-forest/.

19. Antonio Regalado, "Inside the Effort to Print Lungs and Breathe Life into Them with
Stem Cells," *MIT Technology Review*, June 28, 2018, https://www.technologyreview

.com/2018/06/28/240446/inside-the-effort-to-print-lungs-and-breathe-life-into
-them-with-stem-cells.

20. Michael S. Gerber, "One Breath at a Time," *Bethesda Magazine*, March 22, 2020, https://bethesdamagazine.com/bethesda-magazine/march-april-2020/one-breath-at -a-time/.

21. Longevity Technology, "Exclusive Profile: LyGenesis and Growing Ectopic Organs," September 25, 2019, https://www.longevity.technology/exclusive-profile-lygenesis -and-growing-ectopic-organs/.

Chapter 6: The Mighty CAR T Cell:
A Breakthrough Cure for Leukemia

1. American Cancer Society, "Chemotherapy Side Effects," Cancer.Org Treatment and Support, May 1, 2020, https://www.cancer.org/treatment/treatments-and-side-effects /treatment-types/chemotherapy/chemotherapy-side-effects.html.

2. Healio Immuno-Oncology Resource Center, " 'We Have to Cure' Cancer, says CAR T Pioneer Carl H. June, MD," *HemOnc Today*, April 18, 2019, https://www.healio.com /news/hematology-oncology/20190418/we-have-to-cure-cancer-says-car-t-pioneer -carl-h-june-md.

3. Ibid.

4. Rick Weiss and Deborah Nelson, "Teen Dies Underdoing Experimental Gene Therapy," *Washington Post*, September 29, 1999, https://www.washingtonpost.com/wp-srv /WPcap/1999–09/29/060r-092999-idx.html.

5. Rand Alattar, Tawheeda B. H. Ibrahim, Shahd H. Shaar, et al., "Tocilizumab for the Treatment of Severe Coronavirus Disease 2019," *Journal of Medical Virology* 92, no. 10 (October 2020), 2042–49, https://doi.org/10.1002/jmv.25964.

7. Healio Immuno-Oncology Resource Center, " 'We Have to Cure' Cancer, says CAR T Pioneer Carl H. June, M.D.," *HemOnc Today*, April 18, 2019, https://www.healio.com /news/hematology-oncology/20190418/we-have-to-cure-cancer-says-car-t-pioneer -carl-h-june-md.

8. Ibid.

9. Amanda Barrell, "Everything to Know About CAR T-Cell Therapy," *Medical News Today*, March 23, 2021, https://www.medicalnewstoday.com/articles/car-t-cell-therapy.

Chapter 7: Incisionless Brain Surgery:
The Impact of Focused Ultrasound

1. Focused Ultrasound Foundation, "Two Years and Countless Miles Later: Parkinson's Patient Update," November 14, 2017, https://www.fusfoundation.org/news/two-years -and-countless-miles-later-parkinson-s-patient-update.

2. Cleveland Clinic Health Library, "High-Intensity Focused Ultrasound for Prostate Cancer," July 10, 2020, https://my.clevelandclinic.org/health/treatments/16541-high -intensity-focused-ultrasound-hifu-for-prostate-cancer.

3. Maria Syl D. De La Cruz and Edward M. Buchanan, "Uterine Fibroids: Diagnosis and Treatment," *American Family Physician* 95, no. 2 (January 15, 2017), 100–7, https:// pubmed.ncbi.nlm.nih.gov/28084714/.

4. "WVU Addresses Addiction Crisis with Novel Ultrasound Treatment," *WVU Today*,

March 17, 2021, https://wvutoday.wvu.edu/stories/2021/03/17/wvu-addresses-addiction
-crisis-with-novel-ultrasound-treatment.

5. Lenny Bernstein and Joel Achenbach, "Drug Overdoses Soared to a Record 93,000 Last Year," *Washington Post*, July 14, 2021, https://www.washingtonpost.com /health/2021/07/14/drug-overdoses-pandemic-2020/.
6. Focused Ultrasound Foundation, "Kimberly Finds Tremor Relief for her Parkinson's Disease," YouTube channel, April 26, 2016, https://www.youtube.com /watch?v=272TzaUXg_U.
7. Michael J. Fox Foundation, "First U.S. Patients Treated in Dyskinesia Study Using Ultrasound Technology," September 24, 2015, https://www.michaeljfox.org/news/first -us-patients-treated-dyskinesia-study-using-ultrasound-technology.
8. Pam Harrison, "First Trial of Focused Ultrasound in Depression Under Way," *Medscape Medical News*, September 30, 2015, https://www.medscape.com/viewarticle /851906.
9. Focused Ultrasound Foundation, "Two Years and Countless Miles Later."
10. Karl E. Wiedamann, "Back on the Blocks: 'Focused Ultrasound Gave Me Back My Life,' " INSIGHTEC, January 9, 2018, https://usa.essential-tremor.com/back-blocks -focused-ultrasound-gave-back-life/.
11. INSIGHTECH, "Karl Wiedemann is Living Life to the Fullest," INSIGHTECH Facebook Watch page, May 28, 2019, https://www.facebook.com/watch /?v=670271436719081.
12. INSIGHTECH, "Toronto Patient Story," INSIGHTECH Vimeo page, https://vimeo .com/recsf/review/386871134/c82b4a2cac.
13. Meredith Cohn, "University of Maryland Study Uses Tiny Bubbles in Hopes of Getting Cancer-Fighting Drugs Inside the Brain," *Baltimore Sun*, October 2, 2019, https:// www.baltimoresun.com/health/bs-hs-brain-disease-treatment-20191002-asp2ct wabbdqpil2qrm7l6wwei-story.html.
14. Ali Rezai (Principal Investigator for Rockefeller Neuroscience Institute and INSIGHTEC), "Exablate for LIFU Neuromodulation in Patients With Opioid Use Disorder," U.S. National Library of Medicine: ClinicalTrials.gov, August 24, 2021, https:// clinicaltrials.gov/ct2/show/NCT04197921?term=NCT04197921&draw=2&rank=1

Chapter 8: Gene Therapy and CRISPR: The Cure for Disease

1. National Organization for Rare Disorders, "Rare Disease Facts," https://rarediseases .org/wp-content/uploads/2019/02/nord-rareinsights-rd-facts-2019.pdf.
2. Roland W. Herzog, Edmund Y. Yang, Linda B. Couto, et al., "Long-Term Correction of Canine Hemophilia B by Gene Transfer of Blood Coagulation Factor IX Mediated by Adeno-Associated Viral Vector," *Nature Medicine* 5, no. 1 (January 1999), 56–63, https://doi.org/10.1038/4743.
3. Tracy Hampton, "DNA Prime Editing: A New CRISPR-Based Method to Correct Most Disease-Causing Mutations," *Journal of the American Medical Association*, no. 5 (February 2020), 405–06, https://doi.org/10.1001/jama.2019.21827.
4. Buck Institute, "Exploiting a Gene that Protects Against Alzheimer's," Buck Institute blog, January 8, 2019, https://www.buckinstitute.org/news/exploiting-a-gene-that -protects-against-alzheimers/.

Chapter 9: The Wondrous Wnt Pathway: The Ultimate Fountain of Youth?

1. Samumed press release, "Biosplice Therapeutics Closes $120 Million in Equity Financing to Advance Its Alternative Splicing Platform," *Yahoo! Finance*, April 15, 2021, https://finance.yahoo.com/news/biosplice-therapeutics-closes-120-million-1455 00773.html.

2. Samumed press release, "Samumed Closes on $438 Million in Equity Financing," *GlobeNewswire*, August 6, 2018, https://www.globenewswire.com/news-release /2018/08/06/1547385/0/en/Samumed-Closes-on-438-Million-in-Equity-Financing .html.

3. Brittany Meiling, "What's Bigger Than a Unicorn? Samumed Stuns Yet Again as Anti-Aging Pipeline Draws $438M at $12B Valuation," *Endpoints News*, August 6, 2018, https://endpts.com/whats-bigger-than-a-unicorn-samumed-stuns-yet-again-as-anti -aging-pipeline-draws-438m-at-12b-valuation/.

4. Matthew Herper, "Cure Baldness? Health Arthritis? Erase Wrinkles? An Unknown Billionaire's Quest to Reverse Aging," *Forbes*, May 9, 2016, https://www.forbes.com /sites/matthewherper/2016/04/13/the-god-pill/.

5. Breakthrough: The Caltech Campaign, "Winding Back the Clock," https://break through.caltech.edu/story/winding-back-clock/.

6. Y. Yazici, T.E. McAlindon, R. Fleischmann, et al., "A Novel Wnt Pathway Inhibitor, SM04690, for the Treatment of Moderate to Severe Osteoarthritis of the Knee," *Osteoarthritis and Cartilage* 25, no. 10, 1598–1606 (October 1, 2017), https://doi .org/10.1016/j.joca.2017.07.006; Timothy E. McAlindon and Raveendhara R. Bannuru, "Latest Advances in the Management of Knee OA," *Nature Reviews Rheumatology* 14 (January 11, 2018), 73–74, https://doi.org/10.1038/nrrheum.2017.219.

7. Yusuf Yazici (Study Director) for Biosplice Therapeutics, "A Study of the Safety, Tolerability, and Pharmacokinetics of SM04690 Injectable Suspension Following Single Intradiscal Injection in Subjects with Degenerative Disc Disease," U.S. National Library of Medicine: ClinicalTrials.gov, April 23, 2019, https://clinicaltrials.gov/ct2/show /NCT03246399.

8. Darrin Beaupre (Study Chair) for Biosplice Therapeutics, "A Study Evaluating the Safety and Pharmacokinetics of Orally Administered SM08502 in Subjects with Advanced Solid Tumors," U.S. National Library of Medicine: ClinicalTrials.gov, October 15, 2021, https://clinicaltrials.gov/ct2/show/NCT03355066.

9. Canadian Cancer Society, "Chemotherapy for Brain and Spinal Cord Tumors," Cancer Information page, https://cancer.ca/en/cancer-information/cancer-types/brain-and -spinal-cord/treatment/chemotherapy.

10. Alice Melão, "Samumed's SM07883 Can Prevent Tau-Mediated Neuroinflammation, Neurodegeneration in Mice, Study Shows," *Alzheimer's News Today*, July 24, 2019, https://alzheimersnewstoday.com/2019/07/24/sm07883-can-prevent-tau-mediated -brain-damage-mice-suggesting-new-alzheimers-strategy/.

11. Biosplice Therapeutics, "Biosplice Licenses Rights to Lorecivivint, a Novel Phase 3 Osteoarthritis Drug Candidate, to Samil for the Republic of Korea," *Globe Newswire*, April 22, 2021, https://www.globenewswire.com/en/news-release/2021 /04/22/2215363/0/en/Biosplice-Licenses-Rights-to-Lorecivivint-a-Novel-Phase -3-Osteoarthritis-Drug-Candidate-to-Samil-for-the-Republic-of-Korea.html.

Chapter 10: Your Ultimate Vitality Pharmacy

1. Nelson Bulmash, "The Unknown Russian Revolution—Has the Fountain of Youth Already Been Discovered?" *Conscious Life Journal*, July 1, 2018, https://myconscious lifejournal.com/articles/fountain-of-youth-discovered/.

2. Peptides Store, "An Interview with Professor Khavinson," 2011, https://www.pep tidesstore.com/blogs/articles/15207153-an-interview-with-prof-khavinson.

3. Markus Muttenthaler, Glenn F. King, David J. Adams, and Paul F. Alewood, "Trends in Peptide Drug Discovery," *Nature Reviews Drug Discovery* 20 (February 2021), 309–25, https://doi.org/10.1038/s41573-020-00135-8.

4. Andy Chi-Lung Lee, Janelle Louise Harris, Kum Kum Khanna, and Ji-Hong Jong, "A Comprehensive Review on Current Advances in Peptide Drug Development and Design," *International Journal of Molecular Sciences* 20, no. 10, 2383, https://dx.doi .org/10.3390%2Fijms20102383.

5. Technical University of Munich, "Breakthrough for Peptide Medication," *Science Daily*, February 21, 2018, https://www.sciencedaily.com/releases/2018/02/180221122406.htm.

6. Michael Powell, "At the Heart of a Vast Doping Network, an Alias," *New York Times*, March 26, 2018, https://www.nytimes.com/2018/03/26/sports/doping-thomas-mann -peptides.html.

7. Food and Drug Administration, "Impact Story: Developing the Tools to Evalu- ate Complex Drug Products: Peptides," US FDA Regulatory Science Impact Story, February 5, 2019, https://www.fda.gov/drugs/regulatory-science-action/impact-story -developing-tools-evaluate-complex-drug-products-peptides.

8. Yong Qin, Fu-Ding Chen, Liang Zhou, et al., "Proliferative and Anti-Proliferative Effects of Thymosin Alpha1 on Cells Are Associated with Manipulation of Cellular ROS Levels," *Chemico-Biological Interactions*, August 14, 2009, https://doi.org/10.1016/j .cbi.2009.05.006.

9. S. John Weroha and Paul Haluska, "IGF System in Cancer," *Endocrinology and Metabo- lism Clinics of North America* 41, no. 2 (2012), 335–50, https://www.ncbi.nlm.nih.gov /pmc/articles/PMC3614012/.

10. Interview with Ryan Smith, February 2, 2020.

11. Ben Greenfield, "Peptides Unveiled: The Best Peptide Stacks for Anti-Aging, Growth Hormone, Deep Sleep, Hair Loss, Enhanced Cognition, and Much More!", *Ben Greenfield Fitness Podcast* transcript, https://bengreenfieldfitness.com/transcripts/tran script-what-are-peptides/.

12. Sam Apple, "Forget the Blood of Teens. This Pill Promises to Extend Life for a Nickel a Pop," *Wired*, July 1, 2017, https://www.wired.com/story/this-pill-promises-to-extend -life-for-a-nickel-a-pop/.

13. David A. Sinclair, "This Cheap Pill Might Help You Live a Longer, Healthier Life," *Lifespan*, August 15, 2019, https://lifespanbook.com/metformin-pill/.

14. Ibid.

15. Apple, "Forget the Blood of Teens."

16. C. A. Bannister, S. E. Holden, S. Jenkins-Jones, et al., "Can People with Type 2 Dia- betes Live Longer Than Those Without?" *Diabetes, Obesity and Metabolism* 16, no. 11 (November 2014), 1165–1173, https://doi.org/10.1111/dom.12354.

17. Gregory J. Salber, Yu-Bo Wang, John T. Lynch, et al., "Metformin Use in Prac- tice: Compliance with Guidelines for Patients with Diabetes and Preserved Renal

Function," *Clinical Diabetes* 35, no. 3 (July 2017), 154–61, https://doi.org/10.2337/cd15–0045.

18. R. Grace Walton, Cory M. Dungan, Douglas E. Long, et al., "Metformin Blunts Muscle Hypertrophy in Response to Progressive Resistance Exercise Training in Older Adults," *Aging Cell* 18, no. 6 (December 2019), https://doi.org/10.1111/acel.13039.

19. Dana P. Goldman, David Cutler, John W. Rowe, et al., "Substantial Health and Economic Returns from Delayed Aging May Warrant a New Focus for Medical Research," *Health Affairs* 32, no. 10 (October 2013), 1698–1705, https://doi.org/10.1377/hlthaff.2013.0052.

20. Johns Hopkins Medicine, "Hormones and the Endocrine System," https://www.hopkinsmedicine.org/health/conditions-and-diseases/hormones-and-the-endocrine-system.

21. Melinda Ratini, "DHEA Supplements," WebMD Medical Reference, February 5, 2021, https://www.webmd.com/diet/dhea-supplements#1.

22. Max Langridge, "The Truth About Using Peptides and How They Impact Your Health," *DMARGE Health*, June 30, 2021, https://www.dmarge.com/using-peptides.

23. Andy McLarnon, "Tesamoreline Can Improve Cognitive Function," *Nature Reviews Endocrinology* 8, 568 (2012), https://doi.org/10.1038/nrendo.2012.151.

24. Shin-Ichiro Imai and Leonard Guarente, "NAD+ and Sirtuins in Aging and Disease," *Trends in Cell Biology* 24, no. 8 (August 29, 20214), 464–71, https://dx.doi.org/10.1016%2Fj.tcb.2014.04.002.

25. Steve Hill, "NAD+ and the Circadian Rhythm," *Lifespan.io*, May 25, 2020, https://www.lifespan.io/news/nad-and-the-circadian-rhythm/.

26. Hongbo Zhang, Dongryeol Ryu, Yibo Wu, et al., "NAD+ Repletion Improves Mitochondrial and Stem Cell Function and Enhances Life Span in Mice," *Science* 352, no. 6292 (June 17, 2016), 1436–43, https://doi.org/10.1126/science.aaf2693.

27. University of Queensland, "Scientists Reverse Reproductive Clock in Mice," *ScienceDaily*, February 12, 2020, https://www.sciencedaily.com/releases/2020/02/200212103035.htm.

28. Timothy Nacarelli, Lena Lau, Takeshi Fukumoto, et al., "NAD+ Metabolism Governs the Proinflammatory Senescence-Associated Secretome," *Nature Cell Biology* 21 (2019), 397–407, https://www.nature.com/articles/s41556–019–0287–4.

29. Li Chen, Yanbin Dong, Jigar Bhagatwala, et al., "Effects of Vitamin D3 Supplementation on Epigenetic Aging in Overweight and Obese African Americans with Suboptimal Vitamin D Status," *Journals of Gerontology, Series A, Biological Sciences and Medical Sciences* 74, no. 1 (January 2019), 91–98, https://doi.org/10.1093/gerona/gly223.

30. H. Zhu, D. Guo, K. Li, et al., "Increased Telomerase Activity and Vitamin D Supplementation in Overweight African Americans," *International Journal of Obesity* 36, no. 6 (June 2012), https://doi.org/10.1038/ijo.2011.197.

31. E. Patterson, R. Wall, G. F. Fitzgerald, et al., "Health Implications of High Dietary Omega-6 Polyunsaturated Fatty Acids," *Journal of Nutrition and Metabolism* 2012 (2012), https://doi.org/10.1155/2012/539426.

32. Eric B. Rimm, Lawrence J. Appel, Stephanie E. Chiuve, et al., "Seafood Long-Chain n-3 Polyunsaturated Fatty Acids and Cardiovascular Disease," *Circulation* 138, no. 1 (July 3, 2018), e35-e47, https://doi.org/10.1161/cir.0000000000000574.

33. Ake T. Lu, Austin Quach, James G. Wilson, et al., "DNA Methylation GrimAge Strongly Predicts Lifespan and Healthspan," *Aging* 11, no. 2 (January 21, 2019), 303–27, https://doi.org/10.18632/aging.101684.

34. Keith Pearson, "Vitamin K vs K2: What's the Difference?" *Healthline*, September 2017, https://www.healthline.com/nutrition/vitamin-k1-vs-k2.

35. Ryan Raman, "Acetylcholine Supplements," *Healthline*, March 21, 2020, https://www.healthline.com/nutrition/acetylcholine-supplement.

36. Richard B. Kreider, Douglas S. Kalman, Jose Antonio, et al., "International Society of Sports Nutrition Position Stand: Safety and Efficacy of Creatine Supplementation in Exercise, Sport, and Medicine," *Journal of the International Society of Sports Nutrition* 14 (June 13, 2017), 18, https://doi.org/10.1186/s12970-017-0173-z.

37. Jose Antonio, Darren G. Candow, Scott C. Forbes, et al., "Common Questions and Misconceptions about Creatine Supplementation: What Does the Scientific Evidence Really Show?" *Journal of the International Society of Sports Nutrition* 18, no. 1 (February 8, 2021), 13, https://doi.org/10.1186/s12970-021-00412-w.

38. Francis Collins, "Less TOR Protein Extends Mouse Lifespan," *NIH Director's Blog*, September 10, 2013, https://directorsblog.nih.gov/2013/09/10/less-tor-protein-extends-mouse-lifespan/.

39. Bennett G. Childs, Matej Durik, Darren J. Baker, and Jan M. van Deursen, "Cellular Senescence in Aging and Age-Related Disease: From Mechanisms to Therapy," *Nature Medicine* 21, no. 12 (December 2015), 1424–35, https://dx.doi.org/10.1038%2Fnm.4000.

40. University of Texas Health Science Center at San Antonio, "First-in-Human Trial of Senolytic Drugs Encouraging," *ScienceDaily*, January 7, 2019, https://www.sciencedaily.com/releases/2019/01/190107112944.htm.

41. Matthew J. Yousefzadeh, Yi Zhu, Sara J. McGowan, et al., "Fisetin Is a Senotherapeutic That Extends Health and Lifespan," *EBioMedicine* 36 (October 1, 2018), 18–28, https://doi.org/10.1016/j.ebiom.2018.09.015.

42. Richard A. Miller, David E. Harrison, C.M. Astle, et al., "Rapamycin, But Not Resveratrol or Simvastatin, Extends Life Span of Genetically Heterogeneous Mice," *Journals of Gerontology, Series A, Biological Sciences and Medical Sciences* 66A, no. 2 (February 2011), 191–201, https://dx.doi.org/10.1093%2Fgerona%2Fglq178.

43. Alessandro Bitto, Takashi K. Ito, Victor V. Pineda, et al., "Transient Rapamycin Treatment Can Increase Lifespan and Healthspan in Middle-Aged Mice," *eLife* 2016, no. 5 (August 23, 2016), https://doi.org/10.7554/eLife.16351.001.

44. Matt Kaeberlein and Veronica Galvin, "Rapamycin and Alzheimer's Disease: Time for a Clinical Trial?" *Science Translational Medicine* 11, no. 476 (January 23, 2019), https://dx.doi.org/10.1126%2Fscitranslmed.aar4289.

45. Alex Zhavoronkov, "Women in Longevity—Dr. Joan Mannick on Clinical Development for Aging," *Forbes*, June 14, 2021, https://www.forbes.com/sites/alexzhavoronkov/2021/06/14/women-in-longevity—dr-joan-mannick-on-clinical-development-for-aging/.

Chapter 11: Living Pain-Free

1. Eric Yoon, Arooj Babar, Moaz Choudhary, et al., "Acetaminophen-Induced Hepatotoxicity: A Comprehensive Update," *Journal of Clinical and Translational Hepatology* 4, no. 2 (June 28, 2016), 131–42, https://dx.doi.org/10.14218%2FJCTH.2015.00052; Anne M. Larson, Julie Polson, Robert J. Fontana, et al., "Acetaminophen-Induced Acute Liver Failure: Results of a United States Multicenter Prospective Study," *Hepatology* 42, no. 6 (December 2005), 1364–72, https://doi.org/10.1002/hep.20948.

2. Nicole J. Kubat, John Moffett, and Linley M. Fray, "Effect of Pulsed Electromagnetic Field Treatment on Programmed Resolution of Inflammation Pathway Markets in Human Cells in Culture," *Journal of Inflammation Research* 8 (2015), 59–59, https://dx.doi.org/10.2147%2FJIR.S78631; Carlos F. Martino, Dmitry Belchenko, Virginia Ferguson, et al., "The Effects of Pulsed Electromagnetic Fields on the Cellular Activity of SaOS-2 Cells," *Bioelectromagnetics* 29, no. 2 (February 2008), 125–32, https://doi.org/10.1002/bem.20372.

3. Julieta Dascal, Mark Reid, Waguih William IsHak, et al., "Virtual Reality and Medical Inpatients: A Systematic Review of Randomized Controlled Trials," *Innovative Clinical Neuroscience* 14, no. 1–2 (February 2017), 14–21, https://pubmed.ncbi.nlm.nih.gov/28386517/; Brandon Birckhead, Carine Khalil, Xiaoyu Liu, et al., "Recommendations for Methodology of Virtual Reality Clinical Trials in Health Care by an International Working Group," *JMIR Mental Health* 6, no. 1 (2019), https://doi.org/10.2196/11973; Allison Aubrey, "Got Pain? A Virtual Swim With Dolphins May Help Melt It Away," *Shots: Health News From NPR*, August 19, 2019, https://www.npr.org/sections/health-shots/2019/08/19/751495463/got-pain-a-virtual-swim-with-dolphins-may-help-melt-it-away.

4. "Deep Tissue Laser Therapy," Genesis Performance Chiro, https://www.genesisperformancechiro.com/laser.

5. Jeanne Adiwinata Pawitan, "Various Stem Cells in Acupuncture Meridians and Points and Their Putative Roles," *Journal of Traditional and Complementary Medicine* 8(4), October 2018, 437–42, https://doi.org/10.1016/j.jtcme.2017.08.004.

6. Tsung-Jung Ho, Tzu-Min Chan, Li-Ing Ho, Ching-Yuan Lai, Chia-Hsien Lin, Iona Macdonald, et al., "The Possible Role of Stem Cells in Acupuncture Treatment for Neurodegenerative Diseases: A Literature Review of Basic Studies" *Cell Transplant* 23(4–5), 2014, 559–66, https://doi.org/10.3727/096368914X678463.

7. Ying Ding, Qing Yan, Jing-Wen Ruan, Yan-Qing Zhang, et al., "Electroacupuncture Promotes the Differentiation of Transplanted Bone Marrow Mesenchymal Stem Cells Overexpressing TrkC into Neuron-Like Cells in Transected Spinal Cord of Rats," *Cell Transplant* 22(1), 2013, https://doi.org/10.3727/096368912X655037.

8. Ying Ding, Qing Yan, Jing-Wen Ruan, Yan-Qing Zhang, et al., "Electro-Acupuncture Promotes Survival, Differentiation of the Bone Marrow Mesenchymal Stem Cells As Well As Functional Recovery in the Spinal Cord-Transected Rats," *BMC Neuroscience* 10(35), April 20, 2009, doi: 10.1186/1471–2202–10–35.

9. Haibo Yu, Pengidan Chen, Zhouxin Yang, Wenshu Luo, Min Pi, Yonggang Wu, Ling Wang, "Electro-Acupuncture at Conception and Governor Vessels and Transplantation of Umbilical Cord Blood-Derived Mesenchymal Stem Cells for Treating Cerebral Ischemia/Reperfusion Injury," *Natural Regeneration Research* 9(1), January 1, 2014, 84–91, doi: 10.4103/1673–5374.125334.

10. Yu Ri Kim, Sung Min Ahn, Malk Eun Pak, et al., "Potential Benefits of Mesenchymal Stem Cells and Electroacupuncture on the Trophic Factors Associated with Neurogenesis in Mice with Ischemic Stroke," *Scientific Reports* 8(1), February 1, 2010, 2044, doi: 10.1038/s41598–018–20481–3.

11. Genia Dubrovsky, Don Ha, Anne-Laure Thomas, et al., "Electroacupuncture to Increase Neuronal Stem Cell Growth," *Medical Acupuncture* 32(1), February 1, 2020, 16–23, doi: 10.1089/acu.2019.1381.

12. Ya-Yun Chen, Wei Zhang, Yu-Lin Chen, Shui-Jun Chen, Hongxin Dong, Yuan-Shan

Zeng, "Electro-Acupuncture Improves Survival and Migration of Transplanted Neural Stem Cells in Injured Spinal Cord in Rats," *Acupuncture & Electro-Therapeutics Research* 33(1–2), 2008, 19–31, doi: 10.3727/036012908803861212.

13. Qing Yan, Jing-Wen Ruan, Ying Ding, Wen-Jie Li, Yan Li, Yuan-Shan Zeng, "Electro-Acupuncture Promotes Differentiation of Mesenchymal Stem Cells, Regeneration of Nerve Fibers and Partial Functional Recovery After Spinal Cord Injury," *Experimental and Toxicologic Pathology* 63 (1–2), January 2011, 151–56, https://doi.org/10.1016/j.etp.2009.11.002.

14. Yi Zhu, Yaochi Wu, Rong Zhang, "Electro-Acupuncture Promotes the Proliferation of Neural Stem Cells and the Survival of Neurons by Downregulating Mir-449a in Rat with Spinal Cord Injury," *EXCLI Journal* 16 (March 23, 2017), 363–74, doi: 10.17179/excli2017–123.

15. Bin Chen, Jing Tao, Yukun Lin, Ruhui Lin, Weilin Liu, Lidian Chen, "Electro-Acupuncture Exerts Beneficial Effects Against Cerebral Ischemia and Promotes the Proliferation of Neural Progenitor Cells in the Cortical Peri-Infarct Area Through the Wnt/?-Catenin Signaling Pathway," *International Journal of Molecular Medicine* 36(5), November 2015, 1215–22, doi: 10.3892/ijmm.2015.2334.

16. Vyacheslav Ogay and Kwang-Sup Soh, "Identification and Characterization of Small Stem-Like Cells in the Primo Vascular System of Adult Animals," in *The Primo Vascular System: Its Role in Cancer and Regeneration*, Soh K.S., Kang K.A., Harrison D.K., eds. (New York: Springer, 2012) 149–55.

Chapter 12: The Longevity Lifestyle & Diet

1. Dean Ornish, J. Lin, J. Daubenmier, et al., "Increased Telomerase Activity and Comprehensive Lifestyle Changes," *Lancet Oncology* 9 (2008), 1048–57, https://doi.org/10.1016/S1470–2045(13)70366–8.

2. Dean Ornish, J. Lin, J.M. Chan, et al., "Effect of Comprehensive Lifestyle Changes on Telomerase Activity and Telomere Length in Men with Biopsy-Proven Low-Risk Prostate Cancer," *Lancet Oncology* 14, no. 11 (October 2013), 1112–20, http://doi.org/10.1016/S1470–2045(13)70366–8.

3. Larry A. Tucker, "Physical Activity and Telomere Length in U.S. Men and Women: An NHANES Investigation," *Preventive Medicine* 100 (July 2017), 145–51, http://doi.org/10.1016/j.ypmed.2017.04.027.

4. Yanping Li, An Pan, Dong D. Wang, Xiaoran Liu, et al., "Impact of Healthy Lifestyle Factors on Life Expectancies in the US Population," *Circulation* (April 30, 2018), https://doi.org/10.1161/CIRCULATIONAHA.117.032047.

5. X. Zhang, X. O. Shu, Y.B. Xiang, et al., "Cruciferous Vegetable Consumption Is Associated with a Reduced Risk of Total and Cardiovascular Disease Mortality," *American Journal of Clinical Nutrition* 94, no. 1 (July 2011), http://doi.org/10.3945/ajcn.110.009340.

6. H. Arem, S. C. Moore, A. Patel, et al., "Leisure Time Physical Activity and Mortality: A Detailed Pooled Analysis of the Dose-Response Relationship," *JAMA Internal Medicine* 175, no. 6 (2015), 959–67, https://doi.org/10.1001/jamainternmed.2015.0533.

7. I. M. Lee, K. M. Rexrode, N. R. Cook, et al., "Physical Activity and Coronary Heart Disease in Women: Is 'No Pain, No Gain' Passé?" *Journal of the American Medical Association* 285, no. 11 (March 21, 2001), 1447–54, https://doi.org/10.1001/jama.285.11.1447.

8. M. Yang, S. A. Kenfield, E. L. Van Blarigan, et al., "Dietary Patterns After Prostate Cancer Diagnosis in Relation to Disease-Specific and Total Mortality," *Cancer Prevention Research*, June 2015, https://doi.org/10.1158/1940–6207.

9. M.E. Levine, J.A. Suarez, S. Brandhorst, et al., "Low Protein Intake Is Associated with a Major Reduction in IGF-1, Cancer, and Overall Mortality in the 65 and Younger but Not Older Population," *Cell Metabolism* 19, no. 3 (March 4, 2014), 407–17, https://doi.org/10.1016/j.cmet.2014.02.006.

10. M. Wei, S. Brandhorst, M. Shelehchi, et al., "Fasting-mimicking Diet and Markers/Risk Factors for Aging, Diabetes, Cancer, and Cardiovascular Disease," *Science Translational Medicine* 9, no. 377 (February 15, 2017), https://doi.org/ 10.1126/scitranslmed.aai8700.

11. E. Jéquier and F. Constant, "Water as an Essential Nutrient: The Physiological Basis of Hydration," *European Journal of Clinical Nutrition* 64 (2010), 115–23, https://doi.org/10.1038/ejcn.2009.111.

12. E.T. Perrier, L.E. Armstrong, J.H. Bottin, et al., "Hydration for Health Hypothesis: A Narrative Review of Supporting Evidence," *European Journal of Nutrition* 60 (2021), 1167–80, https://doi.org/10.1007/s00394–020–02296-z.

13. Adam Hadhazy, "Fear Factor: Dopamine May Fuel Dread, Too," *Scientific American*, July 14, 2008, https://www.scientificamerican.com/article/fear-factor-dopamine/.

14. Noma Nazish, "How to De-Stress in 5 Minutes or Less, According to a Navy SEAL," *Forbes*, May 30, 2019, https://www.forbes.com/sites/nomanazish/2019/05/30/how-to-de-stress-in-5-minutes-or-less-according-to-a-navy-seal/.

15. Maria Vranceanu, Craig Pickering, Lorena Filip, et al., "A Comparison of a Ketogenic Diet with a Low GI/Nutrigenic Diet Over 6 Months for Weight Loss and 18 Month Follow-Up," *BMC Nutrition* 6 (2020), 53, https://dx.doi.org/10.1186/2Fs40795–020–00370–7.

16. Tanjaniina Laukkanen, Hassan Khan, Francesco Zaccardi, and Jari A. Laukkanen, "Association Between Sauna Bathing and Fatal Cardiovascular and All-Cause Mortality Events," *JAMA Internal Medicine*, 175, no. 4 (April 2015), 542, doi:10.1001/jamainternmed.2014.8187.

17. Setor K. Kunutsor, Hassan Khan, Francesco Zaccardi, Tanjaniina Laukkanen, Peter Willeit, and Jari A. Laukkanen, "Sauna Bathing Reduces The Risk Of Stroke In Finnish Men And Women," *Neurology* 10 (2018), doi: 10.1212/WNL.0000000000005606.

18. Masaki Iguchi, Andrew E. Littmann, Shuo-Hsiu Chang, et al., "Heat Stress and Cardiovascular, Hormonal, and Heat Shock Proteins in Humans," *Journal of Athletic Training* 47, no. 2 (2012), 184–90.

19. Rhonda P. Patrick, "Sauna Use as a Lifestyle Practice to Extend Healthspan," *Experimental Gerontology* 154 (October 2021), 111509, https://doi.org/10.1016/j.exger.2021.111509.

Chapter 13: The Power of Sleep: The Third Pillar of Health

1. Yu Fang, Daniel B. Forger, Elena Frank, et al., "Day-to-Day Variability in Sleep Parameters and Depression Risk," *npj Digital Medicine* 4 (2021), https://doi.org/10.1038/s41746–021–00400-z.

2. "Harvard Research Update," Dental Excellence Integrative Center, https://dentalexcellenceva.com/custom/pdfs/nucalmresearch.pdf.

3. Mike Kruppa, "Wearables Company Whoop Valued at \$3.6bn after SoftBank Investment," *Financial Times*, August 30, 2021, https://www.ft.com/content/f3dde553-0aa1-4137-bc50-093b1003fa71.

4. Lee M. Ritterband, Frances P. Thorndike, Karen S. Ingersoll, et al., "Effect of a Web-Based Cognitive Behavior Therapy for Insomnia Intervention with 1-Year Follow-Up: A Randomized Clinical Trial," *JAMA Psychiatry* 74, no. 1 (January 1, 2017), 68–75, https://doi.org/10.1001/jamapsychiatry.2016.3249.

Chapter 14: Strength, Fitness & Performance: Your Quick Guide to Maximum Results

1. Chi Pang Wen, Jackson Pui Man Wai, Min Kuang Tsai, et al., "Minimum Amount of Physical Activity for Reduced Mortality and Extended Life Expectancy," *Lancet* 378, no. 9798 (October 2011), 1244–1253, http://doi.org/10.1016/S0140-6736(11)60749-6.

2. Press Association, "Brisk Daily Walks Can Increase Lifespan, Research Says," *Guardian*, August 30, 2015, https://www.theguardian.com/society/2015/aug/30/brisk-daily-walks-reduce-ageing-increase-life-span-research.

3. Ross McCammon, "The Grateful Dead's Bob Weir is 72 and Still Working Out Like a Beast," *Men's Health*, October 24, 2019, https://www.menshealth.com/fitness/a29491632/the-grateful-dead-bob-weir-workout/.

4. Susan A. Carlson, E. Kathleen Adams, Zhou Yang, Janet E. Fulton, "Percentage of Deaths Associated with Inadequate Physical Activity in the United States," *CDC Preventing Chronic Disease* 15 (2018),17035, http://dx.doi.org/10.5888/pcd18.170354.

5. "What Women Need to Know," Bone Health and Osteoporosis Foundation: General Facts, https://www.nof.org/preventing-fractures/general-facts/what-women-need-to-know/.

6 Bazil Hunte, John Jaquish, and Corey Huck, Corey, "Axial Bone Osteogenic Loading-Type Resistance Therapy Showing BMD and Functional Bone Performance Musculoskeletal Adaptation Over 24 Weeks with Postmenopausal Female Subjects," *Journal of Osteoporosis and Physical Activity* 3, no. 146 (2015), doi: 10.4172/2329-9509.1000146.

Chapter 15: Beauty: Enhancing Your Visible Health & Vitality

1. Tomas Chamorro-Premuzic, "Attractive People Get Unfair Advantages at Work. AI Can Help," *Harvard Business Review*, October 31, 2019, https://hbr.org/2019/10/attractive-people-get-unfair-advantages-at-work-ai-can-help.

2. Jean Eaglesham, "Mob-Busting Informant Resurfaces in SEC Probe," *Wall Street Journal*, August 17, 2015, https://www.wsj.com/articles/mob-busting-informant-resurfaces-in-sec-probe-1439766192.

3. Venkataram Mysore, "Finasteride and Sexual Side Effects," *Indian Dermatology Online Journal* 3, no. 1 (January-April 2012), 62–65, https://dx.doi.org/10.4103%2F2229-5178.93496.

4. Laura J. Burns, Dina Hagigeorges, Kelly E. Flanagan, et al., "A Pilot Evaluation of Scalp Skin Wounding to Promote Hair Growth in Female Pattern Hair Loss," *International Journal of Women's Dermatology* 7, no. 3 (June 2021), 344–45, https://doi.org/10.1016/j.ijwd.2020.11.006.

5. Glynis Ablon, "Phototherapy with Light Emitting Diodes: Treating a Broad Range of Medical and Aesthetic Conditions in Dermatology," *Journal of Clinical and Aesthetic Dermatology* 11, no. 2 (February 2018), 21–27, https://pubmed.ncbi.nlm.nih.gov/295 52272/.

6. K. E. Karmisholt, C. A. Banzhaf, M. Glud, et al., "Laser Treatments in Early Wound Healing Improve Scar Appearance," *British Journal of Dermatology* 179, no. 6 (December 2018), 1307–14, https://doi.org/10.1111/bjd.17076.

Chapter 16: Women's Health: The Cycle of Life

1. Anne Tergesen, "Is 100 the New Life Expectancy for People Born in the 21st Century?", *Wall Street Journal*, April 16, 2020, https://www.wsj.com/articles/is-100-the-new-life-expectancy-for-people-born-in-the-21st-century-11587041951.

2. W. Hamish B. Wallace and Thomas W. Kelsey, "Human Ovarian Reserve from Conception to the Menopause," *PLOS One* 5, no. 1 (2010), https://doi.org/10.1371/journal.pone.0008772.

3. F. J. Broekmans, M. R. Soules, and B. C. Fauser, "Ovarian Aging: Mechanisms and Clinical Consequences," *Endocrine Reviews* 30, no. 5 (August 2009), 465–93, https://doi.org/10.1210/er.2009–0006.

4. T. J. Mathews and Brady E. Hamilton, "First Births to Older Women Continue to Rise," *National Center for Health Statistics Data Brief* 152 (May 2014), https://www.cdc.gov/nchs/products/databriefs/db152.htm.

5. Vicki Contie, "Egg-Producing Stem Cells Found in Women," *NIH Research Matters*, March 5, 2012, https://www.nih.gov/news-events/nih-research-matters/egg-producing-stem-cells-found-women.

6. Richard J. Fehring, Mary Schneider, and Kathleen Raviele, "Variability in the Phases of the Menstrual Cycle," *Clinical Research* 35, no. 3, 376–84, https://doi.org/10.1111/j.1552–6909.2006.00051.x.

7. Samuel Ellis, Daniel W. Franks, Stuart Nattrass, et al., "Analyses of Ovarian Activity Reveal Repeated Evolution of Post-Reproductive Lifespans in Toothed Whales," *Scientific Reports* 8, no. 1 (August 27, 2018), 12833, https://doi.org/10.1038/s41598-018-31047-8.

8. Margaret L. Walker and James G. Herndon, "Menopause in Nonhuman Primates," *Biology of Reproduction* 79, no. 3 (September 2008), 398–406, https://dx.doi.org/10.1095%2Fbiolreprod.108.068536.

9. Tabitha M. Powledge, "The Origin of Menopause: Why do Women Outlive Fertility?" *Scientific American*, April 3, 2008, https://www.scientificamerican.com/article/the-origin-of-menopause/.

10. Regan L. Bailey, Peishan Zou, Taylor C. Wallace, et al., "Calcium Supplement Use Is Associated with Less Bone Mineral Density Loss, But Does Not Lessen the Risk of Bone Fracture Across the Menopause Transition," *JBMR Plus* 4, no. 1 (January 2020), *https://doi.org/10.1002/jbm4.10246.*

11. Cheryl Karcher and Neil Sadick, "Vaginal Rejuvenation Using Energy-Based Devices," *International Journal of Women's Dermatology* 2, no. 3 (September 2016), 85–88, https://dx.doi.org/10.1016%2Fj.ijwd.2016.05.003.

12. D. Huber, S. Seitz, K. Kast, G. Emons, O. Ortmann, "Use of Oral Contraceptives in BRCA Mutation Carriers and Risk for Ovarian and Breast Cancer: A Systematic

Review," *Archives of Genecology and Obstetrics* 301 (2020), 875–84, https://doi.org/10.1007
/s00404–020–05458-w; Carlo La Vecchia, "Ovarian Cancer: Epidemiology and
Risk Factors," *European Journal of Cancer Prevention* 26(1), January 2017, 55–62, doi:
10.1097/CEJ.0000000000000217.

13. F.M., Helmerhorst, J.P. Vandenbroucke, C.J.M. Doggen, and F.R. Rosendaal. "The
Venous Thrombotic Risk of Oral Contraceptives, Effects of Oestrogen Dose and Progestogen Type: Results of the MEGA Case-Control Study," *BMJ* 339 (August 2009),
doi: https://doi.org/10.1136/bmj.b2921.

14. Mahyar Etminan, Joseph A.C. Delaney, Brian Bressler, James M. Brophy, "Oral
Contraceptives and the Risk of Gallbladder Disease: A Comparative Safety
Study,"*Canadian Medical Association Journal* 183(8), May 17, 2011, 899–904, doi: https://
doi.org/10.1503/cmaj.110161.

Chapter 17: How to Mend a Broken Heart

1. "Left Ventricular Assist Device," Stanford Health Care, https://stanfordhealthcare.org
/medical-treatments/l/lvad.html.
2. Loffredo FS, Wagers AJ, Lee RT. Cell, 2013.
3. "FDA Clears CorMatrix ECM for Vascular Repair," *Diagnostic and Interventional Cardiology*, July 25, 2014, https://www.dicardiology.com/product/fda-clears-cormatrix-ecm
-vascular-repair.
4. Jay H. Traverse, Timothy D. Henry, Nabil Dib, et al., "First-in-Man Study of a
Cardiac Extracellular Matrix Hydrogel in Early and Late Myocardial Infarction Patients," *JACC: Basic to Translational Science* 4, no. 6 (October 2019), 659–69, https://doi
.org/10.1016/j.jacbts.2019.07.012.
5. Barry R. Davis, "Combination of Mesenchymal and C-kit+ Cardiac Stem Cells as Regenerative Therapy for Heart Failure," *U.S. National Library of Medicine:* ClinicalTrials
.gov, April 26, 2021, https://clinicaltrials.gov/ct2/show/results/NCT02501811.6.
6. Doris A. Taylor, B. Zane Akins, Pinata Hungspreugs, et al., "Regenerating Functional
Myocardium: Improved Performance After Skeletal Myoblast Transplantation," *Nature
Medicine* 4 (August 1, 1998), 929–933, https://doi.org/10.1038/nm0898–929.
7. Harald C. Ott, Thomas S. Matthiesen, Saik-Kia Goh, et al., "Perfusion-Decellularized
Matrix: Using Nature's Platform to Engineer a Bioartificial Heart," *Nature Medicine* 14
(January 13, 2008), 213–221, https://doi.org/10.1038/nm1684.

Chapter 18: Your Brain: Treating Strokes

1. Centers for Disease Control and Prevention, "Stroke Facts," https://www.cdc.gov
/stroke/facts.htm.
2. "Good Vibrations: Passive Haptic Learning Could be a Key to Rehabilitation," Georgia Tech School of Interactive Computing, September 20, 2018, https://www.ic.gatech
.edu/news/611757/good-vibrations-passive-haptic-learning-could-be-key-rehabili
tation.
3. "Passive Haptic Learning: Learn to Type or Play Piano Without Attention Using
Wearables," Georgia Tech Research Projects, https://gvu.gatech.edu/research/proj
ects/passive-haptic-learning-learn-type-or-play-piano-without-attention-using-wear
ables.

4. Georgia Institute of Technology, "Wearable Computing Gloves Can Teach Braille, Even if You're Not Paying Attention," *ScienceDaily*, June 23, 2014, https://www.sci encedaily.com/releases/2014/06/140623131329.htm.

5. Loffredo FS, Wagers AJ, Lee RT. Cell, 2013.

6. David Chiu, C. David McCane, Jason Lee, et al., "Multifocal Transcranial Stimulation in Chronic Ischemic Stroke: A Phase 1/2a Randomized Trial," *Journal of Stroke and Cerebrovascular Diseases* 29, no. 6 (June 2020), https://doi.org/10.1016/j.jstrokecerebro vasdis.2020.104816.

Chapter 19: How to Win the War on Cancer

1. National Cancer Institute, "Cancer Statistics," https://www.cancer.gov/about-cancer /understanding/statistics.

2. Peter Moore, "The High Cost of Cancer Treatment," *AARP The Magazine*, June 1, 2018, https://www.aarp.org/money/credit-loans-debt/info-2018/the-high-cost-of-can cer-treatment.html.

3. Pankita H. Pandya, Mary E. Murray, Karen E. Pollok, and Jamie L. Renbarger, "The Immune System in Cancer Pathogenesis: Potential Therapeutic Approaches," *Journal of Immunology Research* (December 26, 2016), https://dx.doi.org /10.1155/2F2016/2F4273943.

4. Philipp Eissmann, "Natural Killer Cells," *British Society for Immunology: Bitesized Immunology*, https://www.immunology.org/public-information/bitesized-immunology /cells/natural-killer-cells.

5. Sara M. Gregory, Beth Parker, and Paul D. Thompson, "Physical Activity, Cognitive Function, and Brain Health: What is the Role of Exercise Training in the Prevention of Dementia?" *Brain Sciences* 2, no. 4 (December 2012), 684–708, https://dx.doi .org/10.3390%2Fbrainsci2040684.

6. Howlader et al., "SEER Cancer Statistics Review, 1975–2018."

7. M.C. Liu, G.R. Oxnard, E.A. Klein, et al., "Sensitive and Specific Multi-Cancer Detection and Localization using Methylation Signatures in Cell-Free DNA," *Annals of Oncology* 31, no. 6 (June 1, 2020), 745–59, https://doi.org/10.1016/j.annonc.2020.02.011.

8. Guy Faulconbridge, "Britain Begins World's Largest Trial of Blood Test for 50 Types of Cancer," *Reuters*, September 12, 2021, https://www.reuters.com/business /healthcare-pharmaceuticals/britain-begins-worlds-largest-trial-blood-test-50-types -cancer-2021–09–12/.

9. "Cancer," World Health Organization, Sept. 12, 2018, https://www.who.int/news -room/fact-sheets/detail/cancer

10. Mokhtari et al., "The Role of Sulforaphane in Cancer Chemoprevention and Health Benefits: A Mini-Review."

11. Fahey et al., "Broccoli Sprouts: An Exceptionally Rich Source of Inducers of Enzymes that Protect Against Chemical Carcinogens."

12. S. Kummel, C. Jackisch, V. Muller, et al., "Can Contemporary Trials of Chemotherapy for HER2-negative Metastatic Breast Cancer Detect Overall Survival Benefit?", *Cancer Management Research* 10 (2018), 5423–31, https://doi.org/10.2147/CMAR.S177240. See Table 2.

13. V. Prasad, "Do Cancer Drugs Improve Survival or Quality of Life?", *BMJ* 359 (2017), 4528, October 4, 2017, https://doi.org/10.1136/bmj.j4528.

14. Eric Benson, "The Iconoclast," *Texas Monthly*, November 2016, https://www.texas monthly.com/articles/jim-allison-and-the-search-for-the-cure-for-cancer/; *Breakthrough* (2019 film), directed by Bill Haney.

15. T.N. Yamamoto, R.J. Kishton, and N.P. Restifo, "Developing Neoantigen-targeted T Cell-Based Treatments for Solid Tumors," *Nature Medicine* 25 (2019), 1488–99, https://doi.org/10.1038/s41591-019-0596-y.

16. Mark Awadalla (Study Director) for Celularity, "Natural Killer Cell (CYNK-001) IV Infusion or IT Administration in Adults with Recurrent GBM (CYNK001GBM01)," U.S. National Library of Medicine: ClinicalTrials.gov, July 14, 2021, https://clinical trials.gov/ct2/show/NCT04489420.

17. S.L. Goff, M.E. Dudley, D.E. Citrin, et al., "Randomized, Prospective Evaluation Comparing Intensity of Lymphodepletion Before Adoptive Transfer of Tumor-Infiltrating Lymphocytes for Patients with Metastatic Melanoma," *Journal of Clinical Oncology* 34, no. 20 (July 10, 2016), 2389–97, https://doi.org/10.1200/JCO.2016 .66.7220.

18. "Prognosis," Hirshberg Foundation for Pancreatic Cancer Research, http://pancreatic .org/pancreatic-cancer/about-the-pancreas/prognosis/.

19. "Exomes in Cancer Therapy," *Grantome*, National Institutes of Health, http://grant ome.com/grant/NIH/R01-CA213233-01.

20. C. Bradley, "iExosomes Target the 'Undruggable,' " *Nature Reviews Cancer* 17, no. 453 (2017), https://doi.org/10.1038/nrc.2017.54.

21. American Cancer Society, "About Prostate Cancer," https://www.cancer.org/content /dam/CRC/PDF/Public/8793.00.pdf.

22. Michael Blanding, "The Prostate Cancer Predicament," *Harvard Public Health Magazine* (Winter 2013), https://www.hsph.harvard.edu/news/magazine/the-prostate-cancer -predicament/.

23. Anna Bill-Axelson, Lars Holmberg, Hans Garmo, et al., "Radical Prostatectomy or Watchful Waiting in Prostate Cancer—29-Year Follow-Up," *New England Journal of Medicine* 379 (December 13, 2018), 2319–29, https://doi.org/ 10.1056/NEJMoa 1807801.

Chapter 20: Conquering Inflammation and Autoimmune Disease: Bringing Peace to the Body

1. Lisa Esposito and Michael O. Schroeder, "How Autoimmune Diseases Affect Life Expectancy," *U.S. News and World Report*, August 30, 2021, https://health.usnews.com /health-care/patient-advice/slideshows/autoimmune-diseases-that-can-be-fatal.

2. Moises Velasquez-Manoff, "An Immune Disorder at the Root of Autism," *New York Times*, August 25, 2012, https://www.nytimes.com/2012/08/26/opinion/sunday/im mune-disorders-and-autism.html.

3. American Autoimmune Related Diseases Association, Autoimmune Facts brochure, December 2019, https://autoimmune.org/wp-content/uploads/2019/12/1-in-5-Bro chure.pdf.

4. Centers for Disease Control and Prevention, "Heart Disease Facts," CDC Heart Disease Home, https://www.cdc.gov/heartdisease/facts.htm.

5. American Cancer Society, "Cancer Prevalence: How Many People Have Cancer?", *Cancer Basics*, https://www.cancer.org/cancer/cancer-basics/cancer-prevalence.html.

6. Fariha Angum, Tahir Khan, Jasndeep Kaler, et al., "The Prevalence of Autoimmune Disorders in Women: A Narrative Review," *Cureus* 12, no. 5 (May 2020), https://dx.doi.org/10.7759%2Fcureus.8094.

7. Anarchy and Autoimmunity, "Flourishing in the Face of Autoimmunity," March 29, 2019, https://anarchyautoimmunity.com/2019/03/29/flourishing-in-the-face-of-auto immunity/.

8. American Autoimmune Related Diseases Association, *Autoimmune Facts brochure*, December 2019, https://autoimmune.org/wp-content/uploads/2019/12/1-in-5-Brochure.pdf.

9. Donna Jackson Nakazawa, *The Autoimmune Epidemic* (New York: Touchstone, 2009).

10. "Autoimmune Diseases," Boston Children's Hospital, https://www.childrenshospital.org/conditions-and-treatments/conditions/a/autoimmune-diseases.

11. Nakazawa, *The Autoimmune Epidemic*.

12. National Cancer Institute, "Chronic Inflammation," Cancer Causes and Prevention, April 29, 2015, https://www.cancer.gov/about-cancer/causes-prevention/risk/chronic-inflammation.

14. Ben Hirschler, "GSK and Google Parent Forge $715 Million Bioelectronic Medicines Firm," Reuters, August 1, 2016, https://www.reuters.com/article/us-gsk-alphabet/gsk-and-google-parent-forge-715-million-bioelectronic-medicines-firm-idUSKCN10C1K8.

15. Michael Behar, "Can the Nervous System Be Hacked?", *New York Times Magazine*, May 23, 2014, https://www.nytimes.com/2014/05/25/magazine/can-the-nervous-system-be-hacked.html.

18. "Biologic Refractory Rheumatoid Arthritis," Mesoblast web page.

19. Mesoblast Limited, "Children Treated with Remestemcel-L Continue to Have Strong Survival Outcomes at Six Months in Mesoblast's Phase 3 Trial for Acute Graft vs Host Disease," *GlobeNewswire*, September 20, 2018, https://www.globenewswire.com/news-release/2018/09/20/1573555/0/en/Children-Treated-With-Remestemcel-L-Continue-to-Have-Strong-Survival-Outcomes-at-Six-Months-in-Mesoblast-s-Phase-3-Trial-for-Acute-Graft-Versus-Host-Disease.html.

20. "Mesoblast Cell Treatment Shows Promise in Rheumatoid Arthritis: Study," Reuters, August 8, 2016, https://www.reuters.com/article/us-mesoblast-arthritis/mesoblast-cell-treatment-shows-promise-in-rheumatoid-arthritis-study-idUSKCN10J2I5.

21. Mesoblast Limited, "FDA Provides Guidance on Clinical Pathway to Marketing Application for Revascor in End-Stage Heart Failure Patients with an LVAD," *GlobeNewswire*, August 27, 2019, https://www.globenewswire.com/news-release/2019/08/27/1906931/0/en/FDA-Provides-Guidance-on-Clinical-Pathway-to-Marketing-Application-for-Revascor-in-End-Stage-Heart-Failure-Patients-With-an-LVAD.html.

22. Jay Greene, "Health Insurers Look for Ways to Cut Costs for Back Surgery," Modern Healthcare, August 27, 2018, https://www.modernhealthcare.com/article/20180827/NEWS/180829918/health-insurers-look-for-ways-to-cut-costs-for-back-surgery.

23. Pat Anson, "Promising Results for Stem Cell Treatment of Degenerative Disc Disease," *Pain News Network*, February 12, 2021, https://www.painnewsnetwork.org/stories/2021/2/12/promising-results-for-stem-cell-treatment-of-degenerative-disc-disease.

24. Mesoblast Limited, "Durable Three-Year Outcomes in Degenerative Disc Disease After a Single Injection of Mesoblast's Cell Therapy," *GlobeNewswire*, March 15, 2017,

https://www.globenewswire.com/news-release/2017/03/15/937833/0/en/Durable
-Three-Year-Outcomes-In-Degenerative-Disc-Disease-After-a-Single-Injection-of
-Mesoblast-s-Cell-Therapy.html.

25. Jessica Lau, "Epidemic of Autoimmune Diseases Calls for Action," *The Harvard Ga-
zette*, January 31, 2019, https://news.harvard.edu/gazette/story/2019/01/epidemic-of
-autoimmune-diseases-pushes-researchers-in-new-direction/.

26. Michael Tenspolde, Katharina Zimmermann, Leonie C. Weber, et al., "Regulatory T
Cells Engineered with a Novel Insulin-Specific Chimeric Antigen Receptor as a Candidate Immunotherapy for Type 1 Diabetes," *Journal of Autoimmunity* 103 (September
2019), https://doi.org/10.1016/j.jaut.2019.05.017.

27. Jane E. Brody, "Virtual Reality as Therapy for Pain," *New York Times*, April 29, 2019,
https://www.nytimes.com/2019/04/29/well/live/virtual-reality-as-therapy-for-pain
.html.

28. Harrison Wein, "Senescent Cells Tied to Health and Longevity in Mice," NIH Research Matters, February 23, 2016, https://www.nih.gov/news-events/nih-research
-matters/senescent-cells-tied-health-longevity-mice.

29. Irina M. Conboy, Michael J. Conboy, Amy J. Wagers, et al., "Rejuvenation of Aged
Progenitor Cells by Exposure to a Young Systemic Environment," *Nature* 433,
no. 7027 (February 17, 2005), 760–764, https://doi.org/10.1038/nature03260.

30. "Plasmapheresis," National Multiple Sclerosis Society: Treating MS, https://www.na
tionalmssociety.org/Treating-MS/Managing-Relapses/Plasmapheresis.

31. David A. Loeffler, "AMBAR, An Encouraging Alzheimer's Trial that Raises Questions," *Frontiers in Neurology* 11 (May 2020), 459, https://dx.doi.org/10.3389/fneur
.2020.00459.

32. Yu Zuo, Srilakshmi Yalavarthi, Hui Shi, et al., "Neutrophil Extracellular Traps in
COVID-19," *JCI Insight* 11, no. 5 (April 24, 2020), https://doi.org/10.1172/jci.in
sight.138999.

33. "Neotrolis Announces Development of Enzyme for Severe COVID-19," Medical
Laboratory Observer Online (LABline), August 7, 2020, https://www.mlo-online
.com/disease/infectious-disease/article/21149323/neutrolis-announces-development
-of-enzyme-for-severe-covid19.

34. Nakazawa, *The Autoimmune Epidemic*.

Chapter 21: Diabetes and Obesity: Defeating a Double Threat

1. Lyudmyla Kompaniyets, Alyson B. Goodman, Brook Belay, et al., "Body Mass Index
and Risk for COVID-19-related Hospitalization, Intensive Care Unit Admission, Invasive Mechanical Ventilation, and Death," *CDC Weekly* 70, no. 10 (March 12, 2021),
355–361, http://dx.doi.org/10.15585/mmwr.mm7010e4.

2. National Institute of Diabetes and Digestive and Kidney Diseases, "Overweight and
Obesity Statistics," NIH Health Information, August 2017, https://www.niddk.nih
.gov/health-information/health-statistics/overweight-obesity.

3. Nicola Davis, "Type 2 Diabetes and Obesity: The Link," Diabetes Self-Management,
April 9, 2018, https://www.diabetesselfmanagement.com/about-diabetes/types-of-dia
betes/type-2-diabetes-and-obesity-the-link/.

4. Centers for Disease Control and Prevention, "Adult Obesity Causes and Consequences," March 22, 2021, https://www.cdc.gov/obesity/adult/causes.html.

5. Harvard T.H. Chan School of Public Health, "Health Risks," Obesity Preven-
    tion Source, https://www.hsph.harvard.edu/obesity-prevention-source/obesity-conse
    quences/health-effects/.
6. Greta M. Massetti, William H. Dietz, and Lisa C. Richardson, "Excessive Weight
    Gain, Obesity, and Cancer: Opportunities for Clinical Intervention," *Journal of
    the American Medical Association* 318, no. 20, 1975–1976, https://doi.org/10.1001
    /jama.2017.15519.
7. Nicholas Jones, Julianna Blagih, Fabio Zani, et al., "Fructose Reprograms Glutamine-
    Dependent Oxidative Metabolism to Support LPS-Induced Inflammation," *Nature
    Communications* 12 (February 2021), https://doi.org/10.1038/s41467–021–21461–4.
8. National Restaurant Association, "Restaurant Sales Surpassed Grocery Store Sales
    for the First Time," *Cision PR Newswire*, May 13, 2015, https://www.prnewswire
    .com/news-releases/restaurant-sales-surpassed-grocery-store-sales-for-the-first-time
    -300082821.html.
9. "Sugary Drinks," Harvard T.H. Chan School of Public Health: The Nutrition Source,
    https://www.hsph.harvard.edu/nutritionsource/healthy-drinks/sugary-drinks/.
10. Bishoy Wassef, Michelle Kohansieh, and Amgad N. Makaryus, "Effects of Energy
    Drinks on the Cardiovascular System," *World Journal of Cardiology* 11, no. 9 (November
    26, 2017), 796–806, https://dx.doi.org/10.4330%2Fwjc.v9.i11.796.
11. The Diabetes Prevention Program Research Group, "The Diabetes Prevention
    Program: Description of Lifestyle Intervention," *Diabetes Care* 12, no. 25 (December
    2002), 2165–2171, https://doi.org/10.2337/diacare.25.12.2165.
12. Frank L. Greenway, Louis J. Aronne, Anne Raben, et al., "A Randomized, Double-
    Blind, Placebo-Controlled Study of Gelesis100: A Novel Nonsystemic Oral Hydrogel
    for Weight Loss," *Obesity* 2, no. 27 (February 2019), 205–216, https://doi.org/10.1002
    /oby.22347.
13. John P.H. Wilding, Rachel L. Batterham, Salvatore Calanna, et al., "Once-Weekly
    Semaglutide in Adults with Overweight or Obesity," *New England Journal of Medicine*
    384 (March 18, 2021), 989–1002, https://doi.org/10.1056/NEJMoa2032183.

Chapter 22: Alzheimer's Disease: Eradicating the Beast

1. "Dementia Fact Sheet," World Health Organization, September 2, 2021, https://www
    .who.int/news-room/fact-sheets/detail/dementia.
2. "As Humanity Ages, the Numbers of People with Dementia Will Surge," *Economist*,
    August 29, 2020, https://www.economist.com/special-report/2020/08/27/as-human
    ity-ages-the-numbers-of-people-with-dementia-will-surge.
3. "Alzheimer's Disease Medications," National Institute on Aging, https://order.nia.nih
    .gov/sites/default/files/2018-03/alzheimers-disease-medications-fact-sheet.pdf.
4. "The Search for a Cure for Dementia is Not Going Well," *Economist*, August 29, 2020,
    https://www.economist.com/special-report/2020/08/27/the-search-for-a-cure-for
    -dementia-is-not-going-well.
5. Bruno P. Imbimbo, Stefania Ippati, Ferdinando Ceravolo, and Mark Watling, "Per-
    spective: Is Therapeutic Plasma Exchange a Viable Option for Treating Alzheimer's
    Disease?" *Alzheimer's and Dementia: Translational Research and Clinical Interventions* 6,
    no. 1 (2020), https://dx.doi.org/10.1002%2Ftrc2.12004.
6. Nicholas Weiler, "Drug Reverses Age-Related Mental Decline Within Days," University

of California San Francisco Research, December 1, 2020, https://www.ucsf.edu /news/2020/12/419201/drug-reverses-age-related-mental-decline-within-days.

7. *"TIME* 100 Next 2019," *Time*, https://time.com/collection/time-100-next-2019/.

8. *Vaxxinity, Inc. Form S-1 Registration Statement Under the Securities Act of 1933*, EDGAR, Securities and Exchange Commission, October 8, 2021, https://www.sec.gov/Archives /edgar/data/1851657/000119312521295612/d142511ds1.htm.

12. Maxime Taquet, John R Geddes, Masud Husain, Sierra Luciano, and Paul J Harrison. "6-Month Neurological and Psychiatric Outcomes in 236,379 Survivors of COVID-19: A Retrospective Cohort Study Using Electronic Health Records," *Lancet*, April 6, 2021, doi: https://doi.org/10.1016/S2215–0366(21)00084–5.

13. Alan K. Davis, Frederick S. Barrett, Darrick G. May, et al., "Effects of Psilocybin-Assisted Therapy on Major Depressive Disorder A Randomized Clinical Trial," *JAMA Psychiatry* 78, no. 5 (2021), 481–89, doi:10.1001/jamapsychiatry.2020.3285.

14. Julia Campbell and Anu Sharma, "Compensatory Changes in Cortical Resource Allocation in Adults with Hearing Loss," *Frontiers in System Neuroscience* 7 (October 25, 2013), https://doi.org/10.3389/fnsys.2013.00071.

15. Sue Hughes, "Twelve Risk Factors Linked to 40% of World's Dementia Cases," Medscape, August 3, 2020, https://www.medscape.com/viewarticle/935013.

16. Betsy Mills, "Does Music Benefit the Brain?" *Cognitive Vitality*, March 5, 2019, https:// www.alzdiscovery.org/cognitive-vitality/blog/does-music-benefit-the-brain.

17. Laura Kurtzman, "FDA Approves Video Game Based on UCSF Brain Research as ADHD Therapy for Kids," University of California San Francisco Patient Care, June 15, 2020, https://www.ucsf.edu/news/2020/06/417841/fda-approves-video-game -based-ucsf-brain-research-adhd-therapy-kids.

18. Tina Meketa, "Intervention Becomes First to Successfully Reduce Risk of Dementia," *University of South Florida Health*, November 13, 2017, https://hscweb3.hsc.usf.edu /blog/2017/11/13/intervention-becomes-first-to-successfully-reduce-risk-of-dementia/.

19. Vance H. Trimble, *The Uncertain Miracle: Hyperbaric Oxygenation* (Garden City, NY: Doubleday and Company, 1974).

20. Genevieve Gabb, Eugene D. Robin, "Hyperbaric Oxygen: A Therapy in Search of Diseases," *Chest Journal* 92, no. 6 (1987), 1074–82, doi: https://doi.org/10.1378/chest .92.6.1074; Cassandra A. Godman, Kousanee P. Chheda, Lawrence E. Hightower, et al., "Hyperbaric Oxygen Induces a Cytoprotective and Angiogenic Response in Human Microvascular Endothelial Cells," *Cell Stress and Chaperones* 15, no. 4 (2010), 2010431–42, doi: 10.1007/s12192–009–0159–0.

21. "Hyperbaric Oxygen Therapy Indications," in *The Hyperbaric Oxygen Therapy Committee Report*, 13th ed., L.K. Weaver, ed. (Durham, NC: Undersea and Hyperbaric Medical Society, 2014).

22. Holbach KH, Wassmann H, Kolberg T. "Verbesserte Reversibilität des Traumatischen Mittelhirnsyndromes bei Anwendung der Hyperbaren Oxygenierung" ("Improved Reversibility of the Traumatic Midbrain Syndrome Following the Use of Hyperbaric Oxygenation"), *Acta Neurochirurgica* 30 (1974), 247–56, https://doi.org/10.1007 /BF01405583.

23. Perng Cheng-Hwang, Chang Yue-Cune, Tzang Ruu-Fen, "The Treatment of Cognitive Dysfunction In Dementia: A Multiple Treatments Meta-Analysis," *Psychopharmacology* 235, no. 5 (2018), 1571–80; Eleanor A. Jacobs, Peter M. Winter, Harry J. Alvis, and Mouchly Small, "Hyperoxygenation effect on cognitive functioning in the aged,"

New England Journal of Medicine 281, no. 14 (1969), 753–7; Amir Hadanny, Malka Daniel-Kotovsky, Gil Suzin, et al., "Cognitive Enhancement of Healthy Older Adults Using Hyperbaric Oxygen: A Randomized Controlled Trial," *Aging* 12, no. 13 (2020), 13740–61.

Chapter 24: Creating an Extraordinary Quality of Life: The Power of Mindset

1. Steve Silberman, "Placebos Are Getting More Effective. Drugmakers Are Desperate to Know Why," *Wired*, August 24, 2009, https://www.wired.com/2009/08/ff-placebo -effect/.

2. Slavenka Kam-Hansen, Moshe Jakubowski, John M. Kelley, et al., "Altered Placebo and Drug Labeling Changes the Outcome of Episodic Migraine Attacks," *Science Translational Medicine* 6, no. 218 (January 8, 2014), https://doi.org/10.1126/scitransl med.3006175.

3. "The Power of the Placebo Effect," *Harvard Health Publishing*, August 9, 2019, https:// www.health.harvard.edu/mental-health/the-power-of-the-placebo-effect.

4. Karrin Meissner and Klaus Linde, "Are Blue Pills Better Than Green? How Treatment Features Modulate Placebo Effects," *International Review of Neurobiology* 139 (2018), 357–78, doi: 10.1016/bs.irn.2018.07.014.

5. Rajesh Srivastava and Aarti T. More, "Some Aesthetic Considerations for Over-the-Counter Pharmaceutical Products," *International Journal of Biotechnology* 11, no. 3 / 4 (November 2010), 267–283, http://dx.doi.org/10.1504/IJBT.2010.036600.

6. Karolina Wartolowska, Andrew Judge, Sally Hopewell, et al., "Use of Placebo Controls in the Evaluation of Surgery: Systematic Review," *BMJ* 2014, no. 348 (May 21, 2014), https://doi.org/10.1136/bmj.g3253.

7. Adam Martin, "The Power of the Placebo Effect," *Pharmacy Times*, February 5, 2018, https://www.pharmacytimes.com/view/the-power-of-the-placebo-effect.

8. J. Bruce Moseley, Kimberley O'Malley, Nancy J. Petersen, et al., "A Controlled Trial of Arthroscopic Surgery for Osteoarthritis of the Knee," *New England Journal of Medicine* 347, no. 2 (July 11, 2002), 81–88, https://doi.org/10.1056/nejmoa013259.

9. Gina Kolata, "VA Suggests Halt to Knee Operation / Arthroscopy's Effectiveness Questioned," *SF Gate*, August 24, 2002, https://www.sfgate.com/health/article/VA -suggests-halt-to-knee-operation-2805822.php.

10. Francesco Pagnini, Cesare Cavalera, Eleonora Volpato, et al., "Ageing as a Mindset: A Study Protocol to Rejuvenate Older Adults with a Counterclockwise Psychological Intervention," *BMJ Open* 9, no. 7 (July 9, 2019), https://doi.org/10.1136/bmjopen -2019-030411.

11. Becca R. Levy, Martin D. Slade, Terrence E. Murphy, et al., "Association between Positive Age Stereotypes and Recovery from Disability in Older Persons," *Journal of the American Medical Association* 308, no. 19 (November 21, 2012), 1972–1973, https://doi .org/ 10.1001/jama.2012.14541

12. "Can We Reverse Aging by Changing How We Think?" *Newsweek*, April 13, 2009, https://www.newsweek.com/can-we-reverse-aging-changing-how-we-think-77669.

13. Francesco Pagnini, Cesare Cavalera, Eleonora Volpato, et al., "Ageing as a Mindset: A Study Protocol to Rejuvenate Older Adults with a Counterclockwise Psychological

Intervention," *BMJ Open* 9, no. 7 (July 9, 2019), https://doi.org/10.1136/bmjopen -2019-030411.

14. Becca R. Levy, Martin D. Slade, Robert H. Pietrzak, and Luigi Ferrucci, "Positive Age Beliefs Protect Against Dementia Even Among Elders with High-Risk Gene," *PLOS One* 13, no. 2 (2018), https://doi.org/10.1371/journal.pone.0191004.

15. Alia J. Crum and Ellen J. Langer, "Mind-Set Matters: Exercise and the Placebo Effect," *Psychological Science* 18, no. 2 (February 2007), 165–71, https://doi.org/10.1111/j.1467 -9280.2007.01867.x.

16. Catherine West, "Mind-Set Matters," *Association for Psychological Science Observer*, March 1, 2007, https://www.psychologicalscience.org/observer/mind-set-matters.

17. Lyudmyla Kompaniyets, Audrey F. Pennington, Alyson B. Goodman, et al., "Underlying Medical Conditions and Severe Illness Among 540,667 Adults Hospitalized with COVID-19," *Preventing Chronic Disease* 18 (July 1, 2021), http://dx.doi.org/10.5888 /pcd18.210123.

18. Ibid.

19. Helen Briggs, "Depression: 'Second Biggest Cause of Disability' in World," BBC News, November 6, 2013, https://www.bbc.com/news/health-24818048.

20. "Suicidality in Children and Adolescents Being Treated with Antidepressant Medications," U.S. Food and Drug Administration Postmarket Drug Safety Information for Patients and Providers, February 5, 2018, https://www.fda.gov/drugs/postmarket -drug-safety-information-patients-and-providers/suicidality-children-and-adoles cents-being-treated-antidepressant-medications.

21. Alan K. Davis, Frederick S. Barrett, Darrick G. May, et al., "Effects of Psilocybin-Assisted Therapy on Major Depressive Disorder," *JAMA Psychiatry* 78, no. 5 (November 4, 2020), 481–489, https://doi.org/ 10.1001/jamapsychiatry.2020.3285.

22. Vanessa McMains, "Psychedelic Treatment with Psilocybin Shown to Relieve Major Depression," *Dome* (November/December 2020), https://www.hopkinsmedicine.org /news/articles/psychedelic-treatment-with-psilocybin-shown-to-relieve-major-depres sion.

24. Jacob M. Wilson, Raad H. Gheith, Ryan P. Lowery, et al., "Non-Traditional Immersive Seminar Enhances Learning by Promoting Greater Physiological and Psychological Engagement Compared to a Traditional Lecture Format," *Physiology and Behavior* 238 (September 1, 2021), https://doi.org/10.1016/j.physbeh.2021.113461.

25. Ibid.

Chapter 25: The Power of Decision: The Gift of Living in a Beautiful State

1. P. Stapleton, G. Crighton, D. Sabot, et al., "Reexamining the Effect of Emotional Freedom Techniques on Stress Biochemistry: A Randomized Controlled Trial," *Psychological Trauma: Theory, Research, Practice, and Policy* 12, no. 8 (2020), 869–77, https://psycnet .apa.org/doi/10.1037/tra0000563.

2. Dawson Church, Peta Stapleton, and Debbie Sabot, "App-Based Delivery of Clinical Emotional Freedom Techniques: Cross-Sectional Study of App User Self-Ratings," *JMIR mHealth and uHealth* 8, no. 10 (October 2020), https://doi.org/10.2196/18545.

3. Peta Stapleton, Evangeline Lilley-Hale, Glenn Mackintosh, and Emma Sparenburg,

"Online Delivery of Emotional Freedom Techniques for Food Cravings and Weight Management: 2-Year Follow-Up," *Journal of Alternative and Complementary Medicine* 26, no. 2 (February 2020), 98–106, https://doi.org/10.1089/acm.2019.0309.

4. Janet Kemp and Robert Bossarte, "Suicide Data Report, 2012," Department of Veteran Affairs Mental Health Services Suicide Prevention Program, 2012, https://www.va .gov/opa/docs/suicide-data-report-2012-final.pdf.

5. "Stellate Ganglion Block," Cleveland Clinic Health Library, https://my.clevelandclinic .org/health/treatments/17507-stellate-ganglion-block.

6. "Stellate Ganglion Block for PTSD," Cornell Pain Clinic blog, December 1, 2019, https://cornellpainclinic.com/stellate-ganglion-block-emerging-treatment-for-ptsd/.

7. Kristine L. Rae Olmsted, Michael Bartoszek, Sean Mulvaney, et al., "Effect of Stellate Ganglion Block Treatment on Posttraumatic Stress Disorder Symptoms," *JAMA Psychiatry* 77, no. 2 (November 6, 2019), https://doi.org/ 10.1001/jamapsychiatry.2019 .3474.

8. The Stellate Institute web page, https://thestellateinstitute.com/.

9. Philip Brickman, Dan Coates, and Ronnie Janoff-Bulman, "Lottery Winners and Accident Victims: Is Happiness Relative?" *Journal of Personality and Social Psychology* 36, no. 8 (September 1978), 917–27, http://dx.doi.org/10.1037/0022–3514.36.8.917.

YOUR 7-STEP ACTION PLAN FOR LASTING RESULTS

Now that you've gone on this extraordinary journey and have been exposed to these incredible tools for strength, healing, vitality, and longevity, you don't want to let your learning lead only to knowledge. As my original teacher Jim Rohn used to say, "Let your learning lead to action, and you'll create an extraordinary life."

To simplify, these 700 pages, let's look at **7 steps** that you can take to create a simple and quick action plan for the things you want to follow through on and transform in your life. Remember, always consult your doctor so that they can help you determine what actions are best for you.

STEP ONE: DECIDE & GET THE INFORMATION YOU NEED

1. **Decide what you truly want for your life physically. What is the result that you're truly after?** Do you want more energy? More vitality? More strength? More flexibility? Do you want to start to rejuvenate your body? Revitalize it? Bring more youth to it?
2. **Get the information that you need.** Get yourself tested, so you can maximize your energy by:

   - Knowing whether there are **toxic metals** in your system that are getting in the way of your well-being.
   - Knowing if your **hormones** are in balance, which can make a giant difference in how you feel day to day.

• And then ideally, do the things that will give you peace of mind for yourself and for your family. Get the GRAIL test plus a full-body MRI so that you can know that there's nothing to be concerned about with cancer. GRAIL can even be done even in your home, with a simple blood test.

• If it's appropriate, I would consider scheduling a **CCTA Test** so that you know exactly where your cardiovascular health is and what needs to be done to stay strong and healthy for years to come.

• Consider getting the **Alzheimer's Test** so that you know if you're genetically predisposed, and also come up with a lifestyle plan that will reduce your risk. If you do this far enough in advance, there are a variety of tools in this book that can make a difference.

• Who's in your family or friendship base whom you would like to also make sure gets tested to look out for their well-being and help them to maximize the quality of their life.

• Last, if you want to have some fun, you can **discover what your true age is.** As I mentioned earlier, I was thrilled to discover that my chronological age of 62 is only 51 years *biologically*. I think you'll be surprised. If it's not where you want it to be, there are so many things within these pages that you can do to change it.

STEP TWO: REVIEW YOUR EDUCATION

If you've read this book, congratulations! You've given yourself a tremendous education. But knowledge isn't power; it's potential power. Decide **what tools do you want to access today. And what do you want to keep track of in the future?**

1. Are **stem cells** something that you want to pursue for some aspect of your life or for someone in your family?
2. Do you want to implement **Dr. Sinclair's Four Vitality Ingredients that help reverse biological aging? Or tap into the energy force of NMN?**

3. Or, are there some technologies that you'll want to keep track of so that you have them when you need them? Perhaps the **Wnt Pathway for Osteoarthritis?**

4. Is there anyone in your family or people you know whom you want to share information with about what you've learned here in **the big 6— heart disease, diabetes/obesity, stroke, cancer, autoimmune disease, and Alzheimer's?**

5. Are you going to keep track of **Gene Therapy and CRISPR** and some of the transformations it's creating?

6. Do you know anyone who has **Parkinson's or severe addiction** who could feel relief from focused Ultrasound without brain surgery?

Make a list of the things that you want to act on and things you want to keep track of, so that if you or anyone you know who needs help, you'll have answers that you can share with them and that they can consider with their doctor. Just create a little **checklist** for yourself. The book is here. It's the ultimate resource you can go back to as often as you need.

STEP THREE: MAXIMIZE YOUR ENERGY & REGENERATION

Consider what aspects of **Vitality Pharmacy (Chapter 10)** might help you accelerate your energy, your strength, your vitality. Or help you to recover from challenges you may be facing.

1. Are you going to **expand your capacity by optimizing your hormones** through **H.O.T. (hormone optimization therapy)?**

2. Would **peptides** be something you may want to consider? Are there any peptides that you'd like to look into that could make a difference in anything from your **immune system to sexual desire and drive?**

3. What are some of the **pharmaceutical-grade supplements** that you might want to have to start your day with energy or to get yourself to sleep at night without side effects?

4. Or would you like to tap into **NAD3** or other **NMN-like products** to maximize your energy and vitality?

STEP FOUR: CREATE A PLAN FOR
SLEEP & LIVING PAIN FREE

Remember, the **third pillar of health** besides diet and exercise is sleep. And it profoundly affects how your diet gets processed or whether you even feel like exercising. So what's your plan? Can you schedule **seven hours and track your sleep with an AI device?** Will you make some of the changes that will make it easier for you to get a **deep and restful sleep** so you feel vital?

And if there's **pain in your body,** or in someone you love, which of the tools do you want to use to free yourself? **PEMF? Pete Egoscue's techniques? Counterstrain? Relief treatment to free up your tissue and nerves?** Are you going to do things to support your back, like a simple **Back Arch?**

STEP FIVE: DEVISE YOUR MAXIMUM
LONGEVITY LIFESTYLE

What are **three to five things** that you want to commit to do? You're not going to do them all. What are the things that you think could make the biggest difference?

1. Is it eating more **live foods? Reducing your sugar?** Perhaps going on a **10-day cleanse** to break the pattern and reset your system?
2. Would you **cut 300 calories** from your daily food intake—one bagel a day—and see a significant change? Would you want to implement one of the new **FDA tools** like **Plenity** to curb your appetite? Or Wegovy to shut off the hormone that creates hunger?
3. If you have **pre-diabetes or diabetes** or know someone who does, what do you want to use out of that chapter to make the changes so that you don't have to live with it anymore?
4. You could even decide to cut back on caffeine and increase your water intake to half your body weight in ounces per day to increase your hydration. Are you going to practice **breathing patterns** that help you to relax and move your lymph, like the **breathing pattern of 1–4–2?**

5. Will you **change your food environment** so you're not triggered by putting fresh foods near you, as opposed to as many packaged and processed foods?

6. **Will you tap into the power of heat and cold to give your body a healthy shock that help protect you from disease and extend your healthspan?**

This is all about designing your lifestyle in a way that's most fulfilling for you.

STEP SIX: MOVEMENT IS LIFE: WHAT IS YOUR FITNESS PLAN?

Given that exercise can reduce your risk of cancer by 40 percent, cut your risk of a stroke by 45 percent, and slash your risk of diabetes by 50 percent . . .

1. Will you just work out ten minutes a week with something like **OsteoStrong**?

2. Will you create a plan with **Billy Beck III,** that you want to act on for free? You'll get your design to start with for free.

3. Do you want to make exercising fun through **VR, by playing through Black box?** You're not even realizing you're working out, because you're playing a game.

STEP SEVEN: TAKE CONTROL OF YOUR MIND

Will you create a daily practice for just 10 minutes per day through priming? Remember, you can visit **TonyRobbins.com/Priming** to supercharge your mind and emotions to set you up for the day?

Do you want to utilize the power of Emotional Freedom Techniques **(EFT) and Tapping? Visit TheTappingMethod.com/Tony to download the app for free and receive a discount on membership.**

Do you know somebody who has **severe anxiety or PTSD** that you can pass along information to on the injection used with great success by vets?

And most importantly, will you become more aware and **not let fear**

take over, knowing that the **mind can make you sick or healthy, frustrated or happy?**

Will you commit to the decision of living in a Beautiful State no matter what? Even when things don't go your way? Will you invoke the **90-second rule** so that you can truly have the freedom you deserve?

WRAP—UP

Whatever you decide to do, these **7 steps** are just a simple way to try to chunk so much of the information that you've learned here. Again, you don't need to do everything in this book, but my hope is that you use it as a **guidebook** that you can come back to for answers for the rest of your life for yourself and for your family. We'll keep updating this on our website, LifeForce.com as well to bring new information as it comes.

Please pick a few things in each of these areas and decide what you're going to take action on, or whom you're going to help. Then, keep expanding your education in these areas as they continue to develop. Your knowledge could not only change a life, in some cases it could save a life.

PERMISSIONS

ACKNOWLEDGMENTS

TONY ROBBINS

How do I limit my acknowledgments when everything here is standing on the shoulders of so many incredible human beings who have gone before me, including **all the extraordinary doctors and research scientists** we've had the privilege of introducing to you in this book?

If you've already read it, I'm sure you've realized by now that most of the characters in these stories are people who are carrying out their lifelong commitments after a trigger of some kind of disaster or personal crisis—the loss of a wife, a child, patients, parents. Something within their heart drove them beyond the standard of care and compelled them to take on all the challenges they surely faced, and persevere—in most cases for decades—before creating a breakthrough that could help so many others. This book must acknowledge those heroes first and foremost. This book is really their story.

For my coauthors, **Peter and Bob**, I simply cannot thank you both enough, not only for the content but also for your vision and life's work. Long before they were writing this book, they were committed to helping, healing, and serving people. I'm so grateful that you were willing to put in the time and effort it took to be able to share all this information with the masses. **A special thanks to you, Dr. Bill Kapp and to Dr. Matt and Dr. G too. I thank you all, my brothers, for your incredible care and committment to help people heal.**

Next, I must acknowledge **the book team** that worked tirelessly on this project with us. Consider the density of this encyclopedia in your hands! No wonder it was a three-year project. In order to get this done in the middle of COVID and get access to interview the very best in the world in the field, we had an army that worked around the clock, and they all played such an important role.

I must acknowledge **Diane Sette Arruza**, who has been the head of my creative department for six years. She was spearheading the team and this enormous undertaking all while our whole company and the way we do business was undergoing a total overhaul in order to reach our audiences digitally during the COVID era. She is able to handle such incredible complexity and is responsible for shepherding this to the finish line and keeping all the pieces together. As if her extraordinary level of intelligence, creativity, and skill weren't enough, her ability to live what I teach in this last chapter of this book—life in a beautiful state—day in and day out, bringing positivity, energy, and solution-orientation is what made this project so enjoyable in the midst of it all. Diane, I can't thank you enough, this book would not be done if it weren't for you.

Mary Buckheit, who is my right arm and bright light that helps me accomplish everything on a day-to-day basis from hardcovers to Henleys. May the life force be with you, Mary B.—you will write the book of our life someday. Your snappy wit, vast depth, and like Diane, a commitment to finding answers all while in the most playful and supportive state anybody could possibly imagine or dream about. I'm truly blessed to have these two women in my life.

Billy Beck III—thank you, buttercup. You are a gift. You're there with me early mornings and late nights, in the dark of time zones all over the world. You round out this family, and I don't know what any of us would do without you in our corner, fixing me up and making me laugh all along. I love you, brother.

I've already acknowledged **my wife, Sage,** in the dedication, because I'm truly dedicated and devoted to her. She has been with me 22 years (and I'm a crazy man). Honey, thank you for your pure love, support, wicked intelligence, and amazing sense of humor. You are nothing but beautiful and bright through it all, because you too know the importance of this mission and live it with me all day, every day. From the very beginning, we said that this book is not just about changing people's lives, this is a book that literally can save people's lives and perhaps the lives of the people they love. I couldn't have made it here without you by my side. I am the happiest man alive, thanks to you.

To the book writing team, my deepest thanks for seeing this through: **Jeff Coplon, Bonnie Rochman, William Green, Dr. Felicia Hsu, Hilary Macht,** and **Mark Healy.**

To Ray Kurzweil, thank you for writing the introduction to this book for us but more important, for your 50 years of prolific contribution, foresight, and the scientific breakthroughs you created. You defied the odds, sequencing the human genome, when everyone else said it wasn't going to happen for another 200 years! Your understanding is unmatched, as is your friendship over the years. Thank you.

I have such deep appreciation for my agent of more than 30 years, **Jan Miller**, and for **Shannon Marven**. Jan, you've been there with me since the beginning. Thank you both for everything, every time.

To my publicist and dear friend, **Jennifer Connelly**, who may never know the esteem and appreciation I have for her instincts, sharp mind, and kind heart (but I'll keep reminding you). Many thanks to you and **Clinton Riley** for your diligence, constancy, and willingness to go wherever we go.

I have the privilege of having more than 100 companies now, about fourteen of which I actively manage, but what allows me to do this is that each and every business I'm in has extraordinary leaders at the helm. The executive teams would be too long a list here, but I'm so grateful for the mindset that all of you have to find a way to do more for others than anybody else does in each of the industries that you all represent, which are as diverse as biotech companies, business and training companies, sports teams, to our resort in Fiji. It gives me joy to be able to work with all of you to find ways to creatively innovate and support our clients in each of these industries all around the world. Special thanks to both the executive teams of Fountain Life and lifeforce.com. I'm humbled to have the privilege to work with each of you and to learn from you. Thank you.

To my core company, **Robbins Research International**, my entire team there, my dear friends, many of whom have been with me 10 to 30-plus years. I can't thank each of you enough for all you do to make this ship fly and especially for your ingenuity during these recent incredible times, all while I had to divert some of my focus to get this book project done. I love you guys.

I want to thank our **CFO, Yogesh Babla**, whose dedication and attention has helped our company continue to touch lives around the world. This company is owned by the employees, and your service to support all of us has been truly extraordinary. Thank you.

And our **CEO, Dean Graziosi,** for your brilliance, because ideas—no matter how good they are—have to find a way to reach people. Even when the work we do was being shut down in these unique times, you found a way to deliver when people needed us most. Your incredible work ethic, crazy genius, and the love we share for serving people truly makes us brothers on the path, and I'm so grateful for you. And that you're a morning person!

To our whole leadership team at RRI, especially my brother, **Scott Humphrey**—love you. bro, and all of your Lions and Platinum Partner family. You guys are the soul of this community.

CCO Kate Austin, whose essence, heart, and intellect impacts us all, and to **CMO Darami Coulter,** who stepped in right when we needed her—thank you for your brilliance and relentless dedication to getting it right. To RRI lifers **Sam Georges, Heather Diem, Shari Wilson, Bruce Levine,** and **Linda Price** for all the years and all the hours. Special thanks to **Joseph McClendon III, Scott Harris, Tad Schinke,** and **Vicki St. George**.

To the road/studio show tech team, especially **John Eberts & Matt Murphy,** everybody in black in the back, and social media sensei **Dani Johnson**—it's a gift to have each of you as partners in it all. I'm forever grateful to you.

And of course, our extraordinary home office team, which makes this world go round eight days a week. The one and only **Bradley Gordon,** our chief of staff, who weaves the web of our life with such insight, grace, thoughtfulness, and spontaneous bouts of laughter. And the incredible **Rhiannon Siegel,** who keenly coordinates each detail of our wild and ever-changing life. Thank you. To **Kacie South,** you late–night warrior, juggler of many milkshakes and mind maps, this book has your fingerprints all over it. To **Matt Vaughn.** whose great taste discovers all our treasures. And to everybody else back home—to **Maria and Tony Rodriguez** for all you do, to **Anna Ahlbom** for all you manage, to **Todd Erickson** and **Darren Walsh** for all you create. Together you're all what makes that house a home and a beautiful place to be. You are all puzzle pieces that make a greater whole. I love you.

To Ajay Gupta, and Joshy, you are incredible friends and partners to me whom I can always bounce ideas off. I love you guys; thank you.

To my own amazing healing team, you keep this big body going. **Jie Chen, James Bowman, Master Stephen Co, Donny Epstein, Brian Tuckey, Tim Hodges, Dr. Daniel Yadegar, Dan Holtz, Dr. Ross Carter, Stephanie Hunter, Mary Ann and Peter Lucarini, John Amaral, Hope and Jen, Bob Cooley, Iris Hernandez**—thanks for the love and care!

To my ongoing role models of true excellence. The men in my life whom I respect most for not only their incredible achievements but for their commitment to make the world a better place. Men who don't just talk a good game but actually walk the talk: my dear friend **Peter Guber**, **Marc Benioff**, **Paul Tudor Jones**, **Steve Wynn**, **Pitbull**, and **Ray Dalio**.

My gratitude goes out to **Feeding America** for their continued partnership in the Feed A Billion challenge. When I first came up with the idea, some of the members of the team were a bit skeptical! But here we are, eight years later, ahead of schedule and **closing in on one billion meals**. Our relationship will continue, and this book will also be another form of support for the great work that you're doing.

And finally to the kind folks at **Simon & Schuster**, including **Dana Canedy, Stuart Roberts, and Jonathan Karp**, I appreciate your sticking with me as this book became larger and larger. You saw the vision and gave me the support it needed.

I give thanks to God, our creator, and to all those named here and unnamed in my life who continue to support me and this mission on my neverending quest to be a blessing in the lives of all those I have the privilege to meet, love, and serve.

PETER H. DIAMANDIS

It's my pleasure to acknowledge my incredible team at PHD Ventures who supported me on this Life Force journey.

First, to **Felicia Hsu, MD**, a member of my personal Strikeforce, whose medical knowledge and incredible writing skills supported Tony and me on so many interviews and drafts. Next, to **Esther Count**, my chief of staff, who juggled my insane schedule and kept all of the trains running on time. Next, **Claire Adair**, the executive director of the Abundance Platinum Longevity trips, whose writing and organizing skills delivered extraordinary content and interviews that appear throughout the book. Thank you to **Derek Dolin** and **AJ Scaramucci**, my past Strikeforce members who helped in the earliest days of Life Force. Finally, it's my pleasure to thank and acknowledge my amazing marketing and audiovisual team, **Tyler Donahue, Cheo Rose-Washington,** and **Greg O'Brien,** whose ninja skills helped us to get our message of a "hopeful, compelling, and abundant-health future" out to the world!

HOW BUSINESS OWNERS CAN CUT HEALTH INSURANCE COSTS

Health insurance is expensive and getting more expensive! Business owners are acutely aware of this line item, and yet, providing robust insurance benefits is a huge factor when attracting and retaining great team members.

Instead of shelling out astronomical premiums for "retail" health insurance, most companies (63 percent, to be exact) will "self-insure" by paying up to a certain dollar amount of claims. They may use a brand name network of doctors, but at the end of the day, they are on the hook. This is why most companies have a vested interested in making their employees more healthy and will attempt to encourage employees to make preventative changes through programs like free fitness watches, cash for quitting smoking, etc.

These are all fine steps to take, but if we want true sea change, a massive reduction in costs, and an improvement of the health of our employees, we need a new kind of health insurance. One where every employee has access to the most advanced diagnostic available that will catch things early AND allow employees to see what's really true about their body and the risks they face. Enter Fountain Health Insurance, a revolutionary platform that can greatly reduce costs by helping to detect disease early and treating it.

Fountain Health Insurance provides employees with access to screening measures using the latest tools in biotechnology. For example . . .

- **Whole Body MRI powered by AI** detects early stage cancer, brain aneurysms, Alzheimer's risk, visceral fat, liver fat, and many other conditions that will rarely be detected by the traditional physical exam.

- **Cleerly Coronary CT angiography powered by AI** finds heart plaque before it ever causes a heart attack, and identifies treatments to reverse your risk of heart attack.

- **Genetic testing can help determine disease risk** and what diet and exercise routine will optimize your health according to your genes.

- **Epigenetic testing assesses how your biologic age compares to your chronologic age** and gives recommendations about how to lower your biologic age.

- **Advanced blood testing measures your organ function, bone marrow status, hormone levels, and inflammatory status.**

- **DEXA scan calculates your bone density, body composition, and muscle mass.**

- **GRAIL blood test recognizes up to fifty different types of cancer by analyzing DNA in your blood plasma.**

By investing in employees through advanced diagnostic testing, Fountain Health believes it can help deliver better care at less cost, while extending health span and improving outcomes for employees!

If you've done what you've always done, you'll get what you've always gotten. If you are a business owner (or c suite executive) and you're interested in learning more, visit www.LifeForce.com, or go to www.FountainHealth.com, where you can inquire about Fountain Health Insurance.

Index

Rothblatt, Martine, 36, 124–133. *See also*
  United Therapeutics (UT)
  accomplishments, 124–126
  carbon-neutral aircraft and, 142–143
  electric vertical aircraft (EVA) and
  EVLP (ex vivo lung perfusion) and,
    134–135
  gender transition, 129–130
  on organ transplants, 134
  personal qualities of, 126–127
  Remodulin drug and, 130–133
  satellite radio and, 127–129
  3D-bioprinting and, 141–142
  United Therapeutics, 124–125
  xenotransplantation and, 137–138
Royer, Tim, 54
Rubin, Lee, 399, 420
Rusk, Howard, 423
Rutan, Burt, 545

Sackler family, 23–24
Sadelain, Michel, 153
safety. *See also* clinical trials; risks
  of cellular medicine, 64
  NAD+ supplements, 233–234
  nutraceuticals, 236
  peptides, 220
Salk Institute, 31, 117, 138
Samikoglu, Cevdet, 197, 202–203, 208, 209
Samumed, 197, 199. *See also* Biosplice
  Therapeutics
Sana Biotechnology, 403
San Francisco 49ers, 255
Sarepta Therapeutics, 189
Satchidananda, Swami, 275
satellite radio (SiriusXM), 125, 127–129
saunas, 297–300
Saunders, Oliver, 346
Scenesse, 224
Schwartz, Erika, 244
science of achievement, 601–602
ScienceOfTonyRobbins.com, 596
Seau, Junior, 255
Section32, 561
Seim, Caitlyn, 416, 417, 418
semaglutide, 221–222, 224, 509–510
senescent cells, 228, 234, 240–241, 368
senolytic medicines, 240–241

sensors, 313, 317, 336, 418, 423, 429, 553
September 11th terrorist attacks, 578–579,
  584–588
Seraya Medical, 421–422
sermorelin, 223, 225
SetPoint Medical, 472, 475
7-Step Action Plan, 649–654
sex hormone binding globulin (SHBG),
  89, 90
sex hormones, 87, 229–230, 377
sexual arousal/satisfaction, peptide for,
  222–223
sexual energy/vitality
  hormonal balance and, 73
  sleep and, 308–309
sexual function, laser technology and, 385,
  386
Shade, Christopher, 91
Shapiro, Roberta, 267
Shaw, Deb, 418–419
Shiseido, 359
sickle cell anemia, 6, 41, 61, 192
Sinclair, David
  accomplishments, 97
  on age-reversal, 566–567
  on anti-aging drugs, 108–109
  biological age of, 99
  Information Theory of Aging, 97–99
  on lifestyle choices, 118–119
  on NAD+ supplements, 233, 234
  NMN mice experiments, 114–116,
    115–116
  NMN supplements and, 233
  rejuvenation recipe, 99–103
  as "science rebel," 119–120
  "Turning Back Time: Reprogramming
    Retinal Cells Can Reverse Age-Related
    Vision Loss," 566
*The Singularity Is Near: When Humans
  Transcend Biology* (Kurzweil), 548
Sirius Satellite Radio (SiriusXM),
  127–129
SiriusXM, 125
siRNA (short interfering RNA), 410, 456
sirtuins, 111, 112–114, 232
Sisco, Peter, 327
sitting, 326, 342
sitting-rising test, 335–336